Unit 1

Unit 2

Unit 3

Unit 4

Unit 5

Unit 6

Unit 7

Unit 8

Unit 9

Unit 10

Unit 11

Unit 12

Unit 13

Unit 14

GENERAL PATHOLOGY
A PROGRAMMED TEXT

Edited by Thomas H. Kent, M.D.
Department of Pathology
University of Iowa College of Medicine

with Joseph A. Buckwalter, Jr.
James D. Nordin
Albert J. Kollasch
Donald M. Cassaday

Little, Brown and Company Boston

First Edition

Fourth Printing

Library of Congress catalog card No. 74-6599

ISBN 0-316-48920-4

Printed in the United States of America

A Note from the Publisher

Since the publication in 1965 of Richard and Murray Sidman's programmed text, *Neuroanatomy*, Little, Brown has known how successful educational programming can be if it is the result of collaboration between experts in subject matter and learning techniques. Because of its excellence, *Neuroanatomy* has carved out a special place as an aid to student learning.

Now we introduce Thomas Kent's programmed text, GENERAL PATHOLOGY. We believe it will have the same high-level acceptance in the field of pathology as Sidman and Sidman has in neuroanatomy.

In Kent's GENERAL PATHOLOGY, both student and instructor will find the subject areas of pathology clearly defined in a way that encourages learning. Each reader will see the impressive attention to careful design which was based on validation of each learning step as well as on overall performance and acceptance by students. Much of the documentation for the learning effectiveness of this text is published in the works cited below. Kent and his colleagues have demonstrated that GENERAL PATHOLOGY works equally well for students both low and high in class standings. He has also determined that six months after learning material in this book by the programmed method, students scored as much as 20 % higher than previous classes learning identical basic material in pathology by traditional methods.

There are 14 units (or chapters) in this text. The extensive evaluation of each unit has included objective tests administered before and after use of the unit. Student attitudes toward the material and ratings of it have been assessed and their suggestions incorporated into subsequent revisions.

At least 80 % of the students studying from this programmed text during four years of testing have indicated a preference for it over other methods of meeting the same objectives. We believe GENERAL PATHOLOGY will prove a unique and valuable teaching and learning tool. We are proud to have a part in making available this new learning resource.

Fred Belliveau, Manager
Medical Book Division

References

1. Buckwalter, J. A., Jr., and Kent, T. H. The Use of Programmed Texts for Efficient Attainment of Competence Levels for Problem Solving in Pathology. In J. P. Lysaught (Ed.), *Instructional Technology in Medical Education, Proceedings of the Fifth Rochester Conference on Self-Instruction in Medical Education.* Rochester: The University of Rochester, 1973. Pp. 77–84.
2. Kent, T. H., and Buckwalter, J. A., Jr. The Effect of Overt vs. Covert Response to Introductory Programmed Texts in Pathology on Scores, Time and Affect. In J. P. Lysaught (Ed.), *Instructional Technology in Medical Education, Proceedings of the Fifth Rochester Conference on Self-Instruction in Medical Education.* Rochester: The University of Rochester, 1973. Pp. 85–89.
3. Kent, T. H., Taylor, D. D., and Buckwalter, J. A., Jr. Field test of programmed texts for teaching general pathology. *J. Med. Educ.* 47:873–878, 1972.
4. Buckwalter, J. A., Jr., and Kent, T. H. Scholastic ability versus attitude, time and performance on programmed instruction. *J. Med. Educ.* 49:584–588, 1974.

Preface

These units were developed to provide the medical student with an efficient means of mastering basic definitions, concepts, and facts of general pathology. They are designed to provide a dependable method of self-instruction on "core" knowledge. It is not our intent that this learning tool replace the traditional lecture or other standard format for teaching pathology. These units provide only a portion of the total learning experience. Indeed, they enable the student to read the textbooks and other materials more critically, to appreciate lectures more fully, and to begin interacting with the faculty at a problem-solving level, through mastery of the basic nomenclature and concepts of pathology. This will give the student knowledge prerequisite to interpreting the essential visual materials of pathology. The content of GENERAL PATHOLOGY: A PROGRAMMED TEXT is based on well-established knowledge and commonly agreed on material. The units are presented in such a form that they will provide a logical framework on which to add more material.

Attention is called to the references listed in the Note from the Publisher on page v, which document the extensive testing and validation of this text from the viewpoint of educational design, and to the Appendix which gives performance and attitude data for the units in this text.

The content of GENERAL PATHOLOGY: A PROGRAMMED TEXT is divided into three general categories. Units in this volume are so indicated; the other topics are planned for a future volume:

I. Introduction to Pathology (Unit 1)

II. Basic Reactions of the Body
- A. Inflammation and Healing (Units 2–6, 8)
- B. Necrosis and Degeneration (Units 7 and 9)
- C. Developmental Abnormalities (Unit 10)
- D. Disturbances of Growth

III. Causes and Pathologic Mechanisms of Disease
- A. Physical Injury
- B. Chemical Injury
- C. Infectious Disease
- D. Hemodynamic Disorders (Units 11–14)
- E. Metabolic Disorders
- F. Immunologic Disorders

Thomas H. Kent

Acknowledgments

Joseph A. Buckwalter, Jr., initiated the development of these programmed text units following his freshman year in medical school. His careful study of the self-instructional process and judgment concerning the learning needs of beginning medical students set the stage for development of succeeding units. Lowell Schoer and Gary Arsham provided valuable technical critique for the early material. D. Dax Taylor field-tested units 1 through 6 at the University of Missouri. James D. Nordin, Donald M. Cassaday, and Albert J. Kollasch developed units 7 through 14 following their freshman years in medical school. The editor bears responsibility for content decisions, the evaluation procedures, and revisions, although many individuals helped in this process.

Ann Bentley did the majority of the typing and along with Joyce Busby, Rose Marr, Barbara Cannon, Marilyn Doty, and others carried out the massive data analysis that made systematic revisions possible. Ronald J. Ervin did the illustrations. The University of Iowa freshman medical classes of 1971, 1972, 1973, and 1974 and the University of Missouri sophomore medical class of 1971 tested and provided the positive response, constructive criticism, and cooperativeness that motivated the completion of this text. Grants from the College of Medicine and University Council on Teaching at the University of Iowa, as well as encouragement and resources provided by Department Heads Emory D. Warner and George D. Penick, made this text possible. Ann L. Kent has been a patient and supportive wife.

T. H. K.

Contents

GENERAL PATHOLOGY
A PROGRAMMED TEXT

Directions

This is a linear programmed text. In each "frame" you will be asked to make one or more responses. After you have responded in your mind or on paper, turn the page and check your response with the recommended response. Proceed through the program in the sequence of frame numbers.

The learning objective and contents are found on the first page of each unit and are repeated in part at the beginning of each section of a unit. An optional pretest is found on the second page of each unit. This may be used as a preview of the material to be covered and for later comparison with posttest answers.

At the end of each section of a unit there are practice true-false questions. These are referenced back to the learning frames in case you wish to review at this point.

The number of frames for a section is indicated at the beginning of the section, so you can judge whether to take a break before continuing.

A multiple-choice posttest for each unit is located at the end of the book. This will help you evaluate what you have learned. The answers to these test questions, in a section following the posttests, are referenced back to the appropriate learning frames.

Unit 1. Introduction to Pathology

Unit 1. INTRODUCTION TO PATHOLOGY

OBJECTIVES

When you complete this unit, you will be able to select correct responses relating to the:

	starting page	frame numbers
A. Definition of Pathology	1.3	1-9

1. definition of pathology and examples of disease.
2. subject matter of pathology compared to other basic medical sciences.

B. Causes of Disease	1.21	10-18

1. three major types of causes of disease and examples of each.
2. correct use of the term *etiology*.

C. Structural and Functional Abnormalities	1.39	19-69

1. recognition of the defining characteristics of the basic responses of the body to injury.
2. classification of examples as cell degeneration and cell death, inflammation and repair, disturbances of growth and abnormal development.
3. identification of examples of the following:

necrosis	inflammation	atrophy	aplasia
cell death	infection	hypertrophy	hypoplasia
somatic death	repair	hyperplasia	malformation
degeneration		neoplasia	

4. distinction between structural and functional abnormalities and correct use of the terms *pathology* and *lesion*.

D. Manifestations of Disease	1.39	70-92

1. differences between signs, symptoms, and laboratory abnormalities.
2. definition of pathogenesis and pathognomonic.
3. information given by a diagnosis.

E. Pathology as a Course and as a Specialty	1.28	93-102

1. specific subjects that are covered in a medical school Pathology course.
2. types of abnormalities which are not included in a medical school Pathology course.
3. activities of pathologists, including subspecialists.

PRETEST
UNIT 1. INTRODUCTION TO PATHOLOGY

SELECT THE SINGLE BEST RESPONSE.

1. Study of which of the following is more germane to Pathology than to other medical science disciplines?
   (A) effects of acid on digestion of meat
   (B) effects of acid on the staining reaction of parietal cells
   (C) effects of acid on esophageal mucosa
   (D) effects of pH on absorption from the intestine

2. A lesion is defined as a
   (A) disease
   (B) structural abnormality
   (C) functional deficit
   (D) area of necrosis
   (E) localized defect

3. Which is classified as a disturbance of growth rather than as abnormal development?
   (A) atrophy
   (B) aplasia
   (C) both
   (D) neither

4. Which of the following is an example of inflammation?
   (A) cellular and vascular response to an electrical burn
   (B) death of tissue surrounding a cut
   (C) enlargement of the left ventricle
   (D) obstruction of the pancreatic duct, causing a decrease in the number of acinar cells

5. An infection is defined as
   (A) invasion of the body by microorganisms
   (B) invasion and multiplication of organisms in the body
   (C) the presence of organisms in the body
   (D) invasion of the body by organisms and reaction of the body to the organisms

6. Which of the following is a sign?
   (A) a patient's report of pain in the abdomen
   (B) high blood glucose levels
   (C) a severe headache
   (D) a physician's observation of abdominal tenderness

7. The term <u>pathogenesis</u> refers to
   (A) the mechanism by which structural abnormalities cause functional abnormalities
   (B) the means by which a disease produces manifestations
   (C) the mechanism by which injurious agents cause structural and functional abnormalities, which in turn cause other abnormalities and manifestations
   (D) the mechanism by which a disease produces functional abnormalities and manifestations

8. Which of the following procedures is performed in a pathologist's laboratory?
   (A) blood glucose determination
   (B) culture of the blood
   (C) both
   (D) neither

GO ON TO NEXT PAGE AND BEGIN THE UNIT.

A. Definition of Pathology (9 frames)

When you complete this section, you will be able to select correct responses relating to the:

1. definition of pathology and examples of disease.

2. subject matter of pathology compared to other basic medical sciences.

1. This section will introduce you to the science of medicine, Pathology. The word comes from the Greek pathes, meaning "disease," and -ology, meaning "the study of." In a strict sense, Pathology is the ______ ______ ______.

---

1. Pathology is the study of disease.

---

2. Diseases are abnormalities of body structure and/or function. Pathology is concerned with the relationship of the abnormalities to the causes of the abnormalities if known, and the manifestations of the abnormalities if present. WHICH OF THE FOLLOWING IS/ARE DISEASES?

   A. structural and functional abnormalities

   B. exposure to an agent which can cause damage to the body

   Are the causes of all diseases known? ☐ yes ☐ no

   Do all diseases have manifestations? ☐ yes ☐ no

---

52. Causal Agent → Basic Response

cyclic hydrocarbons → hyperplasia

---

53. Enlargement of the left ventricle in a person with aortic stenosis (narrowing of aorta valve) is an example of __________. Why?

TURN THE TEXT 180° AND CONTINUE.

---

102. 1. microbiologic analysis
2. chemical analysis
3. hematologic analysis (and blood bank operation)

(or equivalent answers)

THIS IS THE END OF UNIT 1. TAKE THE POSTTEST ON PAGE xiii.

2. Structural and functional abnormalities are disease. Exposure to an agent which can cause damage to the body is not, in itself, disease.

No, the cause of every disease is not known.

No, structural and functional abnormalities are not always manifest to the patient or physician.

---

3. INDICATE WHICH OF THE FOLLOWING ARE DISEASES:

a) high-cholesterol diet

b) Staphylococcus aureus

c) arteriosclerosis (narrowing and hardening of the arteries)

d) exposure to x-rays

e) infectious hepatitis

f) diabetes mellitus

---

53. Hypertrophy. Muscle cells cannot divide, so an increase in tissue size must be hypertrophy.

---

54. Neoplasia is the pathologic growth and proliferation of cells which exceeds and is uncoordinated with the growth of normal cells. Neoplasia, like __________, involves an __________ in the number of cells.

51. Hypertrophy and hyperplasia commonly occur together in enlarging tissues, but in tissues (like skeletal muscle) which are incapable of regeneration hypertrophy can occur but hyperplasia cannot occur.

---

52. The bronchial mucosal cells of a heavy smoker are stimulated to proliferate by the cyclic hydrocarbons in cigarette smoke. FILL IN THE SPECIFIC CAUSAL AGENT AND RESPONSE:

Causal Agent → Basic Response

---

101. A
B
A
B
B

---

102. WHAT THREE MAJOR ACTIVITIES ARE INCLUDED IN CLINICAL PATHOLOGY?

1. ______________________

2. ______________________

3. ______________________

3. c) arteriosclerosis

e) infectious hepatitis
f) diabetes mellitus

---

4. Pathology is the study of disease:
The study of structural and functional abnormalities and their relationship to causes and manifestations of disease. INDICATE WHICH OF THE FOLLOWING IS/ARE INCLUDED IN THE SUBJECT MATTER OF PATHOLOGY:

a) narrowing of the aortic valve (aortic stenosis) and the resultant effects

b) the ultrastructure of liver parenchymal cells

c) the effects of carbon tetrachloride on liver cells

d) the structure of the enzyme necessary for insulin production

---

54. Neoplasia, like hyperplasia, involves an increase in the number of cells.

---

55. There is evidence that cyclic hydrocarbons (as in cigarette smoke), radiation, and viruses can all cause neoplasia. FILL IN POSSIBLE SPECIFIC AGENTS IN THE DIAGRAM BELOW:

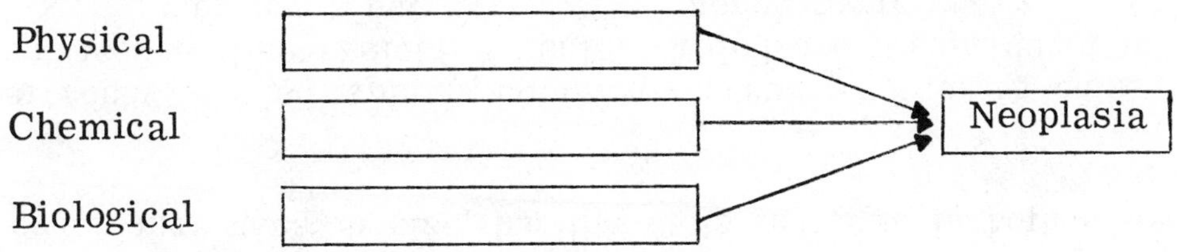

50. B A C

---

51. Hyperplasia and hypertrophy can occur alone but they usually occur together. For example, when one kidney is damaged, the remaining one will greatly increase in size. This process is called compensatory hypertrophy because the organ increases in size, but the cells increase in both size and number.

Hypertrophy and hyperplasia commonly occur together in enlarging tissues, but in tissues (like skeletal muscle) which are incapable of mitotic division __________ can occur but __________ cannot occur.

---

100. A
B
C
C

---

101. MATCH THE FOLLOWING:

____morphologic analysis of tissue

____biochemical analysis of fluids and tissue

____cytologic analysis for evidence of cancer

____microbiological analysis of fluids and tissue

____hematologic analysis of blood and bone marrow

A. Anatomic Pathology

B. Clinical Pathology

4. a) narrowing of the aortic valve (aortic stenosis) and the resultant effects
c) the effects of carbon tetrachloride on liver cells

---

5. Agents which cause disease create structural and functional abnormalities which may produce detectable evidence of disease (manifestations).

Specific diseases are often easily understood if these relationships are schematically diagrammed.

FILL IN THE BOX

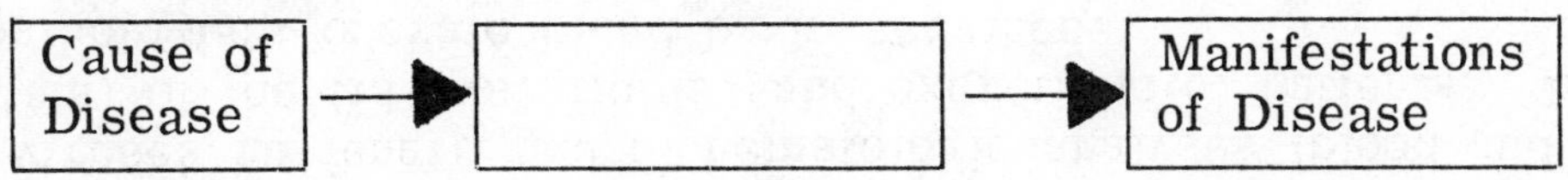

55.

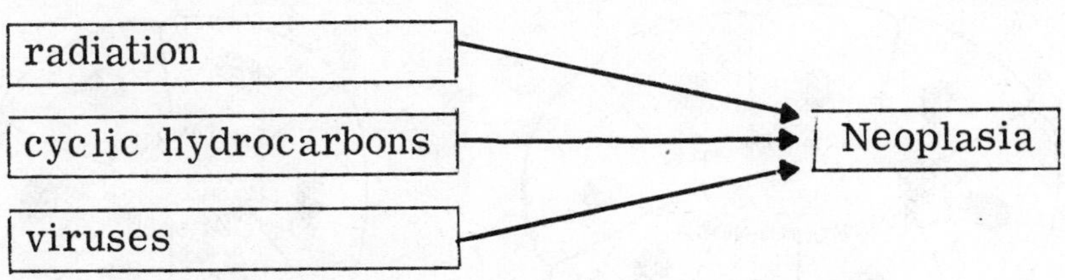

---

56. LIST FOUR ABNORMALITIES OF CELL GROWTH AND PROLIFERATION. WHICH ONE(S) REFER TO A <u>DECREASE</u> IN SIZE?

1. ______________ 3. ______________

2. ______________ 4. ______________

49. __B__ increase in volume due to change in cell size
__A__ increase in volume due to change in cell number
__C__ decrease in volume due to reduced cell size
__C__ decrease in volume due to change in cell number

---

50. Below are three examples of enlarged kidney tubules. MATCH EACH EXAMPLE WITH ITS MECHANISM OF ENLARGEMENT:

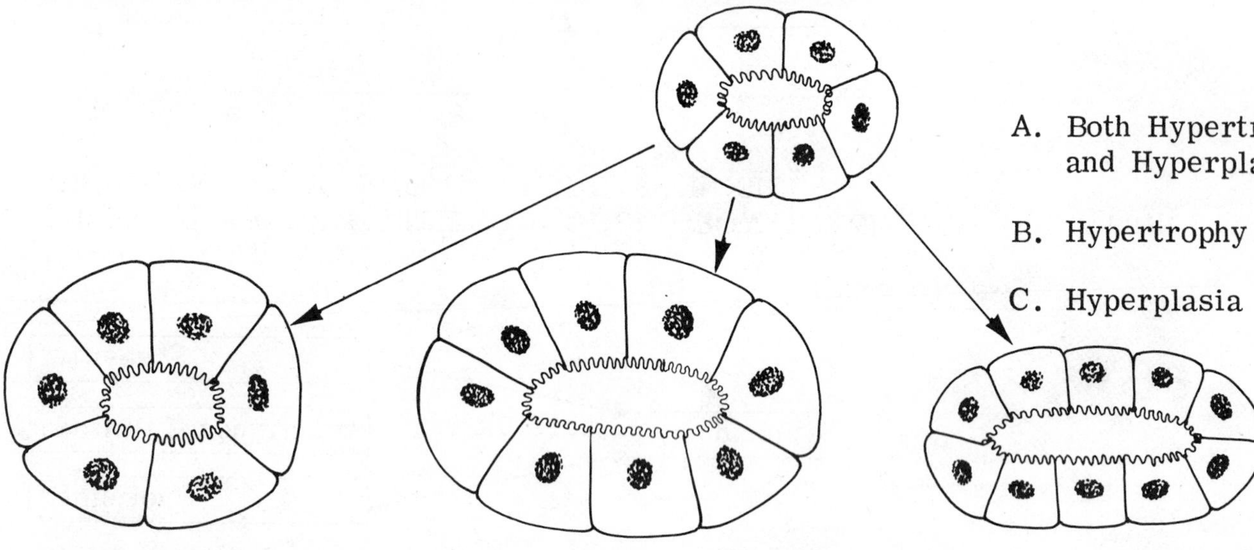

A. Both Hypertrophy and Hyperplasia

B. Hypertrophy only

C. Hyperplasia only

---

99. Surgical Pathology
Cytopathology
Autopsy Pathology [or equivalent]

---

100. The specialty of Pathology is composed of two major divisions, Anatomic Pathology and Clinical Pathology. Clinical pathologists make: a) biochemical analyses (chemical composition); b) microbiological analyses (presence of bacteria, viruses, and fungi); and c) hematologic analyses (blood and bone marrow abnormalities) of the tissues, fluids, and excretions of patients. In addition, clinical pathologists operate blood bank services.

MATCH THE THREE MAJOR AREAS OF CLINICAL PATHOLOGY WITH THEIR FUNCTIONS:

____ culture of urine for bacteria
____ determination of sodium concentration in blood
____ determination of number of white blood cells/cu.mm. of blood
____ matching blood types

A. Clinical microbiology
B. Medical chemistry
C. Hematology and blood bank operation

5. Cause of Disease → Structural and Functional Abnormalities → Manifestations of Disease

---

6. Acid burn of the hand

acid → destruction and inflammation of the skin → pain and redness of the skin

MATCH THE FOLLOWING:

____pain	A. cause
____redness	B. abnormality of structure or function
____destruction and inflammation of the skin	C. manifestation
____acid	

---

56. 1. Neoplasia
2. Hyperplasia
3. Hypertrophy
4. Atrophy (decrease in size)

---

57. Abnormal development includes: 1) aplasia, the complete or almost complete failure of an organ to develop; 2) hypoplasia, the failure of an organ to achieve full size; 3) malformation, the development of a tissue in such a way that it is not within the normal range of structure and/or function. MATCH THE ABNORMAL KIDNEYS WITH THE CORRECT TERM.

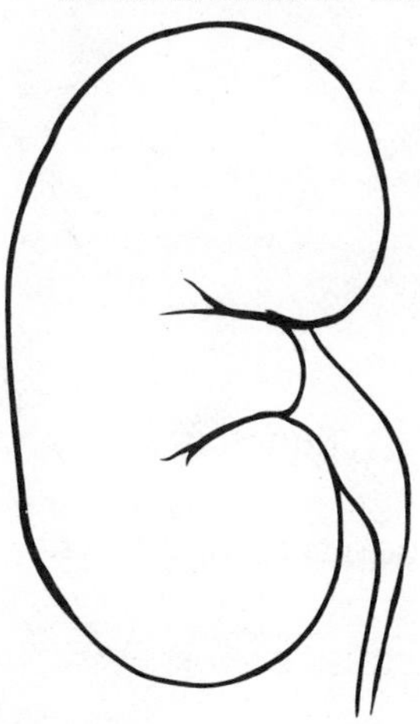

Normal kidney

A. Malformed kidney

B. Hypoplastic kidney

C. Aplastic kidney

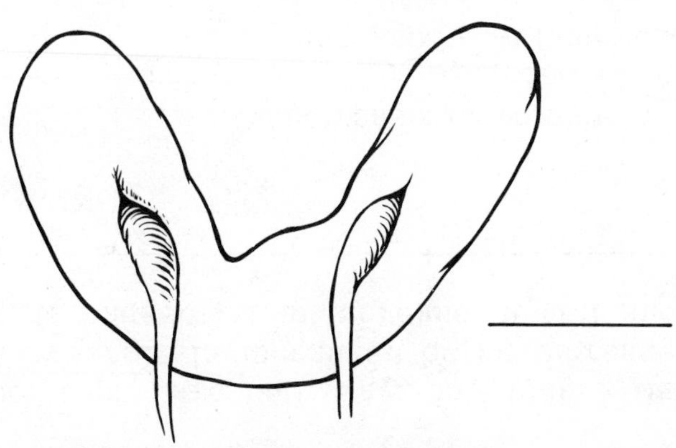

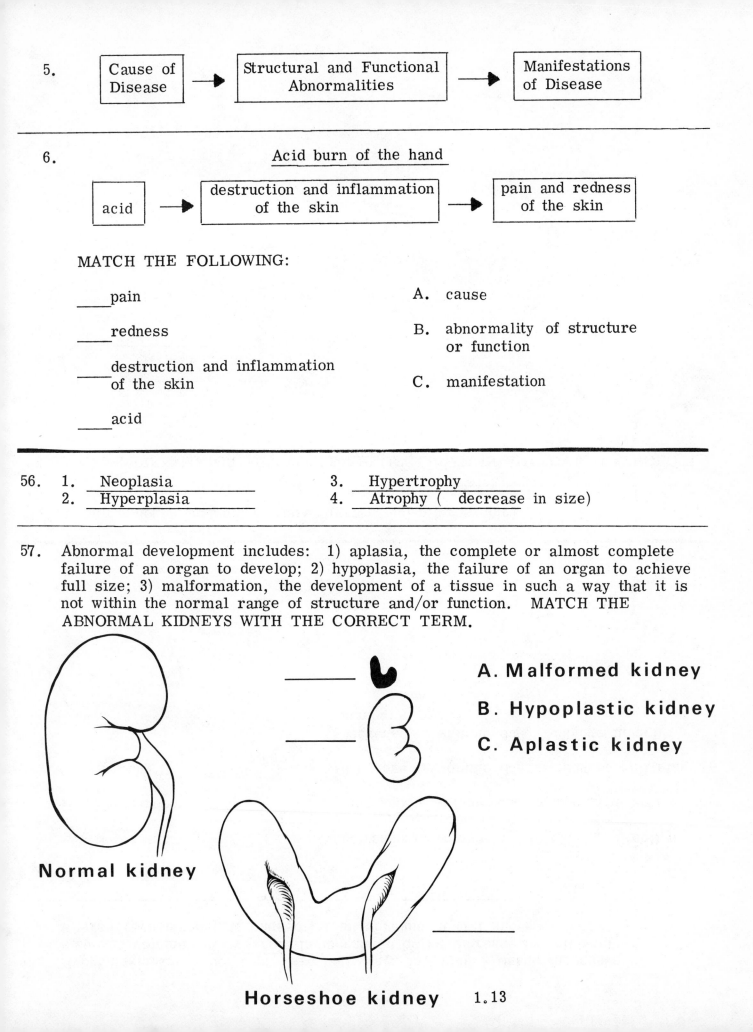

Horseshoe kidney

48. Hyperplasia and hypertrophy are both ways in which a tissue increases in size and volume, but hyperplasia is caused by an increase in cell number whereas hypertrophy is caused by an increase in cell size.

---

49. MATCH THE FOLLOWING:

A. Hyperplasia	___ increase in volume due to change in cell size
B. Hypertrophy	___ increase in volume due to change in cell number
C. Atrophy	___ decrease in volume due to reduced cell size
	___ decrease in volume due to change in cell number

---

98. d) morphologic analysis of tissue (gross and microscopic)

---

99. WHAT THREE MAJOR ACTIVITIES ARE INCLUDED IN ANATOMIC PATHOLOGY?

1. ____________________

2. ____________________

3. ____________________

6. C pain - manifestation
C redness - manifestation
B destruction and inflammation of skin - abnormality of structure or function
A acid - cause

---

7. To recognize and deal with abnormal structure and function of the body, you must first understand the normal structure and function of the body.

MATCH THE SUBJECTS WITH THEIR GENERAL AREA(S) OF STUDY.

____Physiology

____Anatomy

____Histology

____Biochemistry

____Pathology

A. Normal Structure and Function of the Body

B. Abnormal Structure and Function of the Body

---

57. C
B
A

58.

Causes → Developmental Abnormalities → Manifestations

Developmental abnormalities include structural and functional abnormalities resulting from: a) missing or abnormal genes, b) missing or abnormal chromosomes, and c) injuries during embryonic or fetal development. Developmental abnormalities may be caused by ____________, ____________, and ____________ agents. Developmental abnormalities are caused by events that occur ☐ before ☐ after birth.

47. When a tissue decreases in size, it is atrophic, but tissues can also undergo abnormal increases in size. Hypertrophy and hyperplasia are two ways in which a tissue can undergo abnormal increase in size.

---

48. Hyperplasia and __________ are both ways in which a tissue increases in size and volume, but hyperplasia is caused by an increase in cell number whereas hypertrophy is caused by an increase in cell __________.

---

97. b
c

---

98. An autopsy is the postmortem examination of the body to determine the cause of death and in some cases the effect of treatment. The information gained from autopsies contributes to more accurate diagnosis and improved treatment. Performance of autopsies and examination of biopsy and cytopathology specimens are all part of Anatomical Pathology. The primary function of the anatomic pathologist is:

a) biochemical analysis of tissue.

b) immunologic analysis of tissue.

c) microbiological analysis of tissue.

d) morphologic analysis of tissue (gross and microscopic).

7. A Physiology
A Anatomy
A Histology
A Biochemistry
B Pathology

---

8. Pathology is the study of disease with emphasis on structural and functional abnormalities and their relationship to __________ and __________ of disease.

Diseases can be diagrammed in the following manner:

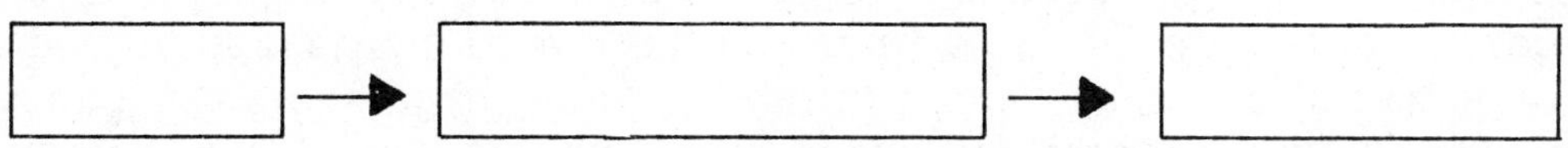

---

58. Developmental abnormalities may be caused by physical, chemical, or biological agents. Developmental abnormalities are caused by events that occur [✓] before birth.

---

59. MATCH THE FOLLOWING:

A. Atrophy	___	an acquired decrease in organ size
B. Hypoplasia	___	agenesis (failure of organ to develop)
C. Aplasia	___	failure of an organ to attain normal size
D. Hyperplasia	___	increase in organ size due to increase in cell number

46. B
C
A

---

47. When a tissue decreases in size, it is ________ic , but tissues can also undergo abnormal increases in size. Hypertrophy and hyperplasia are two ways in which a tissue can undergo abnormal __________ in size.

---

96. C
A
D
B

---

97. Cytopathology (also called exfoliative cytology) is the microscopic examination of cells which have been shed or scraped from an area of the body. This technique is most widely used as a screening test for cancerous and pre-cancerous lesions of the female genital tract, where cells are obtained from the pooled secretions of the vaginal vault or by scraping the cervix. Various collection techniques are used to look for cancer cells at other sites, such as bronchi, stomach, urine, spinal fluid and pleural and peritoneal cavities.

The subspecialty of cytopathology is concerned with

a. ultrastructure of disease.

b. cancer diagnosis using specimens not requiring biopsy.

c. screening for cancer by examining individual cells.

8. causes (and) manifestations

Causes of Disease → Structural and Functional Abnormalities → Manifestations of Disease

---

9. INDICATE FOR THE FOLLOWING TRUE (T) OR FALSE (F):

	frame reference
____ A disease is not necessarily associated with abnormalities of body structure and function.	(2)
____ The accumulation of large amounts of fat in the liver parenchyma, which results in impaired liver function, is an example of a disease.	(2 & 3)
____ Exposure of a person to a virulent virus is an example of a disease.	(2 & 3)
____ Diseases always involve abnormalities of structure or function in the body.	(2 & 3)
____ A disease is not necessarily associated with manifestations.	(2)

---

59. A an acquired decrease in organ size
C agenesis (failure of organ to develop)
B failure of an organ to attain normal size
D increase in organ size due to increase in cell number

---

60. A connection between the esophagus and trachea, called a tracheo-esophageal fistula, is an example of:

a) aplasia

b) hypoplasia

c) malformation

d) neoplasia

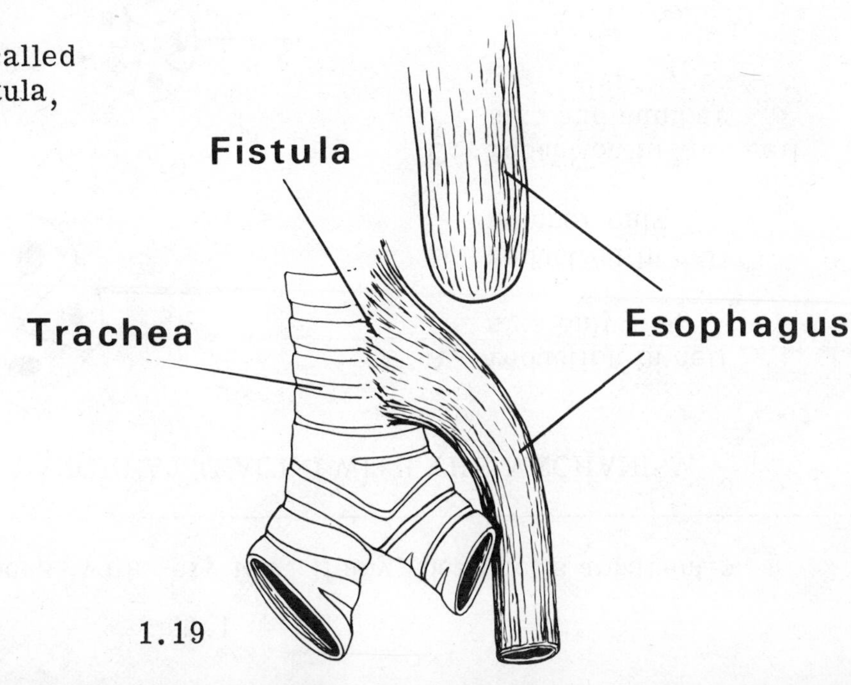

45. b) relatively gradual process with very few, if any, dead cells apparent.

---

46. MATCH THE ATROPHIC PANCREATIC ACINI WITH THE MECHANISM OF THEIR ATROPHY.

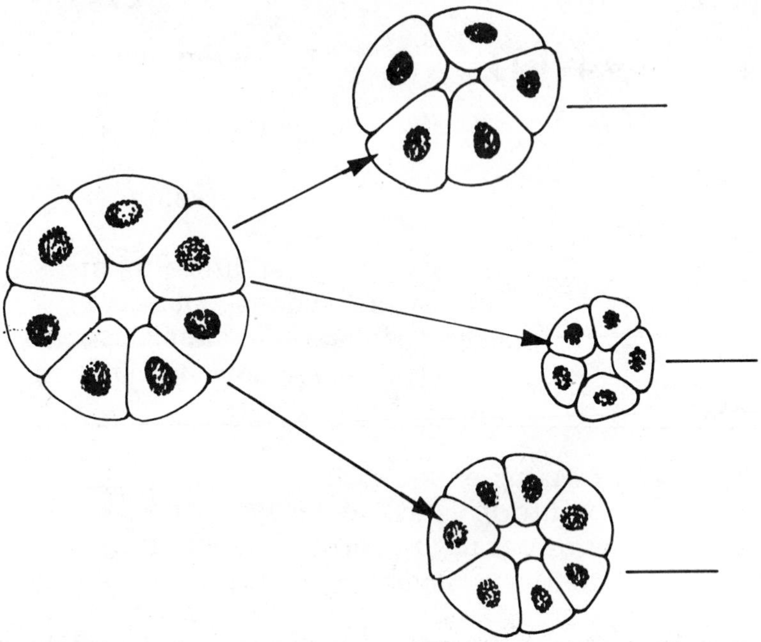

A. reduction in cell size only

B. reduction in cell number only

C. reduction in both cell size and number

---

95. a, b, d, e, f

---

96. Biopsy is the removal of tissue for examination from the living body for the purpose of diagnosis. Biopsy is the procedure by which tissue is removed, and the tissue removed is called the biopsy specimen. The examination of biopsy specimens comprises the subspecialty of surgical pathology.

MATCH THE FOLLOWING:

____the removal of tissue from the body of a living patient

____person who removes tissue from living body

____tissue which has been removed from a living patient

____person who analyzes tissue removed from living body

A. surgeon

B. pathologist

C. biopsy

D. biopsy specimen

9. F
T
F
T
T

B. Causes of Disease (9 frames)

When you complete this section, you will be able to select correct responses relating to the:

1. three major types of causes of disease and examples of each.

2. correct use of the term etiology.

10. Every disease is assumed to have a cause. Understanding of the agents which __________ specific diseases is one of the primary objectives of a course in __________.

---

60. c) malformation

---

61. MATCH THE FOLLOWING:

A. Developmental Abnormality
B. Disturbance of Growth

___ Malformation

___ Atrophy

___ Aplasia

___ Hypertrophy

___ Hyperplasia

___ Hypoplasia

44. Thus, cell degeneration or cell death, or both, may be involved in atrophy.

---

45. Atrophy is usually a

a) very rapid process with many dead cells in the tissue.

b) relatively gradual process with very few, if any, dead cells apparent.

---

94. C stuttering
A diabetes
B neurotic depression

---

95. The aim of the medial specialty of Pathology is to contribute to the prevention, diagnosis, treatment, and understanding of disease through information obtained by morphologic (gross and microscopic), biochemical, microbiologic, serologic, or any other laboratory examination made on specimens obtained from patients. Specimens commonly examined by pathologists include surgically removed solid tissue, blood, urine, feces, spinal fluid, and scrapings from body surfaces. Unlike most other medical specialties, the practice of Pathology does not usually include the treatment and prevention of disease. WHICH OF THE FOLLOWING ACTIVITIES WOULD USUALLY BE PERFORMED BY A PATHOLOGIST?

a) testing serum for antibodies to the organism which causes syphilis

b) examination of material draining from sinuses for the presence of fungi

c) prescribing drugs for the treatment of a fungal infection

d) determining the activity of clotting factor VIII in the blood

e) microscopic examination of liver tissue removed from a patient

f) examination of a body to determine the cause of death

10. Understanding of the agents which cause specific diseases is one of the primary objectives of a course in Pathology.

---

11. Etio- refers to cause, so etiology is the study of causes (of disease). The term cause should be used when referring to a specific agent.

WHICH IS/ARE CORRECT USE (S) OF THE TERM ETIOLOGY?

A. Smoking is the etiology of lung cancer.

B. Sunlight is the etiology of sunburn.

C. Etiology loosely refers to causes of disease.

FILL IN THE BLANKS:

It is more precise to say "What is the __________?" than to say "What is the __________?"

---

61. A Malformation
B Atrophy
A Aplasia
B Hypertrophy
B Hyperplasia
A Hypoplasia

---

62. Abnormal development may be 1) the direct result of chemical, __________, and __________ agents injuring the developing organism, or 2) the result of a(n) __________ defect in the germ cells of the parent.

43. B
A
B
A
A, B

---

44. Growth disturbances that result in a change in organ size are termed atrophy, hypertrophy, or hyperplasia. Atrophy is a gradual decrease in size of a normally developed tissue or organ due to a reduction in cell size or a decrease in cell number, or both. Thus, cell degeneration or cell ________________, or both, may be involved in ________________.

---

93. A / B / C   B / A / C

---

94. By tradition, medical Pathology courses exclude the study of diseases in which functional abnormalities are not accompanied by presently known structural abnormalities. However, the term pathology is still applicable to these abnormalities. MATCH THE FOLLOWING:

A. General Pathology ___ stuttering

B. Psychopathology ___ diabetes

C. Speech Pathology ___ neurotic depression

11. C only
It is more precise to say "What is the cause?" than to say "What is the etiology?"

---

12. Pathology is the study of __________ with emphasis on __________ and __________ abnormalities and their relationship to __________ and __________ manifestations of disease.

---

62. Abnormal development may be 1) the direct result of chemical, physical, and biological agents injuring the developing organism, or 2) the result of a genetic defect in the germ cells of the parent.

---

63. A decrease in size of a normally developed tissue is __________ while the failure of a tissue to develop to full size is __________.

42. A often a direct result of injury to the body
B common response of the body to injury

---

43. Disturbances of growth (the third basic response which may result from biological, chemical, and physical agents) can be divided into two large classes:

1. Diffuse, controlled increases or decreases in organ or tissue size which cease when the initiating stimulus is removed (hyperplasia, hypertrophy, atrophy).
2. Discrete, uncontrolled growths which do not cease when the initiating stimulus is removed (neoplasia).

MATCH THE FOLLOWING:

____ likely to present as a localized tumor
____ diffuse increase or decrease in organ size
____ likely to become manifest long after cause removed
____ reaction in proportion to stimulus
____ caused by physical, chemical, and biological agents

A. Hyperplasia, hypertrophy, or atrophy
B. Neoplasms

---

93. The course in Pathology is organized so that each major section serves as a basis for subsequent sections. The major sections are:

A. Basic structural and functional abnormalities (responses of the body)
B. Causes of disease
C. Diseases by organ systems (because of similarities of manifestations of diseases within an organ)

MATCH THE SECTION OF THE COURSE WITH THE SPECIFIC SUBJECT:

___ Inflammation
___ Injuries produced by chemical and physical agents
___ Kidney diseases
___ Fungus infections
___ Neoplasia
___ Parathyroid diseases

12. Pathology is the study of disease with emphasis on structural and functional abnormalities and their relationship to causes and manifestations of disease.

---

13. Causes

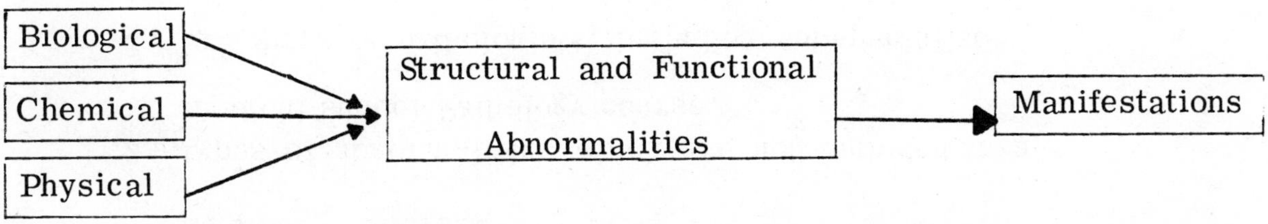

There are many ways to classify the agents which cause injury to the body. MATCH THE CAUSAL AGENTS WITH THE FOLLOWING CLASSIFICATIONS:

P = Physical   C = Chemical   B = Biological

___ bacteria and fungi   ___ radiation and electricity

___ heat and cold   ___ poisons

___ acids and alkalis   ___ viruses and antibodies to the body's own proteins

---

63. A decrease in size of a normally developed tissue is atrophy while the failure of a tissue to develop to full size is hypoplasia.

---

64. MATCH THE FOLLOWING BASIC ABNORMALITIES WITH THE LESIONS.

A. Necrosis or degeneration

B. Growth disturbance or neoplasia

C. Developmental abnormality

a) ___ changes in heart muscle after circulation is blocked

b) ___ spina bifida (failure of dorsal portions of vertebrae to fuse)

c) ___ cancer of the lung

d) ___ having only one kidney

41. inflammation

---

42. MATCH THE FOLLOWING:

A. Cell death and degeneration

B. Inflammation

___ often a direct result of injury to the body

___ common response of the body to injury

---

92. 1) F 2) T 3) T 4) F 5) F 6) T

E. Pathology as a Course and as a Specialty (10 frames)

This section explains briefly how the medical school Pathology course is organized and what the Pathologist, as a medical specialist, does. When you complete this section, you will be able to select correct responses relating to:

1. specific subjects that are covered in a medical school Pathology course.

2. types of abnormalities which are not included in a medical school Pathology course.

3. activities of pathologists, including subspecialists.

GO ON TO NEXT PAGE

13. B bacteria and fungi
P heat and cold
C acids and alkalis
P radiation and electricity
C poisons
B viruses and antibodies to the body's own proteins

---

14. Toxic substances which are harmful in small amounts (less than 50 grams) are classified as poisons. Toxic substances, or poisons, are __________ agents.

---

64. a) A
b) C
c) B
d) C

---

65. MATCH THE FOLLOWING BASIC ABNORMALITIES WITH THE LESIONS.

A. Necrosis or degeneration

B. Growth disturbance

C. Developmental abnormality

a) ___ having a horseshoe-shaped kidney

b) ___ enlargement of left ventricle due to aortic stenosis

c) ___ death of tissue surrounding bullet wound

d) ___ increase in thickness of epithelial layer of skin

40. painful

---

41. A common sequence following injury to the body is cell death and degeneration followed by ______________, which is followed by repair of the injury. This is an oversimplification, as will be seen in later units.

---

91. (1) manifestations of disease (signs, symptoms, and laboratory abnormalities); (2) structural and functional abnormalities; and (3) causes of disease.

---

92. INDICATE "T" TRUE OR "F" FALSE:

	frame reference
___Symptoms are generally apparent during physical examination of a patient.	70-71
___Some manifestations may be both signs and symptoms.	72
___An ideal diagnosis will state the cause of the disease and the structural and functional abnormalities which are likely to be present.	77-78
___Every disease has at least one pathognomonic manifestation.	79-81
___The history given by a patient is the normal source of signs.	70-72
___Once a diagnosis has been made, the physician attempts correction of the abnormalities and/or elimination of the cause, if possible.	86-88

14. chemical

---

15. INDICATE THE CLASSES OF INJURIOUS AGENTS, AND GIVE AN EXAMPLE OF EACH IN THE BLANKS BELOW:

Causes

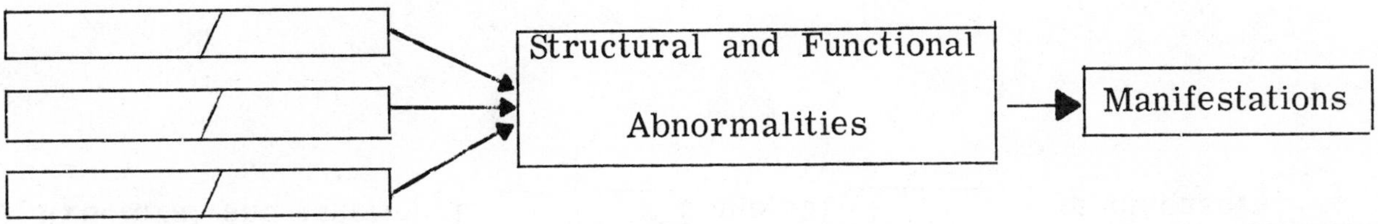

---

65. a) C
b) B
c) A
d) B

---

66. LIST THE FOUR BASIC RESPONSES OF THE BODY TO INJURY:

1. ______________________
2. ______________________
3. ______________________
4. ______________________

39. I bacteria   I radiation
    I heat   I acid
    I cold   I electricity

---

40. If you are stung by a hornet, the area becomes inflamed and appears red; and if you touch the area, it is hot, swollen, and __________.

---

90. Manifestations which might indicate this is a disease of the central nervous system are coma, psychoses, convulsions, and paralysis, but anemia, lead line on the gingivae, and a history of exposure to lead would give the diagnosis of lead poisoning.

---

91. Pathology in a broad sense is the study of the interrelationships among:

(1) manifestations of disease (__________, __________, and __________ __________);
(2) structural and functional __________; and (3) __________ of disease.

15.

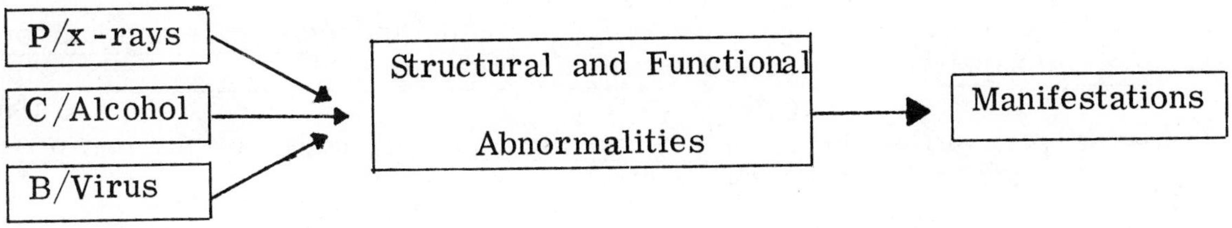

[or equivalent answers]

---

16. IDENTIFY THE TYPE OF AGENT RESPONSIBLE FOR EACH OF THE FOLLOWING AS CHEMICAL, "C," BIOLOGICAL, "B," OR PHYSICAL, "P":

____sunburn

____malaria

____electrocution

____lead poisoning

____athlete's foot

____atomic radiation burns

____syphilis

____common cold

____black eye

____frostbite

---

66. 1. cell degeneration and death
2. inflammation and repair
3. disturbances of growth
4. developmental abnormalities

---

67. MATCH THE FOLLOWING:

A. Inflammation

B. Cell degeneration and cell death

C. Disturbances of growth

D. Developmental abnormalities

___ hyperplasia

___ necrosis

___ immediate vascular and cellular response of body to injury

___ hypoplasia

38. <u>A</u> Capillary dilation
<u>A</u> Increase in capillary permeability
<u>B</u> Migration of leukocytes
<u>B</u> Phagocytosis by leukocytes

---

39. PUT AN "I" IN FRONT OF THE AGENTS WHICH CAN CAUSE INFLAMMATION:

___ bacteria ___ radiation

___ heat ___ acid

___ cold ___ electricity

89.

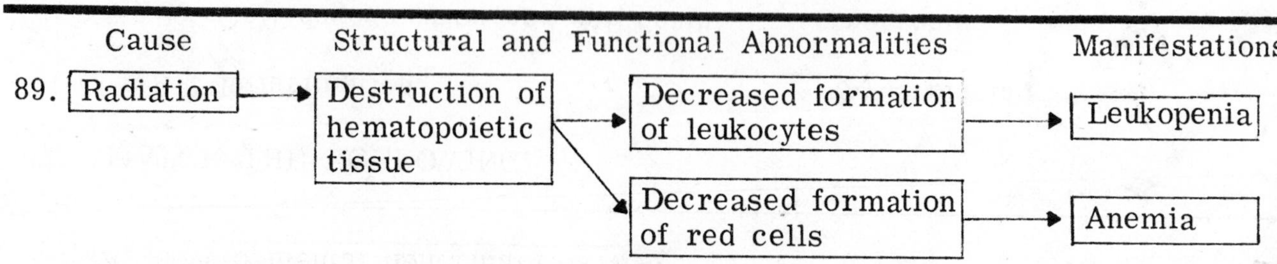

---

90. In some cases the manifestations caused by the action of a single agent are very complex.

Pathogenesis of Lead Poisoning

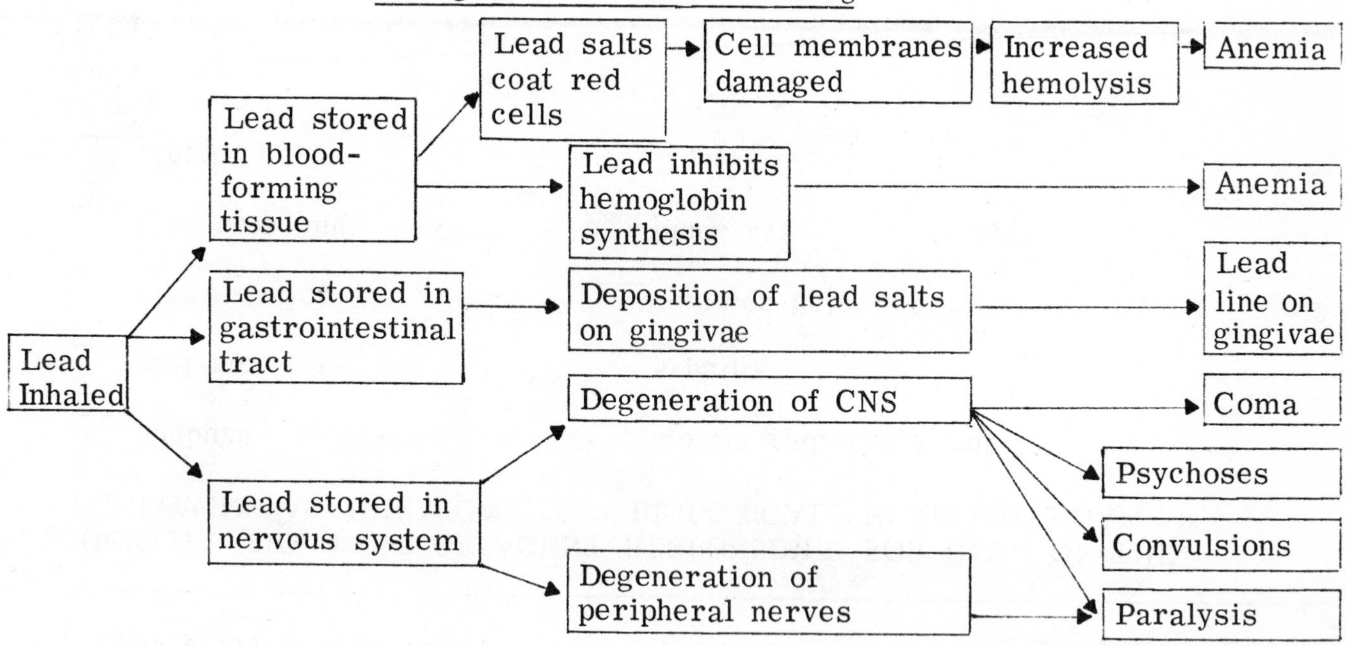

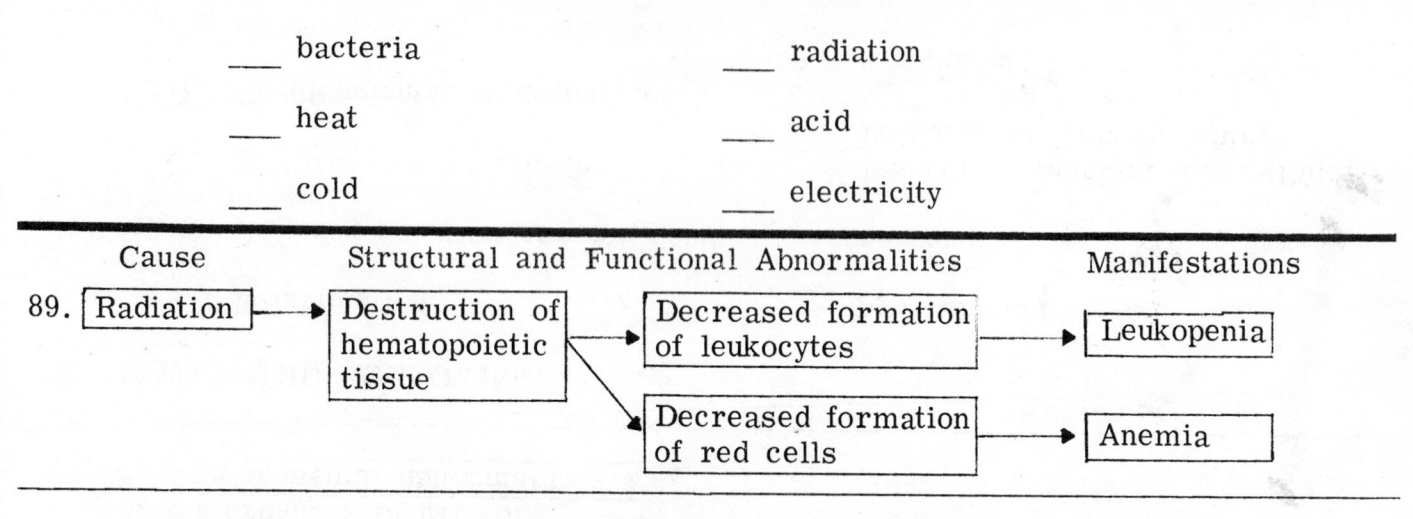

Manifestations which might indicate this is a disease of the central nervous system are ________, ________, ________, and ________, but a ________ ________ on the gingivae and a history of exposure to lead would give the diagnosis of lead poisoning.

16. P sunburn
B malaria
P electrocution
C lead poisoning
B athlete's foot
P atomic radiation burns
B syphilis
B common cold
P black eye
P frostbite

---

17. CLASSIFY THE AGENT IN THE FOLLOWING CASES (C = Chemical; B = Biological; P = Physical):

___ ionizing radiation, producing chromosomal damage

___ virus, causing chromosomal breakage

___ 5-bromouracil, producing increased frequency of chromosomal abnormalities

---

67. C hyperplasia
B necrosis
A immediate vascular and cellular response of body to injury
D hypoplasia

---

68. INDICATE "T" TRUE OR "F" FALSE:

	frame reference
___ The most toxic chemical agents are called poisons.	14
___ Only biological and chemical agents can cause genetic abnormalities.	17
___ Necrosis generally causes somatic death.	32
___ Inflammation usually follows cell injury or cell death.	37,41-42
___ Atrophy is caused only by reduction in cell size.	44

37. Swelling and redness can be seen.
Heat and pain cannot be seen.

---

38. MATCH THE FOLLOWING:

A. Vascular Response	___ Capillary dilation
B. Cellular Response	___ Increase in capillary permeability
	___ Migration of leukocytes
	___ Phagocytosis by leukocytes

---

88. A physician could make a diagnosis of multiple sclerosis on the basis of the manifestations muscle spasticity, sensory loss, and mental changes, but he could do nothing to correct the abnormality or eliminate the cause.

In some cases physicians may try to alleviate some of the manifestations. For example, if a patient has advanced cancer, the physician may be unable to do anything to cure the patient, but he will often try to alleviate the pain.

---

89. A patient is exposed to a large dose of radiation, which leads to destruction of his hematopoietic tissue, causing decreased formation of leukocytes, which leads to the laboratory abnormality of leukopenia (decreased white cells in blood.) The irradiation also causes decreased formation of red cells and leads to anemia (decreased number of red cells). FILL IN THE DIAGRAM BELOW:

Pathogenesis of Irradiation Injury

Cause — Structural and Functional Abnormalities — Manifestations

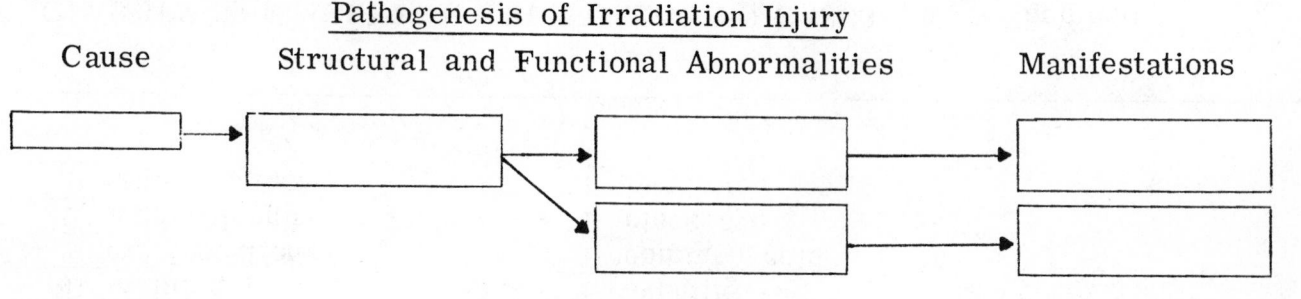

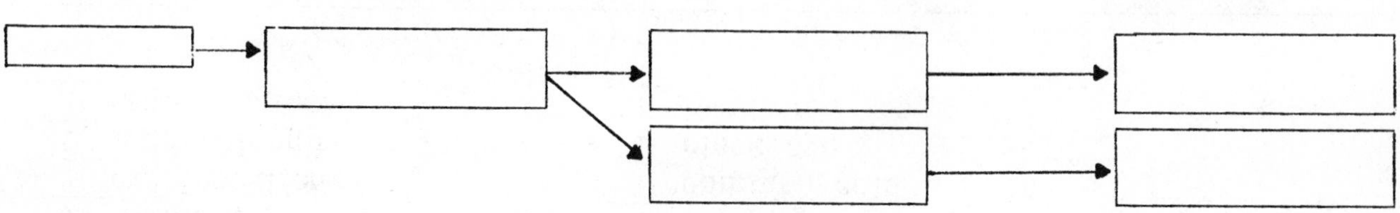

17. P ionizing radiation, producing chromosomal damage
B virus, causing chromosomal breakage
C 5-bromouracil, producing increased frequency of chromosomal abnormalities

---

18. INDICATE FOR THE FOLLOWING TRUE (T) OR FALSE (F):

		frame reference
____	In discussing the agent responsible for a disease, <u>cause</u> is a more precise term than <u>etiology</u>.	11
____	Antibodies to the body's own proteins do not cause disease.	13
____	Poisons are the only chemical substances which can cause injury.	14
____	Burns can be caused by physical agents.	16

---

68. T The most toxic chemical agents are called poisons.
F Only biological and chemical agents can cause genetic abnormalities.
F Necrosis generally causes somatic death.
T Inflammation usually follows cell injury or cell death.
F Atrophy is caused only by reduction in cell size.

---

69. INDICATE "T" TRUE OR "F" FALSE:

		frame reference
____	Neoplasia is only caused by biological agents.	43, 55
____	Malformation, aplasia, and hypoplasia are types of abnormal development.	57
____	Aplasia is an acquired decrease in organ size.	57
____	Atrophy is the complete or almost complete failure of an organ to develop.	44
____	Skeletal muscle can only undergo hyperplasia.	53

36. No. Infection consists of two parts: (1) invasion of the body, and (2) reaction of the body to invasion.

---

37. Inflammation (a vascular and cellular response to injury)

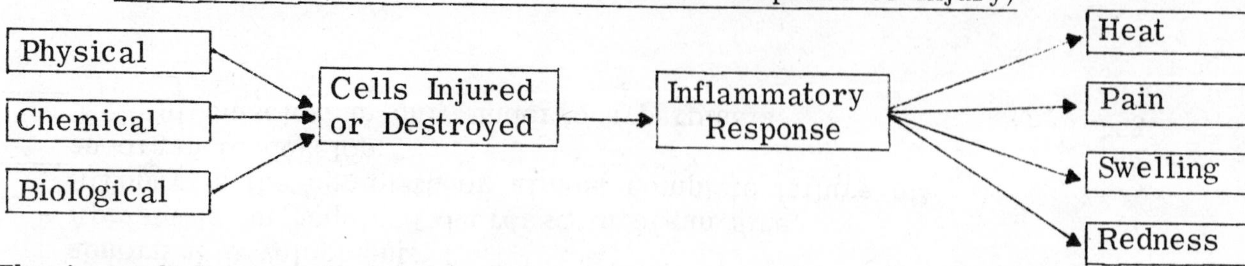

The immediate vascular and cellular response of the body to injury is inflammation, which is manifested by heat, pain, swelling, and redness in the area surrounding the injury.

WHICH MANIFESTATION(S) OF INFLAMMATION CAN BE SEEN?

WHICH CANNOT BE SEEN?

---

87. 1. Determining the manifestations (signs, symptoms, and lab abnormalities) of the disease, and naming it, if possible.
2. Inferring other structural and functional abnormalities that may be present.
3. Determining the causes of the disease.
4. Undertaking treatment (eliminating the causes or correcting structural and functional abnormalities, if possible).

---

88. Unfortunately, with many diseases it is possible to make a diagnosis on the basis of the manifestations and previous knowledge but it is not possible to correct the abnormalities or eliminate the cause.

Multiple Sclerosis

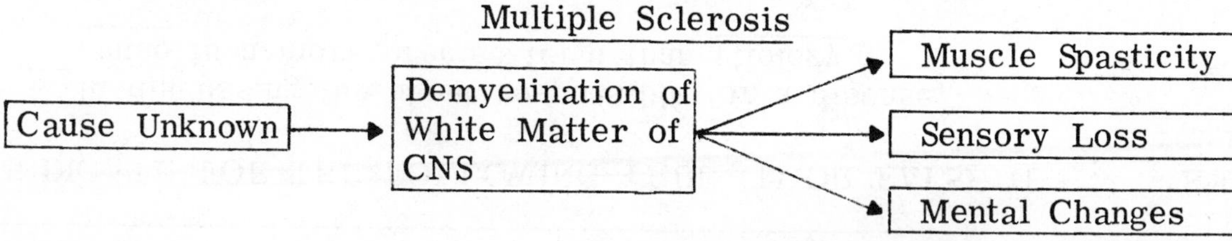

A physician could make a diagnosis of multiple sclerosis on the basis of the manifestations ________ ________, ________ ________, and ________, but he could do nothing to correct the ________ or eliminate the ________.

18. T
F
F
T

C. Structural and Functional Abnormalities (51 frames)

This section deals with the basic structural and functional abnormalities, i.e., the basic responses of the body to injury. When you complete this section, you should be able to select correct responses relating to the:

1. recognition of the defining characteristics of the basic responses of the body to injury.

2. classification of examples as cell degeneration and cell death, inflammation and repair, disturbances of growth and abnormal development.

3. identification of examples of the following:

necrosis	inflammation	atrophy	aplasia
cell death	infection	hypertrophy	hypoplasia
somatic death	repair	hyperplasia	malformation
degeneration		neoplasia	

4. distinction between structural and functional abnormalities and correct use of terms pathology and lesion.

GO ON TO NEXT PAGE

---

69. F Neoplasia is only caused by biological agents.
T Malformation, aplasia, and hypoplasia are types of abnormal development.
F Aplasia is an acquire decrease in organ size.
F Atrophy is the complete or almost complete failure of an organ to develop.
F Skeletal muscle can only undergo hyperplasia.

D. Manifestations of Disease (23 frames)

This section of the program will discuss the classification of manifestations and the relationship of these to basic responses. When you complete this section, you will be able to select correct responses relating to the:

1. differences between signs, symptoms, and laboratory abnormalities.

2. definition of pathogenesis and pathognomonic.

3. information given by a diagnosis

GO ON TO NEXT PAGE

35.

| bacterial invasion |
| cell injury |
| inflammation |

} _____infection_____

---

36. Would the presence of an organism in the body, which did not cause a response, be an infection? ____Yes ____No

EXPLAIN.

---

86. On the basis of accumulated knowledge of the disease, the physician's role is to correct the abnormality or eliminate the cause of the abnormality. However, this is not always possible, and the physician's role may be limited to naming the abnormalities and indicating their likely outcome.

---

87. The major parts of ideal patient care are:

1. Determining the manifestations (__________, __________, and __________ __________) of the disease, and naming it, if possible.
2. Inferring other structural and functional __________ that may be present.
3. Determining the __________ of the disease.
4. Undertaking treatment (eliminating the __________ or correcting __________ and __________ abnormalities, if possible).

19.

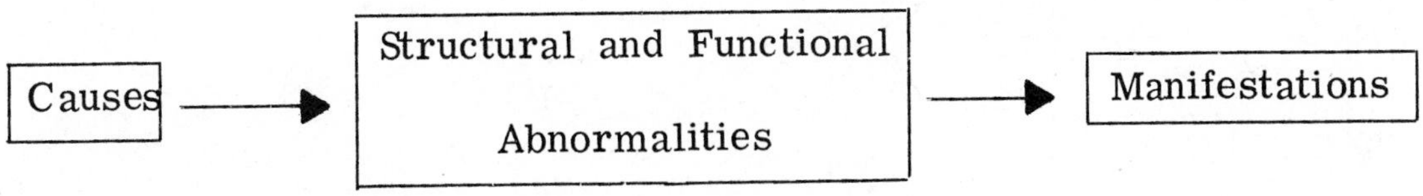

The body, or any part of it, can be abnormal in ______________ and/or ______________.

A disturbance of the normal performance or action of a cell, tissue, or organ is a ________________ abnormality.

A disturbance of the normal anatomic or biochemical conformation of the body is a ______________ abnormality.

70.

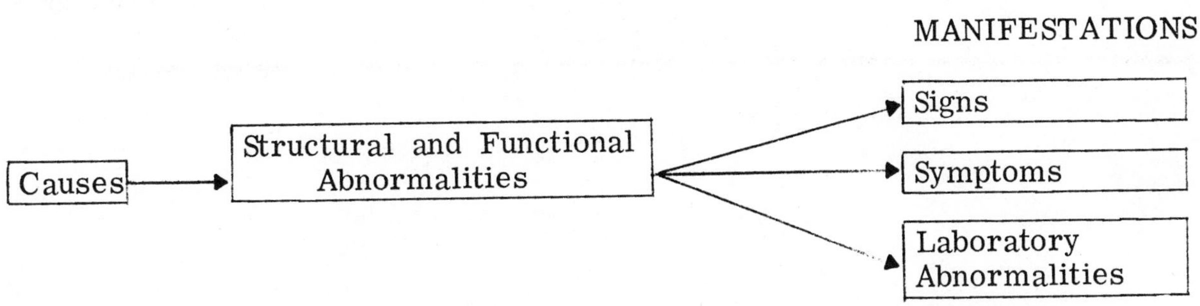

Injurious agents cause abnormalities which lead to the following types of manifestations: a) signs, b) symptoms, and c) laboratory abnormalities.

Signs, which are sometimes called objective symptoms, are direct observations made and recorded by a qualified person examining a patient. CONSIDER THE FOLLOWING:

A. A patient's report of pain in the abdomen.

B. A physician's observation of abdominal tenderness.

WHICH IS CORRECT?

1. Only A is a sign.

2. Only B is a sign.

3. Both A and B are signs.

4. Neither A nor B is a sign.

34. B. septicemia

---

35. LABEL THE TYPE OF DISEASE INDICATED BY THE DIAGRAM.

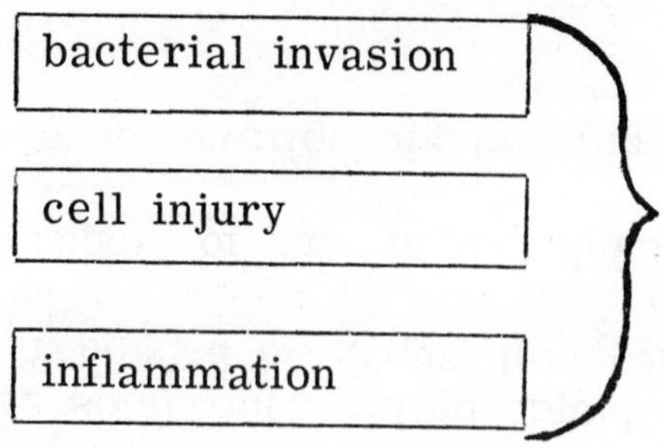

____

---

85. pathogenesis

---

86. On the basis of accumulated knowledge of the disease, the physician's role is to correct the abnormality or eliminate the __________ of the abnormality. However, this is not always possible, and the physician's role may be limited to naming the abnormalities and indicating their likely outcome.

19. The body, or any part of it, can be abnormal in structure and/or function.

A disturbance of the normal performance or action of a cell, tissue, or organ is a functional abnormality.

A disturbance of the normal anatomic or biochemical conformation of the body is a structural abnormality.

20.

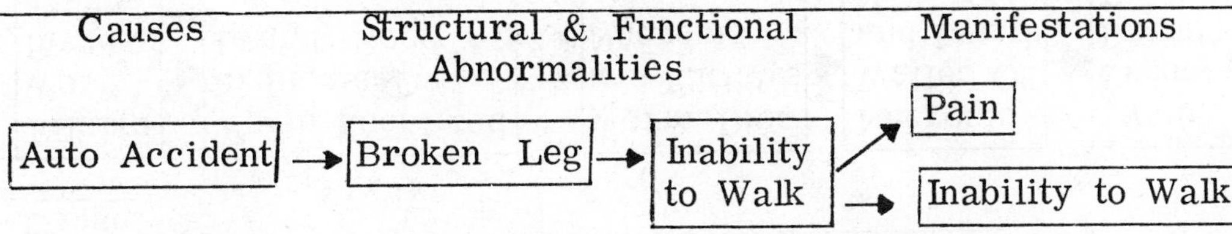

MATCH THE FOLLOWING (letters may be used more than once):

A. cause
B. functional abnormality
C. structural abnormality
D. manifestation

____ auto accident
____ broken leg
____ inability to walk
____ pain

This frame illustrates that a structural or functional abnormality may also be a ________________.

---

70. B. A physician's observation of abdominal tenderness. Pain is only felt by the patient. A physician can observe apparent reaction to pain. If he elicits this reaction by touching the patient, it is called tenderness.

---

71. Symptoms, also called subjective symptoms, are verbalizations by the patient concerning manifestations of a disease. Would a patient who was brought to you in a coma have ☐ symptoms ☐ signs?

33. C. Reaction of the body to microorganisms is an essential component of an infection.

---

34. Bacteremia is the presence of bacteria in the blood. Septicemia is the presence of bacteria in the blood causing fever and tissue damage. WHICH OF THE FOLLOWING IS/ARE INFECTION(S)?

A. bacteremia
B. septicemia
C. both A and B
D. neither A and B

---

84. An 85-lb. scrotum is a structural abnormality and most likely results in several functional abnormalities as well. However, it is also a [✓] sign [✓] symptom [✓] social handicap.

---

85. Pathogenesis of Elephant Scrotum

Cause — Manifestation

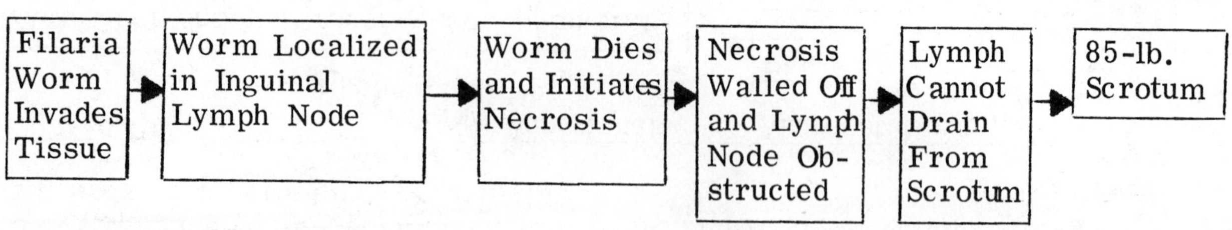

Filaria Worm Invades Tissue
Worm Localized in Inguinal Lymph Node
Worm Dies and Initiates Necrosis
Necrosis Walled Off and Lymph Node Ob-structed
Lymph Cannot Drain From Scrotum
85-lb. Scrotum

The physician makes a diagnosis of elephantiasis of the scrotum and from his diagnosis he is able to infer the structural and functional abnormalities underlying this condition and the cause. In this case the physician could treat the abnormality by removing the scrotum. From his understanding of the ____________ of the lesion, he realizes that any other treatment will not be successful.

20. ___A___ auto accident
___C___ broken leg
B, D inability to walk
___D___ pain

This frame illustrates that a structural or functional abnormality may also be a manifestation.

---

21. Structural abnormalities are referred to as "lesions" and can be either morphologic (or anatomic) or biochemical (or chemical). MATCH THE FOLLOWING:

____ absence of an anatomic structure	B. Biochemical Lesion
____ absence of a molecular structure	M. Morphologic Lesion
____ abnormality of an anatomic structure	
____ abnormality of a molecular structure	

---

71. Signs only, but he could have expressed symptoms before entering coma and related them to you through a relative or friend.

---

72. INDICATE WHETHER THE UNDERLINED WORD IS A SIGN OR A SYMPTOM:

_______ The physician observed the patient vomit.

_______ The patient said he vomited.

_______ The physician observed abdominal tenderness.

_______ The patient complained of abdominal pain.

To generalize from the above, pain is used to describe a ______________ while tenderness is used to describe a ____________. Vomiting is used to describe either a ____________ or a ____________.

32. B. Necrosis is irreversible.
C. Necrosis can be caused by bacteria, x-rays, acids, viruses, and other physical, chemical, and biological agents.

---

33. Infectious diseases (also called infections) are among the most common causes of cell degeneration and death. An infection consists of two steps: a) invasion of the body by pathogenic microorganisms, and b) reaction of the body to the organisms. To fulfill the definition of an infection, these two steps must be causally related. Which of the following is/are true ?

A. The type of agent causing infection is chemical.

B. The presence of microorganisms in the body is diagnostic of an infection.

C. Reaction of the body to microorganisms is an essential component of an infection.

D. Necrosis is unusual in infections.

---

83. F Most diseases produce at least one pathognomonic manifestion.
T Most diseases produce non-specific manifestations.
T Pathognomonic manifestations are uncommon but very valuable.
T A diagnosis can be made on the basis of a single pathognomonic manifestation.

---

84. As an example, assume a physician is faced with a patient who has an 85-lb. scrotum. The patient reveals that he spent some time in the South Pacific a few years previously. An 85-lb. scrotum is a structural ____________ and most likely results in several functional abnormalities as well. Would you consider the 85-lb. scrotum a ☐ sign ☐ symptom ☐ social handicap?

21. M
B
M
B

---

22. INDICATE THE FOLLOWING AS MORPHOLOGIC LESIONS "M" OR BIOCHEMICAL LESIONS "B":

____absence of a lung

____bifid (double) gallbladder

____replacement of adenine by thymine in a DNA molecule

____lack of enzyme necessary for insulin production

____liver with 50% of parenchymal cells dead

____decreased blood glucose

---

72. sign
symptom
sign
symptom

To generalize from the above, pain is used to describe a symptom while tenderness is used to describe a sign. Vomiting is used to describe either a symptom or a sign.

---

73. Laboratory abnormalities are manifestations of disease determined by laboratory procedures. MATCH THE FOLLOWING MANIFESTATIONS WITH THEIR SOURCE:

Manifestation	Source
A. Signs	___ History taken from patient.
B. Symptoms	___ Physical examination of patient.
C. Laboratory Abnormalities	___ Tests on specimens removed from patient.

31. B reversible change
A irreversible change

---

32. Somatic death is the death (cessation of vital functions) of the whole organism. Death of tissue -- individual cells, groups of cells, or small localized areas -- is called necrosis. SELECT THE CORRECT RESPONSE(S):

A. Somatic death always follows necrosis.

B. Necrosis is irreversible.

C. Necrosis can be caused by bacteria, x-rays, acids, viruses, and other physical, chemical, and biological agents.

D. Necrosis does not involve cell death.

---

82. cyanide poisoning

---

83. Unfortunately, most diseases do not produce manifestations which are specific, and the majority have very non-specific manifestations. INDICATE "T" TRUE OR "F" FALSE:

___ Most diseases produce at least one pathognomonic manifestation.

___ Most diseases produce non-specific manifestations.

___ Pathognomonic manifestations are uncommon but very valuable.

___ A diagnosis can be made on the basis of a single pathognomonic manifestation.

22. M absence of a lung
M bifid (double) gallbladder
B replacement of adenine by thymine in a DNA molecule

B lack of enzyme necessary for insulin production
M liver with 50% of parenchymal cells dead
B decreased blood glucose

---

23. Pathology is the study of disease, the study of structural and functional abnormalities and their relationship to ______________ and ______________ of disease. The term pathology should not be used to indicate a structural or functional abnormality. Lesions are ______________ abnormalities.

INDICATE THE CORRECT USE(S) OF THE TERMS PATHOLOGY AND LESION.

A. This patient's pathology is a collapsed lung.
B. Abscess formation is the pathology most often associated with staphylococci.
C. The primary lesion is extensive kidney damage.
D. Morphologic lesions are apparent at the gross or microscopic level.

---

73. B History taken from patient.
A Physical examination of patient.
C Tests on specimens removed from patient.

---

74. It is important to recognize that some manifestations may be both signs and symptoms. For example, discoloration of the skin may be reported by the patient and/or observed by the physician during a physical examination. However, as a general rule, manifestations which can be observed and recorded by the examining physician are called signs. This text will consider manifestations observable by a physician to be signs.

INDICATE WHETHER EACH OF THE FOLLOWING IS A SIGN, SYMPTOM, OR LABORATORY ABNORMALITY:

________ high glucose level in blood
________ low O_2 level in blood
________ redness of skin
________ patient's report of confusion
________ swelling of arm
________ discoloration of gingivae
________ low red cell count (anemia)
________ vague feeling of discomfort (malaise)

30. ☒ reversible

---

31. Cell death is the cessation of vital functions, such as respiration, synthesis of enzymatic and structural proteins, and maintenance of chemical and osmotic homeostasis. MATCH THE FOLLOWING:

A. Cell death ___ reversible change

B. Degeneration ___ irreversible change

---

81. pathognomonic

---

82. Cyanide Poisoning

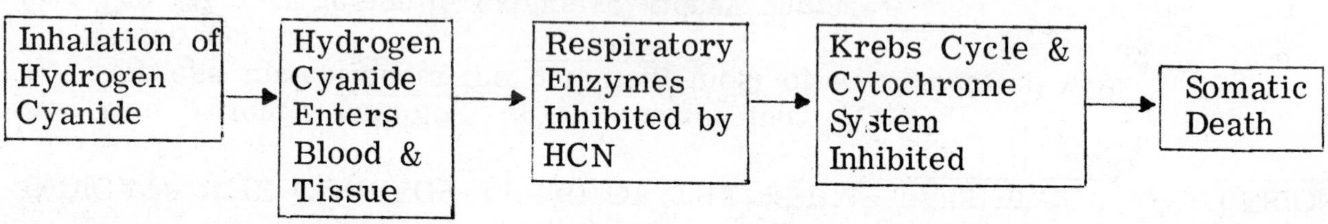

The presence of cyanide in the tissues of a cadaver is pathognomonic for __________ __________.

23. causes (and) manifestations
Lesions are structural abnormalities.
C
D

24.

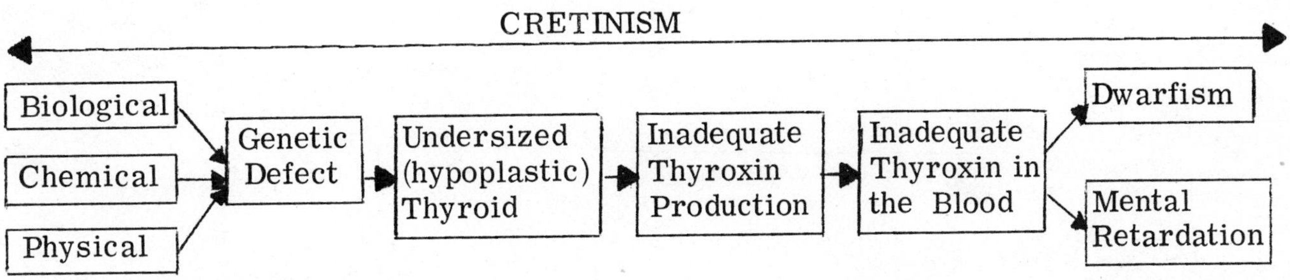

MATCH THE FOLLOWING (LETTERS MAY BE USED MORE THAN ONCE):

____ undersized thyroid		A.	Morphologic abnormality
____ inadequate thyroxin production		B.	Biochemical abnormality
____ inadequate thyroxin in blood		C.	Functional abnormality
____ dwarfism		D.	Manifestation
____ mental retardation			

74.

lab. abn.	high glucose level in blood	sign	swelling of arm
lab. abn.	low O_2 level in blood	sign	discoloration of gingiva
sign	redness of skin	lab. abn.	low red cell count (anemia)
symptom	patient's report of confusion	symptom	vague feeling of discomfort (malaise)

---

75. Path- is a Greek root meaning "__________" and genesis is Greek meaning "to produce or generate." So, in a strict sense, pathogenesis means __________ __________.

29. C. There are a great number of specific agents which can injure the body, and there are a limited number of direct responses the body can make to injury.

---

30. Degeneration refers to the cellular and interstitial changes in which cells are not killed. You would guess that the changes included in degeneration are often ☐ reversible ☐ irreversible.

---

80. pathognomonic

---

81. A white cell count of 1,000,000/cubic millimeter of blood (normal is 5,000 - 10,000/cu.mm.) is __________ for leukemia.

24. A, D undersized thyroid
C inadequate thyroxin production
B, D inadequate thyroxin in blood
A, D dwarfism
C, D mental retardation

---

25. In the example from the previous frame concerning cretinism, WHICH IS TRUE?

A. A structural abnormality has led to a functional abnormality.

B. A functional abnormality has led to a structural abnormality.

C. Both A and B are true.

D. Neither A nor B is true.

---

75. Path- is a Greek root meaning "disease" and genesis is Greek meaning "to produce or generate." So, in a strict sense, pathogenesis means "disease producing (generating)."

---

76. The pathogenesis of a specific disease refers to the mechanism by which structural and functional abnormalities are caused, generate other abnormalities, and produce manifestations of the disease.

Pathogenesis of Cauliflower Ear

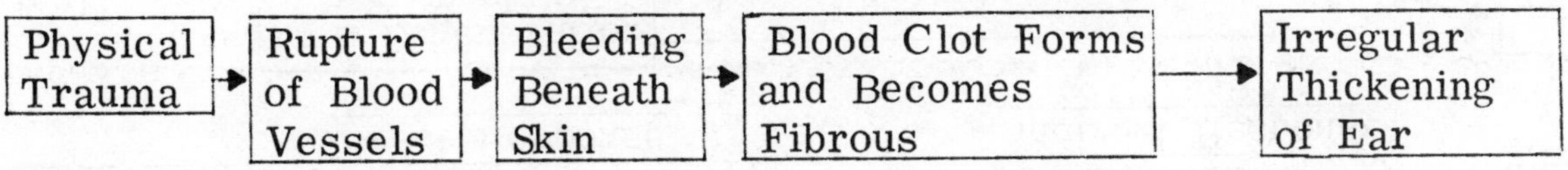

The pathogenesis of a cauliflower ear refers to the events which occur between the cause (__________ __________) and the manifestation (irregular ______________________________).

28. B decreased serum insulin
   F decreased insulin production
   M dead heart muscle
   B increased serum urea nitrogen
   F decreased urine output

---

29. The purpose of this diagram is to illustrate the basic structural and functional abnormalities, i.e., the limited basic responses of the body.

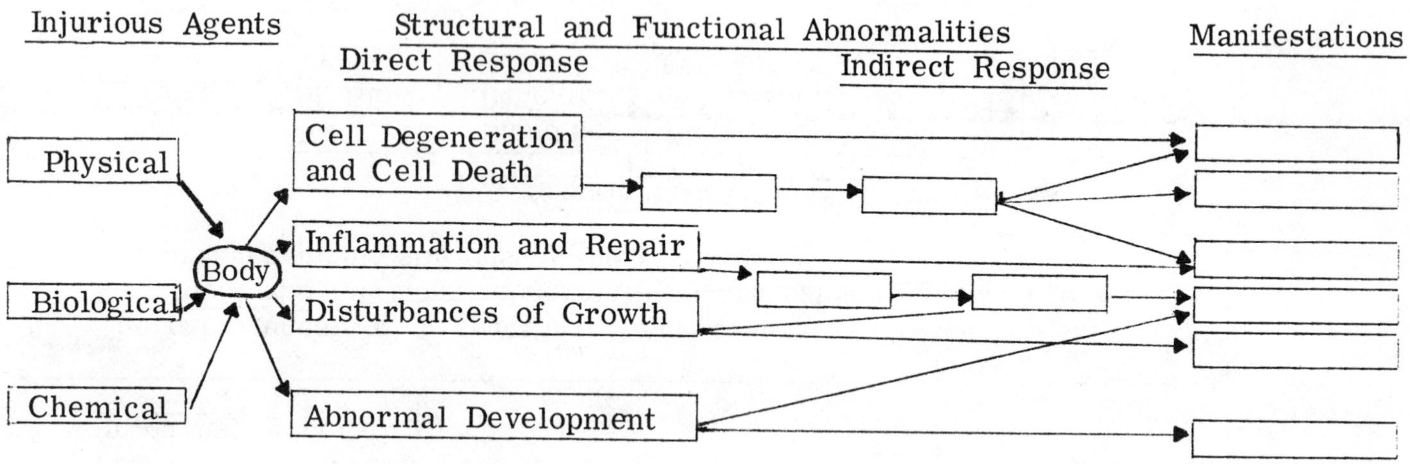

SELECT THE BEST ANSWER:

A. There are a great number of specific agents which can injure the body.

B. There are a limited number of direct responses the body can make to injury.

C. Both A and B are true.

D. Neither A nor B is true.

---

79. F A pathognomonic symptom can be present in several diseases.
   T A pathognomonic sign is present in only one specific disease.
   F A pathognomonic lab abnormality appears mostly as a manifestation of one disease but also appears in others.
   T A diagnosis can be made on the basis of a pathognomonic sign, symptom, or lab abnormality.

---

80. Ragged bone protruding from the leg is a ________ manifestation of a fracture.

25. C Both A and B are true.

undersized thyroid → inadequate thyroxin production → inadequate thyroxin in blood

---

26. WHICH OF THE FOLLOWING IS/ARE TRUE OF MANIFESTATIONS:

A. They are detectable indications of disease.

B. They are present in every disease.

C. They can be either structural or functional abnormalities.

---

76. The pathogenesis of a cauliflower ear refers to the events which occur between the cause (physical trauma) and the manifestation (irregular thickening of the ear).

---

77. A diagnosis is a brief way of saying that a patient has manifestations (________, ________, and ________ ________) similar to those of a group of patients seen in the past and that a specific name has been given to these manifestations.

27. _M_ oversized heart
_B_ lack of enzyme phenylalanine hydroxylase necessary to convert phenylalanine to tyrosine - this condition leads to phenylketonuria
_M_ fluid in interstitial spaces (edema)
_B_ decreased AHG (antihemophilic globulin)
_M_ blood in joint spaces

---

28. MARK EACH OF THE FOLLOWING AS
B = biochemical lesion
M = morphological lesion
F = functional abnormality

____ decreased serum insulin

____ decreased insulin production

____ dead heart muscle

____ increased serum urea nitrogen

____ decreased urine output

---

78. Ideally, an accurate diagnosis will tell the physician what structural and functional abnormalities are producing the manifestations and what is causing the abnormalities.

---

79. In some cases a diagnosis can be made on the basis of one manifestation which is specific for a certain disease. A manifestation on which a diagnosis can be made with certainty is said to be pathognomonic (pa•thog' no mon'ik). INDICATE "T" TRUE OR "F" FALSE:

___ A pathognomonic symptom can be present in several diseases.

___ A pathognomonic sign is present in only one specific disease.

___ A pathognomonic lab abnormality appears mostly as a manifestation of one disease but also appears in others.

___ A diagnosis can be made on the basis of a pathognomonic sign, symptom, or lab abnormality.

26. A and C

---

27. MARK EACH OF THE FOLLOWING AS
B = biochemical lesion
M = morphologic lesion
F = functional abnormality

____oversized heart

____lack of enzyme phenylalanine hydroxylase necessary to convert phenylalanine to tyrosine - this condition leads to phenylketonuria

____fluid in interstitial spaces (edema)

____decreased AHG (antihemophilic globulin)

____blood in joint spaces

TURN TEXT 180° AND CONTINUE.

---

77. A diagnosis is a brief way of saying that a patient has manifestations (signs, symptoms, and laboratory abnormalities) similar to those of a group of patients seen in the past and that a specific name has been given to these manifestations.

---

78. Ideally, an accurate diagnosis will tell the physician what structural and functional __________ are producing the __________ and what is causing the abnormalities.

TURN TEXT 180° AND CONTINUE.

Unit 2. Inflammation: The Vascular and Cellular Response to Injury

Unit 2. INFLAMMATION: THE VASCULAR AND CELLULAR RESPONSE TO INJURY

OBJECTIVES

When you complete this unit, you will be able to select correct responses relating to the:

	starting page	frame numbers
A. Introduction to Inflammation	2.3	1-15

1. signs and symptoms of inflammation.
2. examples of each type of agent (biological, chemical, and physical) that can cause inflammation.
3. components of the inflammatory response.
4. examples of harmful and beneficial inflammatory responses.

B. The Vascular Response	2.33	16-56

1. differentiation of plasma kinins by source, composition, and effect.
2. results of the release of chemical mediators.
3. definitions of capillary dilation and increased capillary permeability.
4. direct causes of the signs of inflammation.
5. differentiation between an exudate and a transudate on basis of composition and probable cause.
6. substances that leave the blood during inflammation.
7. interrelationship between various factors involved in inflammation.

C. The Cellular Response	2.27	57-90

1. steps in the movement of neutrophils and monocytes from vessels to the site of tissue damage.
2. major events of inflammation and their order of occurrence.
3. definition and role of chemotactic.
4. function of the cellular response and role of phagocytosis.
5. definition of debris.

PRETEST

UNIT 2. INFLAMMATION: THE VASCULAR AND CELLULAR RESPONSE TO INJURY

SELECT THE SINGLE BEST RESPONSE.

1. By definition the process of acute inflammation includes
   (A) vascular proliferation
   (B) fibroblastic reaction
   (C) both
   (D) neither

2. Which is capable of causing pain and is a long-acting mediator of the vascular response of inflammation?
   (A) histamine
   (B) negative chemotactic agent
   (C) positive chemotactic agent
   (D) bradykinin

3. Which of the cardinal signs of inflammation results from increased blood volume?
   (A) redness
   (B) redness and heat
   (C) redness, heat, and swelling
   (D) redness, heat, swelling, and pain

4. An exudate is characterized by
   (A) low protein content
   (B) high red blood cell content
   (C) high specific gravity
   (D) brown color

5. Short-acting mediators of inflammation are
   (A) kinins
   (B) produced by polys
   (C) released by mast cells
   (D) activated from blood plasma

6. If the following events were put in sequence as they occur in an inflammatory reaction, which would occur third?
   (A) migration of leukocytes
   (B) margination of leukocytes
   (C) tissue injury
   (D) increased blood volume, leading to heat and redness

7. Which of the following statements concerning debris is FALSE?
   (A) It causes tissue damage.
   (B) It often remains in the tissue long after inflammation has ceased.
   (C) The removal of debris and fluid is called resolution.
   (D) It is dissolved by enzymes released from polys and can then be carried away by plasma fluid.

8. The site of digestion of damaged tissue or injurious agents is
   (A) intracellular
   (B) intercellular
   (C) both
   (D) neither

GO ON TO NEXT PAGE AND BEGIN THE UNIT.

A. <u>Introduction to Inflammation</u> (15 frames)

When you complete this section, you will be able to select correct responses relating to the:

1. signs and symptoms of inflammation.
2. examples of each type of agent (biological, chemical, and physical) that can cause inflammation.
3. components of the inflammatory response.
4. examples of harmful and beneficial inflammatory responses.

1. When cells are injured or destroyed, the vascular and cellular response of the surrounding tissues is __________, which is characterized by the following signs and symptoms: __________, __________, __________, and __________.

---

1. When cells are injured or destroyed, the vascular and cellular response of the surrounding tissues is inflammation, which is characterized by the following signs and symptoms: heat, pain, redness, and swelling. (any order)

---

2. CLASSIFY THE FOLLOWING INFLAMMATORY AGENTS AS BIOLOGICAL (B), CHEMICAL (C), OR PHYSICAL (P):

___ Cold

___ Staphylococcus aureus

___ Sunlight

___ Nitric acid

___ Physical trauma

___ Necrotic tissue

---

45. Increased capillary permeability causes exudation of plasma fluid, proteins, and cells from venules and capillaries.

46.

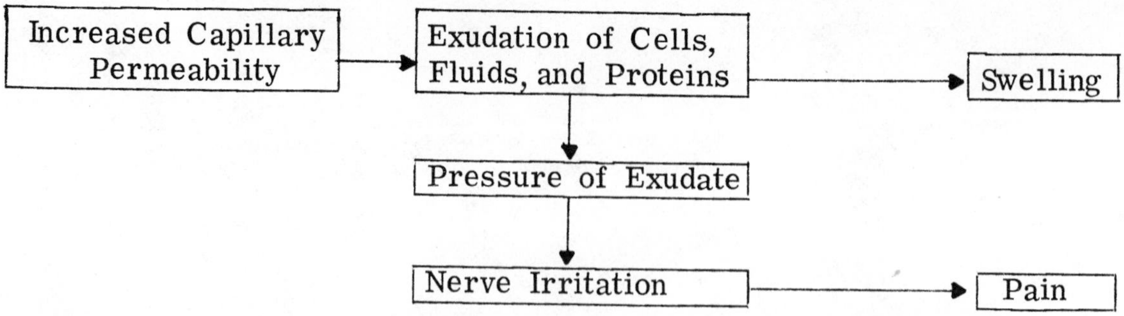

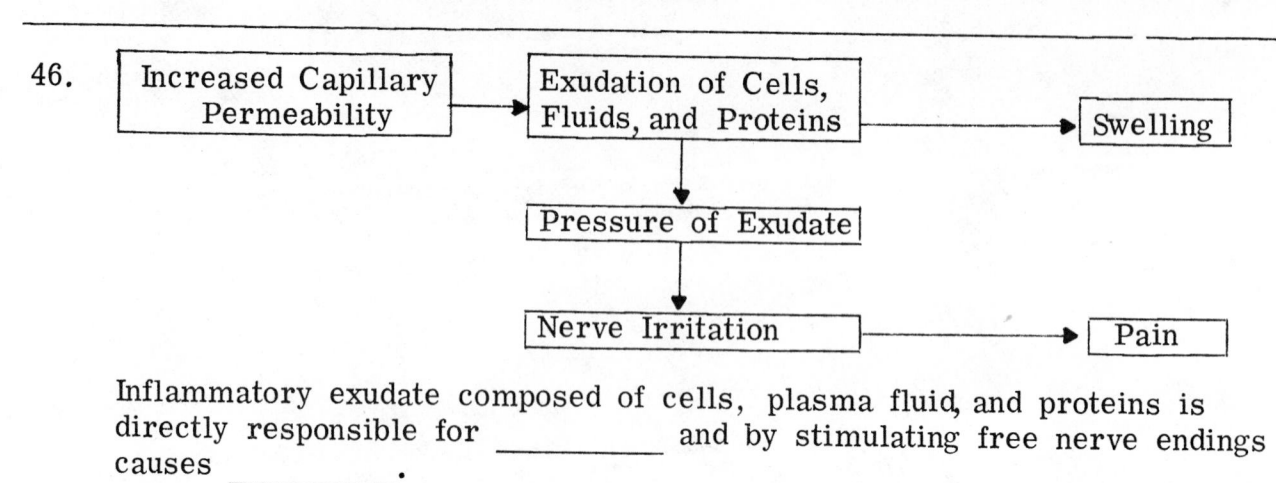

Inflammatory exudate composed of cells, plasma fluid, and proteins is directly responsible for __________ and by stimulating free nerve endings causes __________.

TURN TEXT 180° AND CONTINUE.

2. P B P

C P B

---

3. Agents which cause inflammation are:

a) extremely variable.

b) generally have similar properties.

---

46. Inflammatory exudate composed of cells, plasma fluid, and proteins is directly responsible for swelling and by stimulating free nerve endings causes pain.

47.

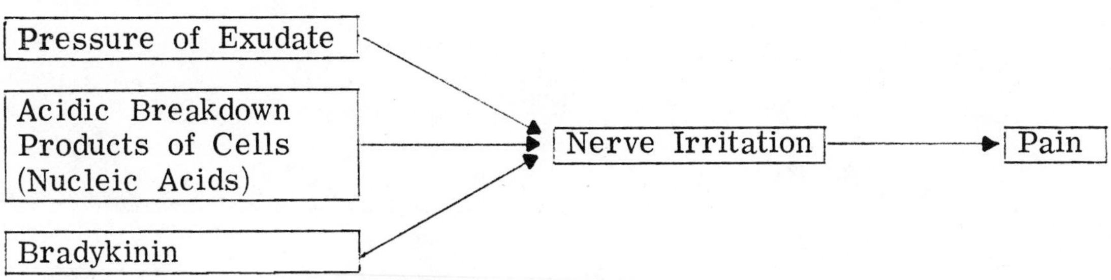

The direct cause of pain in inflammation is __________ __________. Originally it was thought that exudate pressure was the only cause of nerve irritation, but it was discovered that pain often preceded exudation. Experiments have since determined that intradermal injection of __________ breakdown products and at least one of the long-acting chemical mediators, __________, can cause pain. This is not surprising, since bradykinin is one of the major components of wasp venom.

44. c) both a and b.

---

45. Increased capillary permeability causes ______________ of plasma fluid, proteins, and cells from venules and ____________.

---

90. Continuing severe pain indicates inflammation. Since the leg is in a cast, it is impossible to detect any of the other signs and symptoms of inflammation. In this case, the inflammation was due to an infection of the wound.

THIS IS THE END OF UNIT 2. TAKE THE POSTTEST ON PAGE xvi.

3. a) extremely variable.

---

4. Inflammation is a basic response of the body and can occur in any tissue. Regardless of the type of agent or the site of occurrence, the basic nature of the inflammatory response is the same. Although the sequence of events in inflammation is always the same, the ultimate nature, duration, and severity of the inflammatory response is determined by factors related to the host and the injurious agent. (Factors modifying the inflammatory response are covered in a later section.)

IN WHICH ORGAN(S) CAN INFLAMMATION OCCUR?

___ Heart	___ Brain
___ Lung	___ Liver
___ Skin	___ Pancreas

---

47. The direct cause of pain in inflammation is nerve irritation. Originally it was thought that exudate pressure was the only cause of nerve irritation, but it was discovered that pain often preceded exudation. Experiments have since determined that intradermal injection of acidic breakdown products and at least one of the long-acting chemical mediators, bradykinin, can cause pain.

---

48. FILL IN THE BOXES BELOW:

Indirect Causes of Pain

Direct Cause of Pain

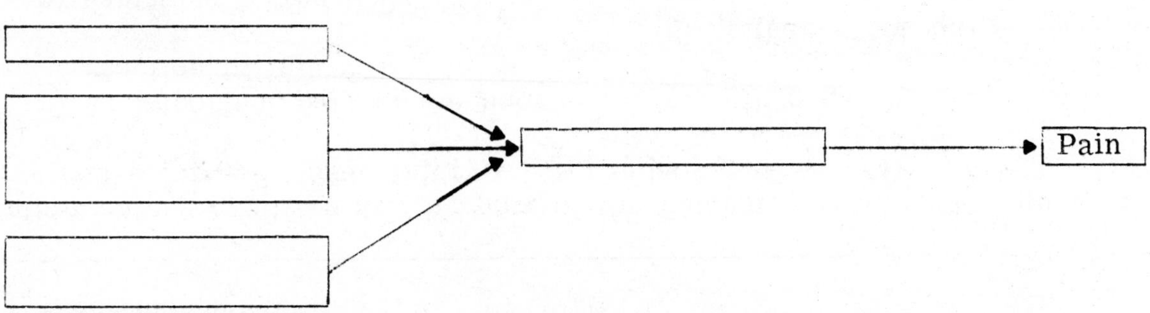

43. 1 transudate
3 fibrinous exudate
2 serous exudate

---

44. Inflammatory exudates may be part of the defensive reaction to injury or they may cause further tissue injury. An exudate may be:

a) an important part of the body's reaction to injury.

b) damaging to the body, as in arthritis.

c) both a and b.

d) neither a nor b.

---

89. Determine whether redness and heat are present. Pain might be present with inflammation, but a neoplasm could also cause pain.

---

90. A 62-year-old woman was in an automobile accident and sustained a compound fracture of her leg. The fracture was reduced and the leg placed in a cast. The woman was known to be extremely neurotic. She complained of great pain. The attending physician ignored her complaints, but two days later she still complained incessantly of extreme pain. What does this indicate?

4. All of the organs listed.

---

5. The sequence of events in inflammation is always the same, but the ultimate nature, duration, and severity of an inflammatory response is determined by factors related to the __________ and __________.

48.

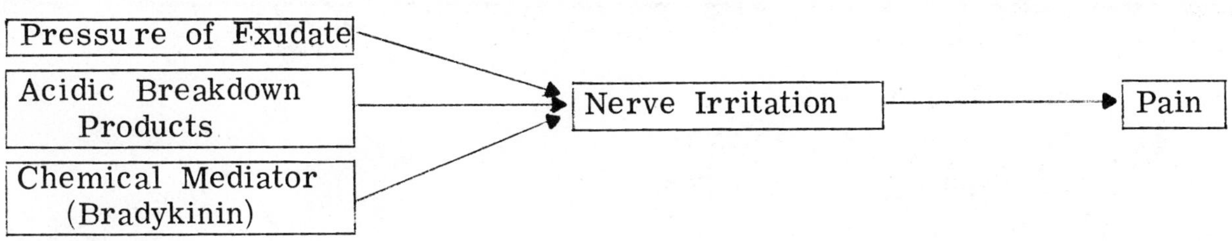

---

49. INDICATE THE DIRECT CAUSES OF THE MANIFESTATIONS OF INFLAMMATION:

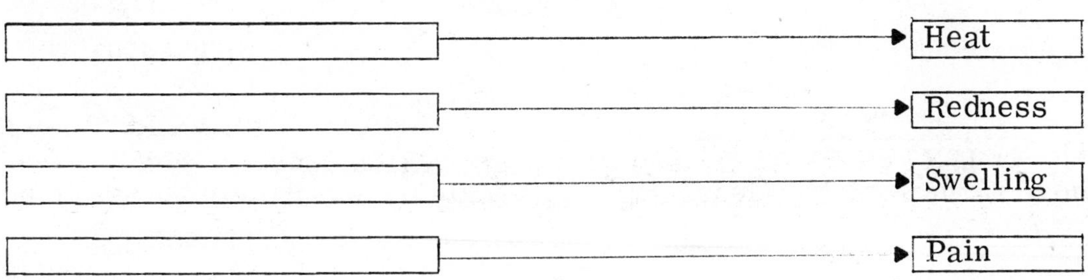

42.

	High Protein Content	Contains the Largest Blood Proteins	Forms Clots in the Tissues	Appears in the Initial Stages of Inflammation
Serous Exudate	☑	☐	☐	☑
Fibrinous Exudate	☑	☑	☑	☐

---

43. The following fluids are all formed by the escape of substances from the blood vessels. RANK THEM FROM LEAST (1) TO GREATEST (3) VESSEL PERMEABILITY.

___ transudate

___ fibrinous exudate

___ serous exudate

---

88. F F
T F
T T

---

89. A man entered his physician's office with a small swelling on the back of his arm. Other than by history, how would you determine if it was a neoplasm or an inflammation?

5. host (and) injurious agent (or equivalent)

---

6. Cell injury or cell death always precedes inflammation. Inflammation is a cellular and vascular response composed of a complex sequence of events. The components of the inflammatory process are:
   1. Blood vessels - primarily venules and capillaries;
   2. Components of the blood - a) plasma fluid, b) plasma solutes, and c) white cells.

Repair is the replacement of dead or injured tissue by new cells. In some tissues, repair may consist of regeneration of parenchymal cells, but in cases where this does not occur, dead and injured cells are replaced by connective tissue cells. Repair often begins during inflammation.

MATCH THE FOLLOWING:

____Vascular response

____Cellular response

____Repair (replacement of dead or injured tissue by new cells)

A. Blood vessels, plasma fluid, plasma solutes

B. Leukocytes

C. Connective tissue cells or parenchymal cells

---

49. Increased Blood Volume → Heat

Increased Blood Volume → Redness

Exudation of Cells, Fluids, and Proteins → Swelling

Nerve Irritation → Pain

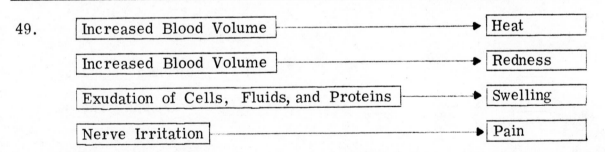

50. COMPLETE THE DIAGRAM:

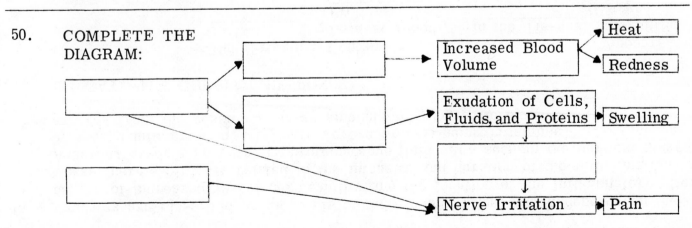

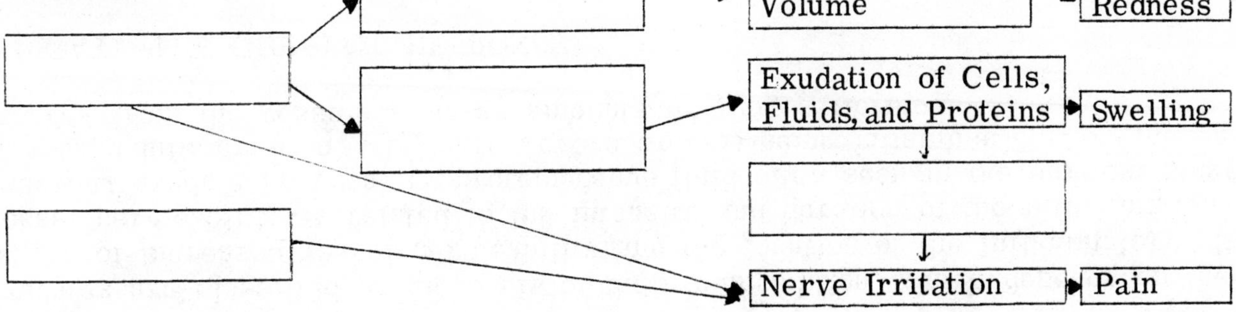

41. a) an exadate. burn (injury) → inflammation → increased permeability to proteins

42. Exudates are classified on the basis of their composition, which depends on the degree of increased vessel permeability and the location of the inflammatory site. Vessel permeability is related to the intensity and duration of the inflammation. A serous exudate is a watery proteinaceous fluid often seen in the earliest stages of a mild inflammation. In more severe or continuing inflammations, fibrinogen escapes from the vessels in large amounts, forming a fibrinous exudate.

INDICATE THE CORRECT RESPONSES:

	High Protein Content	Contains the Largest Blood Proteins	Forms Clots in the Tissues	Appears in the Initial Stages of Inflammation
Serous Exudate	☐	☐	☐	☐
Fibrinous Exudate	☐	☐	☐	☐

---

87. T F
F F
T F

---

88. INDICATE "T" TRUE OR "F" FALSE:

	frame reference
____ In most inflammations, neutrophils accumulate at the inflammatory focus before the signs and symptoms of inflammation appear.	58
____ Dead tissue is often part of the debris of an inflammatory reaction.	75
____ The breakdown or digestion of debris is essential if repair is to take place.	75
____ The emigration of leukocytes through vessel walls requires no active movement on the part of the white cells.	64-66
____ Monocytes are not phagocytic.	77
____ Monocytes and neutrophils respond to chemotactic agents.	67

6. A
B
C

7. 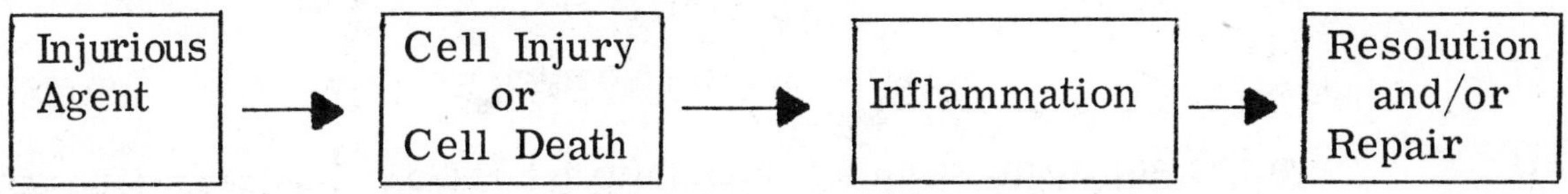

Healing is the process by which the body restores normal structure and function as much as possible. Healing may consist only of resolution -- resorption of liquified dead tissue and material released during inflammation -- or it may also include repair -- replacement by new cells.

MATCH THE FOLLOWING:

____ replacement of dead or injured tissue by connective tissue

____ resorption of liquified dead tissue

____ replacement of dead or injured tissue by parenchymal cells

____ cellular and vascular response of the body to injury

A. Resolution

B. Repair

C. Inflammation

50. 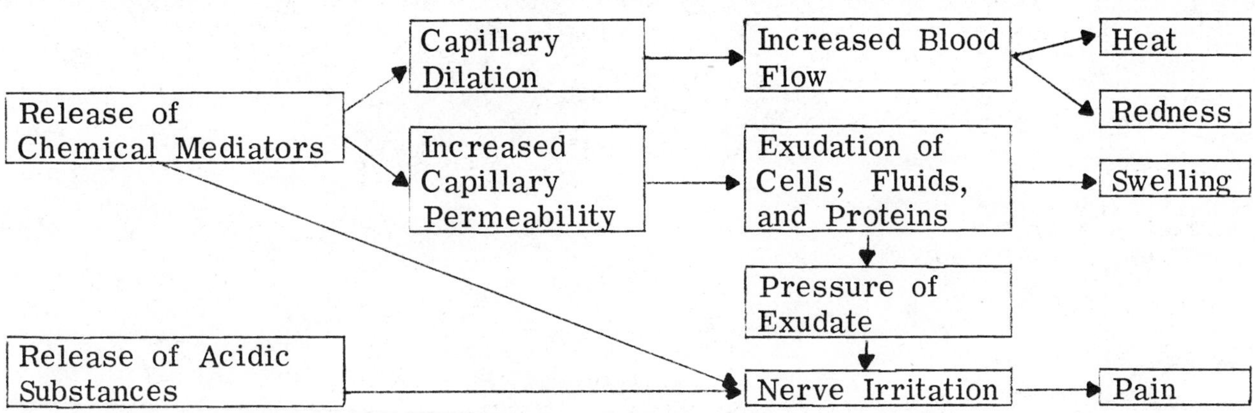

51. What causes release of chemical mediators and acidic breakdown products?

40. fibrinogen

---

41. A patient burned his hand on a hot coffee pot. An analysis of a sample of the blister fluid would reveal that it was:

a) an exudate.

b) a transudate.

c) both a and b.

d) neither a nor b.

---

86. neutrophils and monocytes

---

87. INDICATE "T" TRUE OR "F" FALSE:

	frame reference
____Leukocytes are normally found in the blood although there is always a slight movement from the vessels to the tissue.	58
____Migration of neutrophils is directed by plasma kinins.	67-71
____Margination, adhesion, and emigration are thought to be initiated by kinins.	61
____The chemotactic effect is produced only by the injurious agent.	67
____The chemotactic power of all injurious agents is about the same.	70
____Histamine is a powerful vasoconstrictor.	17,18

7. B
A
B
C

---

8. Inflammation is a complex sequence of events primarily involving which of the following component(s)?

a) blood vessels

b) hormones

c) components of the blood

d) connective tissue

---

51. cell injury

---

52. COMPLETE THE DIAGRAM OF THE INFLAMMATORY PROCESS:

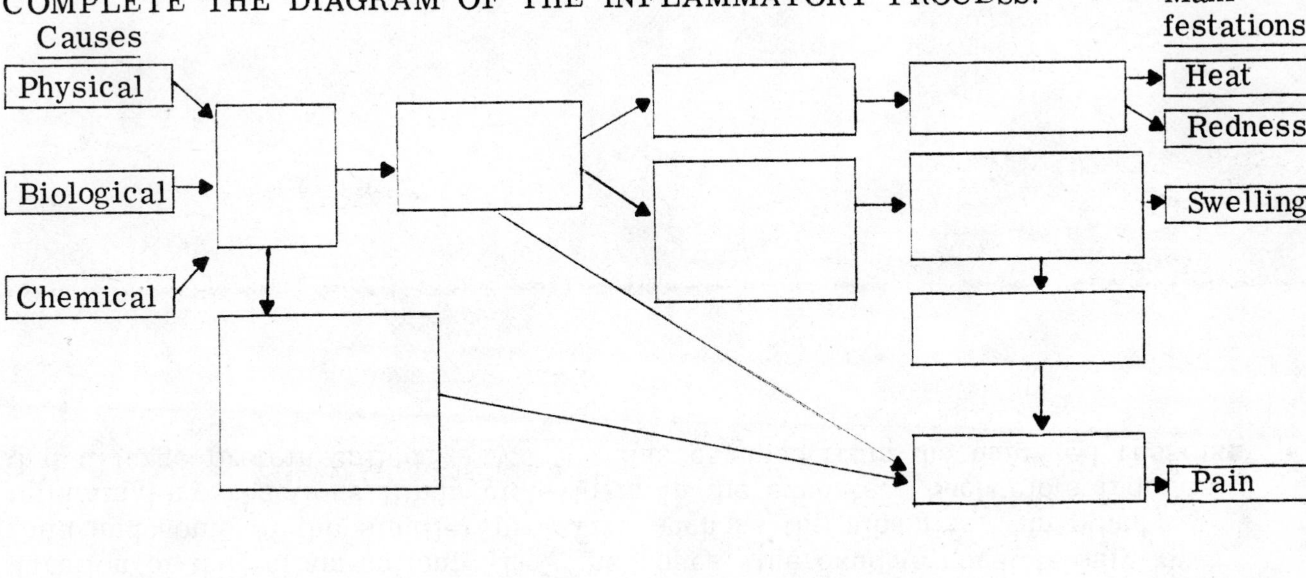

39. exudate
No.

---

40. The degree of increased capillary permeability varies with the intensity and duration of the inflammation. In some cases, the exudate consists only of fluid and some of the smaller proteins, such as the albumins. In other inflammatory reactions, fibrin clots form in the exudate. Such clots indicate that a large protein called __________ has escaped from the damaged vessels.

---

85. 11, 6, 1, 9, 8
4, 7, 5, 2, 10, 3

---

86. A patient used an old wooden-handled shovel and embedded a splinter deep in his hand. Only part of the splinter was removed. A day afterward what cell types would be clustered around the splinter?

8. a)
c)

---

9. Blood vessels, plasma fluid, and proteins are the major elements of the __________ response.

The action of leukocytes (neutrophils and monocytes) is the __________ response of inflammation.

The replacement of dead or injured tissue by new cells is __________ and is carried out by __________ __________ cells or by the parenchymal cells of the injured tissue or organ.

Resorption of liquified dead tissue and material released during inflammation is ______________.

52.

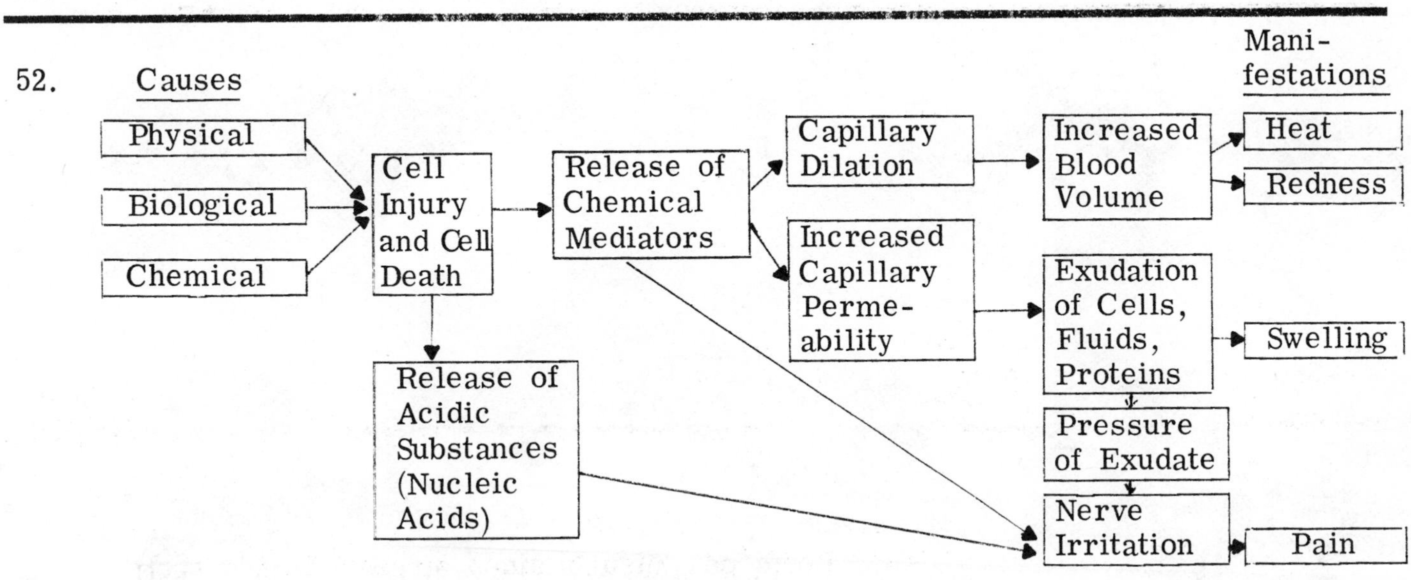

---

53. In a patient with cardiac failure the pleural cavities start to fill with fluid. A sample of this fluid is taken and found to be relatively viscous (a specific gravity of 1.025). Does this indicate the possibility of bacterial pneumonia? EXPLAIN.

38. B
A

---

39. Leukocytes, plasma fluid, and plasma proteins (albumins, globulins, and fibrinogen) are components of an inflammatory ________. A pure exudate is colorless or white, the opacity or whiteness depending on the number of leukocytes present.

Does a pure exudate contain many red blood cells?

---

84. 1. Defensive reaction: destruction or immobilization of the injurious agent
2. Preparation for repair: removal of wreckage

---

85. NUMBER THE FOLLOWING IN ORDER OF THEIR OCCURRENCE:

___ phagocytosis and enzymatic digestion

___ margination of neutrophils and monocytes

___ tissue injury

___ migration of leukocytes to site of damage

___ emigration of leukocytes

___ increased blood volume, leading to heat and redness; exudation, causing swelling and pain

___ adhesion of leukocytes

___ slowing of blood flow; red cell concentration

___ release of chemical mediators and acidic substances

___ accumulation of leukocytes at site of injury

___ capillary dilation and increased permeability

9. vascular
cellular
repair (and is carried out by) connective tissue
resolution

---

10. Inflammation is always preceded by ____________ ____________ or ____________ ____________.

Inflammation is followed by healing, which frequently consists simply of ____________ but may also include ____________.

---

53. Yes, because the high specific gravity indicates that the fluid is an inflammatory exudate, which could result from an infection.

---

54. A patient ran a large splinter into his left big toe. He attempted to remove the splinter. Three days later the toe was still painful and slightly red. What does this indicate?

37. b) exudate

---

38. The specific gravity of a fluid found in body cavities is used to determine whether it is a transudate or an exudate. A simple hygrometer, similar to that used to test antifreeze in an automobile radiator, is used to make this determination.

MATCH THE FOLLOWING:

___ a watery fluid, low in proteins, cells, and solid materials, specific gravity usually less than 1.012	A.	Exudate
___ a fluid rich in plasma proteins with a specific gravity usually greater than 1.020	B.	Transudate

---

83.

Defensive Reaction	Preparation for Repair
✓	✓
✓	✓

---

84. The functions of the cellular response are:

1. ______________________________

2. ______________________________

10. Inflammation is always preceded by cell injury or cell death. Inflammation is followed by healing, which frequently consists simply of resolution but may also include repair.

---

11. Inflammation is a vital part of the body's defense, but it can also be harmful. INDICATE WHETHER THE FOLLOWING ARE HARMFUL EFFECTS OF INFLAMMATION (H) OR BENEFICIAL EFFECTS OF INFLAMMATION (B):

____ rheumatoid arthritis (chronic destructive inflammation of the joints)

____ inflammation limiting the spread of an infection

____ tendonitis (accumulation of fluid and fibrin within a tendon sheath, later resulting in fibrous adhesions and limiting movement)

____ removal of foreign material from a wound by inflammatory cells

---

54. Pain and redness, two of the symptoms and signs of inflammation, are present, so inflammation is probably present. In this case, the wound is probably infected. Remnants of splinter may be present to harbor bacteria from the host's defense.

---

55. INDICATE "T" TRUE OR "F" FALSE:

	frame ref.
____ The release of chemical mediators immediately follows tissue injury.	16
____ Capillary dilation and increased permeability are caused by different substances.	16,18
____ Capillary dilation causes exudation.	28,29
____ Kinins are vasoactive amines.	23
____ Kinins are released from an $alpha_2$ globulin in the plasma.	24,25
____ The same substance activates the plasma kinins and the blood coagulation mechanism.	24,25

36. B
A

37. Considering how they are formed, which do you think would contain larger particles?

a) transudate

b) exudate

82. Mycobacterium tuberculosis can be ingested but not digested by neutrophils.

83. When the foreign material is ingested, digestion takes place inside the cell, or intracellularly, but enzymatic destruction of debris may also be extracellular, or take place outside the cell.

INDICATE THE CORRECT BOXES:

	Defensive Reaction	Preparation for Repair
Phagocytosis and Intracellular Digestion	☐	☐
Extracellular Digestion	☐	☐

11. H
B
H
B

---

12. Repair is the __________ of dead or injured tissue by new solid tissue. The cellular response of inflammation involves ______________________________ whereas, the cellular response of repair involves ____________________ cells and __________ cells.

---

55. T F
F T
F T

---

56. INDICATE "T" TRUE OR "F" FALSE:

	frame reference
____Transudates are more viscous than exudates.	38
____Pure transudates are colorless.	38, 39
____Exudates are colorless or white.	39
____Capillaries are permeable to plasma proteins under normal conditions.	34
____Arterioles greatly increase in permeability during inflammation.	17, 18
____The degree of capillary permeability varies with different inflammatory reactions.	35
____Pain is caused by exudate pressure, acidic substances, and chemical mediators (bradykinin).	47

35.

N	N
I	I
N	I
N	I

36. MATCH THE FOLLOWING:

___ due to osmotic imbalance and/or increased filtration pressure

___ due primarily to increase in permeability

A. Exudate

B. Transudate

81. digestion

82. Most bacteria are enzymatically destroyed after phagocytosis. However, the organism responsible for tuberculosis, Mycobacterium tuberculosis, has a capsule which is resistant to the intracellular enzymes of the phagocytes. Mycobacterium tuberculosis can be ________ but not ________ by neutrophils.

12. Repair is the replacement of dead or injured tissue by new solid tissue. The cellular response of inflammation involves white blood cells (leukocytes); whereas, the cellular response of repair involves connective tissue cells and parenchymal cells.

---

13. INDICATE TRUE "T" OR FALSE "F ":

		frame reference
___	Inflammation can occur only in certain tissues of the body.	4
___	Inflammation can be caused by a wide variety of agents.	2-3
___	The basic sequence of events in an inflammatory reaction varies depending on the agent and host.	4-6
___	The extent, nature, and duration of an inflammatory reaction vary depending on the agent and host.	4-5
___	The components of the inflammatory response are blood vessels and elements of the blood.	1, 6, 8-9
___	Repair follows many but not all inflammations.	7

---

56. F
T
T
F
F
T
T

C. The Cellular Response (34 frames)

When you complete this section, you will be able to select correct responses relating to the:

1. steps in the movement of neutrophils and monocytes from vessels to the site of tissue damage.
2. major events of inflammation and their order of occurrence.
3. definition and role of chemotactic.
4. function of the cellular response and role of phagocytosis.
5. definition of debris.

57. Inflammation is a complex reaction of the body to injury composed of two interrelated responses: a __________ response and a __________ response.

34.

Normal Capillary	Capillary in Inflamed Tissue
☐	☑
☐	☑
☑	☑
☐	☑

---

35. The degree of permeability of vessels varies greatly. In the normal state only molecules smaller than proteins pass through; whereas, in a severe inflammatory reaction large proteins and even cells can escape through pores and intercellular gaps. FOR THE FOLLOWING, INDICATE "N" IF THEY PASS THROUGH VESSEL WALLS UNDER NORMAL CONDITIONS AND "I" IF THEY ESCAPE ONLY WHEN PERMEABILITY IS GREATLY INCREASED:

___ salts	___ amino acids
___ albumin	___ globulins
___ glucose	___ fibrinogen
___ water	___ cells

---

80. phagocytosis
 B engulfing the foreign material by pseudopodia
 A enzymatic destruction of the foreign material

---

81. In some cases the phagocyte does not possess the enzymes necessary to destroy the foreign material. In this case ingestion can take place but __________ cannot.

13. F
T
F
T
T
T

---

14. INDICATE "T" TRUE OR "F" FALSE: frame reference

		frame reference
___	Repair is the replacement of dead or injured tissue by new cells.	6
___	Repair is carried out by connective tissue cells and in some cases by the parenchymal cells of the injured tissue or organ.	6
___	The nervous sytem is an important anatomical component of most inflammatory reactions.	6
___	Inflammation may occur on the surface of the body where the signs and symptoms are readily apparent or internally where they may not be so apparent.	4
___	Inflammation always helps to maintain health and prevent disease.	11
___	Rheumatoid arthritis and tendonitis are examples of harmful inflammations.	11

---

57. Inflammation is a complex reaction of the body to injury composed of two interrelated responses: a cellular response and a vascular response.

---

58. In normal tissue there is a continual slight movement of leukocytes from the blood into the tissue spaces; the great acceleration of this process during inflammation is the cellular response. This movement may begin as early as a few minutes after injury and is quite active within a few hours.

In an inflammatory reaction, tissue injury is followed by release of (1) chemical ________ and (2) ________ breakdown products. These two substances can cause nerve irritation, which causes ________. Capillary ________ and increased capillary ________ are caused by the ________ ________.

	Normal Capillary	Capillary in Inflamed Tissue
Which capillary is larger?	☐	☐
Which capillary has larger pores or gaps?	☐	☐
Which capillary allows salts to pass into the tissues?	☐	☐
Which capillary allows proteins to pass into the tissues?	☐	☐

---

79. neutrophils (and) monocytes
    a)
    b)
    c)

---

80. Ingestion of foreign material by the process of ________ can be followed by intracellular digestion of the foreign material. MATCH THE FOLLOWING:

___ engulfing the foreign material by pseudopodia

___ enzymatic destruction of the foreign material

A. digestion

B. ingestion

14. T
T
F
T
F
T

---

15. MATCH THE FOLLOWING:

A. Inflammation and repair
B. Cell degeneration and death
C. Abnormalities of growth
D. Abnormal development

___ Often direct result of injury to the body.

___ Disturbances of cell maturation and proliferation, for example hyperplasia.

___ The absence, or malformation and/or malfunction of an organ or tissue due to genetic damage.

___ Complex cellular and vascular response of the body to injury.

---

58. In an inflammatory reaction, tissue injury is followed by release of (1) chemical mediators and (2) acidic breakdown products. These two substances can cause nerve irritation, which causes pain. Capillary dilation and increased capillary permeability are caused by the chemical mediators.

---

59. Capillary dilation and increased permeability lead to:
1) increased blood volume, causing __________ and __________;
2) exudation of __________, __________, and plasma __________ (albumin, globulin, and fibrinogen), causing __________ directly and ________ indirectly due to pressure on nerves.

33. In inflammation, the initial increase in vessel permeability is caused by chemical mediators such as histamine.

---

34. Relative Sizes of Substances in Blood

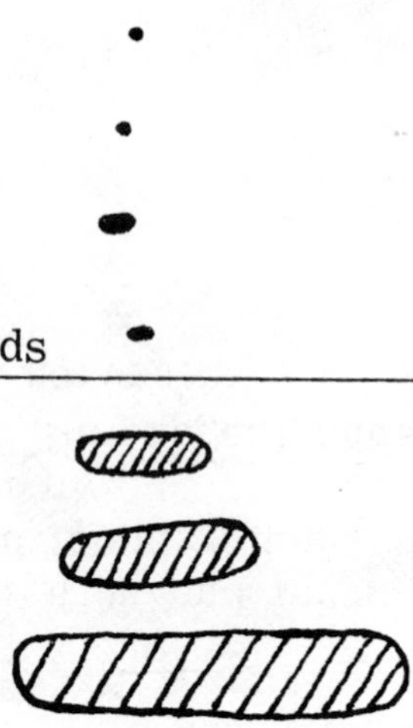

	Molecular Weight	
Na^+		Capillaries and venules normally are permeable to these substances.
Cl^-		
Glucose		
Amino Acids		
Albumin	69,000	These substances pass through capillaries and venules during inflammation.
Globulin	90,000-160,000	
Fibrinogen	400,000	

Capillaries and venules are permeable at all times to water, salts, amino acids, glucose, and other small molecules but not to protein.

GO ON TO THE NEXT PAGE

---

78. In a sterile surgical wound the primary function of phagocytes is preparation for repair, removal of debris (or equivalent answer).

---

79. The cells involved early in the cellular response are ________ and ________. They are:

a) phagocytes
b) leukocytes
c) normally found in the blood
d) normally accumulate in the tissue

15. B
C
D
A

B. The Vascular Response (41 frames)

When you complete this section, you will be able to select correct responses relating to the:

1. differentiation of plasma kinins by source, composition, and effect.
2. results of the release of chemical mediators.
3. definitions of capillary dilation and increased capillary permeability.
4. direct causes of the signs of inflammation.
5. differentiation between an exudate and a transudate on basis of composition and probable cause.
6. substances that leave the blood during inflammation. interrelationship between various factors involved in inflammation.

GO ON TO THE NEXT PAGE

---

59. Capillary dilation and increased permeability lead to: 1) increased blood volume, causing heat and redness; 2) exudation of cells, fluid, and plasma proteins (albumin, globulin, and fibrinogen), causing swelling directly and pain indirectly due to pressure on nerves.

---

60. Following and during exudation, the blood flow in the capillaries slows and the red cells appear to be packed very tightly in the capillaries. NUMBER THE FOLLOWING IN ORDER OF OCCURRENCE:

___ increased blood volume, causing heat and redness; exudation causing swelling

___ release of chemical mediators and acidic breakdown products, causing pain

___ tissue injury

___ slowing or stasis of blood flow in capillaries and concentration of red cells

___ capillary dilation and increased permeability

32. Exudates are usually created by the increased permeability of vessels during inflammation whereas increased filtration pressure or an osmotic imbalance between the blood and the tissue is **n**ormally responsible for a transudate.

[X] exudate. Bacterial inflammations (infections) increase vascular permeability.

---

33. In inflammation, the initial increase in vessel permeability is caused by __________ mediators such as __________. At present the mechanism of increased permeability is thought to be primarily the opening of intercellular gaps.

---

77. cellular
c) both a and b

---

78. In a sterile surgical wound the primary function of phagocytes is __________ ____________________.

16.

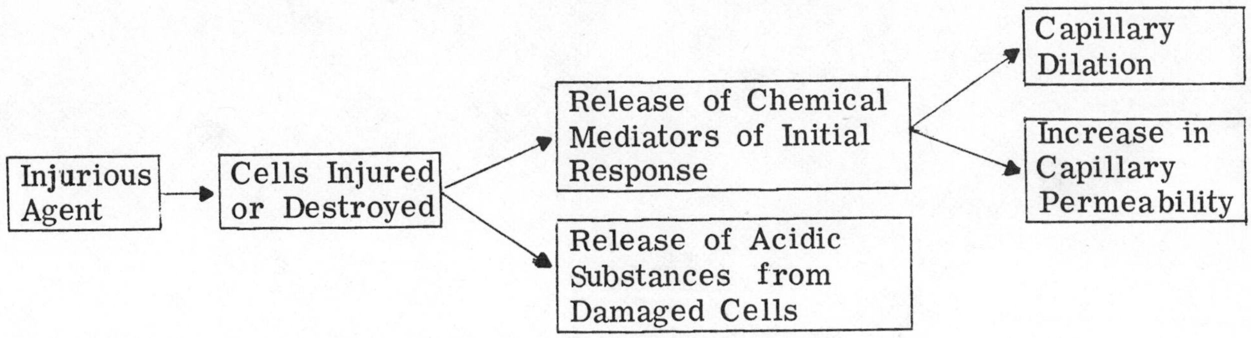

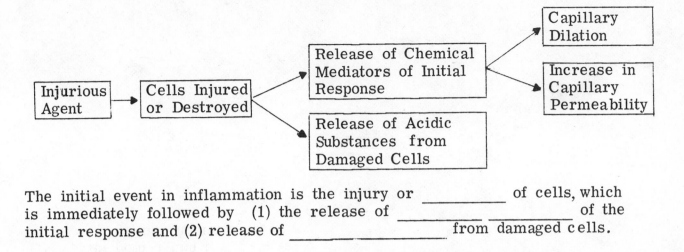

The initial event in inflammation is the injury or __________ of cells, which is immediately followed by (1) the release of __________ __________ of the initial response and (2) release of ___________________ from damaged cells.

---

60. 4
2
1
5
3

---

61. Movement of Leukocytes

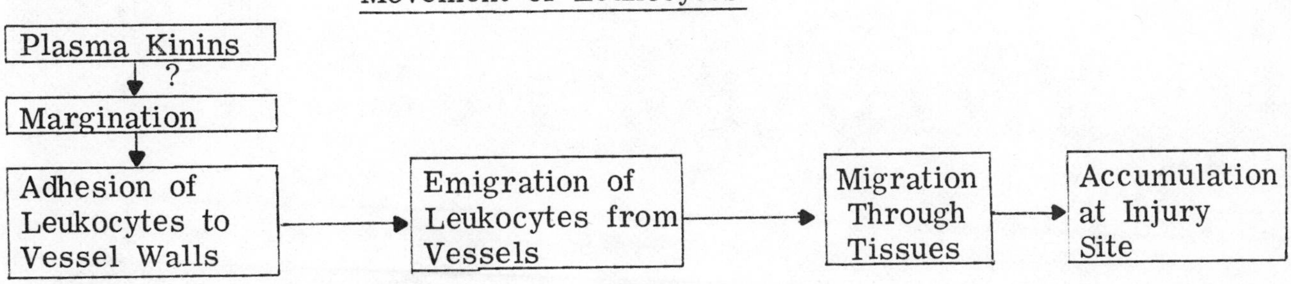

Following slowing of blood flow, leukocytes (neutrophils and monocytes) move peripherally from the center of the capillaries and adhere to the vessel walls. At present this process is thought to be mediated by __________ __________.

31. exudates

---

32. Exudates are usually created by the increased __________ of vessels during inflammation whereas increased filtration pressure or an osmotic imbalance between the blood and the tissue is normally responsible for a __________.

Which would be most likely to contain bacteria? ☐ exudate ☐ transudate. Why?

---

76. yes
resolution

---

77. Phagocytosis (from the Greek phagein, meaning "to eat," and kytos, meaning "hollow vessel," hence "cell") is ingestion of foreign material by cells. Neutrophils and monocytes, the two types of cells involved in the __________ response, both are voracious phagocytes. Phagocytosis is part of:

a) the defensive reaction.
b) the preparation for repair.
c) both a and b
d) neither a nor b

16. The initial event in inflammation is the injury or destruction (or death) of cells, which is immediately followed by (1) the release of chemical mediators of the initial response and (2) release of acidic substances from damaged cells.

---

17. Chemical mediators are released from cells and cause (1) capillary _______ and (2) increased capillary __________.

MATCH THE FOLLOWING:

___ increased transfer of substances through capillary walls into the tissues	A. Capillary dilation
___ increased capillary diameter	B. Increased capillary permeability

NOTE: The term capillary is used throughout this text to refer to small vessels of the microcirculation -- capillaries and small venules.

---

61. plasma kinins

---

62. MATCH THE FOLLOWING:

A. Margination (pavementing) of leukocytes	___ movement of white cells from the axial stream of the capillary to the vessel walls
B. Adhesion of leukocytes	___ sticking by electrochemical forces of leukocytes to vessel walls

30. Increased Capillary Permeability → Exudation → Swelling

---

31. In Latin the word sudare means "to ooze," the prefix ex- means "out of," and the prefix trans- means "through." Fluids which escape from vessels into tissue spaces are called transudates and ______________.

---

75. ✓ dead tissue
✓ fibrin
✓ platelets
✓ dead neutrophils
✓ fragments of foreign material

---

76. Debris causes further inflammation and tissue damage. Is the removal of debris necessary for repair of the injured area?

The resorption of liquified debris and inflammatory exudate is called ______________.

17. (1) capillary dilation and (2) increased capillary permeability.

B
A

---

18. Capillary dilation and increased capillary permeability are the results of the release of chemical mediators. The best understood initial chemical mediator is a vasoactive amine, histamine. Histamine exerts its effects on venules and capillaries, causing __________ and increased __________.

---

62. A
B

---

63. The first step in the movement of leukocytes is __________, followed by __________ to the endothelium of the vessels, which is followed by emigration of leukocytes from the vessels into the tissues.

29. exudation
swelling

---

30. FILL IN THE BOXES BELOW:

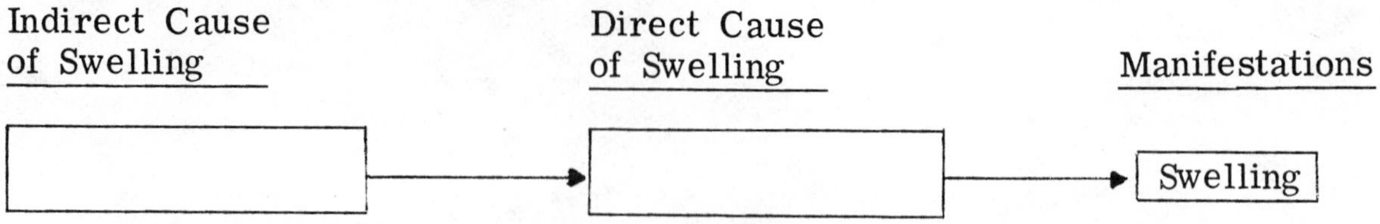

---

74. 9 10
7 5
4 8
3 2
1 6

---

75. The cellular response (the movement of leukocytes) has two functions:
(1) A defensive function: ingestion or immobilization of the injurious agent whether it is biological, chemical, or physical, or dead tissue;
(2) Preparation for repair: removal of debris, by cellular ingestion or release of enzymes. Repair cannot take place until the debris is removed.

Once an inflammatory reaction has started, any materials except live leukocytes, not found in the tissue before injury, are the rubble or wreckage of inflammation called debris. WHICH (IS/ARE) COMPONENTS OF DEBRIS?

___ dead tissue
___ live neutrophils
___ fibrin
___ platelets
___ dead neutrophils
___ viable tissue
___ fragments of foreign material

18. Histamine exerts its effects on venules and capillaries, causing dilation and increased permeability.

---

19. The initial chemical mediator, __________, is present in many different tissues, especially in basophilic leukocytes of the blood and mast cells, which usually are found near small blood vessels.

---

63. The first step in the movement of leukocytes is margination, followed by adhesion to the endothelium of the vessels, which is followed by emigration of leukocytes from the vessels into the tissues.

---

64. MATCH THE FOLLOWING:

A. Emigration of leukocytes	___	cells leaving vessels and entering tissues
B. Migration of leukocytes	___	movement of white cells from the center to the walls of vessels
C. Adhesion of leukocytes	___	sticking of white cells to vessel walls
D. Margination of leukocytes	___	movement of cells from vessel to the site of injury

28.

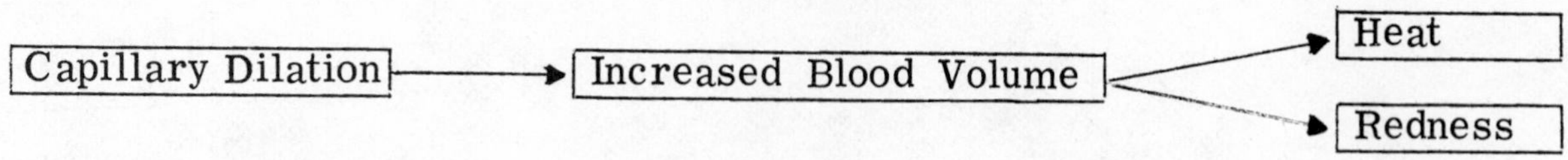

29.

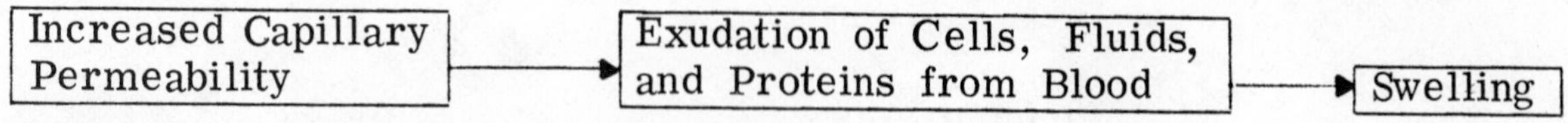

Increased capillary permeability allows ________ of fluids, proteins, and cells from the blood and causes ________ of the surrounding tissues.

73. margination
adhesion
emigration
migration
accumulation

74. NUMBER THE FOLLOWING IN ORDER OF OCCURRENCE:

___ migration of leukocytes

___ adhesion of leukocytes

___ increased blood volume leading to heat and redness; exudation causing swelling and pain

___ capillary dilation and increased permeability

___ tissue injury

___ accumulation of leukocytes at site of damage

___ slowing of blood flow, red cell packing

___ emigration of leukocytes

___ release of chemical mediators and acidic substances

___ margination of leukocytes

19. histamine

---

20. Histamine is found in basophilic _________, which are not considered important in inflammation; however, histamine is also found in ____ ____, which are thought to be the primary source of histamine in the inflammatory response.

---

64. A
D
C
B

---

65. MATCH THE LETTERS ON THE DIAGRAM WITH THE ITEMS BELOW:

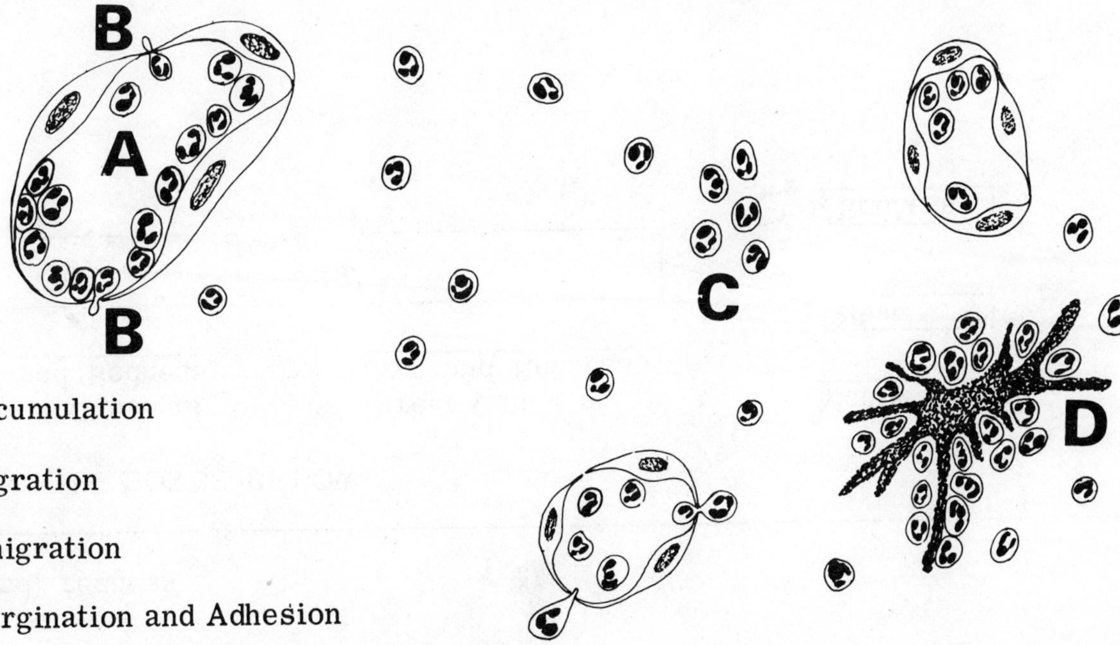

___Accumulation

___Migration

___Emigration

___Margination and Adhesion

27. blood volume
heat (and) redness

---

28. FILL IN THE BOXES BELOW:

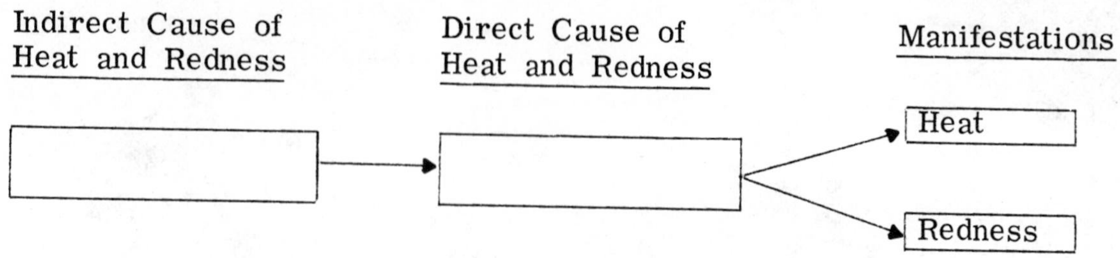

---

72. c) neutrophils (or polys). Neutrophils are easier to identify than protein precipitates. Evaluation of increased tissue space (due to fluid accumulation) in sections may be quite subjective. Red cells are not usually present in exudates.

---

73. NAME THE FOLLOWING:

__________ movement of cells from the axial stream to the walls of vessels

__________ sticking of cells to vessel walls

__________ cells inserting pseudopodia in intercellular junctions and sliding and wriggling through

__________ cells crawling and swimming through and around different tissue structures to arrive at the site of damage

__________ massing of white cells at the site of tissue injury

20. leukocytes
mast cells

---

21. The potent vasoactive properties of histamine have been demonstrated experimentally, and they are responsible for initiating the ☐ vascular ☐ cellular response in inflammation.

---

65. D Accumulation
C Migration
B Emigration
A Margination and Adhesion

---

66. The process by which white cells crawl across and through various structures to arrive at the site of damage is ________.

26. I M / L M / I M / L M   I M / I M / L M

27.

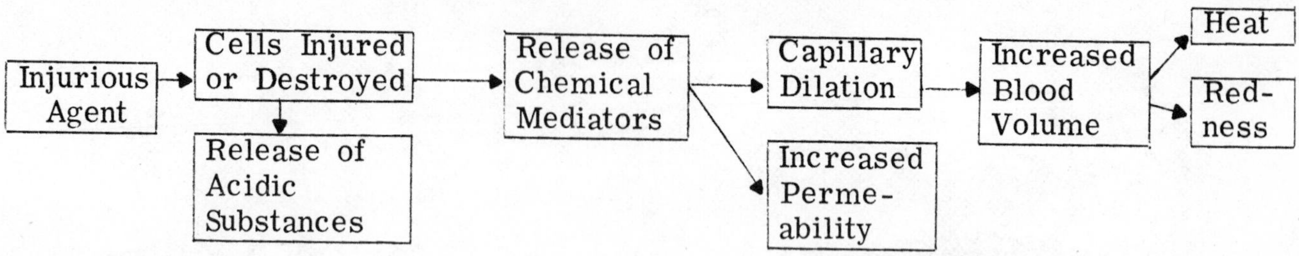

Capillary dilation caused by release of chemical mediators results in increased ________ ________ in the area, which in turn leads to two of the manifestations of inflammation, __________ and __________.

---

71. C
B
A

---

72. One of the most striking microscopic features of inflammation is the accumulation of neutrophils at the site of damage or around foreign material. In the process of preparing histologic sections sometimes blood runs out of dilated vessels and fluid accumulation is indicated only by empty spaces or protein precipitate in the tissue.

Which one of the following would be most evident microscopically in inflamed tissue?

a) enlarged tissue spaces

b) protein precipitate

c) neutrophils (or polys)

d) red cells

21. [✓] vascular

---

22. If histamine is injected intradermally, what happens to the area surrounding the injection site?

---

66. migration

---

67. A positive chemotactic agent is a substance which attracts leukocytes to an injurious agent or to cells damaged by that agent. The chemotactic effect can be produced by: (1) the chemical, biological, or physical agent; (2) by injured cells. The release of a chemotactic agent by injured cells is similar to the release of chemical mediators of the vascular response. Neutrophils respond very actively to chemotactic agents, monocytes respond sluggishly, and lymphocytes respond very little or not at all.

In what order would cells appear in an area of tissue damage due to an agent with high chemotactic activity?

____lymphocytes ____neutrophils ____monocytes

25. kinins

---

26. MARK THE FOLLOWING AS EITHER "I M" INITIAL MEDIATOR OR "L M" LONG-ACTING MEDIATOR:

___ released from mast cells

___ activated from blood plasma

___ initiates vascular response

___ probably maintains inflammatory response for days or weeks

___ maintains inflammation for a few hours

___ an amine

___ polypeptides, e.g., bradykinin and kallidin

---

70. chemotactic

---

71. MATCH THE FOLLOWING:

A. Plasma Kinins

B. Histamine

C. Chemotactic Agent

___ attracts leukocyte from vessel to site of damage

___ potent vasodilator and mediator of initial vascular response

___ capable of causing pain and long-acting mediator of vascular response

22. It becomes inflamed (red, swollen, painful, hot).

---

23. Although histamine can initiate the vascular response, it cannot sustain the reaction. Some inflammations last only a few hours or a day. In these reactions, capillary dilation and increased capillary permeability could be maintained by the vasoactive amine. However, many inflammations go on for days or weeks. The best understood long-acting mediators are polypeptides called plasma kinins.

MATCH THE FOLLOWING:

A. Histamine ___ cannot sustain vascular response

B. Plasma Kinins ___ can sustain vascular response

___ polypeptide structure

---

67. _3_ lymphocytes _1_ neutrophils _2_ monocytes

---

68. A chemotactic agent is a substance which attracts ________ to (1) the site of the injurious agent's action or (2) the site of __________ damaged by that agent.

24. The long-acting mediators called plasma kinins are released from a plasma protein by a mechanism similar to that of: b) blood coagulation.

---

25. The Hageman Factor initiates (a) the release of the plasma (bradykinin and kallidin) from an $alpha_2$ globulin; and (b) the blood clotting mechanism.

---

69. 1. the injurious agent
2. damaged cells

---

70. Some types of bacteria exert a very strong chemotactic influence while others show no effect or possibly repel leukocytes, so there is great variation in ________ power of various agents.

23. A
B
B

---

24. 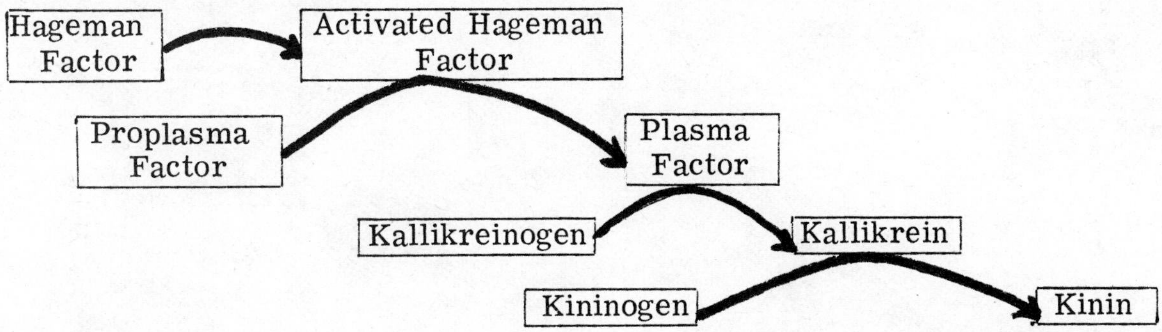

The long-acting mediators called __________ __________ are released from a plasma protein by a mechanism similar to that of:

a) histamine release

b) blood coagulation

TURN TEXT 180° AND CONTINUE.

---

68. A chemotactic agent is a substance which attracts leukocytes to (1) the site of the injurious agent's action or (2) the site of cells damaged by that agent.

---

69. A chemotactic effect can be produced by:

1. ____________________

2. ____________________

TURN TEXT 180° AND CONTINUE.

Unit 3. Inflammatory Cells: Structure and Function

Unit 3. INFLAMMATORY CELLS: STRUCTURE AND FUNCTION

OBJECTIVES

When you complete this unit, you will be able to select correct responses relating to the:

	starting page	frame numbers
A. The Structure of Inflammatory Cells	3.3	1-43

1. shape and size of inflammatory cells.
2. position and morphology of inflammatory cell nuclei.
3. relative amount of cell cytoplasm and type of cytoplasmic granules.
4. normal location and source of inflammatory cells.

B. The Function of Inflammatory Cells	3.16	44-96

1. function of each type of inflammatory cell, if known.
2. time sequence in which polys, mononuclear phagocytes, eosinophils, plasma cells, giant cells, lymphocytes, and fibroblasts appear in an inflammatory site.
3. mechanism of removal of debris.
4. definitions of opsonin and agranulocytosis.

PRETEST

UNIT 3. INFLAMMATORY CELLS: STRUCTURE AND FUNCTION

SELECT THE SINGLE BEST RESPONSE.

1. Aggregates of small, dark-staining (hematoxaphilic) cells with little cytoplasm in an inflammatory site are likely to be
   (A) polys
   (B) macrophages
   (C) eosinophils
   (D) lymphocytes

2. In routine microscopic sections of tissue stained with hematoxylin and eosin, the granules of basophils and mast cells are
   (A) red
   (B) blue
   (C) neutrophilic
   (D) not evident

3. Which inflammatory cells have eccentric nuclei and abundant basophilic cytoplasm?
   (A) lymphocytes
   (B) plasma cells
   (C) both
   (D) neither

4. Cells in an H & E section with one- or two-lobed nuclei and prominent cytoplasmic granules are
   (A) neutrophils
   (B) eosinophils
   (C) basophils
   (D) giant cells

5. Neutrophils
   (A) reproduce rapidly in an inflammatory site
   (B) live for only a few days in the tissues
   (C) are the predominant cell type in prolonged inflammations
   (D) are continually synthesizing and releasing digestive enzymes in an inflammatory site

6. Lymphocytes
   (A) actively migrate from the blood to the tissues early in inflammation
   (B) actively proliferate in the acute stages of inflammation
   (C) appear late in inflammation
   (D) produce digestive enzymes which help remove debris

7. During an inflammatory reaction, the pH of the area
   (A) steadily decreases
   (B) generally increases
   (C) always increases
   (D) may either increase, decrease, or remain about the same

8. Opsonification refers to:
   (A) removal of extracellular debris by specific digestive enzymes
   (B) process by which antibodies make bacteria more susceptible to phagocytosis
   (C) enzymatic destruction of large particles of foreign material over a long period of time
   (D) destruction of the fibrin barrier formed around some bacterial infection sites

GO ON TO NEXT PAGE AND BEGIN THE UNIT.

A. <u>The Structure of Inflammatory Cells</u> (43 frames)

When you complete this section, you will be able to select correct responses relating to the:

1. shape and size of inflammatory cells.
2. position and morphology of inflammatory cell nuclei.
3. relative amount of cell cytoplasm and type of cytoplasmic granules.
4. normal location and source of inflammatory cells.

1. The cells which take part in an inflammatory reaction can be grouped into a) cells which are normally found in the blood and move into the tissues, and b) cells which are normally found in the tissues only.

MATCH THE FOLLOWING:

____plasma cells	A. Normally found in blood only and move into tissue in inflammation.
____neutrophils	B. Normally found in tissues only.

---

48. neutrophils (or polys)

---

49. Neutrophils have an ephemeral moment of glory; their life span in the tissues is very short, at most a few days. Mature polys are end cells like red blood cells; that is, they are incapable of reproduction. In addition, once their granules are formed, protein synthesis ceases. Are mature polys, such as those found in inflammation, capable of repairing themselves or replacing the digestive enzymes they use in the process of phagocytosis? Yes or No. EXPLAIN.

TURN THE TEXT 180° AND CONTINUE.

---

96. F
F
T
T
T
T

THIS IS THE END OF UNIT 3. TAKE THE POSTTEST ON PAGE xviii.

1. B
A

---

2. Leukocytes normally found in the blood are divided into two categories:

GRANULOCYTES or POLYMORPHONUCLEAR LEUKOCYTES

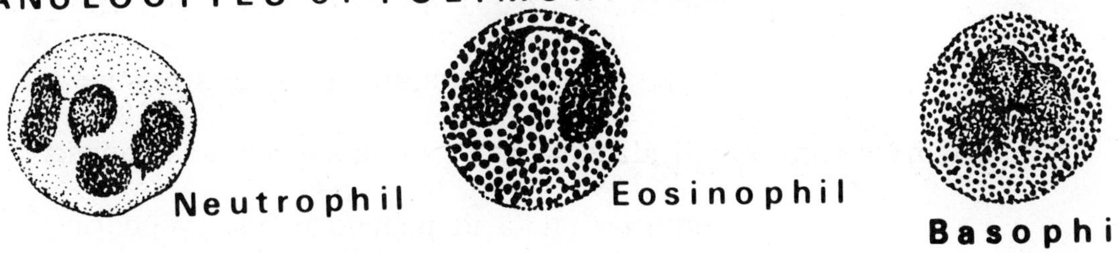

MONONUCLEAR LEUKOCYTES

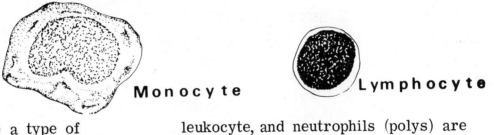

Monocytes are a type of __________ leukocyte, and neutrophils (polys) are __________ or __________ leukocytes.

---

49. No. Since they cannot synthesize protein, they cannot repair damaged structures or replace digestive granules.

---

50. Which is/are true? Once at the inflammatory focus:

a) neutrophils replicate and maintain a constant number.

b) neutrophils decrease in number within a short time unless new cells continue to move from the vessels.

47. chemotactic

---

48. The first cells to arrive at an inflammatory focus are __________, which are followed by mononuclear macrophages.

---

95. T
F
F
F
T
F

---

96. MARK THE FOLLOWING "T" TRUE OR "F" FALSE:

		frame reference
___	Antibodies are effective against physical agents.	85
___	Antibodies are produced in every inflammation.	86
___	Opsonins make bacteria more susceptible to phagocytosis.	88
___	Mast cells release histamine.	90
___	Fibroblasts appear when repair is about to begin.	90
___	Mononuclear phagocytes are found in all but the very first stages of inflammation.	59

2. Monocytes are a type of mononuclear leukocyte, and neutrophils (polys) are polymorphonuclear or granulocytic leukocytes.

---

3. Neutrophils, eosinophils, and basophils are called granulocytes because of the granules in their cytoplasm and polymorphonuclear because of the polymorphous (from the Greek polys, meaning "many," and morphe, meaning "shape or form") segmented form of their nuclei. In the drawing of a blood smear below, WHICH OF THE CELLS (A, B, C, D, E) ARE GRANULOCYTES?

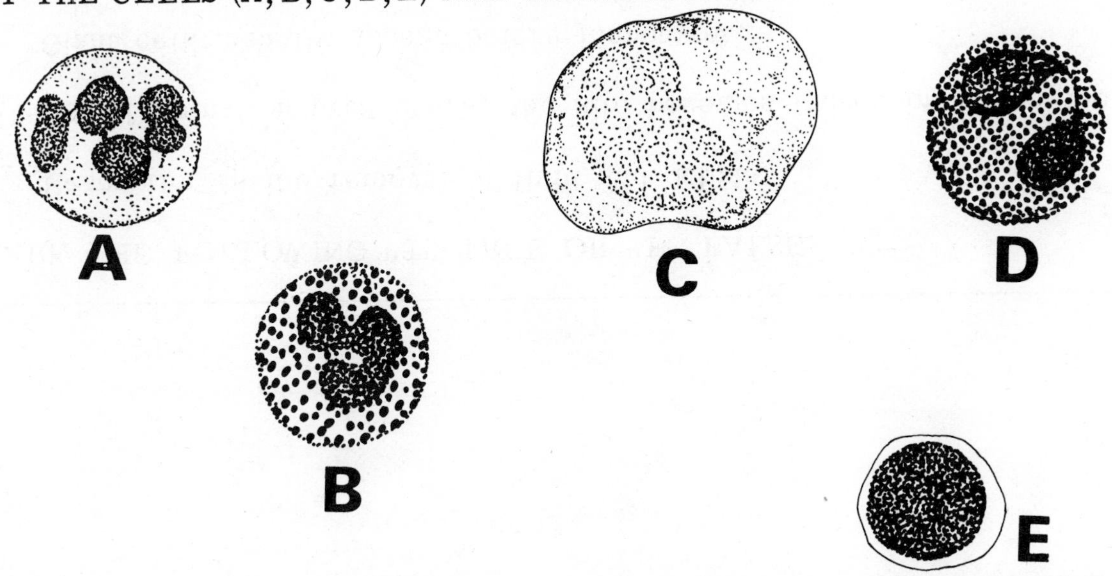

---

50. b

---

51. Neutrophils help destroy injurious agents and remove debris by two mechanisms:
   1) ingestion or phagocytosis and in some cases intracellular digestion,
   2) release of granules containing digestive enzymes from ruptured cell membranes, leading to extracellular digestion.

   Is the destruction or immobilization of the injurious agent necessary to prevent further inflammation? (yes or no)

   Is the removal of debris necessary before repair can take place? (yes or no)

   How does the rupture of neutrophil membranes contribute to the termination of inflammation and preparation for repair? EXPLAIN.

46. c) in less than one hour

---

47. When stimulated by inflammation, polys are active ameboid cells and are chemotropic. A chemotropic cell is a cell which is attracted by a __________ agent.

---

94. F
F
T
T
F
T

---

95. MARK THE FOLLOWING "T" TRUE OR "F" FALSE:

		frame reference
___	Resorption is the removal of fluid and debris.	57
___	As inflammation progresses, the site becomes increasingly alkaline.	64
___	Giant cells usually appear before monocytes.	67
___	Destruction of microbial invaders by polys is a function of little importance.	70
___	Eosinophils are thought to be important in the removal of antigen-antibody complexes.	76
___	The presence of plasma cells and lymphocytes indicates that the reaction is about a day old.	78, 80

3. A, B, D

---

4. Based on the staining reactions of their granules, polymorphonuclear leukocytes or __________ are divided into three types:

   1) Eosinophils - granules stain red-pink with eosin, an acidic dye.

   2) Basophils - granules stain blue-black with some basic dyes but not hematoxylin.

   3) __________ - granules are usually inconspicuous but may stain slightly.

---

51. yes
yes
The rupture of neutrophil membranes releases granules containing digestive enzymes which can inactivate injurious agents and dissolve debris.

---

52. A short time after arriving at an inflammatory focus, neutrophils begin to degenerate and the cell membrane ruptures, pouring granules containing __________ __________ into the area.

45. blood
tissues

---

46. In the initial stages of inflammation polys are the predominant cell type. They move from the blood vessels to the inflammatory focus:

a) immediately.

b) before the signs and symptoms of inflammation appear.

c) in less than one hour.

d) in several hours.

e) in a few days.

---

93. A. eosinophil
B. neutrophil
C. mast cell
D. plasma cell
E. mononuclear phagocyte
F. lymphocyte

---

94. INDICATE "T" TRUE OR "F" FALSE:

	frame reference
___ The most numerous and important of the granulocytes are the eosinophils.	45
___ Polys arrive at the inflammatory focus a few days after injury.	46
___ Polys are like kamikazes. Once they take off from the vessels for the battle site, they never return.	49
___ The dissolution of debris is an important function of polys.	51
___ Once they enter the inflammatory zone, monocytes cannot replace the digestive enzymes they use.	62
___ Monocytes arrive in large numbers at the inflammatory focus a few hours after the polys.	59

4. granulocytes
   neutrophils

---

5. The primary distinguishing characteristics of granulocytes are:

   1) the __________ shape of their nuclei.

   2) the __________ in their cytoplasm.

---

52. digestive enzymes

---

53. Can accumulation of debris cause tissue damage and continuing inflammation? Yes or No.

44. 1) polymorphonuclear leukocytes (neutrophils)
2) mononuclear phagocytes
3) giant cells

---

45. Neutrophilic polymorphonuclear leukocytes, often called "polys" or "polymorphs," are the most numerous and important of the granulocytes. Polys, along with monocytes, are normally found in the __________ and move into the __________ during inflammation.

---

92. A	C
A, C	C (sometimes A)
C	C
C	

---

93. IDENTIFY THE CELLS BELOW:

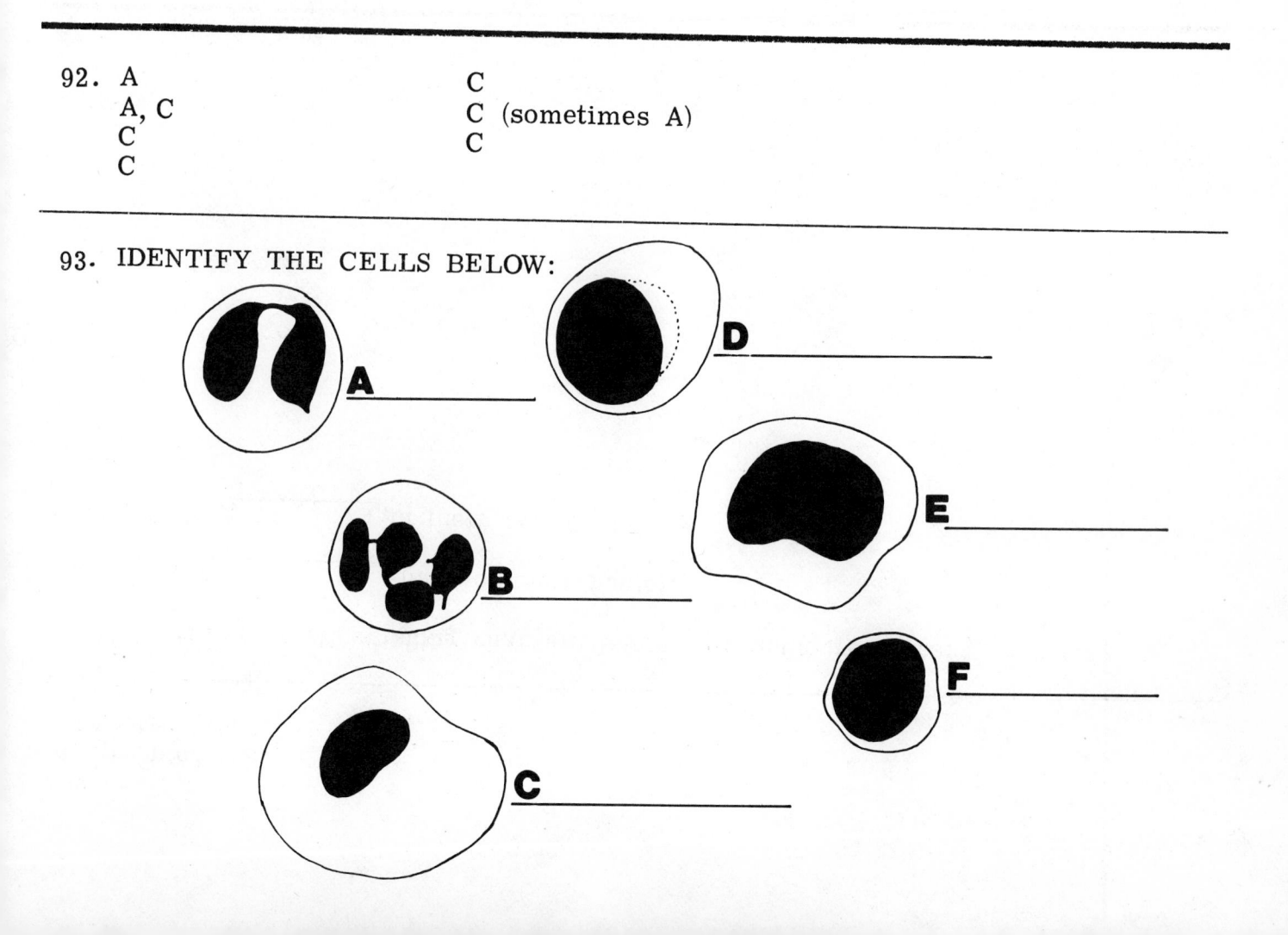

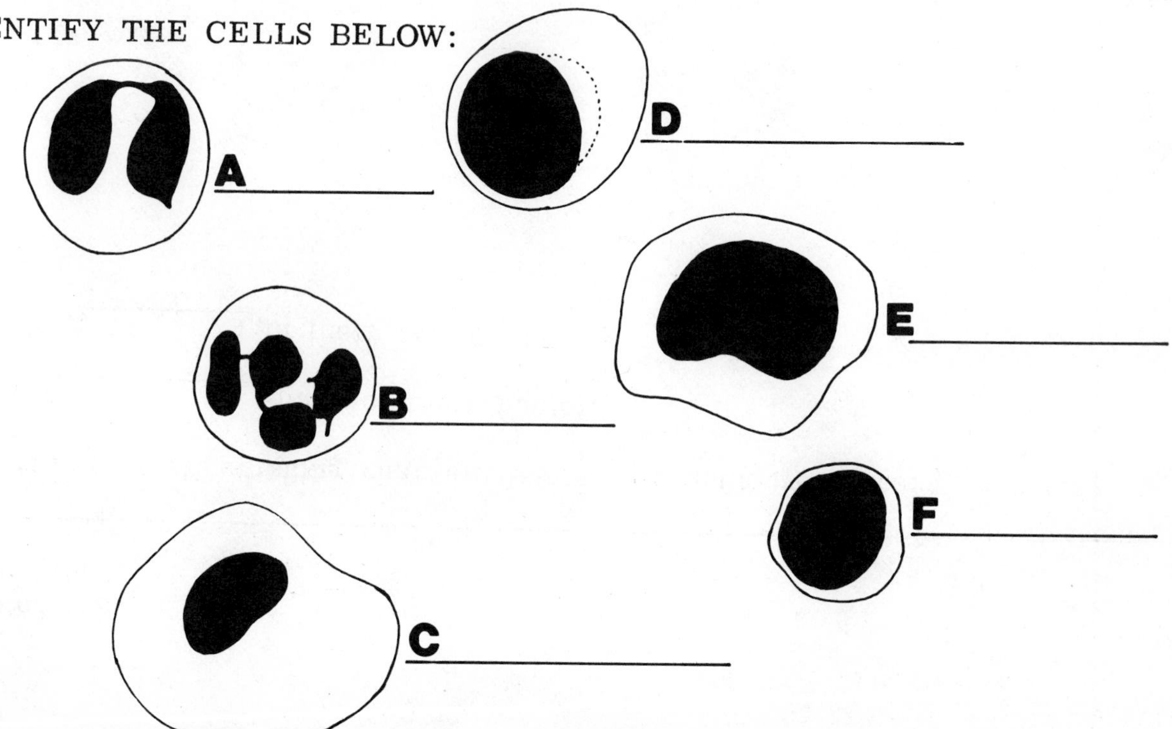

5. polymorphous or segmented granules

---

6. MATCH THE FOLLOWING CELLS WITH THE STAINING REACTIONS OF THEIR GRANULES:

Cell	Staining Reactions
___ neutrophils	A. large, irregular, coarse granules stain blue-black with stains used for blood smears but not in ordinary tissue stains
___ eosinophils	B. large, closely packed granules stain bright red-pink with acidic dyes in ordinary tissue stains and blood smear stains
___ basophils	C. fine, inconspicuous granules give neither acidophilic nor basophilic reaction with ordinary tissue stains

---

53. Yes.

---

54. Which of the following do polys help remove by phagocytosis or release of enzymes?

a) active lymphocytes

b) fibrin

c) dead neutrophils

d) dead tissue

e) dead lymphocytes

f) live tissue

43. T
F
T
F
F
T

B. The Function of Inflammatory Cells (53 frames)

When you complete this section, you will be able to select correct responses relating to the:

1. function of each type of inflammatory cell, if known.
2. time sequence in which polys, mononuclear phagocytes, eosinophils, plasma cells, giant cells, lymphocytes, and fibroblasts appear in an inflammatory site.
3. mechanism of removal of debris.
4. definitions of opsonin and agranulocytosis.

44. The cells described in the preceding section have four known functions in inflammation and repair and removal of debris: 1) phagocytosis; 2) production and release of antibodies; 3) histamine release; and 4) repair. The three types of phagocytic cells are:

1) ____________ 2) ____________ 3) ____________

---

91. D
A
C
C
B
B

---

92. MARK THE CELLS WHICH ARE CHARACTERISTIC OF ACUTE STAGES OF INFLAMMATION "A" AND THOSE WHICH ARE CHARACTERISTIC OF CHRONIC INFLAMMATION "C ":

___ neutrophils

___ mononuclear phagocytes

___ plasma cells

___ lymphocytes

___ giant cells

___ eosinophils

___ fibroblasts

6. C
B
A

---

7. There is also some difference in nuclear morphology between the three types of granulocytes, which is helpful in distinguishing neutrophils and eosinophils in tissue. MATCH THE FOLLOWING:

Nuclear Morphology

___ nucleus dark-staining, centrally placed, segmented into two to six lobes (usually three or four)

___ nucleus often situated on the circumference of the cell with the lobes extending centrally, usually only two lobes

___ nucleus centrally placed; usually two or three lobes; often lobes are not distinctly separated

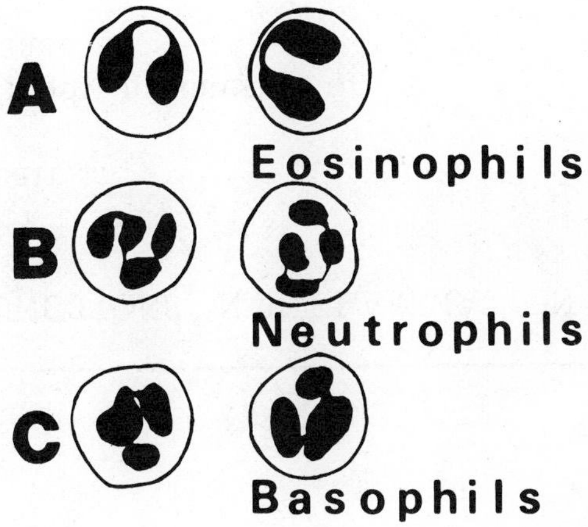

---

54. b, c, d, e

---

55. Debris is any material, except live leukocytes, not found in the tissue before injury. For the most part debris is ☐ soluble ☐ insoluble in the plasma fluid.

42. T
F
F
F
T
F

---

43. INDICATE "T" TRUE OR "F" FALSE:

		frame ref.
___	Monocytes can turn into macrophages in the tissue.	29
___	Mast cell granules stain with normal tissue stains.	4
___	Many tissue macrophages are normally inactive but can become mobile and phagocytic when stimulated by an inflammatory reaction.	22
___	Foreign-body giant cells are often found in tuberculosis.	34
___	Plasma cells are normally found in the blood and move into the tissues during inflammation.	17
___	The three types of polymorphonuclear leukocytes are distinguished primarily by the staining reactions of their granules.	4

---

90. dilation
permeability

[✓] do not

repair

---

91. MATCH THE FOLLOWING CELLS WITH THEIR FUNCTIONS IN INFLAMMATION AND REPAIR:

___ mast cells

___ fibroblasts

___ polys

___ mononuclear phagocytes

___ plasma cells

___ lymphocytes

A. repair

B. antibody production or release

C. phagocytosis and preparation for repair

D. histamine release

7. B
A
C

---

8. MATCH THE FOLLOWING:

Cell	Nuclear Morphology and Location
___ and ___ Eosinophil	A. nucleus centrally placed
___ and ___ Basophil	B. nucleus peripherally placed
___ and ___ Neutrophil	C. two- or three-lobed nucleus
	D. two- to six-lobed nucleus, highly segmented

---

55. [✓] insoluble

---

56. The release of digestive enzymes by polys helps make debris __________ so that it can be carried away by the plasma fluid.

41.

	Diameter			Nucleus Shape		Normal Location	
	<10μ	10-15μ	>15μ	segmented	round or indented	blood	tissue
Polymorphonuclear Neutrophils		✓		✓		✓	
Lymphocytes	✓				✓	✓	✓
Monocytes		✓	✓		✓	✓	
Mast Cells		✓			✓		✓
Plasma Cells		✓			✓		✓
Macrophages		✓	✓		✓		✓
Giant Cells			✓		✓		✓

---

42. INDICATE "T" TRUE OR "F" FALSE:

	frame reference
___ Neutrophils, eosinophils, and basophils are the only inflammatory cells with segmented nuclei.	2-3
___ The monocyte is the smallest of the inflammatory cells.	14
___ Lymphocytes have granular cytoplasm.	2-3
___ Granulocytes often vary greatly in shape and size.	14
___ Plasma cells are usually oval.	18
___ Giant cells are formed by fusion or amitotic division of polymorphonuclear neutrophils.	32

---

89. a, c, d

---

90. Histamine release is believed to result from lysis of mast cell membranes, releasing mast cell granules, which, in turn, release histamine. Histamine causes capillary __________ and increased capillary __________.

Basophils also contain histamine. Basophils ☐ do ☐ do not play an important role in inflammation.

Late in the inflammatory reaction, fibroblasts begin to appear. Fibroblasts proliferate and secrete procollagen and protein-polysaccharide complexes (ground substance). Their primary function is the replacement of dead and injured tissue with new cells and connective tissue fibers. This process is one type of __________.

8. B and C
A and C
A and D

---

9. IDENTIFY THE FOLLOWING GRANULOCYTES:

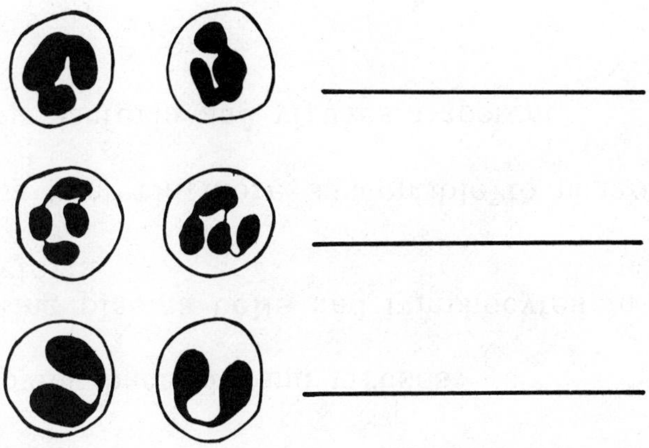

---

56. soluble

---

57. The removal of debris and fluid is called resolution. Is resolution necessary for complete repair to occur?

40. No Stain (colorless)
No Stain (colorless)
Red-Pink
No Stain or Very Faint

41.

	Diameter			Nucleus Shape		Normal Location	
	$<10\mu$	$10-15\mu$	$>15\mu$	segmented	round or indented	blood	tissue
Polymorphonuclear Neutrophils							
Lymphocytes							
Monocytes							
Mast Cells							
Plasma Cells							
Macrophages							
Giant Cells							

---

88. b

---

89. INDICATE THE CORRECT RESPONSE(S). Antibodies act by:

a) destroying bacteria and viruses.

b) assisting plasma cells and lymphocytes in the enzymatic destruction of bacteria.

c) making bacteria more susceptible to phagocytosis.

d) making bacteria and viruses impotent.

9. basophil
neutrophil
eosinophil

---

10. Because of the complex morphology of their nuclei, the appearance of granulocytes in blood smears and in tissue sections differs. In blood smears cells are simply flattened and cell lobes of their nuclei are apparent, while in tissue sections the nuclei may be cut so that the bulk of the nucleus is not included in the section.

MATCH THE FOLLOWING:

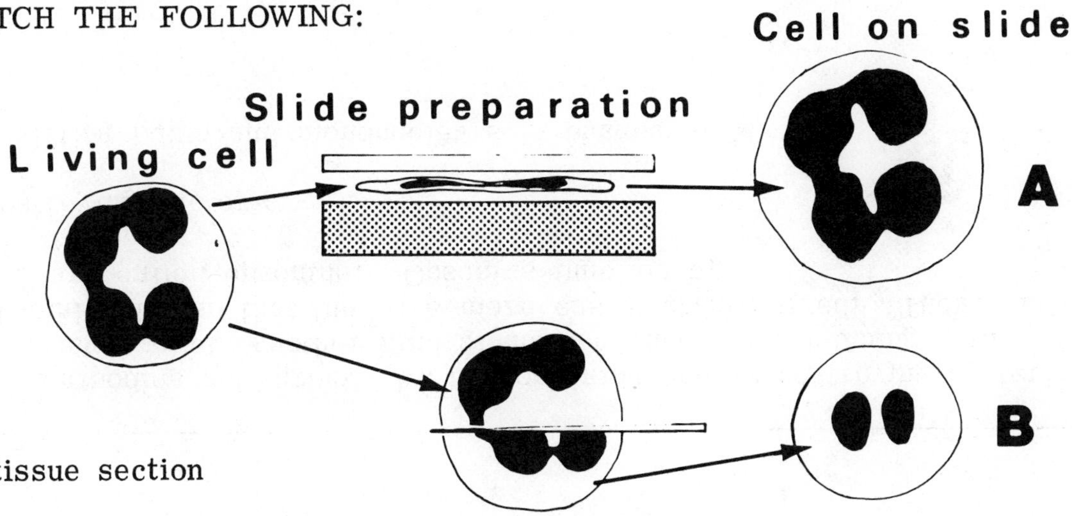

___tissue section

___smear

In addition to the differences in the appearance of the nuclei, a cell 11 μ in diameter in the blood might be 13 μ in diameter in a blood smear and 9 μ in diameter in a tissue section. WHY?

---

57. Yes.

---

58. Once the debris has been broken down by __________ __________ so that it is soluble in the plasma fluid, it can be carried away by the capillaries and lymphatics.

39. 1) eosinophil
2) macrophage
3) mast cell
4) Langhans' cell
5) foreign-body giant cell
6) fibroblast

---

40. With an ordinary tissue stain such as H&E, what is the color of the granules of the cells below?

Cell	Color of Granules
Mast Cell	________
Basophil	________
Eosinophil	________
Neutrophil	________

---

87. a

---

88. Many antibodies act directly by immobilizing and/or destroying bacteria and viruses. But another kind of antibody acts by combining with microbial cells so that they are more easily phagocytized. These antibodies are called opsonins. Opsonins function by:

a) destroying bacteria.

b) assisting polys and mononuclears in phagocytosis.

10. B
A

The slices of cells in tissue cannot exceed the largest diameter of the entire cell and most often are smaller, while the cells in blood smears are simply flattened cells and therefore are slightly larger than their original diameter.

11.

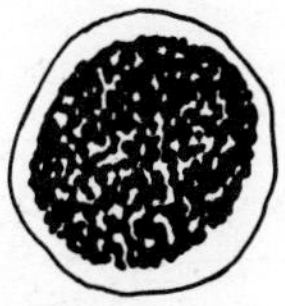

Lymphocyte

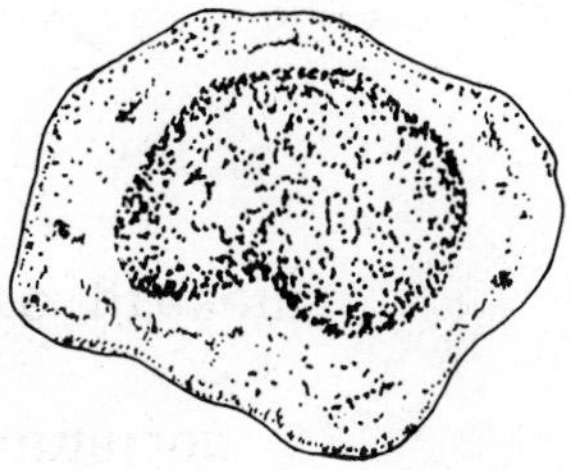

Monocyte

Mononuclear leukocytes, unlike granulocytes, have rounded or indented nuclei and lack conspicuous granules in their cytoplasm.
INDICATE THE APPROPRIATE BOXES:

	Cytoplasmic Granules	Segmented Nucleus	Rounded or Indented Nucleus	Normally Found in the Blood
Polymorphonuclear Leukocytes	☐	☐	☐	☐
Mononuclear Leukocytes	☐	☐	☐	☐

---

58. digestive enzymes

---

59. Shortly after the arrival of the polys, monocytes begin to appear in the inflamed area. After entering the tissue, a monocyte becomes a _____________.

38. A. monocyte
B. lymphocyte
C. neutrophil
D. eosinophil
E. plasma cell

---

39. IDENTIFY THE FOLLOWING CELLS:

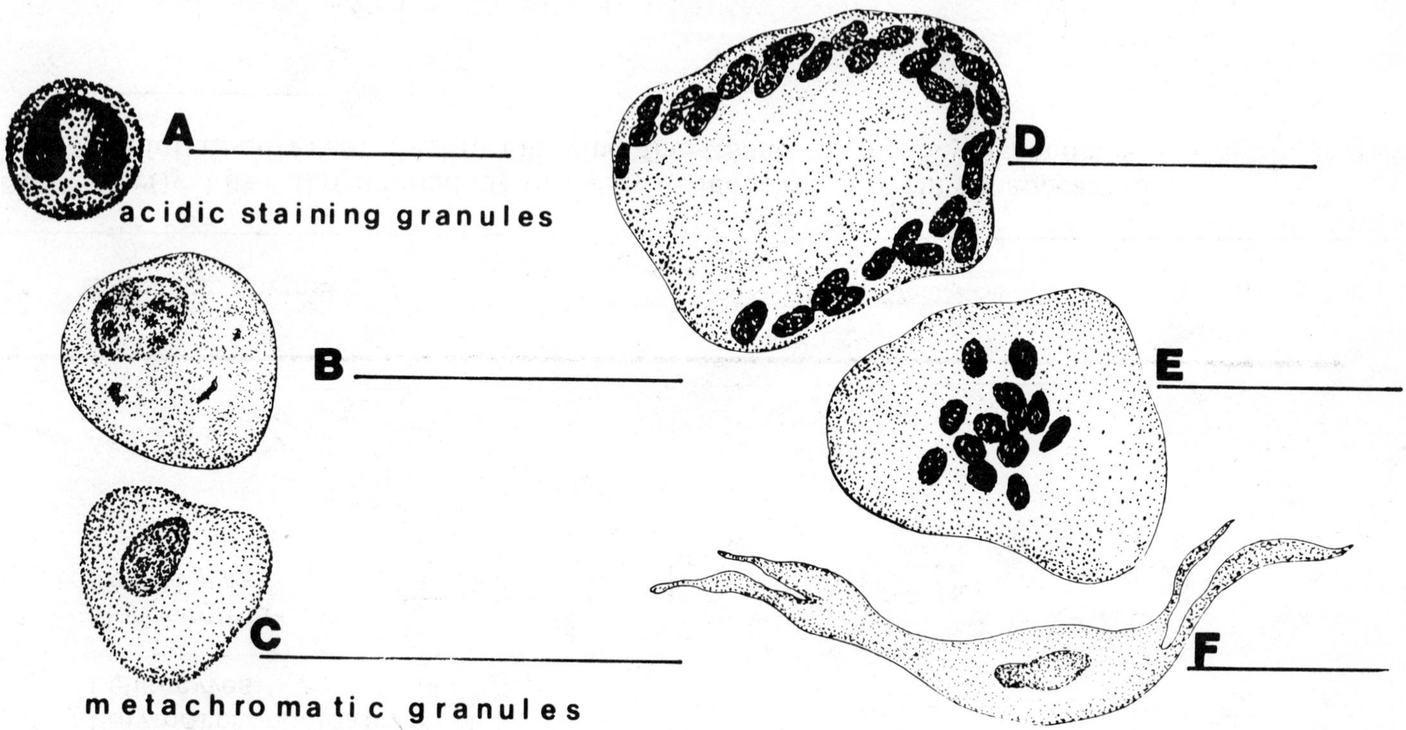

---

86. b

---

87. Lymphocytes and plasma cells appear:

a) in almost every long-term inflammation.

b) only when bacteria or viruses are present.

11.

Polymorphonuclear Leukocytes	☑	☑	☐	☑
Mononuclear Leukocytes	☐	☐	☑	☑

---

12. MATCH THE FOLLOWING:

___ dark-staining polymorphous nuclei

___ rounded or indented nuclei

___ large granules in cytoplasm

___ homogeneous cytoplasm

A. granulocytes

B. mononuclear leukocytes

---

59. macrophage (mononuclear phagocyte)

---

60. Monocytes appear at the inflammatory focus:

a) immediately.

b) within 12 hours.

c) within a few days.

37. E
D
C
F
G
A

38. IDENTIFY THE FOLLOWING CELLS:

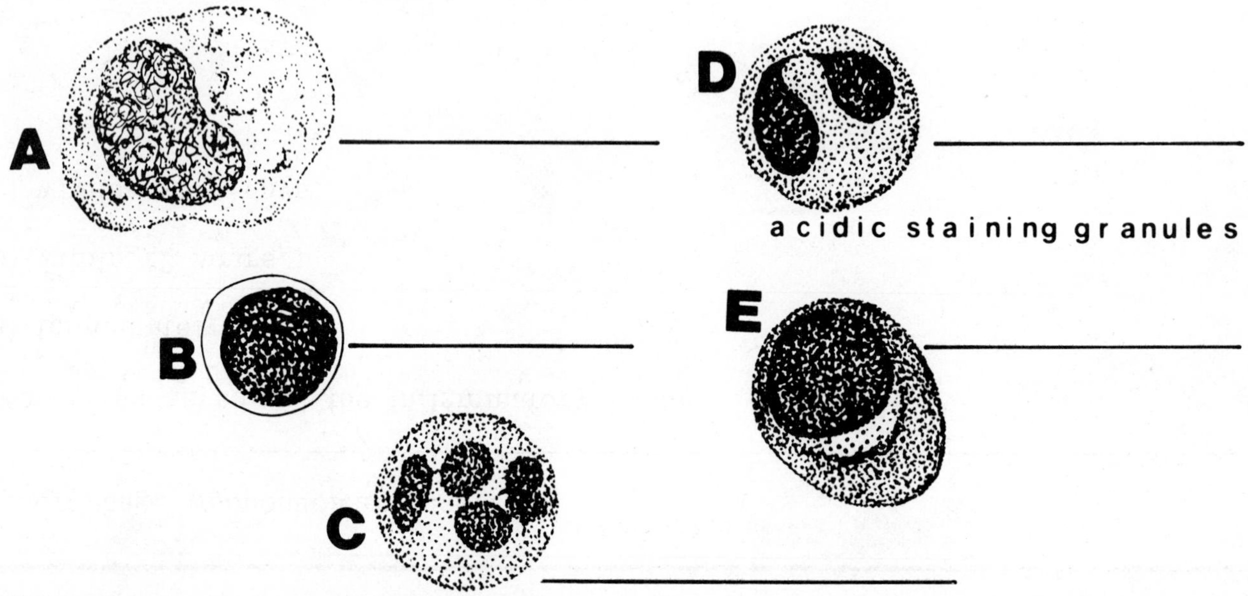

85. b

86. Antibodies are produced when the causal agent remains in the tissue, but lymphocytes and plasma cells are present in most all long-term inflammations regardless of cause. Antibodies are commonly measurable:

a) in every inflammation.

b) when bacteria or viruses are present.

12. A
B
A
B

---

13. Lymphocytes are small (8 μ in diam.) round cells, slightly larger than a red blood cell. The nucleus is round, stains deeply, and occupies almost the entire cell. The cytoplasm is a thin rim around the nucleus. MATCH THE FOLLOWING:

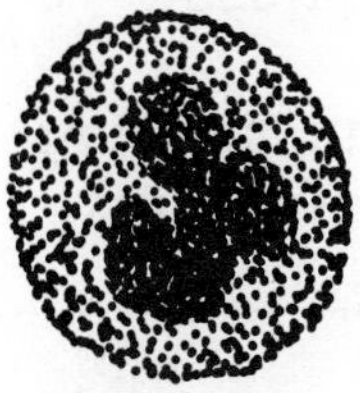 ______ 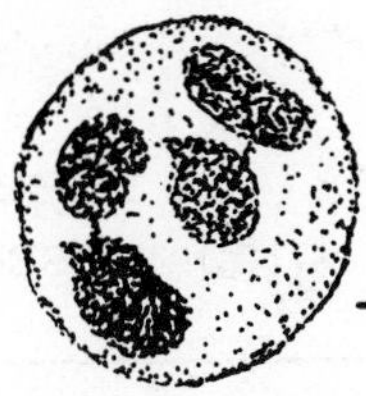 ______

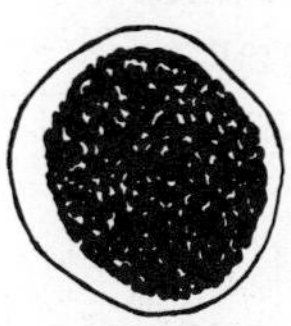 ______ 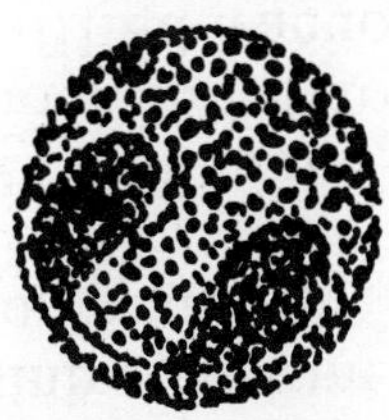 ______

A. Eosinophil

B. Basophil

C. Neutrophil

D. Lymphocyte

---

60. b

---

61. Like polys, mononuclears are actively mobile, respond to chemotactic agents, are phagocytic, and release digestive enzymes when they die. Extracellular digestion of debris occurs as a result of the release of ______ ______ from polys and mononuclears.

The removal of debris and fluid is called ______.

36. fibroblast
lymphocyte
mononuclear phagocyte
giant cell

[✓] repair

---

37. MATCH THE FOLLOWING:

___ an oval cell with a round, eccentrically placed nucleus containing dark-staining clumps of chromatin

___ a small round cell with a dark-staining round nucleus which takes up almost the entire cell

___ an irregularly shaped cell with small oval nucleus and many large metachromatic granules in the cytoplasm

___ a round cell, approximately 12 μ in diameter, with an oval nucleus and granular cytoplasm due to ingested debris

___ a round cell, approximately 12 μ in diameter, with a dark - staining, segmented nucleus and granular cytoplasm

___ a very large cell with many nuclei scattered throughout the cytoplasm and numerous debris-filled vacuoles

A. foreign-body giant cell
B. Langhans' cell
C. mast cell
D. lymphocyte
E. plasma cell
F. macrophage
G. neutrophil

---

84. b, c, e

---

85. Lymphocytes and plasma cells produce and release antibodies. Antibodies function in inflammation by:

a) dissolving debris.

b) helping to immobilize or inactivate some biological agents.

13. B C

D A

---

14. Monocytes are usually the largest of the leukocytes, varying from 12 to 20 μ in diameter. Often the light-staining nucleus is horseshoe-shaped or indented. The cytoplasm is abundant. MATCH THE FOLLOWING (letters may be used more than once):

___	dark-staining, segmented nucleus	A.	Eosinophil
___	slightly larger than a red blood cell	B.	Basophil
___	dark-staining round nucleus	C.	Neutrophil
___	thin rim of cytoplasm	D.	Lymphocyte
___	cell which varies in size (12μ-20μ)	E.	Monocyte
___	granules in cytoplasm		
___	indented, light-staining nucleus		

---

61. digestive enzymes
resolution

---

62. Unlike polys, monocytes live for weeks or months, are probably not end cells, and can synthesize proteins, especially the enzymes used in phagocytosis. MATCH THE FOLLOWING:

___	the first cell to appear at the inflammatory site	A.	neutrophil
___	the second cell to appear	B.	monocyte
___	incapable of protein synthesis		
___	remains active in latter part of inflammation		
___	lives for a few days at most		
___	disintegrates shortly after arrival, releasing digestive granules		

35. Langhans' Cell
Foreign-body giant cell

---

36. Fibroblasts are large fusiform or spindle-shaped cells, but they occasionally have several slender branching processes. Their oval nuclei are the largest of any tissue cell and usually have prominent nucleoli. Fibroblast cytoplasm is nearly homogeneous and stains faintly. In tissue slides the cytoplasm is often so faint that only the nuclei are apparent. Fibroblasts are the connective tissue cells responsible for the production of connective tissue fibers and ground substance. LABEL THE CELLS IN THE DIAGRAM BELOW:

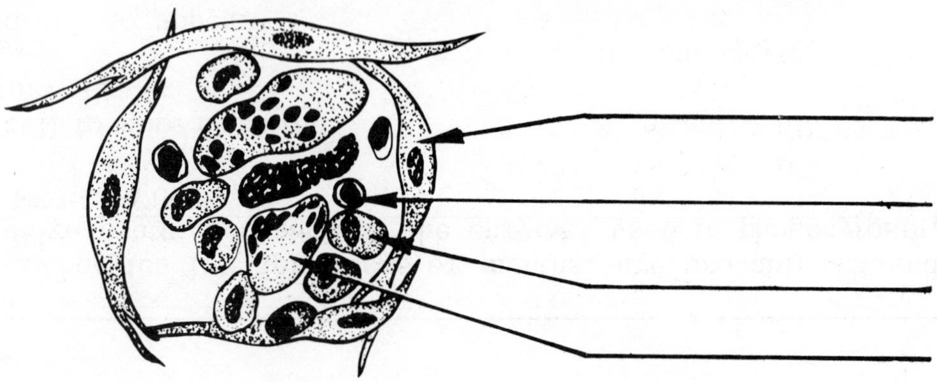

Fibroblasts are usually the primary cell of: ▱ inflammation ▱ repair

---

83. B
A
A
A, B
B A

---

84. There is considerable evidence that lymphocytes can become fibroblasts, mononuclear phagocytes, and stem cells. Which of the following are potential sources of mononuclear phagocytes during inflammation?

a) plasma cells

b) monocytes

c) tissue macrophages

d) neutrophils

e) lymphocytes

14. A, B, C
D
D
D
E
A, B, C
E

---

15. IDENTIFY THE CELLS BELOW:

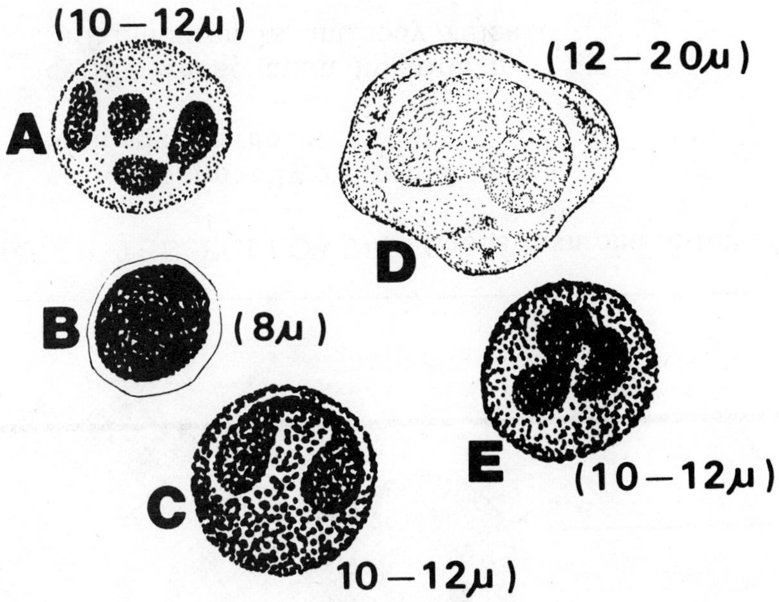

A ____________

B ____________

C ____________

D ____________

E ____________

---

62. A
B
A
B
A
A

---

63. Polys are capable of either aerobic metabolism with production of CO_2 or anaerobic metabolism with production of lactic acid. Anaerobic metabolism enables the poly to carry on its phagocytic activity when the circulation is poor and in necrotic areas. Glycolysis causes the surrounding area to become more ☐ acidic ☐ basic.

34. foreign-body giant cell

---

35. The Langhans' cell has many nuclei around the periphery of the cell arranged in the form of an incomplete circle. Foreign-body giant cells have nuclei scattered throughout their cytoplasm but are otherwise the same as Langhans' cells. IDENTIFY THE CELLS BELOW:

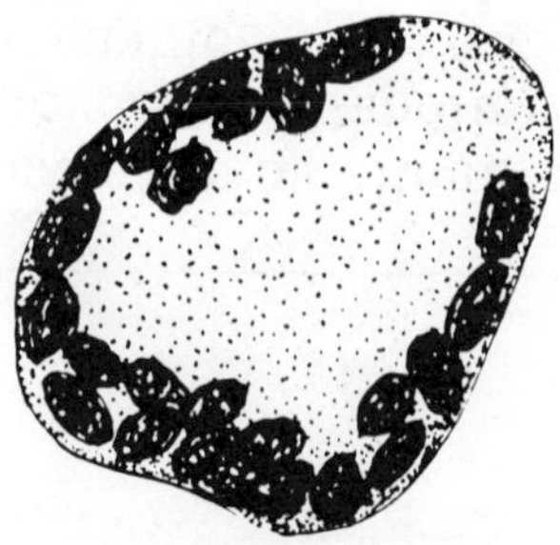

____

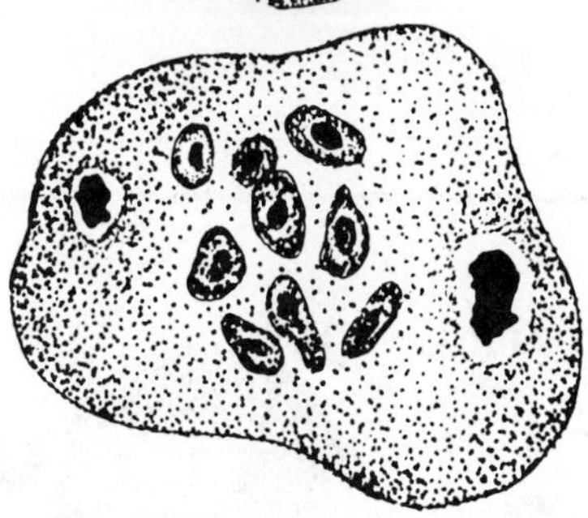

____

---

82. b

---

83. MATCH THE FOLLOWING (more than one letter may apply):

___ cell(s) primarily responsible for antibody synthesis	A. lymphocyte
___ cell(s) whose main function in inflammation is antibody release	B. plasma cell
___ cell(s) normally found in the blood	
___ cell(s) whose presence indicates a long-lasting inflammation	

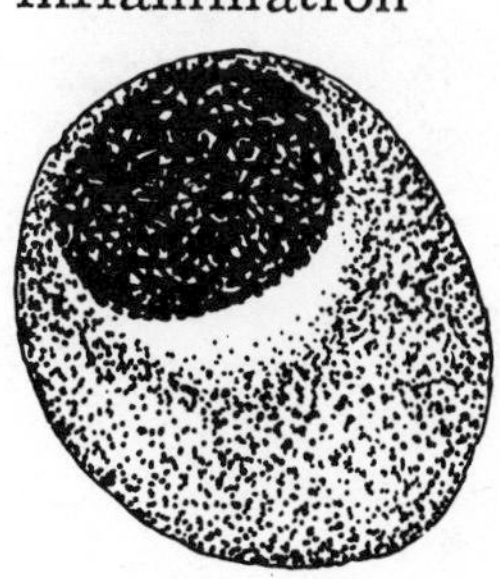

____

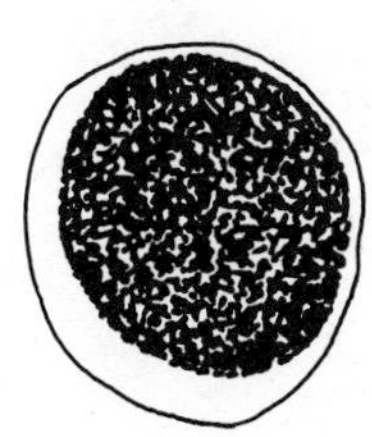

____

15. A. neutrophil
B. lymphocyte
C. eosinophil
D. monocyte
E. basophil

---

16. INDICATE THE CORRECT BOXES:

	Diameter			Nuclear Shape		Granules in Cytoplasm		Nuclear Staining	
	8 μ	10-12μ	12-20μ	segmented	rounded or indented	yes	no	dark	light
Eosinophils									
Basophils									
Neutrophils									
Lymphocytes									
Monocytes									

---

63. [✓] acidic

---

64. In its initial stage the pH of an inflammatory site is usually in the range of 7.2 to 7.4, but as the reaction continues acid metabolites accumulate and the pH [ ] increases [ ] decreases. When the pH is reduced below 7.0, the polys begin to die and release their enzymes; in contrast, mononuclear phagocytes remain active at a pH below 6.8.

33. mononuclear phagocytes (macrophages)

---

34. Giant cells derived from mononuclear phagocytes are often classified into two types: Langhans' giant cells and foreign-body giant cells.

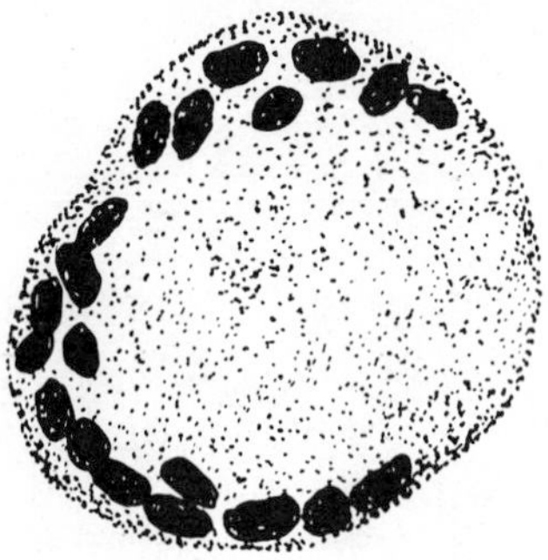

Langhans'
Giant Cell

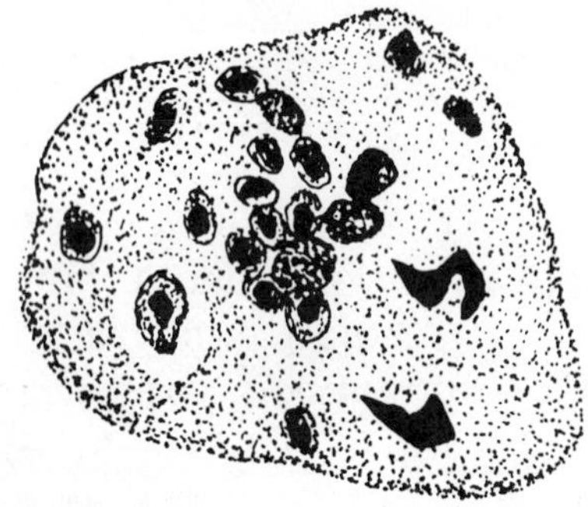

Foreign-Body
Giant Cell

Langhans' cells are "classically" formed in tuberculosis while foreign-body giant cells are formed in an inflammatory area containing debris too large to be phagocytized by a single mononuclear cell. Which type of cell is commonly found surrounding suture material left from an operation?

____

---

81. b

---

82. The primary function of lymphocytes in inflammation is probably the release of antibodies. It is not known whether lymphocytes produce antibodies or simply transport them to the inflammatory focus. However, when the lymphocytes clustered in an inflammatory zone are lysed, a high concentration of antibody is released. In an inflammatory response lymphocytes and plasma cells are concerned with:

a) removal of debris.

b) production and release of antibodies.

c) histamine release.

d) repair.

16.

	Diameter			Nuclear Shape		Granules in Cytoplasm		Nuclear Staining	
	8μ	$10\text{-}12\mu$	$12\text{-}20\mu$	segmented	rounded or indented	yes	no	dark	light
Eosinophils		✓		✓		✓		✓	
Basophils		✓		✓		✓		✓	
Neutrophils		✓		✓		✓		✓	
Lymphocytes	✓				✓		✓	✓	
Monocytes			✓		✓		✓		✓

---

17. Granulocytes and mononuclears are normally found in the __________ and can migrate into the tissues. Inflammatory cells normally found in the tissues are:

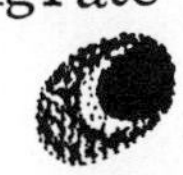
Plasma cells

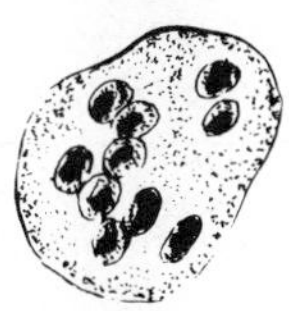
Giant cells

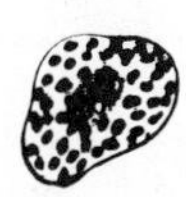
Mast cell (metachromatic stain)

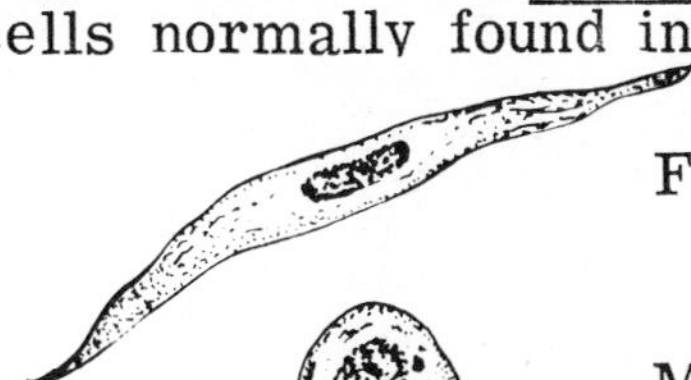
Fibroblast

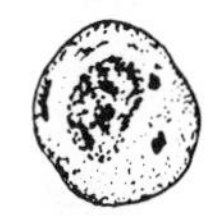
Macrophage

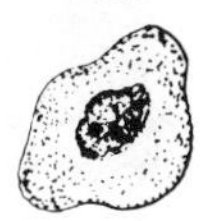
Mast cell (tissue stain)

Which of the cells above most closely resembles a monocyte? __________

---

64. [✓] decreases

---

65. Progressively increasing acidity first destroys the __________, releasing their enzymes. In the later stages of inflammation dead polys are phagocytized by __________.

32. C
A, B, C
B
A
A, B, C

---

33. Giant cells originate by fusion or amitotic division of _________.

---

80. blood and some tissues

---

81. Plasma cells mixed with lymphocytes on the periphery of an active inflammatory zone indicates that the reaction:

a) is a few hours old (acute).

b) has been continuing for a long time (chronic).

17. Granulocytes and mononuclears are normally found in the blood and can migrate into the tissues.

Tissue macrophages closely resemble monocytes.

---

18. Plasma cells may superficially resemble lymphocytes, but they are larger (approximately 10 μ in diameter). They have much more cytoplasm, which is distinctly basophilic, and an eccentrically placed nucleus. Lymphocytes are round and plasma cells are usually oval. The eccentrically placed nucleus often contains deeply staining clumps of chromatin arranged peripherally so the nucleus resembles a watch dial. LABEL THE CELLS BELOW:

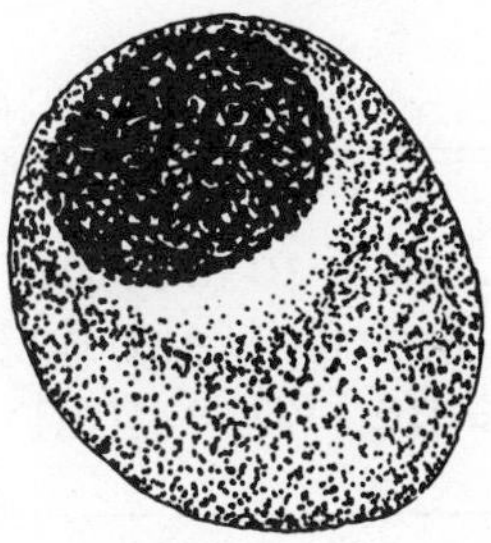

______

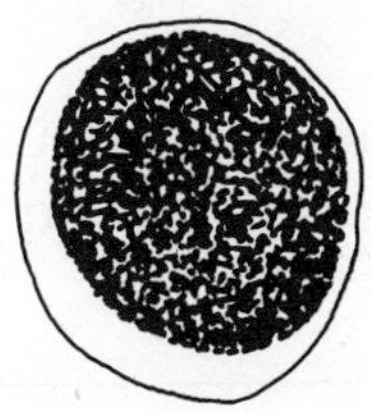

______

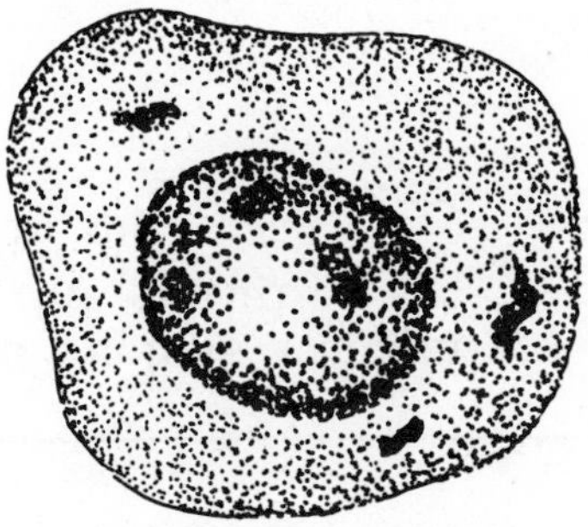

______

---

65. polys
mononuclear phagocytes

---

66. MATCH THE FOLLOWING:

___ cell which forms digestive granules on arrival at the inflammatory focus	A. neutrophil
___ cell which lives for weeks or months	B. monocyte or macrophage
___ cell which is active at a pH below 6.8	
___ an end cell, like a red blood cell	
___ cell with a centrally located, segmented nucleus	
___ first line of defense at the site of injury	

31. neutrophils
large mononuclear phagocytes
giant cells

---

32. Giant cells arise from fusion of many mononuclear phagocytes or by amitotic division of cells which fail to separate. MATCH THE FOLLOWING (letters may be used more than once):

___ many nuclei	A.	neutrophils
___ often have vacuoles containing debris	B.	mononuclear phagocytes
___ single oval rucleus	C.	giant cells
___ normally found in the blood		
___ found during inflammation in the tissues		

---

79. eosinophils

---

80. Unlike the other blood leukocytes, lymphocytes move more or less randomly, so they rarely accumulate in an inflammatory zone during the initial stages of the reaction. Lymphocytes are normally found in the __________ and ______________.

18. plasma cell lymphocyte macrophage

---

19. MATCH THE FOLLOWING:

___ oval cell with basophilic cytoplasm

___ a thin rim of cytoplasm

___ a uniformly dark-staining nucleus

___ a small round cell

___ eccentrically placed nucleus

A. Lymphocyte

B. Plasma Cell

---

66. B
B
B
A
A
A

---

67. Giant cells are formed by the fusion or amitotic division of __________ __________.

30. B
    A

---

31. The three general types of active phagocytic cells in inflammation are:

    1) __________

    2) __________

    3) __________

---

78. [✓] chronic

---

79. Cells which appear late in inflammation and are thought to specialize in the removal of antigen-antibody complexes are __________.

19. B
A
A
A
B

---

20. Mast cells are about 12 μ in diameter and vary widely in shape. They have small oval nuclei and their cytoplasm is filled with large granules which can be seen only with metachromatic stains. Mast cell granules contain the chemical mediator of inflammation, ____________.

MATCH THE CELLS WITH THEIR STAINS:

Stain

___metachromatic stain

___normal tissue stain

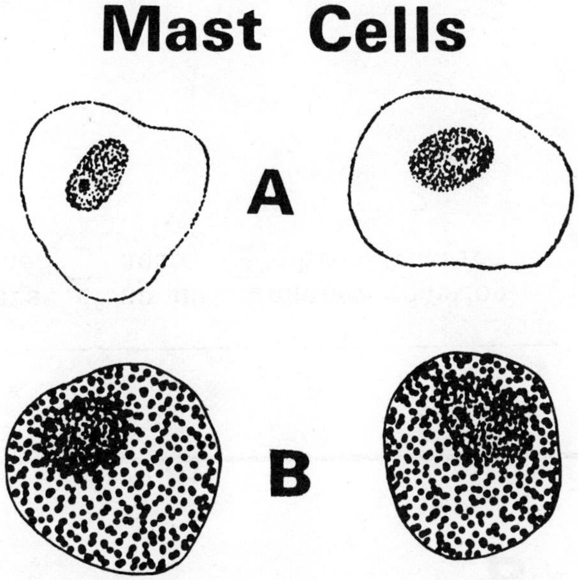

Do eosinophil granules stain with normal tissue stains? ▱ yes ▱ no.

---

67. mononuclear phagocytes

---

68. What type of cell is formed in an inflammatory area containing debris too large to be phagocytized by individual mononuclear cells?

29. macrophages

---

30. Mononuclear phagocytes form giant cells during some inflammations. Giant cells are very large, up to 60-100 μ in diameter, many times as large as the mononuclear phagocytes. Their shape is round to oval but they are usually distorted by the debris they have engulfed.

MATCH THE FOLLOWING:

___nucleus of giant cell

___crystalline debris in giant cell

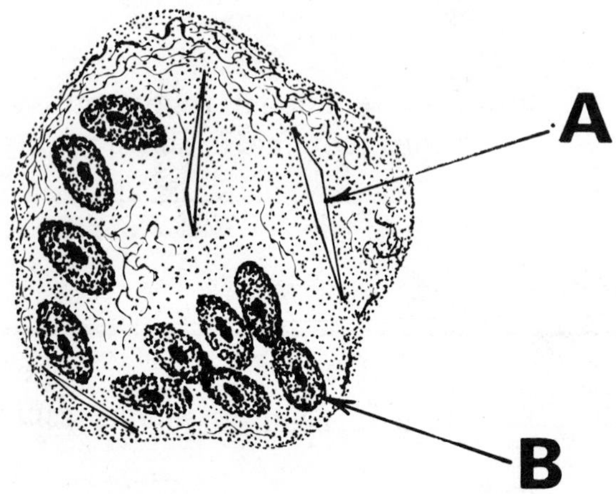

---

77. tissues

---

78. Plasma cells appear late in the course of an inflammatory reaction and are therefore an indication of the ☐ acute ☐ chronic nature of an inflammation.

20. histamine
B
A
☑ yes

---

21. LABEL THE FOLLOWING CELLS:

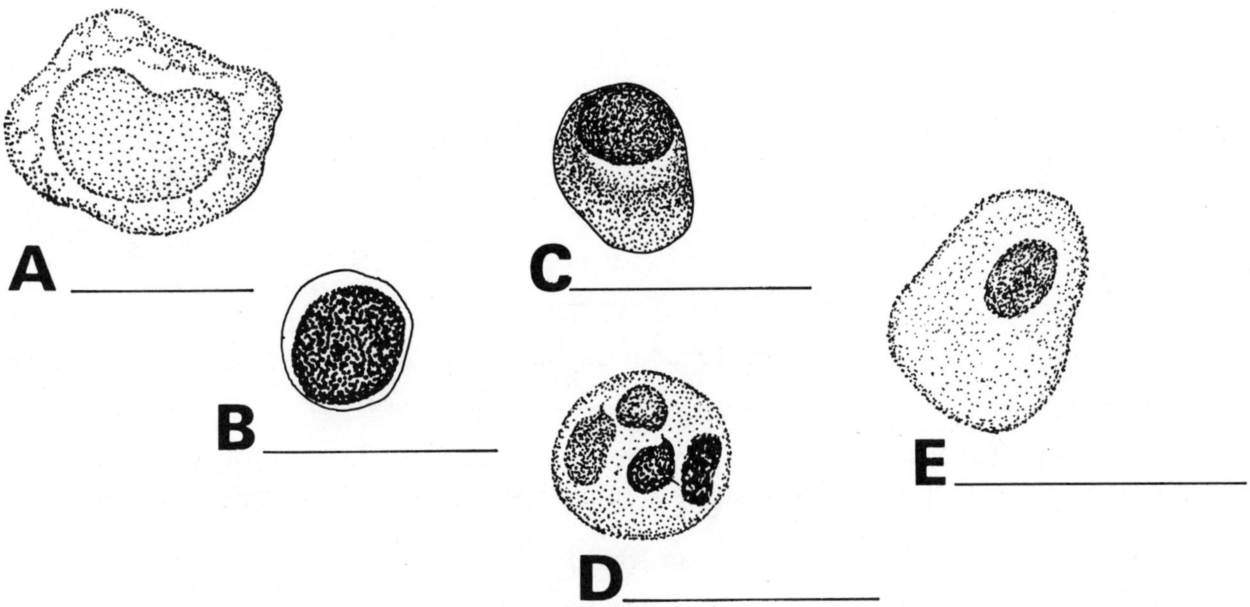

---

68. foreign-body giant cell

---

69. NUMBER THE FOLLOWING IN THE ORDER OF THEIR APPEARANCE AT THE INFLAMMATORY SITE:

___ giant cells

___ fluid of inflammatory exudate

___ polys

___ mononuclear phagocytes

28. tissue
blood

---

29. Under the stimulation of inflammation, monocytes turn into ________ and are indistinguishable microscopically from macrophages derived from tissue.

---

76. [✓] late OR [✓] early
[✓] support [✓] weaken

Either choice is correct. Although we think of eosinophils as arriving late in inflammation, they sometimes make an early appearance.

---

77. Plasma cells are the primary source of antibodies and are normally found in the ________.

21. A. monocyte
B. lymphocyte
C. plasma cell
D. neutrophil
E. mast cell

---

22. Tissue macrophages (also called histiocytes or large mononuclears) are phagocytic and actively migrate toward inflammatory foci. When inactive, they are small (about 12 μ), widely scattered, and inconspicuous. In an inflammatory focus, they proliferate, accumulate, and become more conspicuous because of increased cytoplasm.

MATCH THE FOLLOWING (more than one letter may apply):

____normally found in the tissues	A. Monocytes
____phagocytic	B. Tissue Macrophages
____diameter of 12 μ or more	
____travel toward inflammatory foci	
____normally found in the blood	

---

69. 4
1
2
3

---

70. The importance of polys for protection of the host from microbial invaders is well established. Persons afflicted with agranulocytosis (a clinical condition in which neutrophils are almost completely absent):

a) are unaffected as long as the other leukocytes are present in normal numbers.

b) are extremely susceptible to infections.

27. polymorpho

---

28. Macrophages (histiocytes) and monocytes are similar in structure and function but are normally found in different sites-- macrophages in the __________ and monocytes in the __________.

---

75. b

---

76. The best-supported hypothesis concerning eosinophil function is that they are specialized for the phagocytosis of antigen-antibody complexes. Since in most cases antibodies are not formed until the inflammatory reaction has persisted for some time, the ☐ late ☐ early appearance of eosinophils at the inflammatory site tends to ☐ support ☐ weaken the hypothesis.

22. B
A, B
A, B
A, B
A

23. The nuclei of tissue macrophages are oval or indented, and their cytoplasm often contains debris they have ingested. IDENTIFY THE CELLS BELOW:

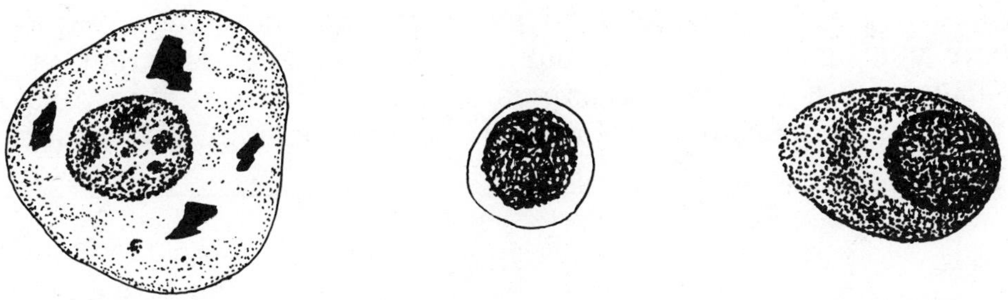

____________ ____________ ____________

70. b

71. Which curve (A or B) would most likely be characteristic of a person with agranulocytosis?

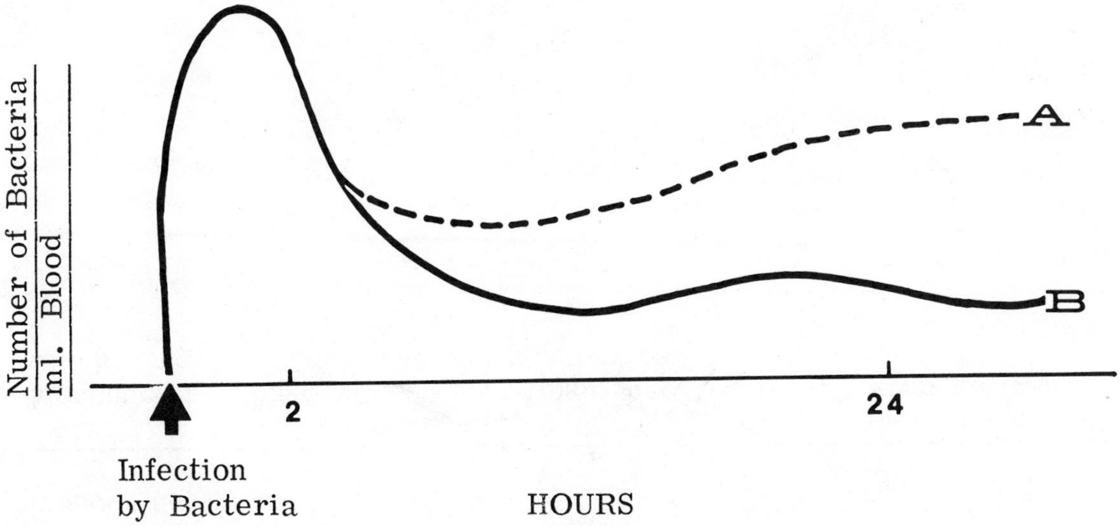

26. macrophages
monocytes

---

27. Mononuclear phagocytes are distinguished from cells such as neutrophils which are __________ nuclear phagocytes.

---

74. A. neutrophil
B. basophil
C. monocyte
D. eosinophil
E. lymphocyte.

---

75. Eosinophils are thought to have phagocytic capabilities, but they do not contribute significantly to the defensive reaction. They move from the blood in increasing numbers when the healing process has already begun. Like polys, they are end cells and probably only live for a few days. Their primary function is not known for certain. The presence of large numbers of eosinophils at an inflammatory site probably indicates which of the following?

a) The reaction is only a few hours old.

b) Resolution has begun.

23. macrophage lymphocyte plasma cell

---

24. MATCH THE FOLLOWING (letters may be used more than once):

___ oval cell slightly larger than a red cell and smaller than a neutrophil	A. plasma cell
___ round nucleus with chromatin distribution resembling the spokes of a wheel	B. neutrophil
___ a narrow rim of cytoplasm surrounding a dark - staining nucleus	C. macrophage
___ a dark - staining, segmented nucleus	D. lymphocyte

---

71. A

---

72. Using the same graph, MATCH THE CURVES WITH THEIR PROBABLE RESULTS:

Result	Curve
___ sepsis and somatic death	A
___ localization of infection	B

25. A
B

26. Inflammation

Tissue Macrophages → Mononuclear Phagocytes
Monocytes → Mononuclear Phagocytes

Under the stimulation of inflammation the number of phagocytic cells at the inflammatory focus is greatly increased. The number of mononuclear phagocytes is increased in several ways:
1) fixed tissue macrophages become active and move to the inflammatory focus;
2) macrophages divide;
3) monocytes leave the blood vessels and become macrophages;
4) there is some evidence that lymphocytes may become macrophages.

Mononuclear phagocytes are derived from tissue __________ and blood __________.

73.

Polys	✓	✓	✓	✓	
Monocytes	✓	✓	✓	✓	✓

74.

IDENTIFY THE CELLS BELOW:

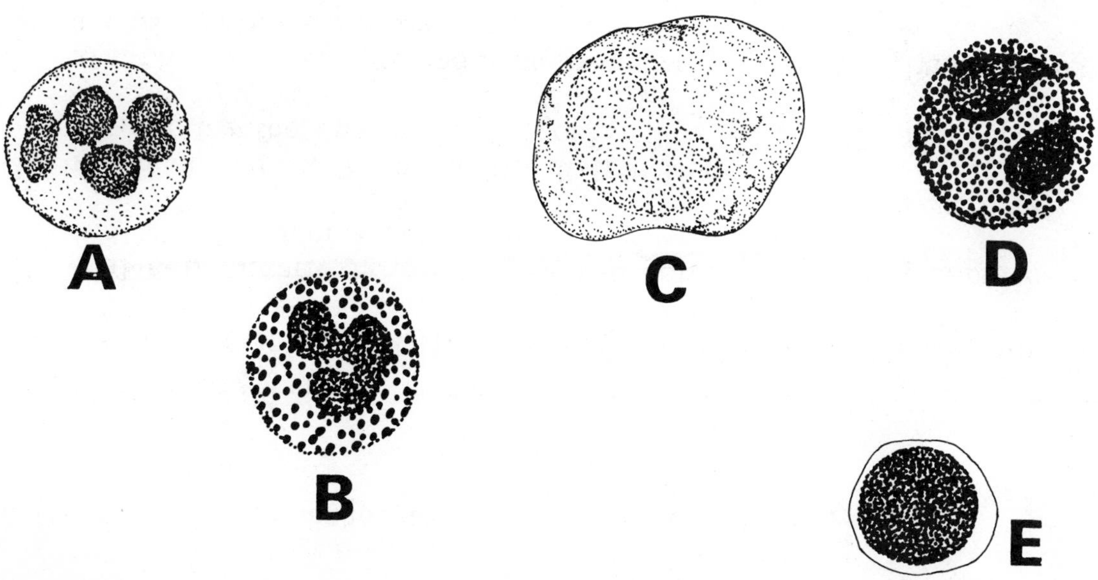

24. A
A
D
B

---

25. MATCH THE CELLS WITH THEIR GENERAL SHAPE:

Cell	Shape
___ plasma cell	A. oval
___ lymphocyte	B. round

TURN TEXT 180° AND CONTINUE.

---

72. A
B

---

73. CHECK THE APPROPRIATE BOXES:

	Normally Found in the Blood	Phagocytic	Ameboid Mobile	Chemotropic	Active in Acidic Media
Polys	☐	☐	☐	☐	☐
Monocytes	☐	☐	☐	☐	☐

TURN TEXT 180° AND CONTINUE.

Unit 4. Factors Which Modify Inflammation

Unit 4. FACTORS WHICH MODIFY INFLAMMATION

OBJECTIVES

When you complete this unit, you will be able to select correct responses relating to the:

	starting page	frame numbers
A. Factors Relating to the Causative Agent	4.3	1-34

1. factors related to the causative agent which influence the nature, extent, site, and duration of inflammation.
2. definition of pathogenicity, invasiveness, toxicity, pyogenic, and pus.

B. Factors Relating to the Host	4.17	35-55

1. factors which determine the physiologic condition of the host.
2. local and systemic host factors which influence inflammation.
3. importance of location to the nature of inflammation.

PRETEST

UNIT 4. FACTORS WHICH MODIFY INFLAMMATION

SELECT THE SINGLE BEST RESPONSE

1. Which of the following does not ordinarily affect the invasiveness of bacteria?
   (A) stimulation of fibrin formation in blood vessels and lymphatics
   (B) production of spreading factors
   (C) production of toxins
   (D) susceptibility of phagocytosis

2. Which of the following is FALSE?
   (A) Viruses are potent pyogenic agents.
   (B) Pathogenic bacteria which enter the blood often cause severe infections.
   (C) Some bacteria can be ingested by phagocytes but not digested.
   (D) The amount, duration of exposure, and pathogenicity of an agent modify the inflammatory response.

3. An agent which the body's defenses cannot overcome will always cause
   (A) serous exudation
   (B) fibrinous exudation
   (C) acute inflammation
   (D) chronic inflammation

4. The term pyogenic refers to the ability of certain substances to cause
   (A) fever
   (B) increased poly production
   (C) both
   (D) neither

5. In the list below, select the pair of injurious agents which differ in pathogenicity.
   (A) ultraviolet light and x-rays
   (B) 10^2 staphylococci and 10^7 staphylococci
   (C) 1 hour of sunlight and 3 hours of sunlight
   (D) an iron at 200° and boiling water

6. Which is LEAST predictable in its influence on inflammation reactions?
   (A) physiologic condition of the host
   (B) location in the body
   (C) toxicity of agent
   (D) invasiveness of agent

7. The general physiologic condition of a host
   (A) does not generally influence the pattern of an inflammatory reaction to a noticeable degree
   (B) is determined by age, nutrition, and presence or absence of disease
   (C) is an important factor only in inflammations due to pyogenic agents
   (D) is important only when it influences the efficiency of the cellular defensive response

8. An injurious agent would cause the most extensive damage in
   (A) muscle tissue
   (B) a joint space
   (C) dense connective tissue
   (D) loose connective tissue

GO ON TO NEXT PAGE AND BEGIN THE UNIT.

A. Factors Relating to the Causative Agent (34 frames)

When you complete this section, you will be able to select correct responses relating to the:

1. factors related to the causative agent which influence the nature, extent, site, and duration of inflammation.

2. definition of pathogenicity, invasiveness, toxicity, pyogenic, and pus.

GO ON TO NEXT PAGE

---

1. Scale Indicates the Nature of the Inflammatory Response

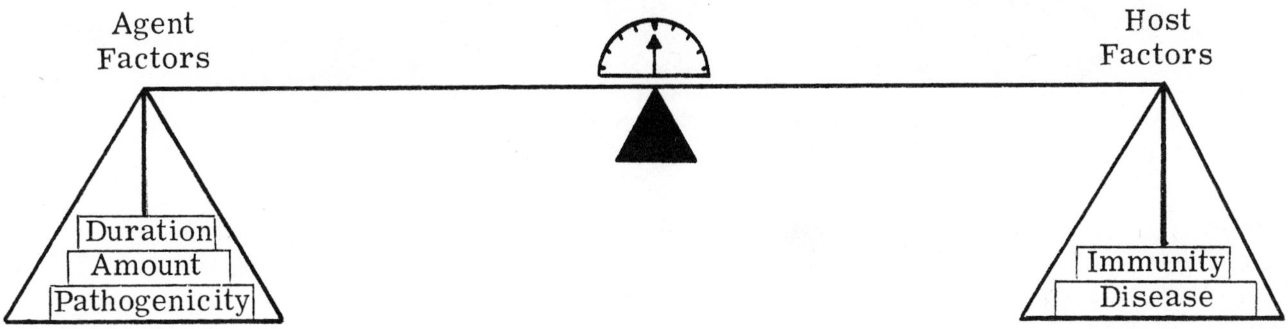

Inflammation is a conflict between injurious agent and host, and the outcome is determined by variables which are related to both. An abdominal knife wound with accompanying bacterial contamination of the peritoneal cavity may result in a short-lived inflammation with rapid repair or a massive infection causing death, depending on factors related to the host and bacteria.

The sequence of cellular and vascular changes in the initial inflammatory reactions are:

☐ always the same.
☐ determined by factors related to the host and injurious agent.

The ultimate nature, duration, and severity of the inflammatory response is:

☐ always the same.
☐ determined by factors related to the host and injurious agent.

28.

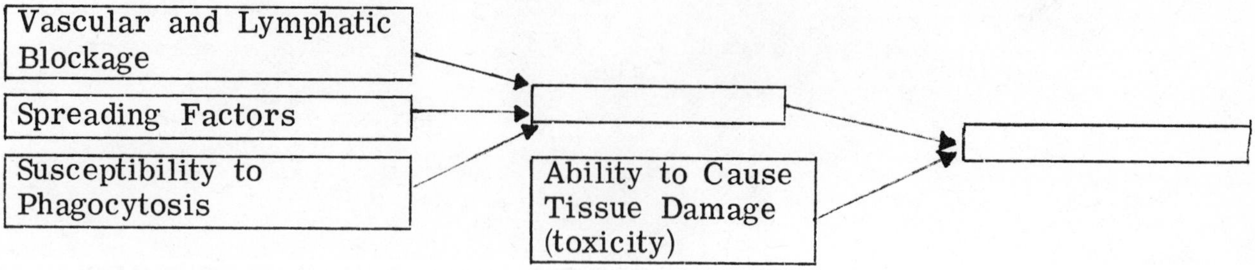

---

29. In reference to bacteria, the ability to cause tissue damage is often called toxicity. Organisms which are very toxic and highly invasive are extremely __________.

TURN TEXT 180° AND CONTINUE.

---

55. T
F
F
F
F

THIS IS THE END OF UNIT 4. TAKE THE POSTTEST ON PAGE xx.

1. [✓] always the same

[✓] determined by factors related to the host and injurious agent.

---

2. Inflammations vary in:
   1) duration: from short-lived acute responses lasting a few hours to long-lasting chronic reactions that persist for months or years;
   2) exudate: serous, fibrinous, and others;
   3) degree of localization: from small focal areas to widespread;
   4) the type of tissue affected: liver, lung, skin, and any others.

An inflammation in which the injurious agent persisted over a period of time would necessarily:

a) be widespread.

b) have a fibrinous exudate.

c) be in solid tissue.

d) become chronic.

---

29. pathogenic

---

30. An invasive organism is not necessarily toxic, and some highly toxic organisms are not invasive. Of course, some are both. Other organisms may be invasive but not pathogenic. INDICATE "T" TRUE OR "F" FALSE:

___ Invasive organisms are all highly toxic.

___ All toxic organisms are highly invasive.

___ Invasive organisms are often, but not always, pathogenic.

___ Toxic organisms are not highly invasive.

27. spreading factors

---

28. FILL IN THE BOXES BELOW:

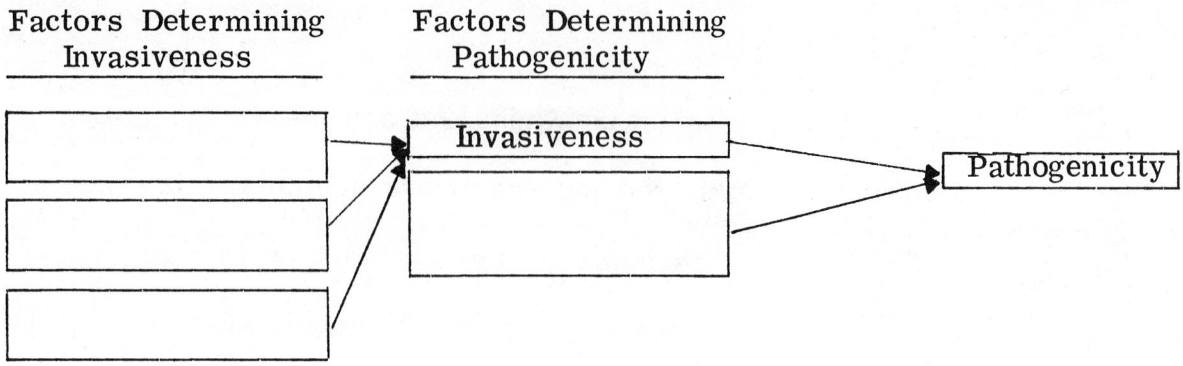

---

54. T
F
T
T
F
F

---

55. INDICATE "T" TRUE OR "F" FALSE: — frame ref.

		frame ref.
___	Age, nutrition, and disease influence the physiologic condition of an individual.	37
___	As an individual ages, his defensive reactions become increasingly efficient.	37
___	A person who has been exposed to prolonged thermal stress (extreme heat or cold) generally is more resistant to infection.	41
___	Poorly vascularized tissues have the most rapid inflammatory reaction.	46
___	Once a microorganism is ingested by a phagocyte, it is always destroyed.	26

2. d)

---

3. An inflammation may be spread widely through the tissue or it may be localized. Inflammation also differs depending on the tissue affected. INFLAMMATIONS VARY IN WHICH OF THE FOLLOWING WAYS?

a) duration (a few hours to months or years)

b) sequence of events in the cellular response

c) type of exudate

d) degree of localization

e) order of events in the vascular response

f) the type of tissue affected

---

30. F
F
T
F

---

31. The organism responsible for tetanus (Clostridium tetani) does not spread far from its site of entry, but it does produce a very powerful poison which causes violent convulsions. Which of the following (is/are) true of Clostridium tetani?

a) highly toxic and highly invasive
b) highly toxic but not invasive
c) not toxic or invasive
d) pathogenic

26. invasive (virulent, pathogenic)

---

27. Bacteria which dissolve clots produce ____________ or lysins.

53.

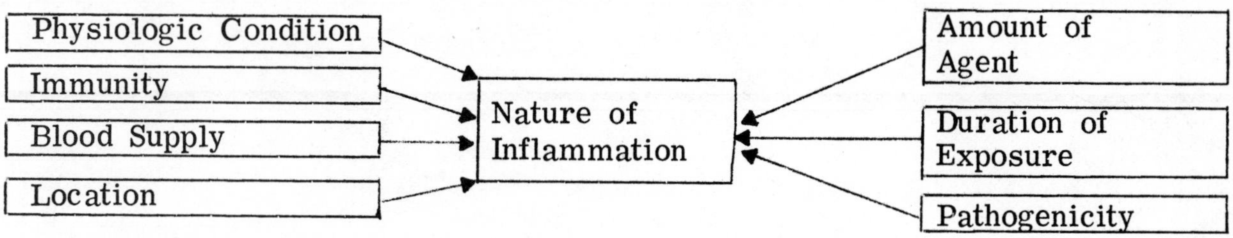

---

54. INDICATE "T" TRUE OR "F" FALSE:

	frame ref.
___ An organ with an impaired blood supply is more susceptible to infection than normal.	46, 47
___ Infections are usually sharply localized in loose tissue.	48
___ Inflammations on body surfaces usually have a shorter duration than those deep in the tissues.	52
___ Pus formation is usually but not always caused by pyogenic bacteria.	15
___ Bacteria which spread widely through the body are universally very toxic.	30
___ Clostridium tetani is very invasive.	31

3. a, c, d, f

4.

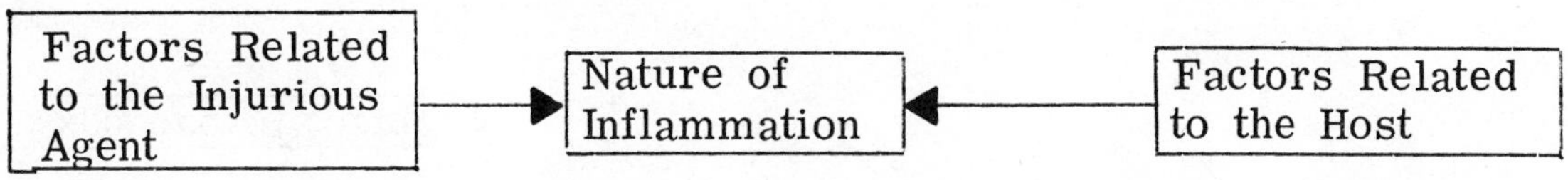

The final outcome of any inflammation hinges on the balance between agent and host factors. In what ways does inflammation vary depending on the agent and the host?

1. ______________________________

2. ______________________________

3. ______________________________

4. ______________________________

---

31. b and d

---

32. FILL IN THE BOXES BELOW:

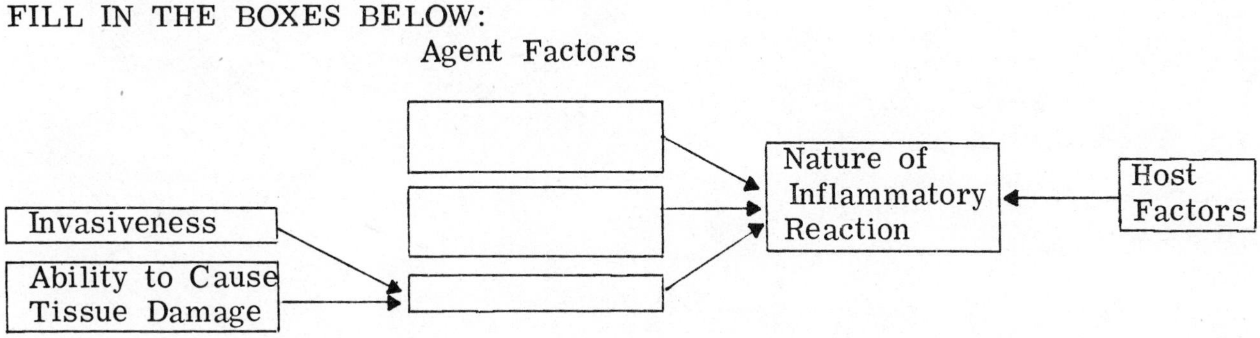

25. [✓] are not

---

26. Some organisms are susceptible to phagocytosis but cannot be digested by the white cell. These bacteria may remain alive and even proliferate within the leukocyte. Organisms which resist intracellular digestion or repel phagocytes are often highly __________.

---

52. b) Exudate and debris are discharged into the lumen of the esophagus, carrying the agent with them, and are removed from the body by the GI tract.

---

53. FILL IN THE BOXES BELOW:

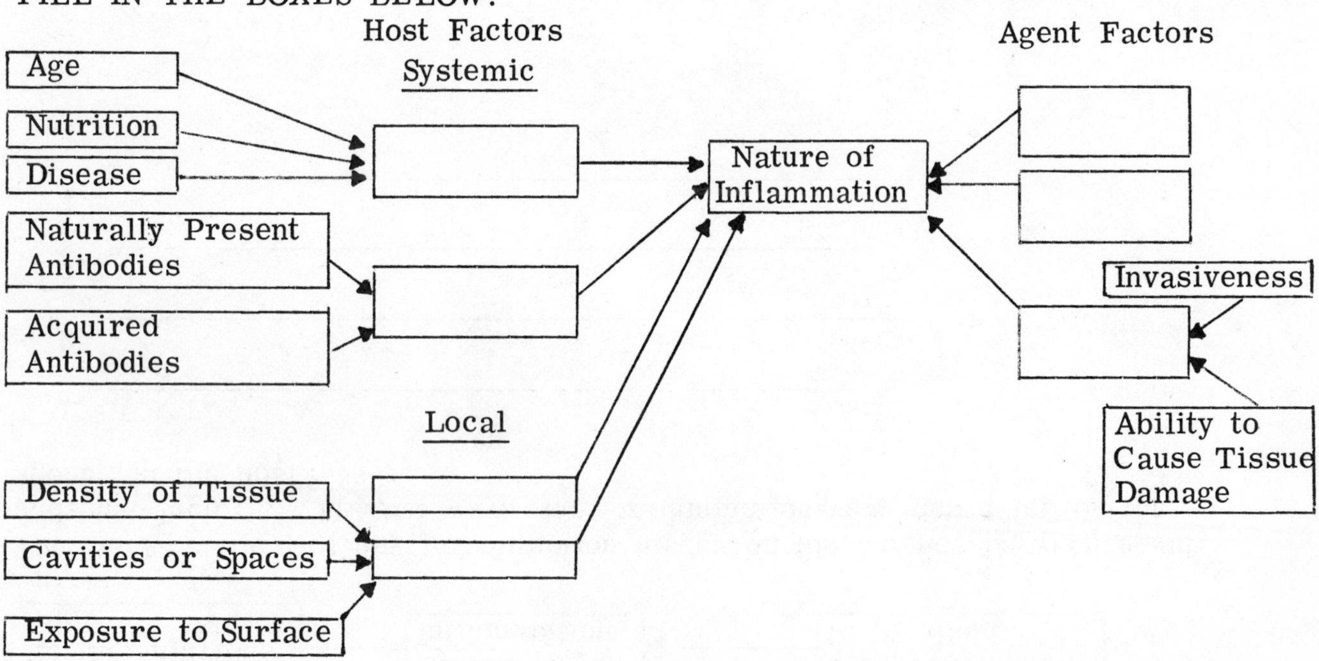

4. 1. duration
2. type of exudate
3. degree of localization
4. type of tissue affected

---

5. Inflammation is caused by:

a) a limited number of specific biological, chemical, and physical agents.

b) all types of biological and physical agents.

c) only chemical agents.

d) a wide variety of biological, chemical, and physical agents.

32.

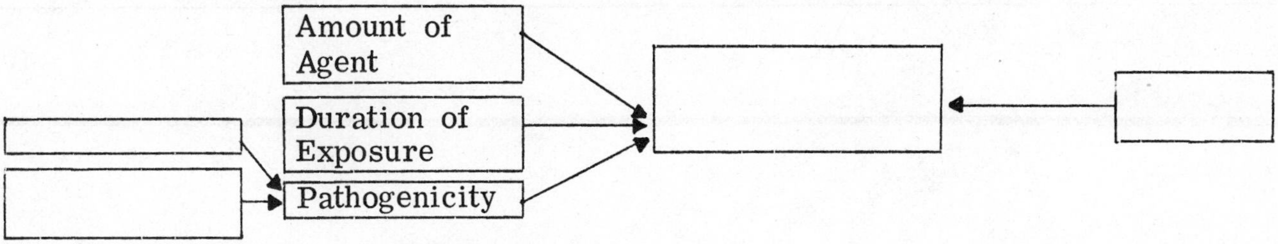

---

33. INDICATE "T" TRUE OR "F" FALSE:

	frame reference
____The sequence of cellular and vascular changes in acute inflammation is always the same.	1
____The amount, duration of exposure, and pathogenicity of an agent influence the nature of the inflammatory response.	6
____The pathogenicity of an agent is determined only by its invasiveness.	9
____Toxicity is the ability of the agent to cause tissue damage.	29
____Pus is composed of dead and living polys and debris.	13

24. A
B

---

25. Microorganisms vary in their ability to attract or repel leukocytes and in their susceptibility to phagocytosis. Organisms which are easily phagocytized and killed by phagocytes ☐ are ☐ are not highly invasive.

---

51. c)

---

52. Inflammations on body surfaces, such as the skin or mucosa of the intestinal tract, tend to discharge exudate and necrotic debris, and therefore remove injurious agents. In deeper inflammations, the injurious agent cannot be removed in this manner, and the inflammatory reaction often persists due to the continuating presence of the agent. Other factors being equal, which inflammation will probably be of the shortest duration?

a) inflamed liver

b) inflamed esophageal mucosa

c) inflammation of pleural cavity

d) inflammation of meninges

WHY?

5. d)

---

6. Factors Relating to the Injurious Agent

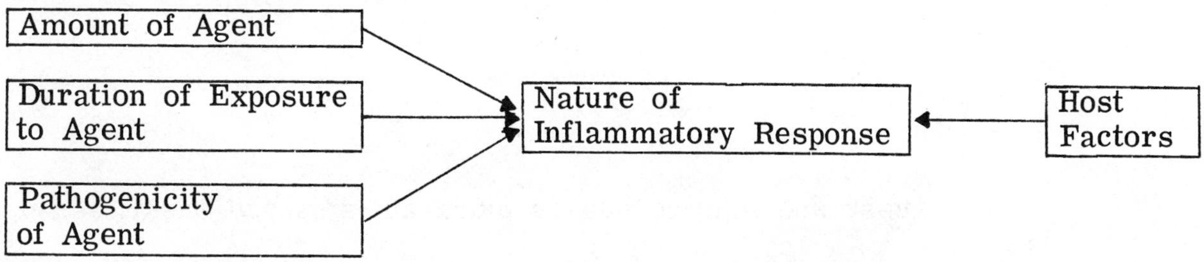

The amount, duration of exposure, and pathogenicity of an agent influence the severity of the resulting inflammation. In the list of injurious agents INDICATE THE PAIRS WHICH DIFFER IN DURATION OF EXPOSURE "D" AND THE PAIRS WHICH DIFFER IN AMOUNT "A":

___ 100 ml. of HCl vs. 500 ml. HCl
___ 1 hour in sunlight vs. 5 hours in sunlight
___ 10^2 staphylococci vs. 10^7 staphylococci
___ holding dry ice for 30 seconds vs. 3 minutes

---

33. T F
T T
T

---

34. MARK THE FOLLOWING "T" TRUE OR "F" FALSE:

	frame reference
____Pus formation is often caused by viruses.	16
____Pathogenic bacteria which enter the lymphatics or blood vessels can cause severe generalized infection.	22
____Bacteria which produce spreading factors are always very toxic.	30
____Organisms which are easily phagocytized are not very invasive.	25
____Some bacteria can be ingested by phagocytes but not digested.	26
____In reference to biological agents, invasiveness means the ability of the agent to enter the host, multiply, and spread through the body.	19

23. c)

---

24. In contrast to organisms which evoke fibrin formation, some bacteria, such as streptococci, produce lysins or spreading factors which dissolve fibrin or the ground substance of the tissue. These organisms cannot be trapped in the tissue by fibrin.

MATCH THE FOLLOWING:

____bacterial production of fibrinolysin	A. spreading factor
____bacterial enhancement of fibrin formation	B. anti-spreading factor

---

50. T
F
T
F

---

51. Injurious agents generally do not cause severe damage in dense tissue because:

a) the defensive reaction is more rapid in dense tissue.

b) inflammation is more extensive in dense tissue.

c) dense tissue prevents the rapid spread of injurious agents.

6. A
D
A
D

---

7. Silica dust is a low grade inflammatory agent and cannot be destroyed or inactivated by any of the body's defenses. Silica is often inhaled in large concentrations by industrial workers and over a period of years causes slow, progressive, insidious inflammation of the lungs. Initially the inflammation may be minor, but the inability of the body to inactivate the silica is an example of severity of inflammation being influenced by the _________ of _________ to the injurious agent.

---

34. F	T
T	T
F	T

B. Factors Relating to the Host (21 frames)

When you complete this section, you will be able to select correct responses relating to the:

1. factors which determine the physiologic condition of the host.
2. local and systemic host factors which influence inflammation.
3. importance of location to the nature of inflammation.

35. The factors which modify an inflammatory reaction can be classified into two groups: those relating to the _________ and those relating to the _________.

22. B.
A.

---

23. In almost any inflammation there is sufficient damage to the vessels in the area to allow bacteria to enter the blood. Therefore, obstruction of vessels by fibrin formation helps prevent the spread of bacteria.

Organisms which stimulate the formation of fibrin walls around the lesions they cause prevent their dissemination but they also protect the bacteria from the body's defenses and drugs. Fibrin formation is:

a) beneficial in an inflammation because it prevents the spread of organisms.

b) detrimental because it protects the organisms from destruction by antibodies, phagocytes, or drugs.

c) both a and b.

d) neither a nor b.

---

49. Because the lung is composed of very loose tissue through which bacteria can spread rapidly.

---

50. Infections in the peritoneal, pericardial, and pleural cavities, and the joint spaces are even more severe than those in loose tissue because the injurious agent is extremely difficult to localize and contain in open areas. INDICATE "T" TRUE OR "F" FALSE:

___ An inflammation in a joint space often spreads rapidly through the entire space.

___ Infections of the peritoneal cavity are rarely severe and are easy to contain.

___ An injurious agent is often difficult to contain in loose subcutaneous tissue.

___ Other factors being equal, an infection usually spreads at the same rate whether it is in muscle or lung.

7. duration (of) exposure

---

8. The pathogenicity of an agent is the ability of the agent to cause disease. Ability to cause disease is determined by fwo factors: 1) the inherent ability of the agent to cause tissue damage; 2) the invasiveness or penetration of the agent. In the list of agents, SELECT THE ONES WHICH DIFFER IN INHERENT ABILITY TO CAUSE INJURY:

a) sunlight vs. x-rays

b) an hour of sunlight vs. three hours

c) hydrochloric acid vs. acetic acid

d) 100 ml. nitric acid vs. 500 ml. nitric acid

e) Staphylococcus aureus vs. Streptococcus viridans

f) 10^1 tubercle bacilli vs. 10^3 tubercle bacilli

---

35. The factors which modify an inflammatory reaction can be classified into two groups: those relating to the host and those relating to the agent.

---

36. Host factors can be classified as systemic or local. In the list below INDICATE THE SYSTEMIC FACTORS "S" AND THE LOCAL FACTORS "L":

___ density of the tissue

___ vascular supply of the tissue

___ state of health

___ immunity

21.

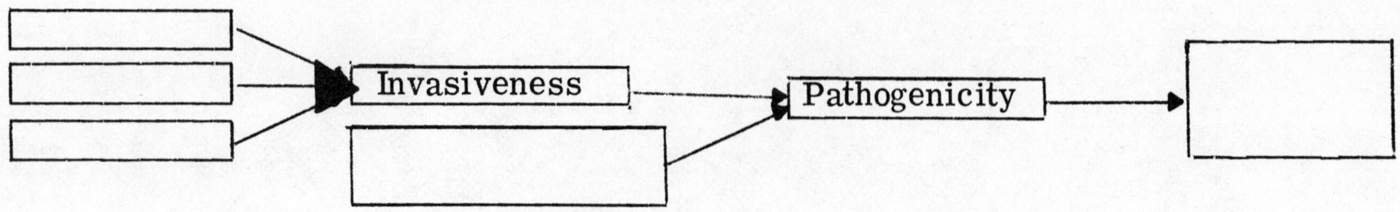

22. One of the most important factors determining whether an infection will remain localized is the ability of the organisms to enter blood vessels and lymphatics and spread through the body. Staphylococcus aureus frequently causes fibrin formation in the lymphatics whereas beta hemolytic streptococci do not. MATCH THE FOLLOWING:

___	remains localized	A.	beta hemolytic streptococci
___	spreads widely	B.	Staphylococcus aureus

48. c) lung

49. Loose tissue generally has open spaces and potential cleavage planes which allow the rapid spread of injurious agents, often resulting in large areas of tissue damage and extensive inflammation. Why do lung infections spread quickly?

8. a, c, e

---

9. 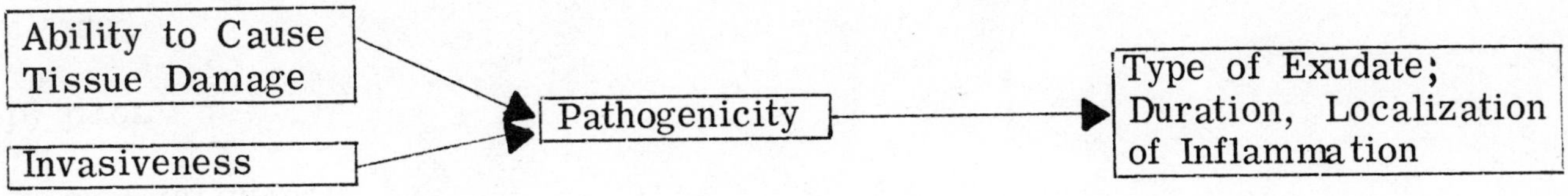

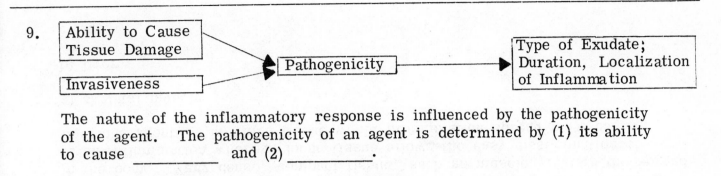

The nature of the inflammatory response is influenced by the pathogenicity of the agent. The pathogenicity of an agent is determined by (1) its ability to cause __________ and (2) __________.

---

36. L L
S S

---

37. 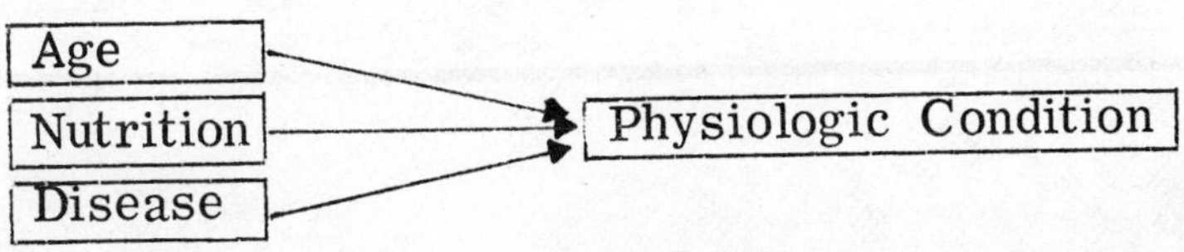

One of the variables influencing the outcome of an inflammation is the health or general physiologic condition of the host. Although the precise relationships are not understood, it is generally accepted that age, nutrition, and the presence or absence of disease influence the physiologic condition of the host and, therefore, the nature of the inflammatory response. Statistically, people who are older do not receive adequate nutrition and/or suffer from a chronic disease, and have more frequent and more severe inflammatory diseases. Which of the following people are most likely to develop a severe inflammatory disease? SELECT ONE RESPONSE FOR EACH OF a, b, and c.

a) ☐ healthy 80-year-old or ☐ healthy 35-year-old

b) ☐ 18-year-old male or ☐ 18-year-old diabetic

c) ☐ healthy 5-year-old or ☐ 5-year-old with protein deficiency

20. b)

---

21. Three factors which affect the invasiveness (ability to spread) of bacteria are 1) ability to produce vascular and lymphatic obstruction; 2) production of spreading factors; and 3) the susceptibility of the organism to phagocytosis. FILL IN THE BOXES BELOW:

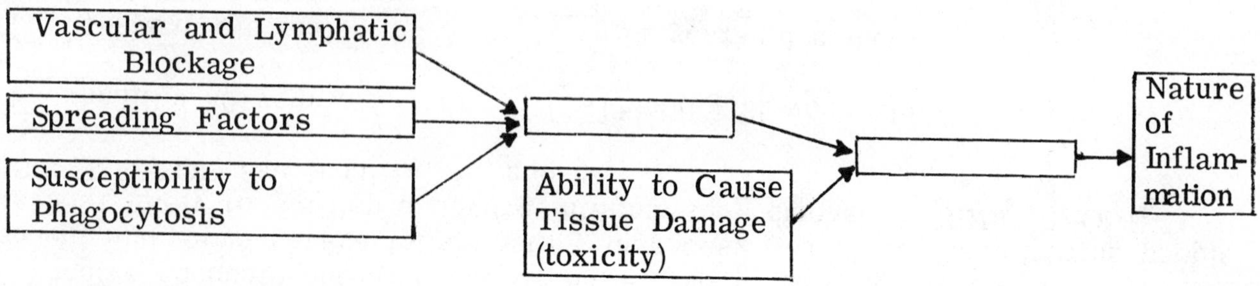

---

47. ✓ more

48.

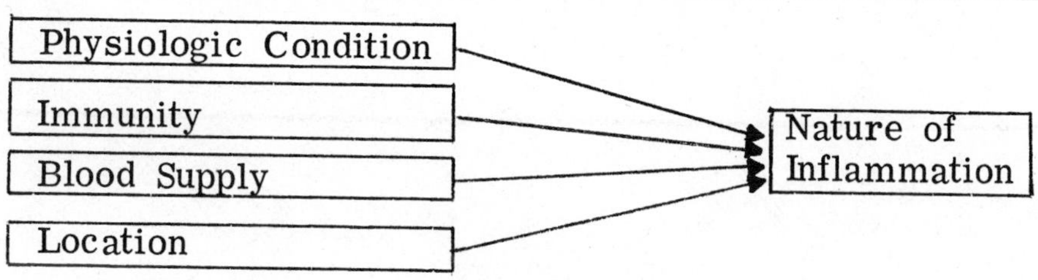

The local host factors influencing the inflammatory reaction are the vascularity of the tissue and the location of the injury.

The pattern of an inflammatory response varies considerably with its location in the body. Very dense, compact tissue, such as muscle, resists the spread of an inflammation, whereas loose tissue allows the easy dissemination of injurious agents. In which tissue would inflammation spread most easily?

a) skeletal muscle

b) liver

c) lung

9. 1) tissue damage
2) invasiveness

---

10. The pathogenicity of an agent is the ability of that agent to cause ________.

---

37. a) [✓] or [ ]
b) [ ] or [✓]
c) [ ] or [✓]

---

38. Which factor(s) might be involved in making older people more susceptible to inflammatory diseases?

___ poor circulation

___ decreased antibody response

___ alterations of tissue structure leading to loss of physiologic tone

19. penetration

---

20. Microorganisms differ from inanimate injurious agents in that they are capable of aggressive action. They can strengthen their forces by proliferating. Some types produce toxins which damage the host; others are capable of assisting their spread by dissolving the ground substance of the tissue. Some can even prevent their own destruction by phagocytes. Inflammation resulting from bacterial infection:

a) is very similar to that caused by chemical and physical agents.

b) is a dynamic battle between host and microorganism, each with its own offensive and defensive mechanisms.

---

46. a)
Vascularity is very poor; therefore, the inflammatory response is less effective.

---

47. If the blood supply to the appendix is obstructed, it is ☐ more ☐ less susceptible to infection than normally.

10. disease (injury)

---

11. Pathogenicity is usually used in reference to biological agents. Some types of bacteria can be present in large numbers without causing any ill effects to the host. By contrast, only a few very virulent bacteria are necessary to cause an infection. When only a few bacteria are necessary to cause a disease, they are highly __________.

---

38. All of them could possibly be part of the aging process.

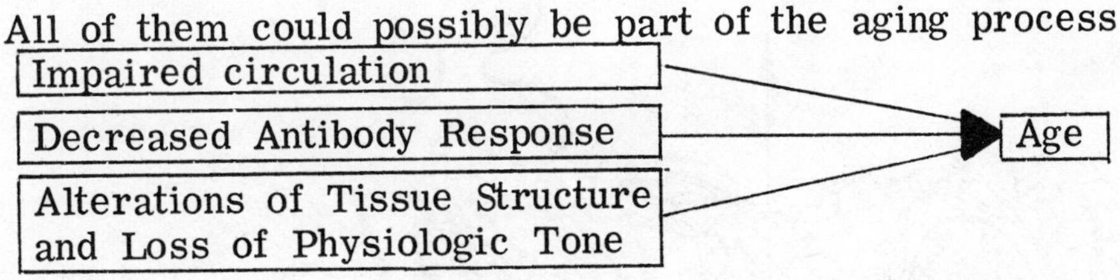

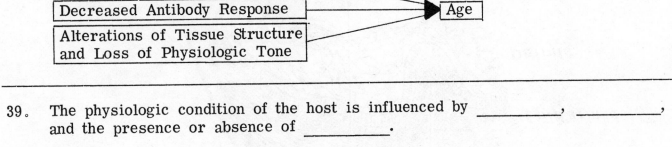

39. The physiologic condition of the host is influenced by __________, __________, and the presence or absence of __________.

18. 1. the inherent ability of the agent to cause tissue damage
    2. the invasiveness or penetration of the agent

---

19. Invasiveness and penetration generally refer to the ability of organisms to enter the host, multiply, and spread. However, they also apply to non-biological agents. Some types of radiation affect only the skin while others produce injury in deeper structures. This is an example of variation in __________.

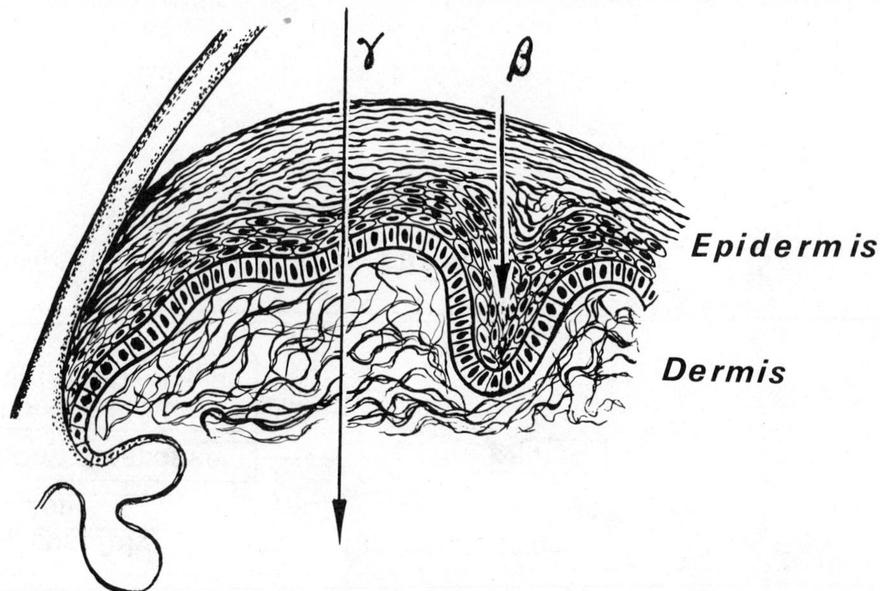

---

45. local

---

46. When injury occurs far from blood vessels, more time is needed for white cells to reach the inflammatory site. Poor circulation also limits the development of an inflammatory reaction sufficient to localize or destroy the injurious agent. Other factors being equal, which is more susceptible to extensive tissue damage?

a) the leg of a 78-year-old woman with arteriosclerosis (narrowing and hardening of the vessels)

b) the leg of a 22-year-old athlete

WHY?

11. pathogenic (or virulent)

---

12. Many agents have specific inherent pathogenic properties that produce distinctive reactions. Pyogenic (from the Greek roots pyo- meaning "pus" and gen- meaning "to produce") bacteria cause the formation of _______________.

---

39. The physiologic condition of the host is influenced by age, nutrition, and the presence or absence of disease.

---

40. INDICATE WHICH DIETARY FACTOR(S) MIGHT BE INVOLVED IN MAKING A PERSON MORE SUSCEPTIBLE TO INFLAMMATORY DISEASE:

___ vitamin C deficiency

___ protein deficiency

___ vitamin B complex deficiency

17. a)

18. INDICATE WHICH TWO FACTORS DETERMINE THE PATHOGENICITY OF AN AGENT.

1.

2.

44. opsonin (review from Unit 3)

45.

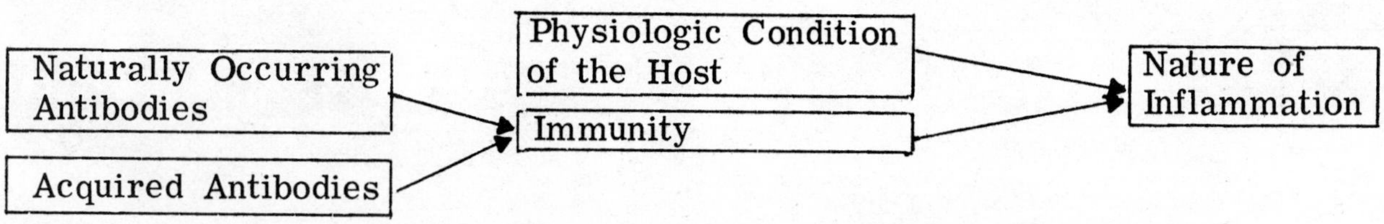

Two systemic host factors which influence the inflammatory reaction are:
1) Physiologic condition, and
2) Immunity.

Immunity and physiologic condition are systemic host factors; the vascularity of the injured tissue is a __________ factor.

12. pus

---

13. Some bacteria produce toxic substances which kill cells and leukocytes. The dead leukocytes release digestive enzymes which breakdown necrotic tissue and debris. The yellow or greenish fluid produced by this process is pus. Pus is a viscous liquid composed of (1) large numbers of dead and living polys, and (2) necrotic tissue and debris partially liquified by the enzymes released from dead polys. What type of bacteria cause the formation of pus?

---

40. All of them.

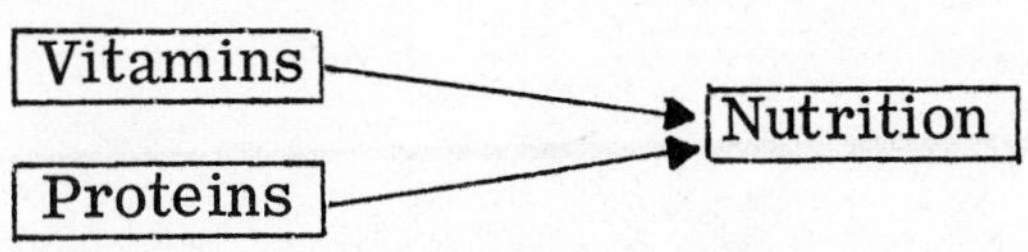

---

41. Metabolic diseases (e.g. diabetes mellitus) and previous exposure to physical agents, such as extreme heat or cold, or chemical agents like alcohol, generally decrease resistance to injury. INDICATE "T" TRUE OR "F" FALSE:

___ A severe infection usually decreases host resistance to a second infection.

___ A severe infection usually strengthens host defenses for a second infection.

___ Bacterial infections in diabetics generally evoke the same degree of response as in non-diabetics.

___ Extensive burns can weaken host resistance to infection.

16. A
B
A
B

---

17. The patterns of inflammatory reactions:

a) are often similar but may give a clue as to the class of specific agent responsible.

b) are usually quite distinctive, often enabling the physician to determine the specific causative agent.

---

43. ☐ less severe

---

44. An antibody which coats bacteria, making them more susceptible to phagocytosis, is a(n) ________.

13. Pyogenic Bacteria

---

14. Which of the following can be a component of pus?

a) live polys
b) dead polys
c) cholesterol
d) fats
e) proteins
f) deoxyribonucleoprotein

---

41. T
F
F
T

---

42. FILL IN THE BOXES BELOW:

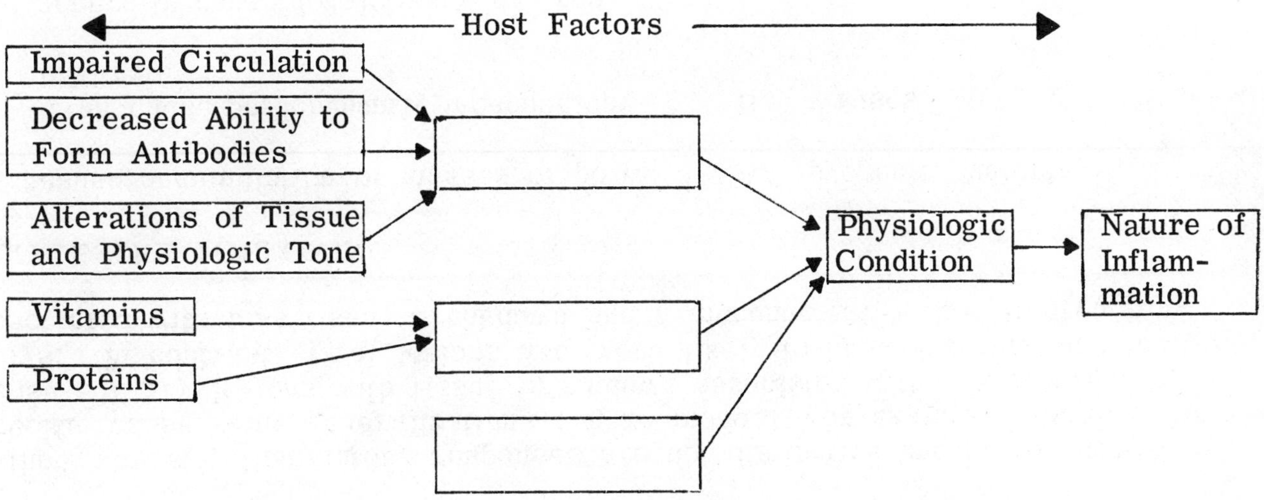

15. pyogenic bacteria

---

16. Although most inflammatory responses are not distinctive enough to suggest a specific cause, some generalizations can be made. For example, bacteria often cause solitary lesions, with tissue breakdown associated with the presence of polys. In contrast, viral lesions are more likely to be widespread and multiple, associated with less tissue breakdown and a mononuclear leukocytic reaction.

MATCH THE FOLLOWING:

___ cause accumulation of masses of polys	A. pyogenic bacteria
___ often cause predominantly mononuclear infiltrate	B. viruses
___ generally cause focal tissue damage	
___ rarely cause pus formation	

---

43. Most individuals have naturally occurring humoral substances which act against inflammatory agents, especially microorganisms. In addition, previous exposure to specific microorganisms can cause the formation of powerful antibodies which attack the organism which led to their formation.

Invasion | Microorganisms Attacked by Naturally Occurring Antibodies | Formation of Specific Antibodies

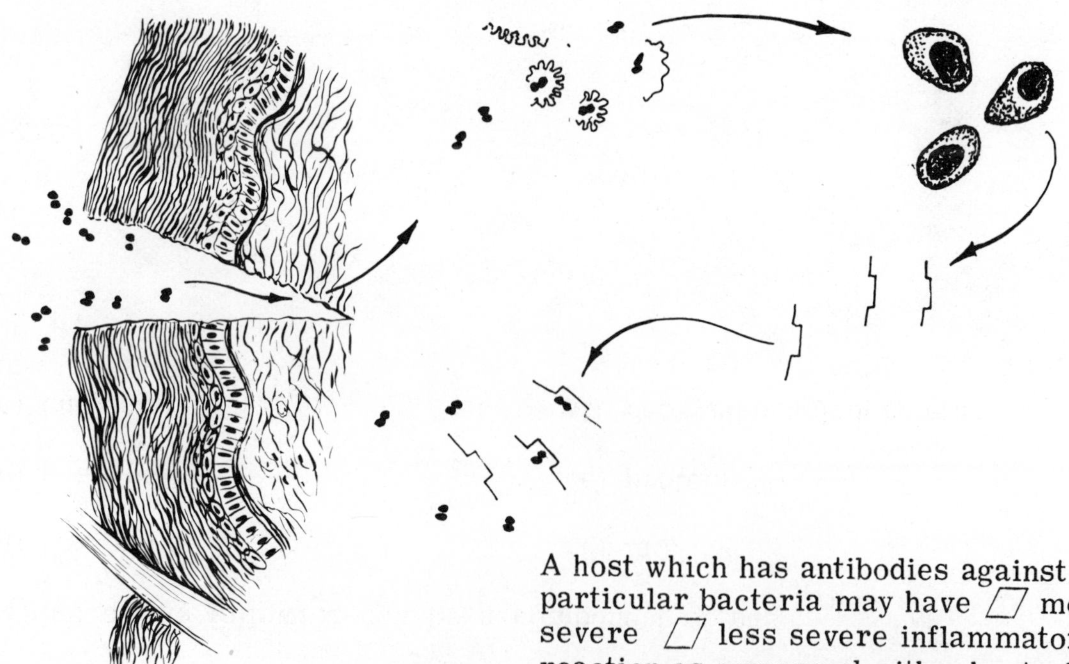

A host which has antibodies against a particular bacteria may have ☐ more severe ☐ less severe inflammatory reaction as compared with a host which does not have those antibodies.

14. All of them.

15.

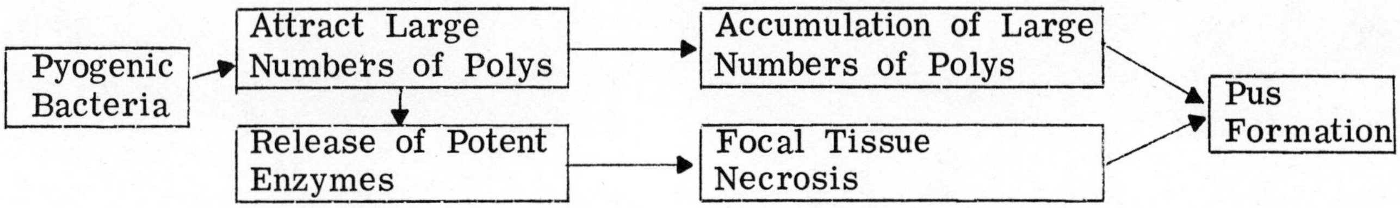

Pus formation can be caused by a few chemical agents, such as turpentine, but the appearance of pus in an inflammation usually indicates that the reaction is caused by ____________ ____________.

TURN TEXT 180° AND CONTINUE.

42.

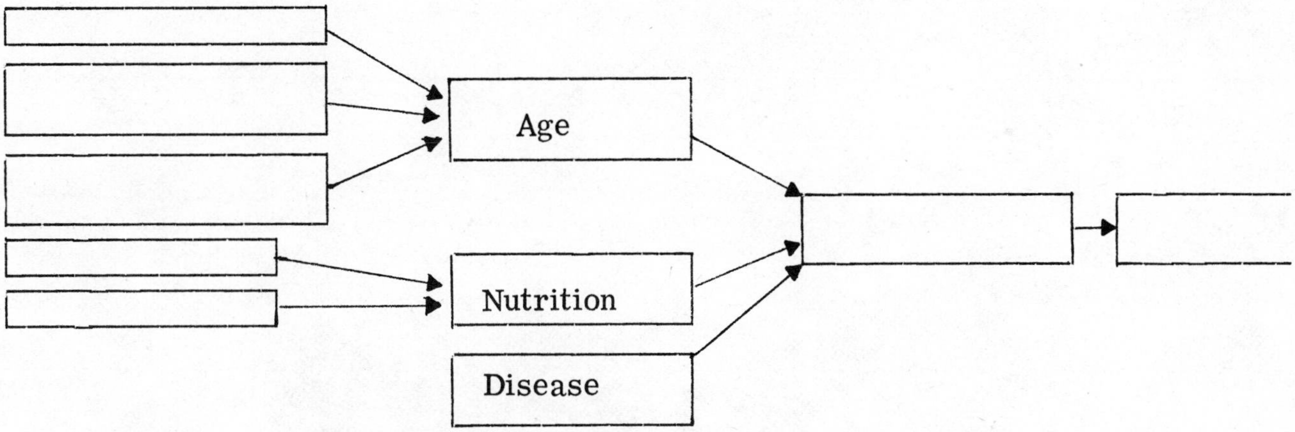

TURN TEXT 180° AND CONTINUE.

Unit 5. Classification and Complications of Inflammation

Unit 5. CLASSIFICATION AND COMPLICATIONS OF INFLAMMATION

OBJECTIVES

When you complete this unit, you will be able to select correct responses relating to the:

	starting page	frame numbers
A. Variation in Duration and Complications of Inflammation	5.3	1-56

1. classification of inflammations as acute, subacute, and chronic on the basis of (a) duration, and (b) predominant cell types.
2. agent and host factors responsible for chronic inflammation.
3. complications of chronic inflammation.
4. definition of granuloma, epitheliod cell, and granulation tissue.
5. mechanism of granuloma formation and the type of agents responsible.

B. Variation in Exudate	5.20	57-89

1. composition and examples of serous, fibrinous, purulent, catarrhal, hemorrhagic, and mixed exudates.
2. definition and mechanism of serous, fibrinous, purulent, catarrhal, and hemorrhagic exudates and pseudomembranous inflammation.

C. Variation in Degree of Localization and Location	5.57	90-126

1. definition of abscess, empyema, furuncle, carbuncle, phlegmon, cellulitis, ulcer, and erosion.
2. mechanism of formation and location of abscesses, empyemas, furuncles, carbuncles, phlegmons, cellulitis, ulcers, and erosions.
3. ways of naming inflammations.

PRETEST

UNIT 5. CLASSIFICATION AND COMPLICATIONS OF INFLAMMATION

SELECT THE SINGLE BEST RESPONSE.

1. Which is/are generally associated with an inflammation becoming chronic?
   (A) increasing prominence of the cardinal signs
   (B) fibroblastic proliferation
   (C) both
   (D) neither

2. Acute inflammations are by definition always of
   (A) short duration
   (B) severe intensity
   (C) both
   (D) neither

3. Epitheliod cells are
   (A) transformed epithelial cells
   (B) the primary cell of epithelial tumors
   (C) transformed macrophages
   (D) outer layer cells of an eosinophilic granuloma

4. Which of the following most closely resembles blood plasma?
   (A) serous exudate
   (B) sanguinous exudate
   (C) fibrinous exudate
   (D) catarrhal exudate

5. Which type of exudate is associated with leakage of the smallest particles from vessels?
   (A) catarrhal
   (B) serous
   (C) fibrinous
   (D) purulent

6. A pseudomembranous inflammation is characterized by a
   (A) defect in an epithelial lined surface
   (B) diffuse mixture of dead mucosal cells, bacteria, and inflammatory exudate on a mucosal surface
   (C) spherical defect containing dead tissue and leukocytes
   (D) ramifying defect containing dead tissue and leukocytes

7. Carbuncles
   (A) usually develop in internal organs
   (B) involve hemorrhagic exudation
   (C) have multiple points of discharge
   (D) generally develop into granulomatous inflammations

8. In which of the following areas could pseudomembranous inflammation take place?
   (A) pleural cavity
   (B) intestinal tract
   (C) skin
   (D) meninges

GO ON TO NEXT PAGE AND BEGIN THE UNIT.

A. Variation in Duration and Complications of Inflammation (56 frames)

When you complete this section, you will be able to select correct responses relating to the:

1. classification of inflammations as acute, subacute, and chronic on the basis of (a) duration, and (b) predominant cell types.
2. agent and host factors responsible for chronic inflammation.
3. complications of chronic inflammation.
4. definition of granuloma, epithelioid cell, and granulation tissue.
5. mechanism of granuloma formation and the type of agents responsible.

1. Inflammations vary in which of the following ways?

a) location

b) degree of localization

c) sequence of events in the initial cellular response

d) duration

e) sequence of events in the initial vascular response

f) type of exudate

---

126. F
T
T
T
T
F

THIS IS THE END OF UNIT 5. TAKE THE POSTTEST ON PAGE xxii.

1. a) location
   b) degree of localization
   d) duration
   f) type of exudate

---

2. Inflammations are classified as acute, subacute, and chronic on the basis of duration. There are no clear distinctions between these divisions, so classification on the basis of duration is arbitrary. MATCH THE FOLLOWING:

Duration of Inflammation	Classification
___ months to years	A. acute
___ weeks to a month	B. subacute
___ days or hours to weeks	C. chronic

---

63. fibrinous

---

64. Serous and fibrinous exudates contain very few inflammatory cells and are distinguished by the composition of their fluid. CHECK THE CORRECT BOXES:

	Present in Mild Inflammations	High Specific Gravity >1.020	Can Occur in Any Tissue	Responsible for Formation of Fibrin Masses	Closely Resembles Blood Serum	Closely Resembles Blood Plasma
Serous Exudate						
Fibrinous Exudate						

TURN TEXT 180° AND CONTINUE.

---

125. T
F
T
T
F
T

---

126. INDICATE "T" TRUE OR "F" FALSE:

		frame ref.
___	Carbuncles have a single point of discharge while furuncles have several.	104
___	Carbuncles are more deeply located than furuncles.	104
___	Phlegmon and cellulitis are widespread inflammations without definite limits.	109
___	Ulceration always involves the loss of tissue.	112
___	Exudation may be present in chronic ulcers.	117
___	The suffix -itis indicates inflammation due to microorganisms.	123

2. C
B
A

3. Acute, subacute, and chronic refer not only to duration but to the morphologic character of the reaction. SELECT THE CORRECT ANSWER:

a) Acute reactions are indistinguishable from chronic reactions and are differentiated only by duration.

b) Acute, subacute, and chronic reactions differ in character as well as in duration.

64.

	Present in Mild Inflammations	High Specific Gravity 1.020	Can Occur in Any Tissue	Responsible for Formation of Fibrin Masses	Closely Resembles Blood Serum	Closely Resembles Blood Plasma
Serous Exudate	X	X	X		X	
Fibrinous Exudate		X	X	X		X

65. Which of the following is/are correct concerning serous and fibrinous exudates?

a) They contain high concentrations of polys.

b) They contain large numbers of red blood cells.

c) They are mostly high-protein fluid with a few inflammatory cells.

d) They are watery, low-protein fluids with large numbers of inflammatory cells.

62. serous exudate

---

63. Many inflammations begin with serous exudation, and as the reaction becomes more severe, capillary permeability increases further and the large plasma protein fibrinogen escapes. When this occurs, a serous exudate becomes a __________ exudate.

---

124. -itis
chronic suppurative (or purulent) myositis
abscess
empyema

---

125. INDICATE "T" TRUE OR "F" FALSE:

		frame ref.
___	Abscesses can be caused by some chemical agents (e.g.,turpentine).	review
___	Abscesses are very poorly localized inflammations.	91
___	Abscesses may become nodules of fibrous tissue.	95,97
___	The pus must be removed from an abscess before it can heal.	98,99
___	Empyema is an accumulation of pus within the tissues or within a body cavity.	102
___	Both carbuncles and furuncles frequently begin as folliculitis.	104

3. b) Acute, subacute and chronic reactions differ in character as well as in duration.

---

4. Which reaction is more likely to have a preponderance of polys?

a) acute

b) subacute

c) chronic

---

65. c)

---

66. During rheumatic fever the pericardial cavity may become filled with large masses of fibrin, which may cause the epicardium to rub against the pericardium, producing a sound called "friction rub." If the epicardium is stripped away from the pericardium, the fibrin covers both surfaces, resembling two slices of buttered bread which have been pulled apart (bread-and-butter pericarditis). If in a case of suspected rheumatic fever you hear a friction rub, it is probably due to the presence of a __________ exudate.

A ☐ fibrous ☐ fibrinous exudate contains a large amount of fibrin; whereas, ☐ fibrous ☐ fibrinous tissue contains a large amount of collagen.

61. c)

62.

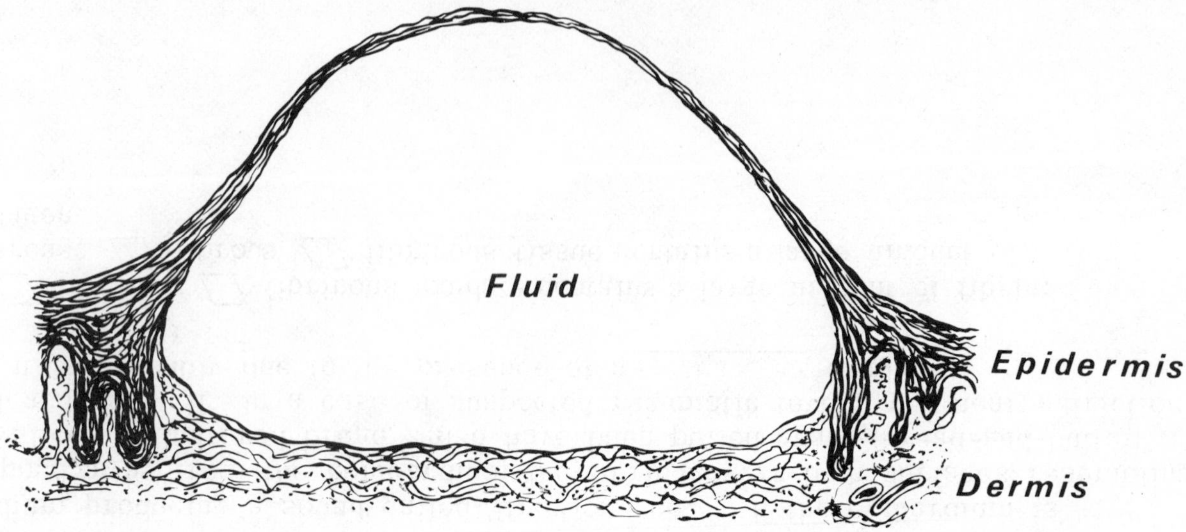

The fluid which fills blisters like the one above is called _______ _______.

---

123. cholecystitis - <u>inflammation of the gallbladder</u>
hepatitis - <u>inflammation of the liver</u>
myositis - <u>inflammation of the muscles</u>
enteritis - <u>inflammation of the intestines</u>
pneumonia - <u>inflammation of the lungs</u>
carditis - <u>inflammation of the heart</u>

---

124. In describing a specific inflammation, the duration and location are usually mentioned and occasionally the type of exudate.

The suffix for inflammation is -______.

A purulent inflammation of skeletal muscle which lasted for three months would be called __________ __________ myos__________.
(duration) (type of exudate) (location) (inflammation)

The terms for the localization are usually specific enough that no further specification is needed except for location.

A focal accumulation of pus within the liver is called a liver __________.

A suppurative inflammation of the pleural cavities is called pleural __________.

4. a)

---

5. It is important to recognize that subacute and chronic inflammations do not always begin as acute reactions. Many subacute and chronic inflammations are caused by relatively mild injurious agents and never have an acute stage. MARK THE FOLLOWING "T" TRUE OR "F" FALSE:

___ All inflammations begin as acute reactions.

___ All inflammations pass through acute, subacute, and chronic stages before they subside.

___ Some inflammations begin and end as acute reactions.

___ Chronic reactions may persist for years.

---

66. fibrinous
[✓] fibrinous
[✓] fibrous

---

67. Suppuration is the formation of pus. It may occur within the tissues, on a body surface, or within a body cavity. Suppuration may occur in which of the following locations?

a) within the spinal cord

b) in the epidural space

c) in the pericardial cavity

d) within the gallbladder

60. c) and d)

---

61. Serous exudates contain very few inflammatory cells and, in general, closely resemble plasma except for a low concentration of which of the following?

a) albumin

b) lipoprotein

c) fibrinogen

d) globulin

---

122. 1. cellulitis
2. ulcer
3. phlegmon
4. erosion

---

123. In addition to duration, type of exudate, and localization, inflammation is also classified by the specific tissue involved. The suffix -itis denotes inflammation of the tissue indicated by the word stem to which it is added. Unfortunately, this rule is not strictly adhered to. For example, pneumonia means inflammation of the lungs. WRITE OUT THE MEANING OF THE WORDS BELOW:

cholecystitis ______________________________

hepatitis (hepat-, liver) ______________________________

myositis (myo-, muscle) ______________________________

enteritis (enter-, intestine) ______________________________

pneumonia ______________________________

carditis (card-, heart) ______________________________

5. F
F
T
T

---

6. Acute generally refers to the duration of a reaction, but it is also used to indicate the severity of a response. A painful inflamed appendix is often called a very __________ appendicitis.

---

67. a, b, c, d (all locations)

---

68. Suppurative (purulent) exudation is the production of large amounts of pus (purulent exudate), which is a thick fluid composed of large numbers of dead and living polys and tissue debris. The primary components of a purulent exudate are produced when degenerating polys release enzymes which digest the dead cells, necrotic tissue, and other debris. Certain chemicals, such as turpentine and silver nitrate, can cause purulent exudation, but the most common cause is a group of bacteria called __________ bacteria.

59. serous
Blood serum contains (among other things) [✓] albumin
Blood plasma contains (among other things) [✓] albumin [✓] fibrinogen

---

60. Serous exudate forms from the blood serum or from the secretions of serosal cells lining serous cavities. A serous exudate may occur: (More than one answer may be correct.)

a) only in serous cavities, as in the pleural cavities during a lung infection.

b) only in response to a few specific agents.

c) in response to almost any agent.

d) anywhere in the body.

---

121. 1. abscess
2. carbuncle
3. empyema
4. furuncle

---

122. NAME THE FOLLOWING TYPES OF INFLAMMATION:

1. A widely spread irregular inflammation without a definite limit which occurs most frequently in loose tissue. __________

2. A cavity in the surface of an organ or tissue surrounded by inflammation and caused by the loss of necrotic tissue. __________

3. A diffuse inflammation without distinct limit which takes the form of layers and occurs in relatively dense tissue. __________

4. Destruction of the epithelial layer of a membrane. __________

6. acute

---

7. Acute reactions are always of short duration but are often not severe. In reference to inflammation, acute always indicates the __________ of the reaction and sometimes indicates the __________.

---

68. pyogenic

---

69. Suppurative inflammation differs from other types of inflammation:

a) because polys migrate to the inflammatory focus in a suppurative inflammation but not in the others

b) because of the formation of relatively large quantities of pus in suppurative inflammation in comparison to the others

c) both a and b

d) neither a nor b

58. c)

---

59. Inflammations can be classified on the basis of their exudates, which vary in the types of cells and fluid they contain. Composition of exudates is determined by the duration of the reaction, the agent, the severity of the damage, and the tissue affected.

Because of its resemblance to blood serum, the watery fluid which appears in mild inflammatory reactions and in the early stages of most others is called ________ exudate.

Blood serum is the watery part of blood left after clotting. Clotting is caused by conversion of the soluble protein, fibrinogen, to insoluble protein, fibrin. Before the fibrin has been precipitated and removed, the watery part of blood is called plasma.
Blood serum contains ☐ red blood cells ☐ albumin ☐ fibrinogen ☐ fibrin
Blood plasma contains ☐ red blood cells ☐ albumin ☐ fibrinogen ☐ fibrin

---

120. G B
F D
A C
E

---

121. NAME THE FOLLOWING TYPES OF INFLAMMATION:

1. A localized accumulation of pus within the tissue or in a natural space. ________
2. A deeply located, multicentric, suppurative inflammation of the skin, usually located on the posterior part of the neck and back. ________
3. The accumulation of pus within a body cavity (given a special name). ________
4. A localized suppurative inflammation of the skin with a single point of discharge. ________

7. duration
severity

---

8. Most inflammations run a short definite course; they are ________.
Some reactions go on for months or years; they are called ________.

---

69. b)

---

70. Pus contains which of the following?

a) viable polys

b) dead polys

c) tissue breakdown products such as cholesterol, fats

d) proteins, DNA and RNA

57. 1. duration
2. type of exudate
3. location
4. degree of localization

---

58. Exudates are:

a) usually most prominent in chronic inflammation.

b) present only in subacute and chronic inflammation.

c) most characteristic of acute inflammations.

d) present only in acute inflammation.

---

119. 5 regeneration of epithelium
3 sloughing of necrotic tissue to form a cavity
2 exudation and infiltration by polys
1 focal necrosis of tissue
4 proliferation of connective tissue

---

120. MATCH THE FOLLOWING:

____Phlegmon
____Cellulitis
____Empyema
____Erosion

____Furuncle
____Carbuncle
____Ulcer

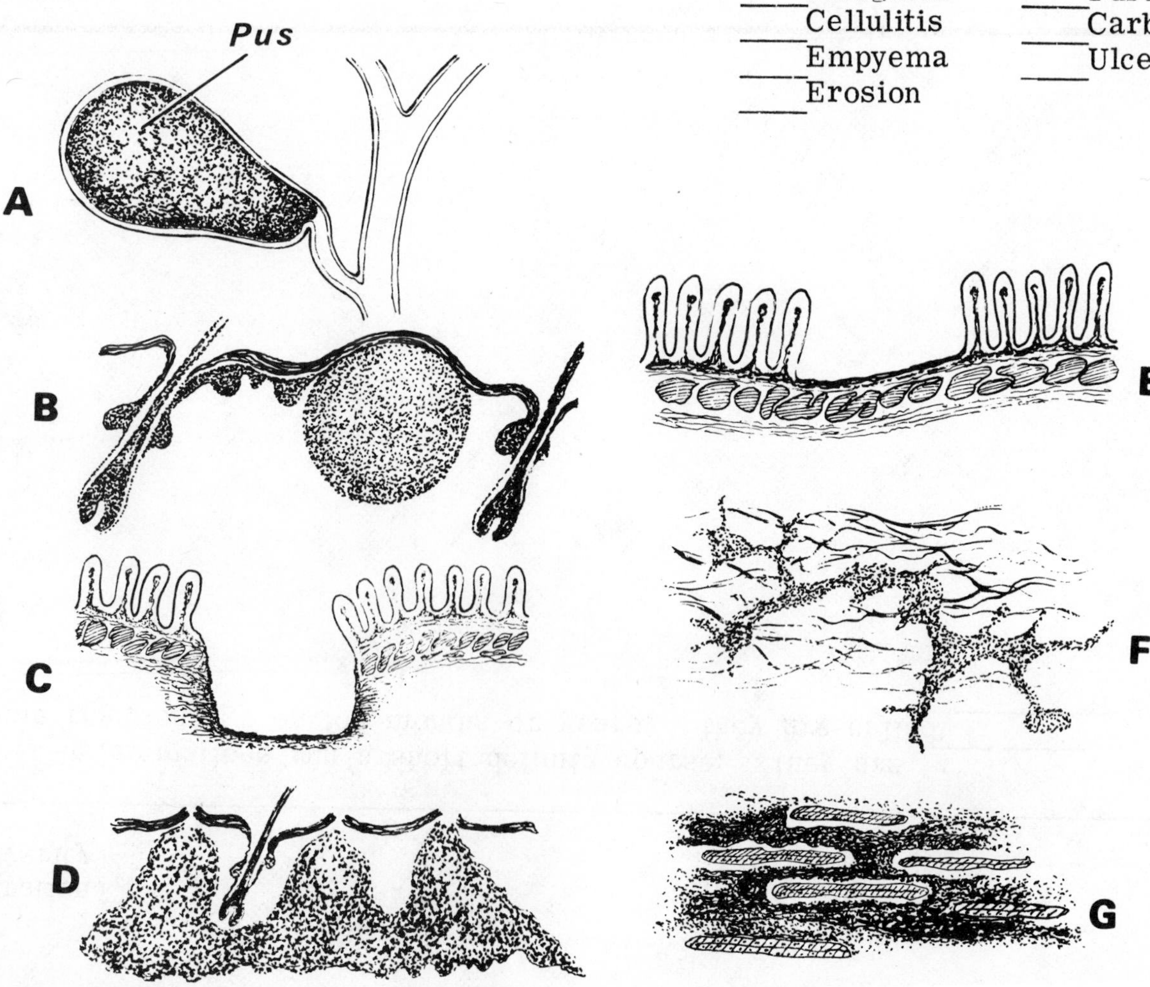

8. acute
chronic

---

9. Inflammation continues only as long as an inflammatory agent is present. Chronic inflammation occurs when:

a) the injurious agent or debris remains in the tissue.

b) an acute inflammation is unusually severe.

---

70. a, b, c, d

---

71. Which of the following would be required for the formation of a purulent exudate ?

a) accumulation of macrophages

b) accumulation of polys

c) fibrinous exudation

56. F
T
F
F
F
F

B. Variation in Exudate (33 frames)

When you complete this section, you will be able to select correct responses relating to the:

1. composition and examples of serous, fibrinous, purulent, catarrhal, hemorrhagic, and mixed exudates.
2. definition and mechanism of serous, fibrinous, purulent, catarrhal, and hemorrhagic exudates and pseudomembranous inflammation.

57. Inflammations vary in four basic ways:

1. ____________________
2. ____________________
3. ____________________
4. ____________________

---

118. a, b, c

---

119. Generally, ulcers heal by filling the crater with connective tissue, followed by regeneration of epithelium over the scar tissue. Like any inflammation, ulceration is not a rigid sequence of discrete occurrences but a series of overlapping events which can be placed in a logical order. In the example below, NUMBER THE EVENTS OF FORMATION AND HEALING OF AN ULCER IN THE ORDER OF THEIR OCCURRENCE:

___ regeneration of epithelium

___ sloughing of necrotic tissue to form a cavity

___ exudation and infiltration by polys

___ focal necrosis of tissue

___ proliferation of connective tissue

9. a) the injurious agent or debris remains in the tissue.

---

10. 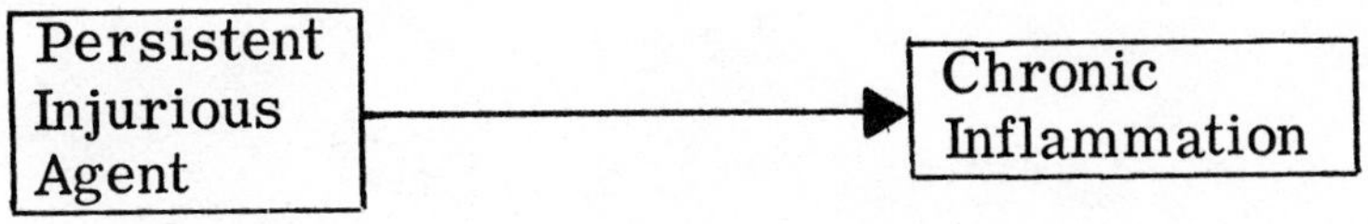

Chronic inflammation depends on the persistence of an injurious agent.

Inflammatory agents persist when:

1) the agent has properties which make it persistent, and/or

2) the host's defense mechanisms are impaired and unable to overcome the agent.

Chronic inflammation is due either to factors relating to the __________ or to the injurious __________.

---

71. b)

---

72. Suppuration (formation of pus) generally occurs within the tissues, interstitially. Is the accumulation of large numbers of polys always indicative of suppuration? ☐ Yes ☐ No

EXPLAIN.

55. F
F
T
F
T
T

---

56. INDICATE "T" TRUE OR "F" FALSE:

		frame reference
___	Chronic granulomatous inflammation occurs only when the body's defenses are weakened.	38,39
___	Macrophages are the predominant cell type of infectious and foreign-body granulomas.	39
___	The macrophages associated with a tubercle are called epithelioid cells because they are derived from epithelium.	39,42
___	Granulomas are only formed in response to inanimate foreign bodies.	39
___	Granulomas develop in any prolonged inflammation.	40
___	Granulomas have the same structure and function as granulation tissue.	51

---

117. B
A
C

---

118. Chronic reflux of gastric juices into the esophagus could cause:

a) esophagitis.

b) ulceration of esophageal mucosa.

c) fibrosis and striction of the esophagus.

d) granuloma formation.

10. host
agent

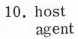

11. Mechanisms of Chronic Inflammation

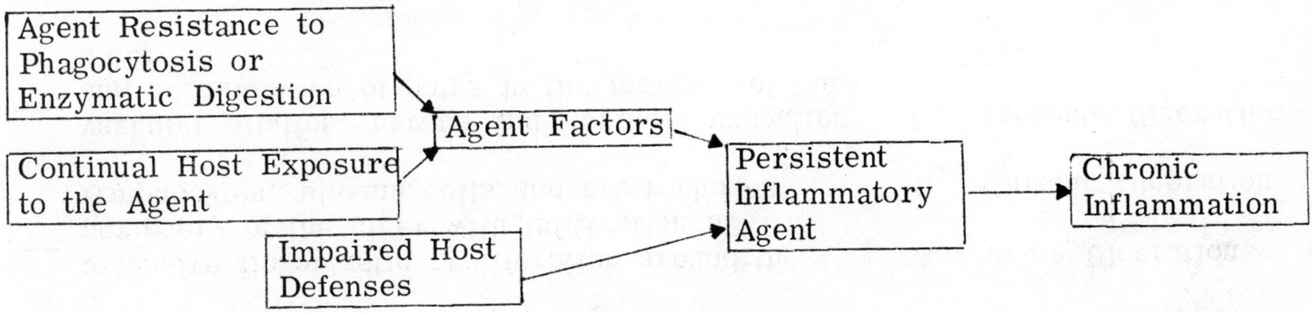

Many chronic inflammations are due to agents which are resistant to phagocytosis or enzymatic digestion. Agents such as mineral oil, asbestos, silica, wood, many fungi, and the bacteria which cause tuberculosis, leprosy, and syphilis are very resistant to phagocytosis or enzymatic digestion and are common causes of ________ ________.

---

72. [✓] No. Suppurative exudate (pus) is also composed of liquefied debris which is created by the release of enzymes from the dying polys.

---

73. Catarrhal exudates are very similar to serous exudates except for the large quantities of mucus. Mild inflammation of a mucous membrane usually causes a catarrhal inflammation. MATCH THE FOLLOWING:

___ serous exudate

___ fibrinous exudate

___ purulent exudate

___ catarrhal exudate

A. Occurs in or on any type of tissue.

B. Occurs on mucous membrane.

54. F
T
F
F
T
T

---

55. INDICATE "T" TRUE OR "F" FALSE:

		frame reference
___	Inflammation is always beneficial to the host.	34
___	The cardinal signs are usually more pronounced in a chronic inflammation than in an acute reaction.	33
___	Mononuclear phagocytes are usually present in acute, subacute, and chronic inflammation.	30
___	Polys proliferate in the tissues whereas macrophages must be continually supplied from the blood.	28
___	The presence of plasma cells, lymphocytes, mononuclears, and fibroblasts indicate that an inflammation is chronic.	29
___	Inflammation may cause more damage to the host than the injurious agent.	34-37

---

116. All locations.

---

117. A classic ulcer of the stomach is a distinct oval or circular excavation of the mucosa with nearly straight walls and a level base which may be covered with necrotic debris. Inflammation takes place around the periphery of the ulcer and, like other inflammations, varies with the duration of the reaction. However, in chronic ulcerations, some acute reaction may persist in the area encircling the sides and base of the ulcer, surrounded by chronic inflammation. MATCH THE FOLLOWING:

___ extensive fibroblastic proliferation around the periphery of the ulcer with infiltration of lymphocytes, plasma cells, and macrophages

___ vascular dilation, serous and fibrinous exudation, and accumulation of polys in the margins of the ulcer

___ an ulcer surrounded by polys, with serous and/or fibrinous exudation, enveloped by fibroblastic proliferation

A. Acute Ulceration

B. Chronic Ulceration

C. Subacute Ulceration

11. chronic inflammation

---

12. Microorganisms, such as fungi or the bacteria responsible for tuberculosis, leprosy, and syphilis, and inanimate substances such as asbestos cause inflammation because they are resistant to _________ or ____________.

---

73. A
A
A
B

---

74. The slimy stage of a runny nose which usually accompanies the common cold is an example of a _________ exudate.

53. T
F
F
T
F
T

54. INDICATE "T" TRUE OR "F" FALSE:

		frame reference
___	All chronic inflammations pass through an acute stage.	5
___	An acute reaction is always short but not always severe.	7
___	Inflammation can continue long after the removal or neutralization of any inflammatory agent.	9
___	Chronic inflammation develops only when the host's defenses are weakened and are unable to overcome the agent.	11
___	Recurring exposure to an agent can cause chronic inflammation.	14
___	Agents which are usually resistant to host defenses often cause chronic inflammation.	11

115. F
T
T
F

116. Ulceration occurs in which of the following locations?

a) oral mucosa

b) skin

c) cervix of the uterus

d) mucosa of the stomach and intestine

12. digestion (enzymatic degradation)
phagocytosis

13.

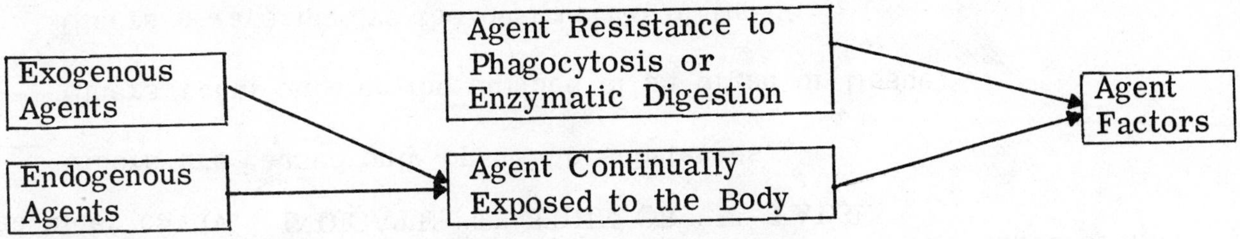

Chronic inflammation is also caused by agents which:

a) can be rapidly neutralized by the body.

b) are continually produced within the body (endogenous).

c) are present in the environment (exogenous) to which the host is continually exposed.

d) live within the host for long periods of time but do not cause any tissue damage.

---

74. catarrhal

---

75. In which of the following tissues would you expect a mild inflammation to produce a catarrhal exudate?

a) pericardial cavity

b) nasopharynx

c) subcutaneous tissue

d) intestinal tract

e) lungs

f) mucus-secreting glands

52. B A

53. INDICATE "T" TRUE OR "F" FALSE:

		frame reference
___	Chronic inflammation never occurs unless an inflammatory agent persists in the tissues.	9
___	Polys are present only in acute inflammations.	27
___	The predominant feature of acute inflammation is fibroblastic proliferation.	28, 30
___	Polys are the predominant cell of acute inflammation.	28
___	Subacute inflammation is clearly distinguished by predominance of plasma cells.	30
___	Replacement of the parenchymal cells of the liver by connecting tissue may be the result of chronic inflammation of the liver.	34

114. A, B
A
B
A, B

115.

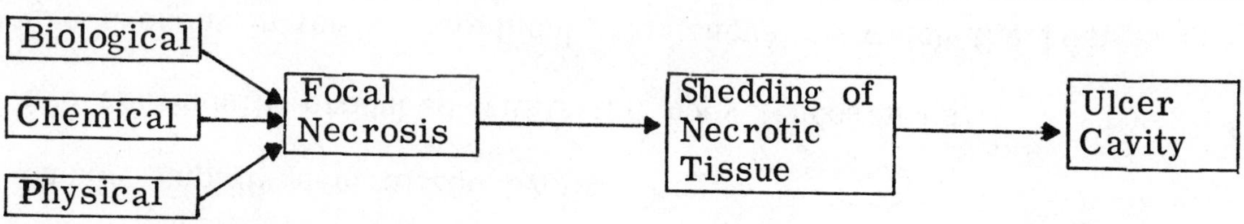

Focal necrosis of tissue followed by shedding of the necrotic tissue creates an ulcer cavity. INDICATE "T" TRUE OR "F" FALSE:

___ Ulcers are caused only by acidic substances.

___ Ulcers occur only on the surface of an organ or tissue.

___ Ulcers always involve the destruction of tissue.

___ Ulcer formation is limited to the stomach and duodenum.

13. b) and c)

---

14. Recurring exposure to endogenous and exogenous agents is one cause of ________ ________. MATCH THE FOLLOWING:

___ an agent produced within the body — A. endogenous

___ an agent present in the environment — B. exogenous

---

75. b, d, e, f

---

76. When a mucous membrane is attacked by a very toxic agent (diphtheria toxin, poison gas, acid, or alkali), the superficial epithelium is destroyed and the agent penetrates into the deeper tissues, where it causes a great increase in vessel permeability and therefore in fibrinous exudation. The exudate spreads over the eroded surface, where it coagulates to form a false membrane composed of (1) fibrin, (2) necrotic epithelium, and (3) a few inflammatory cells. Formation of this gray-white false membrane over an inflamed mucous surface is called pseudomembranous inflammation. MATCH THE FOLLOWING:

___ response of a mucous membrane to a mild agent — A. Pseudomembranous inflammation

___ response of a mucous membrane to a very toxic agent — B. Catarrhal exudation

51. B
A
A
B
B
A

---

52. IDENTIFY THE FOLLOWING:

A. Granulation Tissue

B. Granuloma

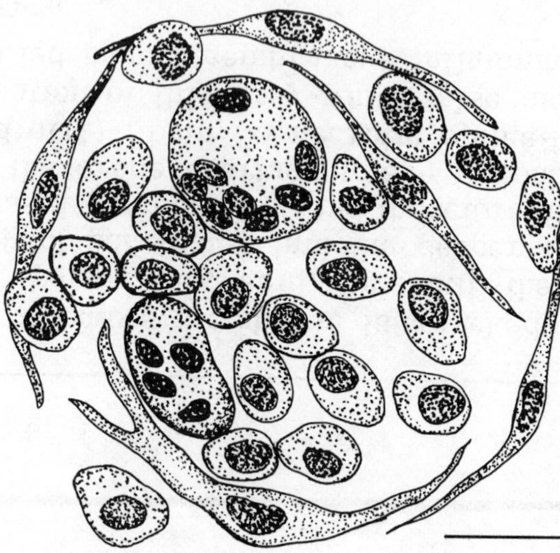

___

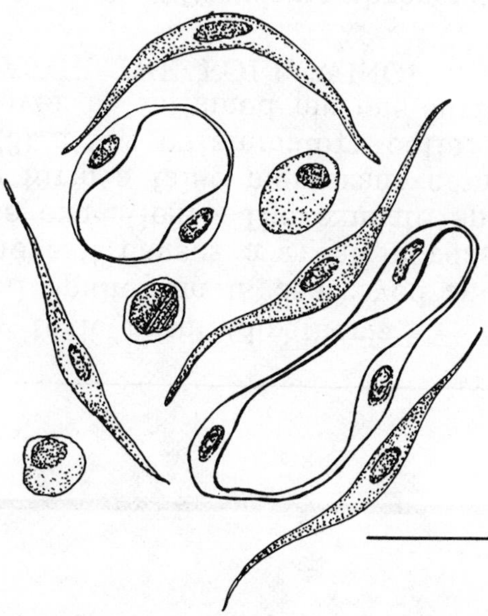

___

---

113. c)

---

114. Ulceration and erosion differ primarily in their depth. MATCH THE FOLLOWING:

___ occurs on an epithelial lined surface of an organ

___ usually only involves the epithelial layer

___ forms a cavity which extends well beneath the epithelium

___ cannot heal until the injurious agent is removed or neutralized

A. Erosion

B. Ulceration

14. chronic inflammation
A
B

---

15. Auto-immune reactions where the inflammatory agents are antigenic material within the host's own tissues are examples of a(n) __________ agent causing chronic inflammation.

Inflammations caused by allergic reactions, such as pollen causing hay fever, are examples of a(n) __________ agent causing chronic inflammation.

---

76. B
A

---

77. Formation of a pseudomembrane in the nasopharynx is highly suggestive of diphtheria. Which of the following are necessary for pseudomembranous inflammation to take place?

a) accumulation of polys

b) necrosis of epithelium

c) catarrhal exudation

d) fibrinous exudation

e) accumulation of macrophages

f) proliferation of fibroblasts

50. d)

51. Granulation tissue is new connective tissue consisting of capillary buds and fibroblasts, often with many inflammatory cells, and it is responsible for wound healing in many situations. The appearance of granulation tissue and granulomas may be very similar. Some authors consider granulomas as nodules of granulation tissue; however, they are considered basically different reactions by most. MATCH THE FOLLOWING:

A. granulation tissue

B. granulomas

___ small, firm nodules composed predominantly of macrophages

___ masses of capillary buds and fibroblasts which are extremely variable in size and shape

___ consists of many fibroblasts, newly formed blood vessels, lymphocytes, plasma cells, mononuclear phagocytes, and occasional polys

___ predominantly mononuclear phagocytes with some giant cells and fibroblasts

___ walls off agents which cannot be phagocytized or enzymatically digested

___ responsible for wound healing

---

112. C
A
B

---

113. Which of the following necessarily involves erosion of a membrane?

a) hemorrhagic inflammation

b) granulomatous inflammation

c) pseudomembranous inflammation

d) suppurative inflammation

15. endogenous
exogenous

---

16. The agents responsible for chronic inflammation can be divided into two major categories:

1. agents which are continually exposed to the body (either endogenous or exogenous)

2. ______________________________

---

77. b) and d)

---

78. NAME THE TWO TYPES OF EXUDATE WHICH ONLY OCCUR ON MUCOUS MEMBRANES:

1. ______________

2. ______________

49. b, c, e, f

---

50. Granulomatous inflammation is:

a) a relatively non-specific form of inflammation which occurs whenever an inflammatory reaction persists for a long time.

b) a distinctive form of inflammation which indicates the specific agent responsible.

c) the response of the body to specific agents, which can be acute, subacute, or chronic.

d) a distinctive form of inflammation which allows recognition of a group of diseases.

---

111. abscess
phlegmon
cellulitis

---

112. In contrast to the diffuse, widespread inflammations, ulceration and erosion are localized, destructive inflammations. Ulceration is an excavation of an epithelial surface of an organ, resulting in a localized defect surrounded by an inflammatory reaction. Erosion, on the other hand, is a more superficial process: the loss of tissue does not involve the underlying layers but is limited to the epithelial layer. Of course, many ulcers begin with an erosion. (Note: This semantic difference between erosion and ulcer is commonly used, but you will not find this distinction clearly made in a textbook or dictionary.) MATCH THE FOLLOWING:

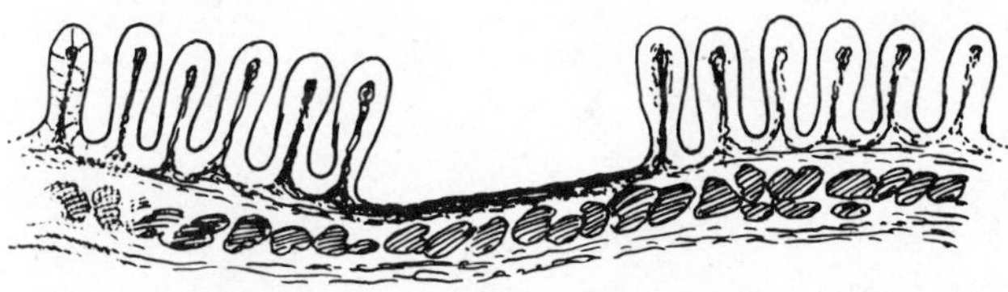

A

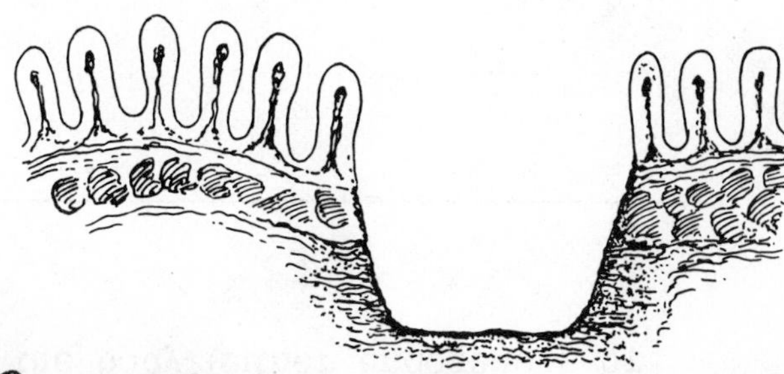

B

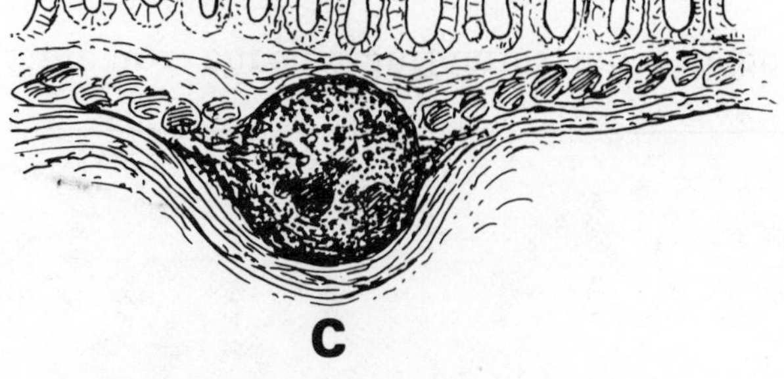

C

____Abscess
____Erosion
____Ulcer

16. 2. agents which are resistant to phagocytosis or enzymatic digestion

---

17. Agents cause chronic inflammation by two mechanisms: a) resistance to host defenses; b) repeated exposure to the body. MATCH THE FOLLOWING:

Inflammations

___ chronic inflammation of the lung due to aspiration of mineral oil

___ chronic contact dermatitis caused by prolonged exposure to industrial detergents

___ inflammation of the larynx due to continual exposure to SO_2 in New York City air

___ berylliosis (lung inflammation due to inhalation of beryllium dust)

___ chronic inflammatory response surrounding suture material

Causes

A. agent which is continually produced or exposed to the body

B. agent which is usually resistant to phagocytosis or enzymatic digestion

---

78. 1. catarrhal
    2. pseudomembranous

---

79. Suppuration (formation of pus) occurs most frequently:

☐ interstitially. ☐ on free surfaces.

Catarrhal exudation occurs most frequently:

☐ interstitially. ☐ on free surfaces.

48. a, b, c, d, e, f

---

49. Which of the following diseases produce chronic granulomatous inflammation?

   a) measles

   b) tuberculosis

   c) syphilis

   d) tetanus

   e) parasitic infections (e.g., trichinosis)

   f) lymphogranuloma venereum

---

110. A
B
B
A

---

111. A focal suppurative inflammation in subcutaneous tissue or muscle would be a(n) __________.

A diffuse, spreading suppurative inflammation in skeletal muscle would be a(n) __________.

A diffuse, spreading non-suppurative inflammation of loose subcutaneous tissue would be a(n) __________.

17. B
A

A
B
B

---

18. Chronic inflammation results when an inflammatory agent persists. The persistence of an agent can be due to either __________ or __________ factors.

---

79. [✓] interstitially
[✓] on free surfaces

---

80. Although the various types of exudate may occur separately, they often are mixed. For example, a reaction may initially produce a serous exudate, and, as it becomes more severe, fibrin may escape from the vessels, forming a serofibrinous exudate. Eventually, the exudate may become predominantly fibrinous but the response may progress to suppuration, forming a __________-purulent exudate.

On a mucous membrane the response may begin as a serous exudation and then progress to catarrhal exudation, forming a __________-mucinous exudate.

Suppuration following catarrhal exudation may create a __________-purulent exudate.

Rupture of a small blood vessel in the area of a blister filled with watery fluid would produce a __________-sanguinous (bloody) exudate.

47. macrophage

---

48. Sarcoidosis is a granulomatous disease of unknown cause which can affect many tissues in the body. Giant cells and epithelioid cells are present in sarcoid granulomas, which makes them difficult to distinguish from tuberculous granulomas. As a general rule, sarcoidosis is diagnosed by eliminating the other granulomatous diseases. Which of the following cause granuloma formation?

a) fungi

b) bacteria

c) viruses

d) unknown agents

e) silica

f) asbestos

---

109. A
C
B

---

110. Cellulitis and phlegmon are two types of diffuse, spreading inflammation differing only in their manner of expansion, which is influenced by the tissue in which they are located. MATCH THE FOLLOWING:

___ occurs in tissues which have few barriers to diffusion of an infection	A. cellulitis
___ commonly occurs in dense tissues, such as skeletal muscles, which direct the spread of infection	B. phlegmon
___ usually spreads in thin sheets confined by tissue planes	
___ spreads in an indiscriminate, undirected fashion	

18. agent (or) host

---

19. Which two major classes of inflammatory agents persist in the tissues and cause chronic inflammation?

    1. ______________________________

    2. ______________________________

---

80. fibrino-purulent
    sero-mucinous
    muco-purulent
    sero-sanguinous

---

81. Some specific agents cause extensive vascular damage, which leads to the loss of blood from the vessels (hemorrhage). When large numbers of erythrocytes escape from damaged vessels and are found in an exudate, it is called a hemorrhagic exudate and the process is called hemorrhagic inflammation. Which of the following are hemorrhagic exudates?

    a) serous exudate with a large number of erythrocytes

    b) fibrinous exudate with a large number of erythrocytes

    c) hemorrhage into a purulent exudate

    d) hemorrhage interstitially

46. A
B
C

---

47. The most numerous cell in the foreign-body reaction is the ________.

---

108. C
B
C
A

---

109. In contrast to abscesses, which are localized inflammations, cellulitis and phlegmon are very diffuse, widespread inflammations. Loose areolar tissue, such as loose subcutaneous tissue, has very few physical barriers to the spread of infection and, therefore, is susceptible to widely disseminated, non-suppurative inflammation called cellulitis. Dense tissues, on the other hand, may contain and regulate the expansion of an infection. An inflammation which spreads under these conditions often takes the form of thin layers separated by elements of the dense tissue; such an infection is called phlegmon. MATCH THE FOLLOWING:

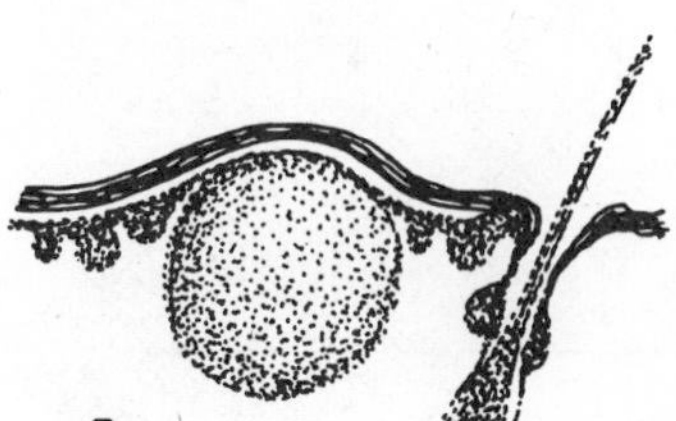

A

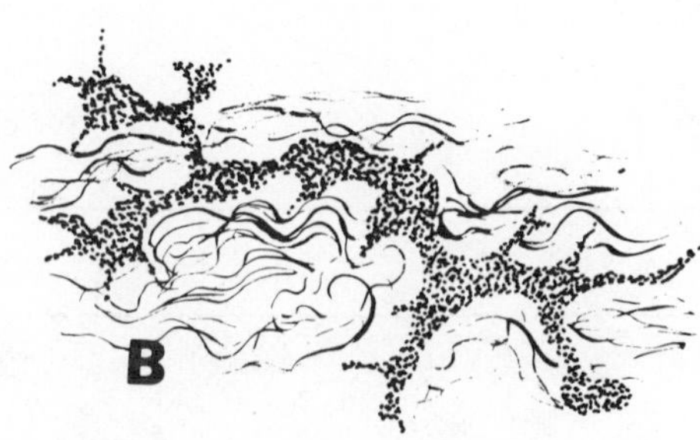

B

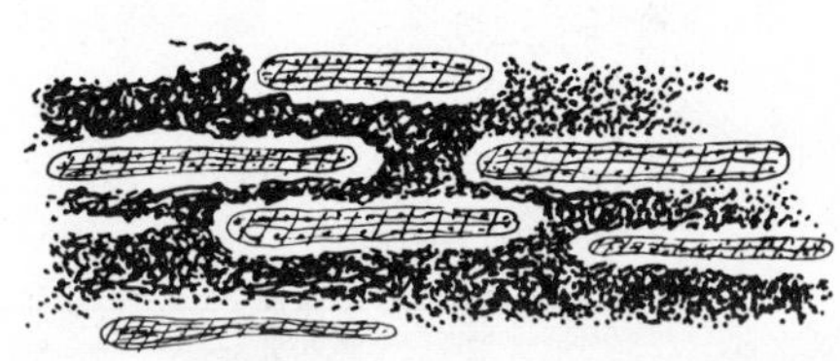

C

____Abscess
____Phlegmon
____Cellulitis

19. 1. agents which are continually exposed to the body (exogenous or endogenous)
2. agents which are resistant to phagocytosis or enzymatic digestion

---

20. Agents which are continually replaced at the inflammatory focus can be either ________ or ________.

---

81. a, b, c

---

82. The organism responsible for Rocky Mountain spotted fever causes damage to small blood vessels, which leads to focal hemorrhages. Often the focal hemorrhages occur all over the body, producing a prominent hemorrhagic rash or spotted appearance. More severe cases of bubonic plague have widely disseminated overwhelming hemorrhage, which produces discoloration of the skin, giving rise to the name "black death." Which of the following (is/are) true?

a) Vascular damage is rarely part of hemorrhagic inflammation.

b) Any exudate plus a large number of red blood cells is a hemorrhagic exudate.

c) The loss of large numbers of erythrocytes from the blood vessels is hemorrhagic exudation.

d) Certain specific agents, like plague bacillus, characteristically produce hemorrhagic inflammation.

45. T
F
F
T

---

46. Silicosis is an example of a foreign-body granulomatous reaction with progressive destructive effects. Silica (SiO_2) is a major component of quartz and sand, and is very common in nature. The reaction of the body to inhalation of silica dust is very similar to that in tuberculosis. Macrophages and giant cells appear around the silica, and there is slow, progressive fibroblastic proliferation over a period of years. And if there is sufficient exposure, eventually the lungs may become almost completely fibrous, with only small islands of normal tissue.

MATCH THE FOLLOWING:

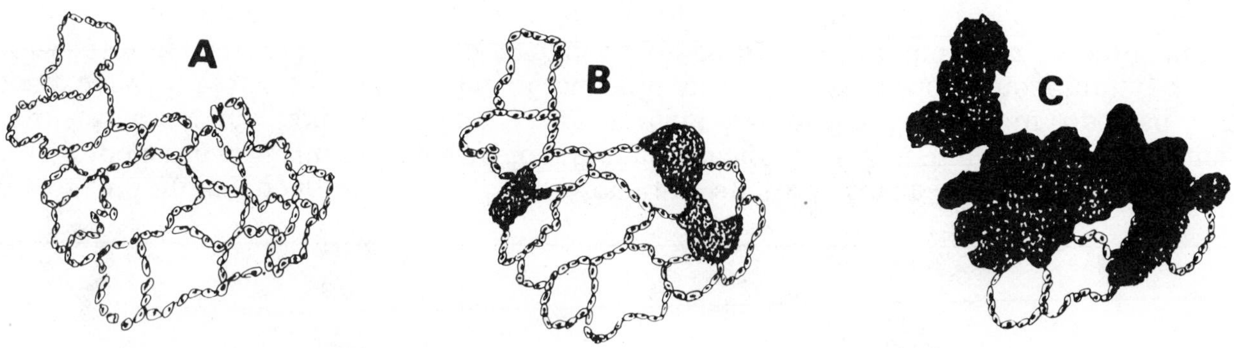

____Normal lung tissue
____7 years work as a sandblaster
____20 years work as a sandblaster

---

107. [✓] greater than

---

108. The suppurative inflammations discussed so far are all abscesses and therefore cause focal tissue damage and consist of localized accumulations of pus within the tissues or natural spaces of the body. However, depending on their location and special features, some types of abscess have been given specific names. MATCH THE FOLLOWING:

___ found in body cavities	A. furuncle
___ located deep in the subcutaneous fascia with multiple sinuses	B. carbuncle
___ found in the pleural cavities	C. empyema
___ occurs superficially in the subcutaneous tissue with a single point of discharge	

20. exogenous (or) endogenous

---

21. Primary Gout

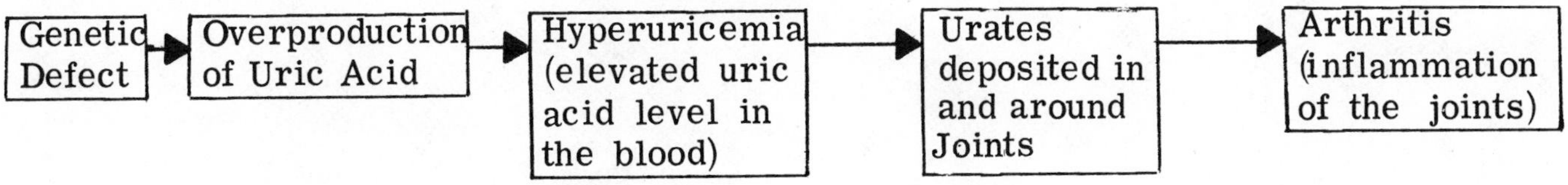

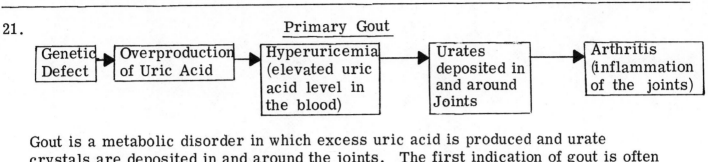

Gout is a metabolic disorder in which excess uric acid is produced and urate crystals are deposited in and around the joints. The first indication of gout is often acute inflammation of affected joints. Later, the formation of tophi (gross deposits of urates) begins. The body is relatively ineffective in removing the tophi, so, as more urate is deposited, the inflammation becomes chronic.

MATCH THE FOLLOWING:

___ Genetic defect	A. Causative factor
___ Overproduction of uric acid	B. Laboratory abnormality
___ Hyperuricemia	C. Sign or morphologic finding
___ Tophi	
___ Arthritis	

---

82. b) and d)

---

83. Some inflammations are distinctive and, along with other manifestations, may suggest the causative agents. But, most inflammations are very non-specific. INDICATE THE THREE TYPES OF INFLAMMATION WHICH MOST LIKELY WOULD HELP YOU NARROW THE LIST OF POSSIBLE CAUSES:

___ Hemorrhagic

___ Chronic

___ Chronic granulomatous

___ Pseudomembranous

___ Acute

___ Subacute

44. tuberculosis
B
A

---

45. Lymphogranuloma venereum is a disease of long chronicity, often lasting for months. The agent is a virus which is usually transmitted by sexual intercourse. Swollen regional lymph nodes are frequently the most prominent sign. Within the affected lymph nodes, aggregates of macrophages develop into small granulomas. INDICATE "T" TRUE OR "F" FALSE:

___ A late complication of lymphogranuloma venereum is fibroblastic proliferation, causing scarring of the lymph nodes.

___ Lymphogranuloma venereum is an example of a disease in which foreign-body granulomas are formed.

___ The granulomas of tuberculosis are radically different from those of lymphogranuloma venereum.

___ Elephantiasis of the scrotum may develop in the late stages of lymphogranuloma venereum due to scarring and obstruction of the lymph nodes.

---

106. The fascial planes in these areas allow the lateral spread characteristic of a carbuncle.

---

107. Furuncles and carbuncles can cause considerable pain and tissue damage, but their biggest threat is the spread of infection to other parts of the body. Threat of spreading infection from a carbuncle or furuncle in a diabetic is ☐ greater than ☐ equal to ☐ less than than in a normal person.

21. A
A
B
C
C

---

22. Urate is an ☐ endogenous ☐ exogenous inflammatory agent which is:

a) continually being produced and thus exposed to the host.

b) relatively resistant to phagocytosis and enzymatic digestion.

c) both a and b.

d) neither a nor b.

---

83. ✓ Hemorrhagic
✓ Chronic granulomatous
✓ Pseudomembranous

---

84. In some cases the type of inflammation can be helpful in making a diagnosis.
MATCH THE FOLLOWING:

Disease		Type of Inflammation
___ Bubonic Plague	A.	Pseudomembranous Inflammation
___ Rocky Mountain Spotted Fever	B.	Chronic Granulomatous Inflammation
___ Tuberculosis	C.	Hemorrhagic Inflammation
___ Diphtheria	D.	Suppurative Inflammation
___ Sarcoidosis		
___ Pyogenic Infection		

43. c)

---

44. Langhans' cells are found in several different granulomatous diseases, but they are most often associated with what disease? ________

MATCH THE FOLLOWING:

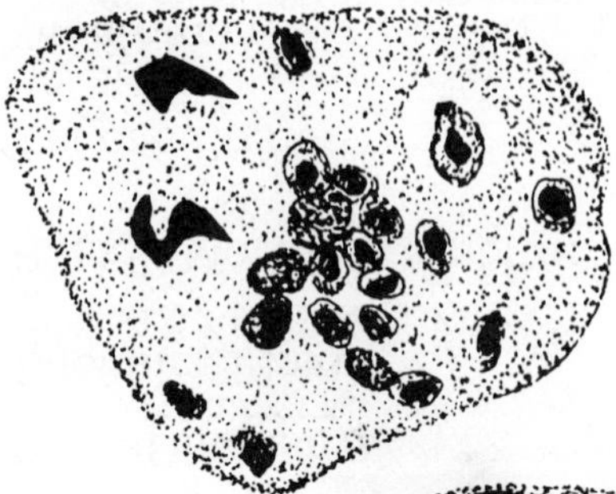 ____

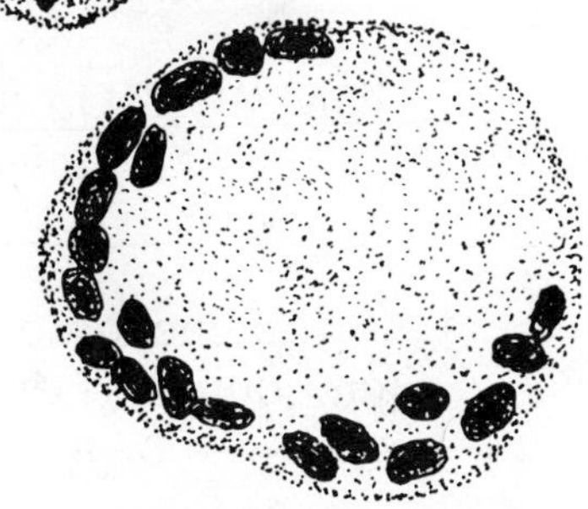 ____

A. Langhans' Cell

B. Foreign-Body Giant Cell

105.

	Location				Points of Discharge	
	Deep, Beneath Subcutaneous Fascia	Shallow	Hairy, Moist Areas	Back and Nape of the Neck	Single	Multiple
F		X	X	X	X	
C	X			X		X

---

106. Why do carbuncles occur most frequently on the back and the nape of the neck?

22. [✓] endogenous
c) both a and b

---

23. 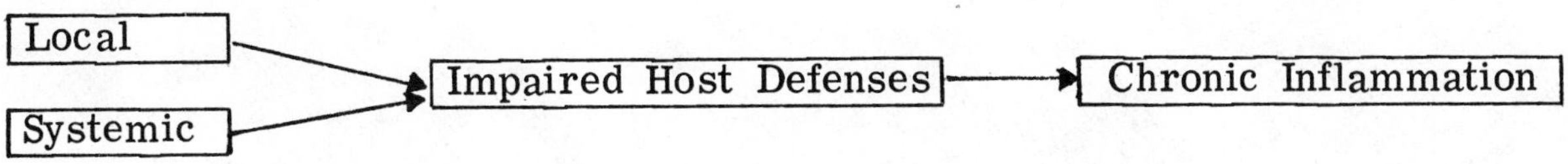

In chronic inflammation, where impaired host defense mechanisms are the primary cause, the defect may be local or systemic. For the following INDICATE "L" LOCAL IMPAIRMENT OR "S" SYSTEMIC IMPAIRMENT:

___ impaired blood supply to an organ or tissue

___ obstruction of bronchi by mucus, preventing normal cleansing of the pathway

___ impaired immunologic capability

___ agranulocytosis

---

84. C Bubonic Plague
C Rocky Mountain Spotted Fever
B Tuberculosis
A Diphtheria
B Sarcoidosis
D Pyogenic Infection

---

85. Exudates vary in the type of cells and fluids of which they are composed. MATCH THE FOLLOWING:

___ serous exudate

___ fibrinous exudate

___ purulent exudate

___ catarrhal exudate

___ hemorrhagic exudate

A. contains a few inflammatory cells but closely resembles blood plasma

B. contains large numbers of polys

C. contains a few inflammatory cells and closely resembles blood serum

D. resembles blood serum except for a high mucus content

E. contains red blood cells

42. C tubercle
D epithelioid cell

---

43. One of the problems in the treatment of tuberculosis is that drugs cannot easily reach the bacteria encapsulated within the granuloma. SELECT THE CORRECT RESPONSE:

a) Granulomas may protect the host by preventing further spread of an organism.

b) Granulomas may protect the invading organism.

c) Both a and b.

d) Neither a nor b.

---

104. B
A

---

105. The distinction between furuncles and carbuncles is based on their location and the presence of one or multiple sinuses. INDICATE THE CORRECT BOXES (F = Furuncle; C = Carbuncle):

	Location				Points of Discharge	
	Deep, Beneath Subcutaneous Fascia	Shallow	Hairy, Moist Areas	Back and Nape of the Neck	Single	Multiple
F						
C						

23. L
L
S
S

---

24. Impaired physiologic condition may predispose an individual to chronic inflammation. Physiologic condition is influenced by age, __________, and the presence or absence of __________.

---

85. C serous exudate
A fibrinous exudate
B purulent exudate
D catarrhal exudate
E hemorrhagic exudate

---

86. Although exudates are often mixed, they do occur separately, and it is easier to remember their composition if you can remember an example of each one. MATCH THE FOLLOWING:

___	common cold	A.	Serous Exudate
___	black plague	B.	Fibrinous Exudate
___	bread-and-butter pericarditis	C.	Purulent Exudate
___	blister	D.	Catarrhal Exudate
___	pyogenic infection	E.	Hemorrhagic Exudate

41. d) macrophage

---

42. Tuberculosis is a chronic infection which usually affects the lungs but can involve any tissue in the body. Tuberculous granulomas are often called tubercles and consist of round, plump mononuclear phagocytes and often Langhans' cells. The enlarged macrophages are called epithelioid cells because their abundant cytoplasm and their tendency to arrange themselves very closely together makes them resemble epithelial cells. MATCH THE FOLLOWING:

___ tubercle	A. small neoplasm
___ epithelioid cell	B. transformed epithelial cell
	C. granuloma
	D. transformed macrophage

---

103. empyema

---

104. Many abscesses of the skin begin as infected hair follicles (folliculitis) and are given special names. Furuncles, commonly called boils, are focal suppurative inflammations of the skin and subcutaneous tissue; they may be single or multiple but are not contiguous. They can occur anywhere but most frequently occur in moist, hairy areas of the skin, such as the face, neck, groin, and axilla. Carbuncles are more deeply located suppurative inflammations which spread laterally beneath the deep subcutaneous fascia and then burrow to the surface to produce multiple points of discharge. The most frequent sites of carbuncles are the back and the nape of the neck where the fascial planes allow their characteristic lateral spread. MATCH THE FOLLOWING:

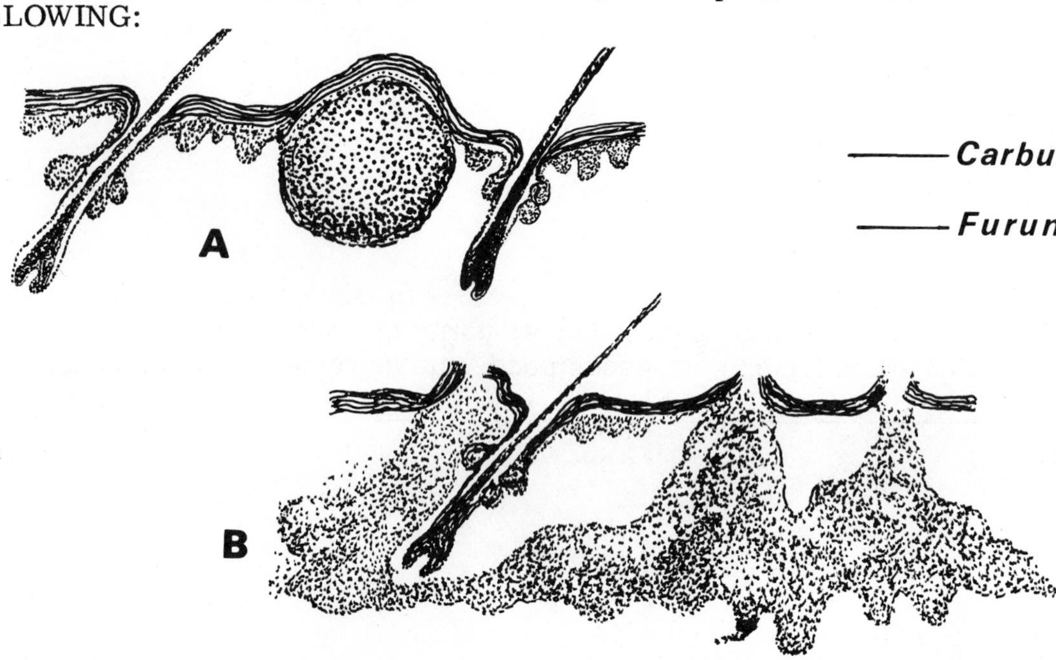

——— Carbuncle

——— Furuncle

24. nutrition
disease

---

25. FILL IN THE BOXES BELOW:

Mechanism of Chronic Inflammation

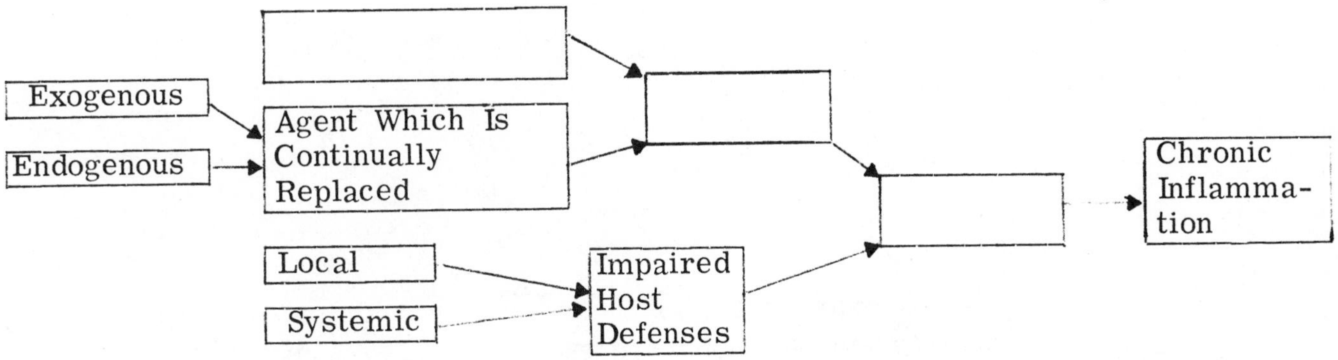

---

86. D common cold
E black plague
B bread-and-butter pericarditis
A blister
C pyogenic infection

---

87. The presence of different types of fluid in the pericardial cavity indicate different diseases. MATCH THE FOLLOWING:

Cause		Fluid
___ a fulminating infection causes exudation and bleeding into the pericardial cavity	A.	Hemopericardium (hemorrhage into the pericardial cavity)
___ a low blood protein level causes accumulation of a clear fluid in the pericardial cavity	B.	Serous exudate
___ a rupture of the intrapericardial segment of the aorta causes rapid accumulation of blood	C.	Transudate
___ a non-bacterial inflammation is accompanied by the accumulation of a clear, protein-rich fluid (specific gravity 1.027) with a few inflammatory cells	D.	Hemorrhagic exudate

40. c)

---

41. The most characteristic cell of chronic granulomatous inflammation is the:

a) lymphocyte.

b) plasma cell.

c) eosinophil.

d) macrophage.

---

102. F
F
T
T
F

---

103. When the gallbladder is inflamed (cholecystitis, from the Greek chole-, meaning bile, and kystis, meaning bladder; and -itis, meaning inflammation), it may become almost filled with purulent exudate. This condition is called ______________ of the gallbladder.

25. 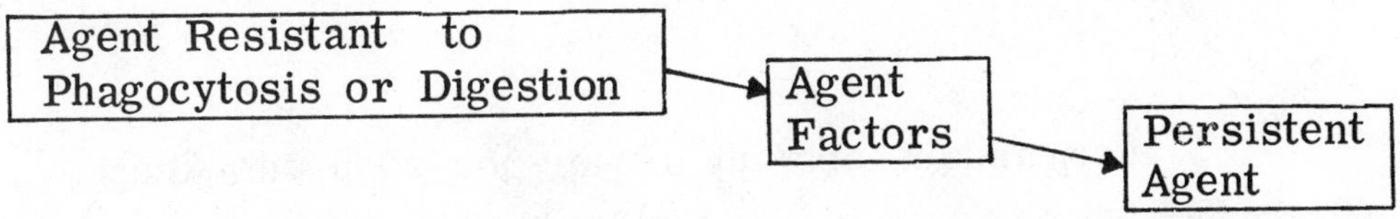

---

26. Chronic inflammation occurs when the inflammatory agent remains in the tissue. Inflammatory agents persist when (1) the agent has properties which make it persistent, and (2) the host's defense mechanisms are impaired and are unable to overcome the agent.

___ depression of the reticuloendothelial system by a toxic drug

___ allergy to clothing material

___ inhalation of asbestos

___ impaired circulation to the leg

___ wood splinters

___ host antibodies formed to host kidney tissue

A. Agent which is resistant to host defenses

B. Agent to which the host is continually exposed (exogenous or endogenous)

C. Impaired local host defenses

D. Impaired systemic host defenses

---

87. D
C
A
B

---

88. INDICATE "T" TRUE OR "F" FALSE:

	frame reference
___ Inflammations vary only in location and duration.	57
___ Exudates are most prominent in chronic inflammations.	58
___ Blood plasma and serous exudate are nearly identical.	63, 64
___ Fibrinous exudates are most common in very mild inflammations.	63, 64
___ Polys accumulate only at the inflammatory focus in pyogenic infections.	68
___ Suppuration rarely causes tissue damage.	68

39. B Fungi
B Mycobacterium tuberculosis
B Spirochete responsible for syphilis
A Dust
A Silica
A Suture material

---

40. Granuloma formation indicates that the body cannot easily overcome the agent responsible and has tried to wall it off and contain it. Chronic granulomatous inflammation occurs only when:

a) the host's defenses are weakened.

b) the agent is insoluble in body fluids.

c) specific agents which are resistant to the body's defenses enter the tissue.

d) any inflammatory agent persists in the tissue for more than a few months.

---

101. Yes, because it probably contains enough of the pyogenic bacteria to spread the infection.

---

102. Spontaneous rupture of an internal abscess is potentially very harmful. When an abscess ruptures into a normally existing space, the space will become a large abscess, which is extremely difficult to drain, and therefore inflammation may continue indefinitely. Accumulation of pus in a natural body cavity (due to primary infection or the rupture of an abscess) is called empyema. For example, pus in the pericardial cavity would be pericardial empyema; however, the term usually refers to suppuration in the pleural cavity or pyothorax. INDICATE "T" TRUE OR "F" FALSE:

___Empyema necessarily begins with the rupture of an abscess.

___Empyema can occur within the tissue or in a natural body cavity.

___Empyema can be considered a type of abscess.

___Prolonged empyema of the pleural cavities often causes fibrous adhesions between the lungs and parietal surface.

___Empyema does not always include suppuration.

26. D
B
A
C
A
B

---

27. Although polys may be present even in chronic inflammatory reactions, an inflammatory lesion can often be classified as acute, subacute, or chronic on the basis of the predominant cell types. MATCH THE FOLLOWING:

___	polys	A.	acute
___	mononuclear phagocytes	C.	chronic
___	fibroblasts		
___	plasma cells		
___	lymphocytes		

---

88. F
F
F
F
F
F

---

89. INDICATE "T" TRUE OR "F" FALSE:

		frame reference
___	Catarrhal exudates are very similar to serous exudates except for the large concentration of mucus.	73
___	Catarrhal exudates and pseudomembranous inflammation occur only on mucus membranes.	76
___	Serous exudation is an important part of pseudomembrane formation.	76
___	The various types of exudate are frequently mixed.	80
___	Vascular damage is usually a part of hemorrhagic inflammation.	81
___	Most inflammations are very distinctive and usually are of value in making a diagnosis.	83

38. a) are resistant to the host's defenses

---

39. GRANULOMA FORMATION

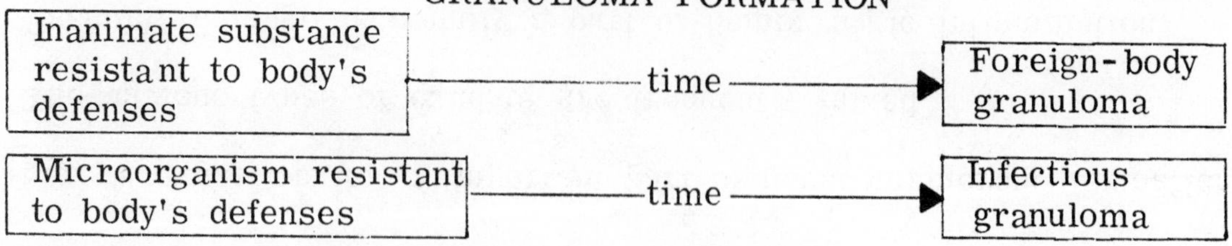

Granulomas are small, firm nodules composed primarily of plump macrophages often called epithelioid cells because of their resemblance to epithelial cells. They are caused by two types of agents which are resistant to phagocytosis or enzymatic digestion: 1) microorganisms and parasites; and 2) foreign material. The corresponding reactions are infectious granulomas and foreign-body granulomas. MATCH THE FOLLOWING:

Agents	Granulomas
___ Fungi	A. Foreign-Body Granulomas
___ Mycobacterium tuberculosis	B. Infectious Granulomas
___ Spirochete responsible for syphilis	
___ Dust	
___ Silica	
___ Suture material	

---

100. 4
1
2
3

---

101. Would you guess that purulent exudate from a pyogenic infection would be infective ?

27. A
A, C
C
C
C

---

28. In acute inflammations the predominant features are exudation and the accumulation of neutrophils. Polys are the primary cell of acute inflammation. SELECT THE CORRECT RESPONSE(S): Polys

a) proliferate in the inflammatory focus.

b) live for weeks or months in the tissue.

c) live for at most a few days in the tissue.

d) must be continually replaced from the marrow.

---

89. T	T
T	T
F	F

C. Variation in Degree of Localization and Location (37 frames)

When you complete this section, you will be able to select correct responses relating to the:-

1. definition of abscess, empyema, furuncle, carbuncle, phlegmon, cellulitis, ulcer, and erosion.
2. mechanism of formation and location of abscesses, empyemas, furuncles, carbuncles, phlegmons, cellulitis, ulcers, and erosions.
3. ways of naming inflammations.

90. The nature and outcome of an inflammatory reaction is greatly influenced by its location in the tissues and the degree to which it is localized. For example, what type of inflammation can occur only on mucous membranes?

37. c)

38. Although most chronic inflammations follow the same pattern of cell proliferation and increased fibrous tissue, some agents produce a distinctive reaction called chronic granulomatous inflammation. The agents which cause chronic granulomatous inflammation

a) are resistant to the host's defenses.

b) are susceptible to host defenses.

---

99. c)

---

100. Complex interactions between agent and host govern the changing structure of an abscess during its formation and healing. NUMBER THE EVENTS BELOW IN ORDER OF THEIR OCCURRENCE:

___ Polys die in large numbers and release their enzymes, which liquify more tissue.

___ A pyogenic agent enters the tissue or a body cavity.

___ Polys accumulate and indulge in extensive phagocytosis.

___ Accumulation of acid metabolites reduces the pH below 7.0.

28. c) and d)

---

29. Chronic inflammation is characterized more by cell proliferation than by exudation. The principle cells of chronic inflammation are mononuclear phagocytes, plasma cells, lymphocytes, and fibroblasts, although polys may also be present. MATCH THE FOLLOWING:

___ proliferation of fibroblasts and production of collagen

___ exudation

___ proliferation of capillary buds

___ movement of leukocytes from the vessels in large numbers

A. acute inflammation

B. chronic inflammation

---

90. pseudomembranous inflammation

---

91. An abscess is a localized accumulation of purulent exudate interstitially associated with localized tissue damage. In forming an abscess, polys accumulate around a pyogenic agent and as they degenerate release enzymes which digest the cells and debris. Usually an abscess consists of a central mass of pus surrounded by viable polys with a zone of fibroblastic proliferation peripherally. MATCH THE LABELS WITH THE DESCRIPTIONS:

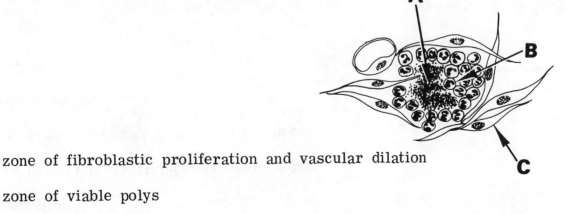

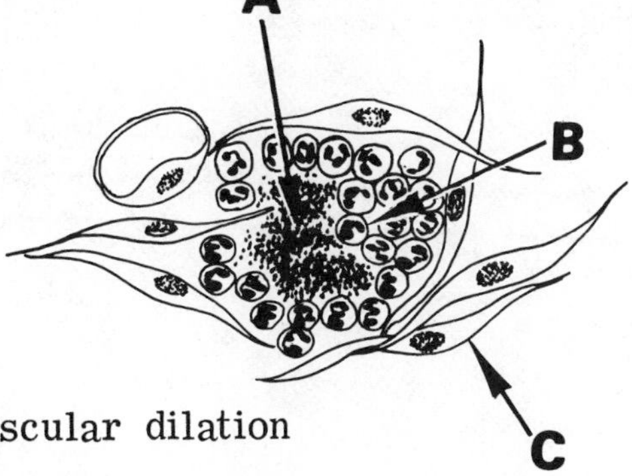

___ zone of fibroblastic proliferation and vascular dilation

___ zone of viable polys

___ central mass of pus

36. b, c, d

---

37. Inflammation

a) can protect the host from microorganisms.

b) can cause extensive damage to the host.

c) both a and b.

d) neither a nor b.

---

98. No. Because exudate and the debris can provoke inflammation themselves.

---

99. Why is it normally desirable to drain an abscess surgically?

a) It speeds up healing since inflammation will continue until the purulent exudate, the necrotic debris, and the agent are removed.

b) It prevents spontaneous rupture, which is dangerous because the abscess may spread internally and disseminate the infection.

c) Both a and b.

d) Neither a nor b.

29. B
A
B
A

---

30. Subacute inflammation is poorly defined, but it is usually thought of as an intergrade between acute and chronic. In subacute inflammation polys and exudate are not as prominent as in acute inflammation, and lymphocytes and plasma cells are often apparent. Characteristically, there is some fibroblastic proliferation in subacute inflammation, although dense fibrous tissue does not develop until the reaction becomes chronic. MATCH THE FOLLOWING:

Predominant Cell Types

___ polys and mononuclears

___ plasma cells, lymphocytes, mononuclears, and fibroblasts

___ polys, plasma cells, lymphocytes, and mononuclears

Duration

___ up to a few weeks

___ months or years

___ weeks to months

Classification

A. Acute

B. Subacute

C. Chronic

---

91. C
B
A

---

92. An abscess is a focal accumulation of ________ within tissue.

35. c)
Chronic inflammation of the urethra would cause fibroblastic proliferation and eventual obstruction.

---

36. Which of the following is/are generally consistent with an inflammation becoming chronic ?

a) increasing exudation

b) increasing cell proliferation

c) disappearance of the cardinal signs

d) fibroblastic proliferation

---

97. C
B
A

---

98. Can the inflammatory reaction of an abscess cease before the suppurative exudate and necrotic debris are removed? Yes or No. EXPLAIN.

30. A
C
B
A
C
B

---

31. The cardinal signs of inflammation are heat, __________, __________, and __________.

---

92. pus

---

93. Abscesses may form in which of the following locations?

a) within the lung

b) on a serous membrane

c) within the liver

d) on mucous membranes

e) within the subcutaneous tissue

f) within the brain

34. chronic
chronic

35. The results of an inflammatory reaction are not always beneficial and may cause extensive damage to the host. Which of the following would be the most likely complication of chronic gonorrhea in a male?

a) redness of the skin

b) loss of libido

c) difficult urination

d) discharge of serous exudate

WHY?

96. ☑ decreases
a)

97.

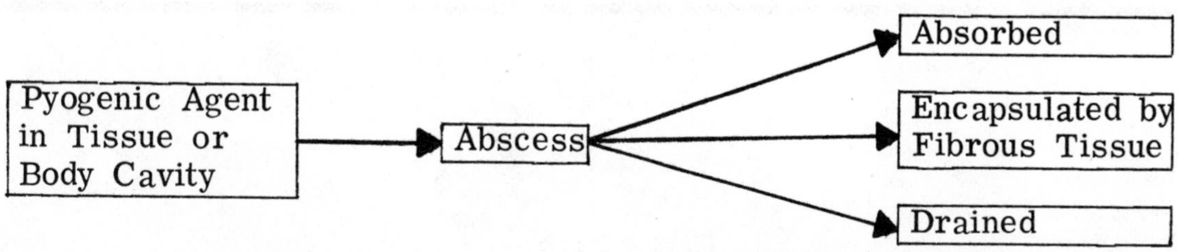

Several possible fates are open to any given abscess. Smaller abscesses are often absorbed while larger ones may be walled off by connective tissue and even become calcified (impregnated with calcium salts). Frequently, abscesses rupture, which is very beneficial if it occurs on a body surface. However, if an abscess ruptures internally, it may cause a widespread infection. MATCH THE FOLLOWING:

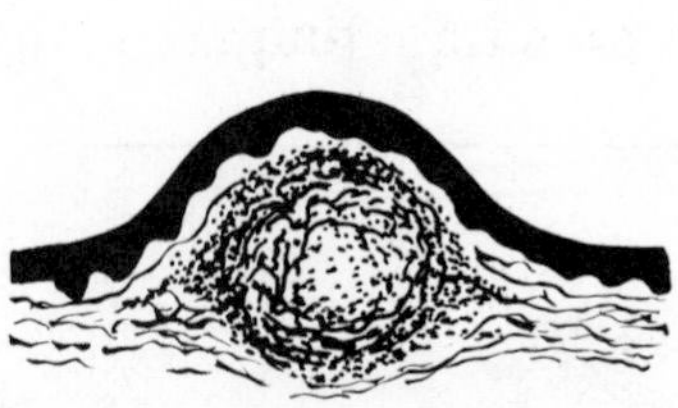

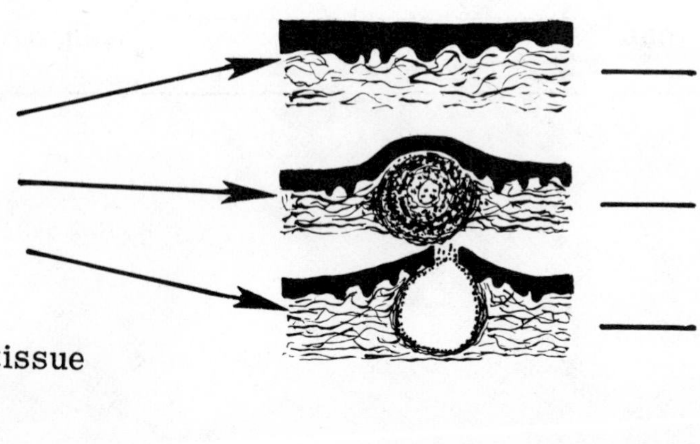

A. draining abscess
B. abscess encapsulated by fibrous tissue
C. abscess absorbed

31. The cardinal signs of inflammation are heat, pain, redness, and swelling.

32. FILL IN THE BOXES BELOW:

Mechanism of the Vascular Response

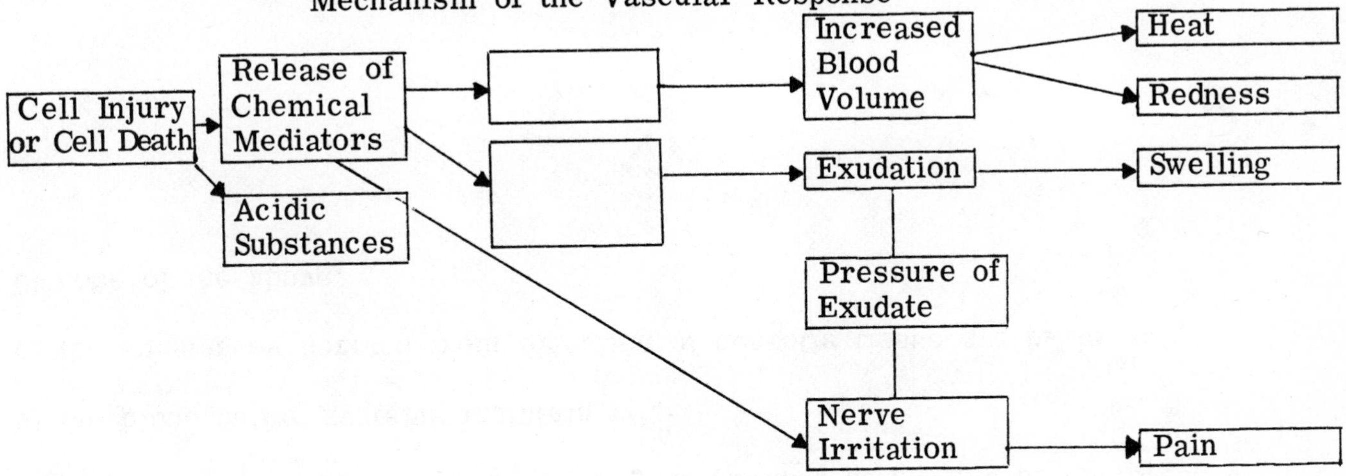

93. a, c, e, f

94. Does the formation of an abscess involve destruction of tissue? Yes or No. EXPLAIN.

33. [✓] less obvious than

---

34. The fibroblastic proliferation characteristic of __________ inflammation often causes extensive scarring with resultant deformities, such as (1) fibrous adhesions between serosal surfaces; (2) obstruction of the bowel or urethra; and (3) fibrous replacement of functional parenchymal elements. Scarring and permanent damage often result from __________ inflammation.

---

95. c)

---

96. Usually, as an abscess matures, the pH of the area [ ] decreases [ ] increases [ ] remains constant, in part because:

a) polys perform anaerobic respiration and produce acidic end products.

b) the blood buffer systems maintain pH.

c) the substances derived from digestion of necrotic tissue are basic.

d) none of the above.

32.

Capillary Dilation

Increased Capillary Permeability

---

33. In chronic inflammation the vascular response is less pronounced than in acute inflammation, so in a chronic reaction the cardinal signs are:

- [ ] the same as
- [ ] more pronounced than
- [ ] less obvious than

in an acute response.

TURN TEXT 180° AND CONTINUE.

---

94. Yes. Suppuration involves necrosis and the liquifaction of the necrotic tissue.

---

95. As an abscess matures the proliferating fibroblasts produce a connective tissue wall, which limits further spread.

a) The connective tissue barrier around an abscess performs a beneficial function by preventing the spread of infections.

b) The connective tissue barrier around an abscess performs a harmful function by preventing the host defenses and drugs from reaching the bacteria effectively.

c) Both a and b.

d) Neither a nor b.

TURN TEXT 180° AND CONTINUE.

Unit 6. Systemic Manifestations of Inflammation

Unit 6. SYSTEMIC MANIFESTATIONS OF INFLAMMATION

OBJECTIVES

When you complete this unit, you will be able to select correct responses relating to the :

	starting page	frame numbers
A. Fever	6.3	1-68

1. definition of fever
2. mechanisms of increased heat production, reduced heat loss, and increased heat loss.
3. normal mechanisms of body temperature regulation.
4. definition of a pyrogen.
5. mechanisms and stages of fever.
6. manifestations associated with fever.

B. Leukocytosis	6.11	69-98

1. definition of leukocytosis and leukopenia in terms of white cells per cubic millimeter of blood.
2. mechanisms of leukocytosis and leukopenia.
3. significance of a differential count.

C. Increased Serum Gamma Globulin and Erythrocyte Sedimentation Rate	6.62	99-115

1. significance of elevated gamma globulin and fibrinogen levels.
2. definition and mechanism of erythrocyte sedimentation rate.

D. Lymphadenitis	6.63	116-126

1. definition, mechanism, and manifestations of lymphadenitis.

PRETEST

UNIT 6. SYSTEMIC MANIFESTATIONS OF INFLAMMATION

SELECT THE SINGLE BEST RESPONSE.

1. By definition, fever occurs when
   (A) body temperature rises due to stimuli reaching the thermoregulatory center
   (B) oral temperature exceeds 37.7° C
   (C) body heat production exceeds heat loss
   (D) a patient notices symptoms associated with elevated temperature

2. Which is true?
   (A) The thermoregulatory center increases or decreases body temperature in response to pyrogens.
   (B) The effect of pyrogens on the thermoregulatory center is similar to that of heat.
   (C) During the cold stage of fever, heat production is less than heat loss.
   (D) Deep thermal receptors in the hypothalamus are influenced by blood temperature.

3. Which cells are associated with pyrogen production?
   (A) lymphocytes
   (B) plasma cells
   (C) eosinophils
   (D) neutrophils

4. Which is a systemic manifestation of inflammation resulting from fever?
   (A) alkalosis
   (B) ketosis
   (C) high blood glucose
   (D) positive nitrogen balance

5. A white cell count of 25,000/cu. mm. is
   (A) within the normal range
   (B) pathognomonic for leukemia
   (C) leukocytosis
   (D) leukopenia

6. Prolonged leukocytosis is associated with
   (A) necrosis of the bone marrow
   (B) inflammation of the bone marrow
   (C) release of immature cells from bone marrow
   (D) the release of leukocytosis-promoting factor

7. Erythrocyte sedimentation rate is increased in association with
   (A) elevated plasma fibrinogen and gamma globulin levels
   (B) decreased plasma fibrinogen and gamma globulin levels
   (C) acute inflammation but not with chronic inflammation
   (D) chronic inflammation but not with acute inflammation

8. Elevated fibrinogen levels are
   (A) not related to erythrocyte sedimentation rate
   (B) associated with increased erythrocyte sedimentation rate
   (C) often used to diagnose internal inflammation
   (D) usually preceded by elevated gamma globulin levels

GO ON TO NEXT PAGE AND BEGIN THE UNIT

A. Fever (68 frames)

When you complete this section, you will be able to select correct responses relating to the:

1. definition of fever.
2. mechanisms of increased heat production, reduced heat loss, and increased heat loss.
3. normal mechanisms of body temperature regulation.
4. definition of a pyrogen.
5. mechanisms and stages of fever.
6. manifestations associated with fever.

1. The preceding sections of this program have dealt with local manifestations of inflammation. This section deals with the general or systemic manifestations of inflammation. Local signs, symptoms, and laboratory abnormalities are limited to the area surrounding the inflammatory site. General manifestations affect body systems or the entire body.

IN THE LIST BELOW, INDICATE SYSTEMIC MANIFESTATIONS "S" AND LOCAL MANIFESTATIONS "L":

_____ swelling

_____ oral temperature of 41°C

_____ leukocytosis (increase of white cells in blood)

_____ redness

_____ pain

_____ accumulation of polys in tissue

_____ malaise (vague feeling of discomfort)

_____ elevated fibrinogen level in blood

---

64. c)

---

65. The preceding frames have illustrated how profoundly body processes can be disturbed by fever and that fever:

a) always is present in inflammation.

b) is associated with inflammation alone.

c) is a manifestation of many different diseases.

TURN TEXT 180° AND CONTINUE.

1. L L
S L
S S
L S

---

2. Fever (or pyrexia) is an abnormally high body temperature due to a disturbance of the body's temperature-regulating mechanism. Control of body temperature is associated with a cluster of nerve cells in the hypothalamus called the thermoregulatory center. Stimuli which affect the thermoregulatory center can cause:

a) fever

b) a decrease in body temperature

c) both a and b

d) neither a nor b

---

65. c) is a manifestation of many different diseases

---

66. INDICATE "T" TRUE OR "F" FALSE:

		frame reference
___	Pyrexia is caused by a resetting of the body's thermostat at a higher level.	2
___	Fever occurs in most inflammations which last more than a few hours.	33
___	The elevation of body temperature due to exercise is fever.	2-6
___	Heat production depends on metabolic activity.	7
___	Vasoconstriction and shivering are the primary mechanisms of increased heat loss.	13
___	Vasodilation is manifested by a drop in skin temperature.	18-22

63. ✓ negative nitrogen balance
✓ ketosis
✓ dehydration and salt loss
✓ rapid breathing

---

64. Mild or short-lived fevers produce no serious effects, but prolonged high fevers or hyperpyrexia can cause dehydration, circulatory and renal failure, wasting of fat and muscle, and brain damage. There are no known beneficial effects of fever. Fever:

a) is always harmful.
b) is an important part of the body's defenses against disease.
c) may be harmful or innocuous.

---

126. F
T
F
T
T
T

THIS IS THE END OF UNIT 6. TAKE THE POSTTEST ON PAGE xxiv.

2. c) both a and b

---

3. Whenever body heat production exceeds heat loss, body temperature:

a) rises.

b) drops.

c) remains the same.

---

66. T
T
F
T
F
F

---

67. MARK THE FOLLOWING "T" TRUE OR "F" FALSE:

		frame reference
___	The thermoregulatory center either increases or decreases body temperature in response to pyrogens.	27
___	The effect of pyrogens on the thermoregulatory center is similar to that of heat.	27
___	The mechanism by which pyrogens influence the thermoregulatory center is not understood.	27
___	During the cold stage of fever, heat production is less than heat loss.	40
___	Deep thermal receptors in the hypothalamus are influenced by blood temperature.	24
___	Some malignant neoplasms can cause fever.	33

62. fever →
- increased metabolic rate
- increased cardiac output
- increased pulmonary ventilation
- increased insensible fluid loss

---

63. CHECK THE ITEMS IN THE LIST BELOW THAT CAN BE THE RESULT OF FEVER:

___ decreased heart rate

___ negative nitrogen balance

___ ketosis

___ dehydration and salt loss

___ rapid breathing

___ drop in the metabolic rate

---

125. cervical
It would indicate a very widespread infection or infection by an organism which produces a toxic substance which has spread throughout the body.

---

126. INDICATE "T" TRUE OR "F" FALSE:

	frame reference
____The most apparent manifestations of lymphadenitis are redness and heat.	119
____Lymph flow is greatly increased in inflamed areas.	121
____The removal of bacteria and toxic substances from the lymph is purely a mechanical filtration process.	123
____Inflamed lymph nodes are very effective in removing bacteria from the lymph, but some types of bacteria pass through the nodes.	172
____Polys infiltrate inflamed lymph nodes just like any other tissue.	170
____The lymph nodes draining an infected area undergo reactive hyperplasia of their reticular phagocytes.	136

3. a) rises

---

4. During vigorous exercise, heat __________ exceeds heat __________ and body temperature __________.

---

67. F
F
T
F
T
T

---

68. INDICATE "T" TRUE OR "F" FALSE:

		frame reference
___	Granulocytes generate pyrogen in response to endotoxin, exudates, and phagocytosis.	36, 37
___	During the hot stage of fever, heat production equals heat loss.	40
___	The first sign of fever is cutaneous vasoconstriction.	42
___	During the cold stage, central body temperature rises and skin temperature falls.	43-46
___	Dehydration, tachycardia (rapid heartbeat), and tachypnea (rapid breathing) can be manifestations of prolonged inflammation.	61-62
___	Ketosis, acidosis, and negative nitrogen balance can be manifestations	55

61. 1) increasing cardiac output
2) increasing pulmonary ventilation

62.

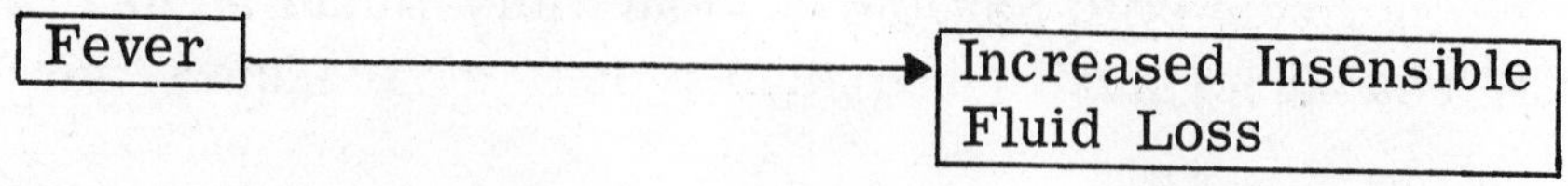

Although sweating does not usually occur during fastigium, there is a large increase in insensible fluid loss. If the fever is prolonged, there may be great losses of water and salt. Severe dehydration in prolonged fevers can cause circulatory and renal failure. FILL IN THE RESULTS OF FEVER:

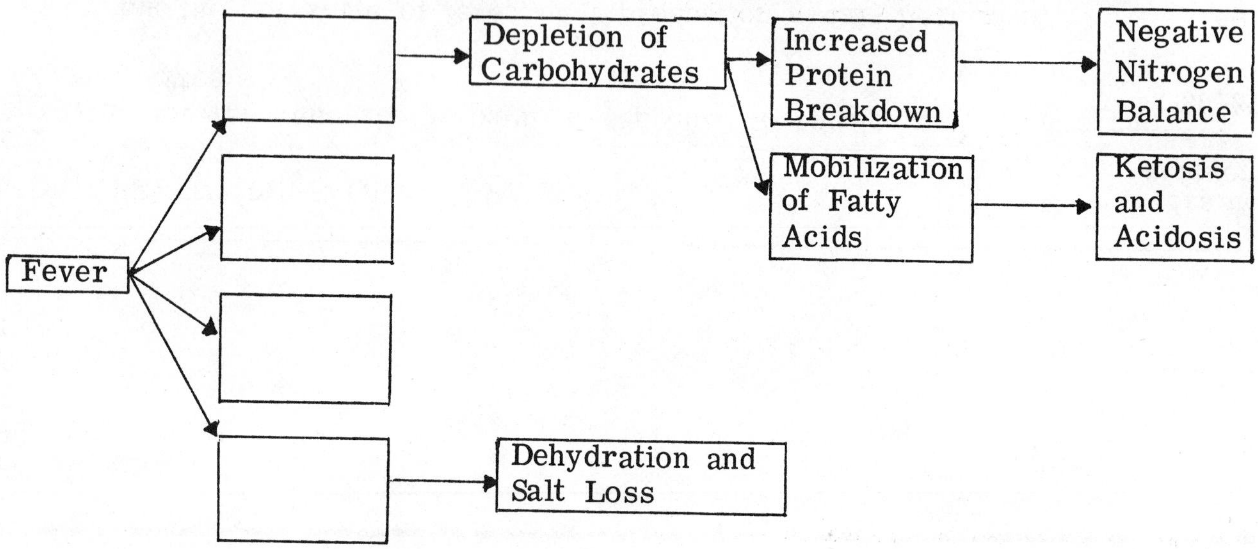

---

124. swollen
painful

---

125. An infection of a tooth socket would most likely cause lymphadenitis of the __________ nodes.

What would lymphadenitis involving inguinal, axillary, cervical, and mediastinal nodes indicate?

4. During vigorous exercise, heat production exceeds heat loss and body temperature rises.

---

5. Is every elevation of body temperature a fever? EXPLAIN.

---

68. T
T
T
T
T
T

B. Leukocytosis (30 frames)

When you complete this section, you will be able to select correct responses relating to the:

1. definition of leukocytosis and leukopenia in terms of white cells per cubic millimeter of blood.
2. mechanisms of leukocytosis and leukopenia.
3. significance of a differential count.

69. Leukocytosis (an increase in the number of circulating leukocytes) is a
☐ local ☐ systemic manifestation of some inflammations.

60. ketosis

loss of appetite
acidosis

61.

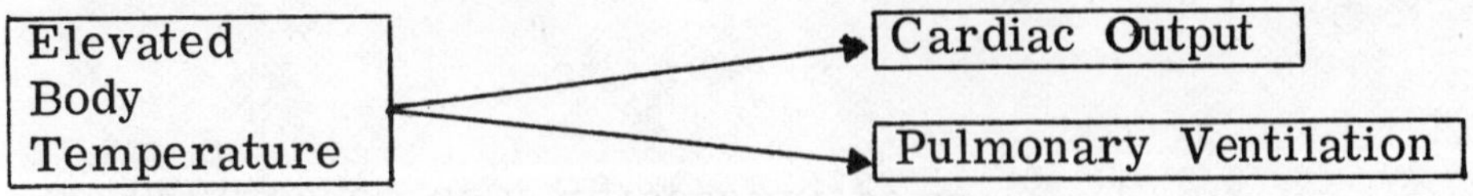

Fever often appears to affect the cardiovascular and respiratory systems by:

1) ____________________
2) ____________________

---

123. This indicates spreading infection. (or equivalent)

---

124. In some cases inflamed lymph nodes may cause the overlying skin to appear red and feel warm, but, in almost every case, inflamed nodes are __________ and __________.

5. No. A fever is caused by a disturbance of the thermoregulatory center.

---

6. When environmental temperature and humidity are high, the body cannot dissipate its own heat efficiently and it gains heat from the environment. A person working outside on a very warm, humid day may have an elevated body temperature. Is this a fever? Explain.

---

69. ☑ systemic

---

70. Normally, the number of circulating leukocytes varies between 5,000 and 10,000 per cubic millimeter of blood. A white cell count of 30,000/cu.mm. is called ________________.

59. [✓] symptoms

---

60. Which of the following can be systemic manifestations of fever and thus of inflammation?

___ alkalosis

___ ketosis

___ high blood glucose

___ positive nitrogen balance

___ loss of appetite

___ acidosis

---

122. b)

---

123. Lymph nodes can be very effective filters, up to 99% effective against some bacteria; but the strategic defensive function of lymph nodes makes them very vulnerable to secondary involvement in almost every infectious disease and many neoplastic growths.

A 26-year-old female go-go dancer suffered a laceration of the left hand while two burly construction workers were competing for her attention. Unfortunately, she did not have an opportunity to cleanse and bandage the wound properly. Afterward she noticed small, tender lumps around her elbow, and soon after that the same kind of funny, painful little lumps appeared on her neck. What does this indicate?

6. No. Fever involves a disturbance of the body's internal temperature-regulating mechanism.

---

7. Heat production in the body is due to the metabolic activity of its tissues. If the metabolic rate is increased by exercise, alcohol, food, or hyperthyroidism (excess production of thyroid hormone) and not compensated by increased heat loss, body temperature will _________.

---

70. leukocytosis

---

71. Leukocytosis commonly refers to an increase in the number of circulating neutrophils. These cells:

    a) live for weeks or months.

    b) reproduce themselves in the tissues by mitotic division.

    c) live for a very short time and must be continually replaced.

58. acidosis

---

59. Loss of appetite, malaise (vague feeling of discomfort), and headache are ☐ signs ☐ symptoms ☐ lab abnormalities related to fever.

---

121. lymphadenitis

---

122. Inflamed lymph nodes have been demonstrated to be more effective than non-inflamed lymph nodes in removing bacteria from the lymph. From what you have learned in the text so far, SELECT THE BEST REASON FOR THE INCREASED EFFECTIVENESS:

a) Swelling of the lymph node allows for greater filtration area.

b) Hyperplasia of the reticular phagocytic cells and infiltration of the node by polys greatly increases the phagocytosis of bacteria.

c) Increased blood supply to the lymph node allows the cells to work more efficiently.

7. rise (increase)

8.

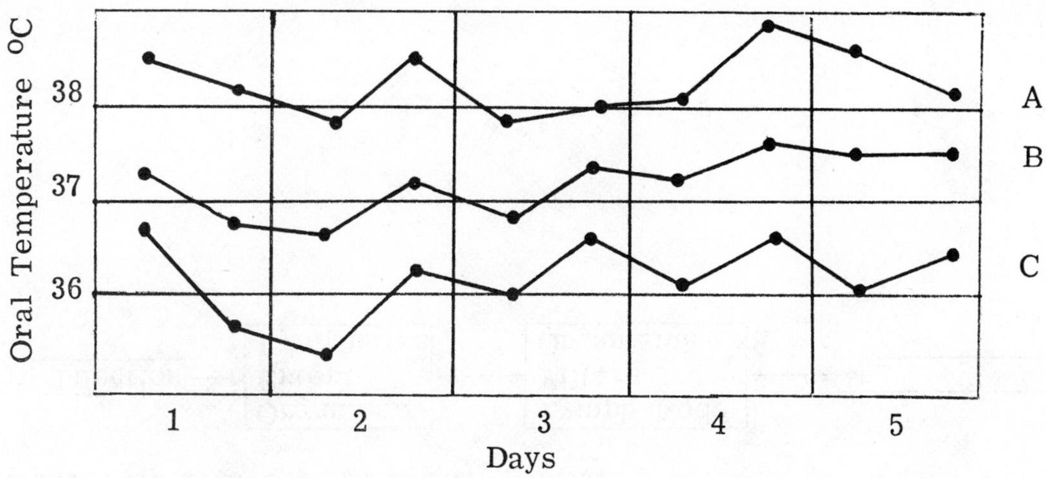

Above are typical temperature charts which show the normal diurnal temperature variation. The nurses mixed up the temperature charts of three patients. You know that one patient is normal, one has hyper-thyroidism, and one has hypothyroidism (deficiency of thyroid hormone). MAKE THE BEST GUESS YOU CAN AS TO WHICH CHART BELONGS TO EACH PATIENT:

___ normal ___ hypothyroidism ___ hyperthyroidism

EXPLAIN.

---

71. c

---

72. In a healthy individual at rest, billions of polys are circulating in the blood and an equal number are marginated on vessel walls or are sequestered in shut-down capillaries. During exercise, blood flows rapidly through the capillaries and washes the marginated and sequestered polys into the general circulation. After violent exercise, the white cell count may be as high as 25,000/cu.mm. or more. This is called ________________.

57. ketosis

---

58. Ketones are moderately strong acids, and their continual formation exhausts the buffer capacity of the blood and causes __________.

---

120. A
B
C

---

121. FILL IN THE EMPTY BOX:

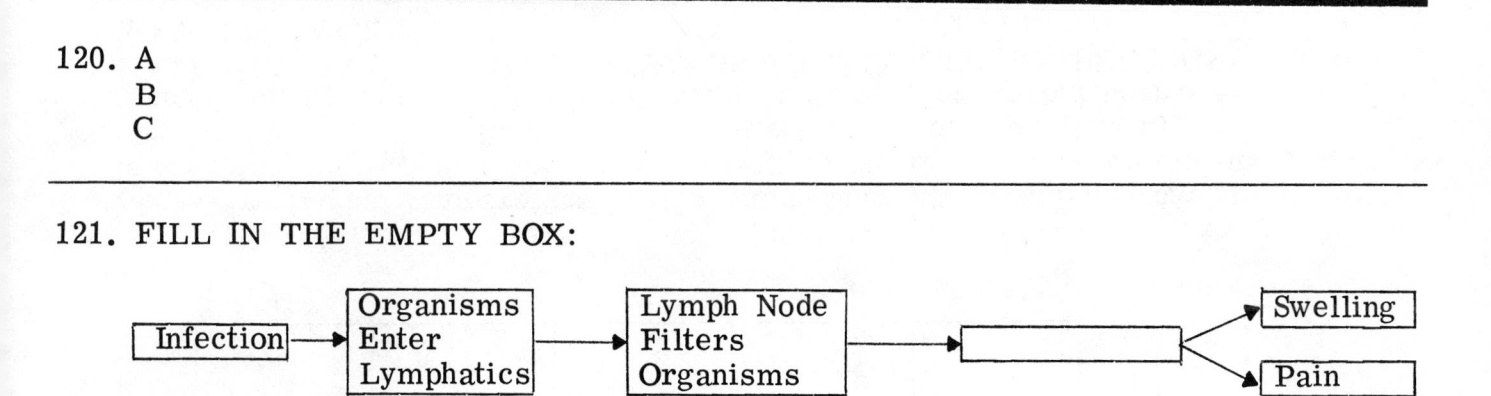

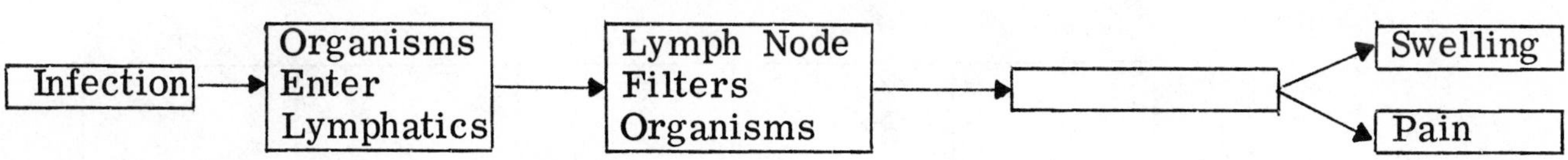

8. B normal
C hypothyroidism
A hyperthyroidism

Thyroid hormone influences metabolic rate (see frame 7). Therefore, excess or deficiency of thyroid hormone causes slight corresponding elevation or depression of body temperature.

9.

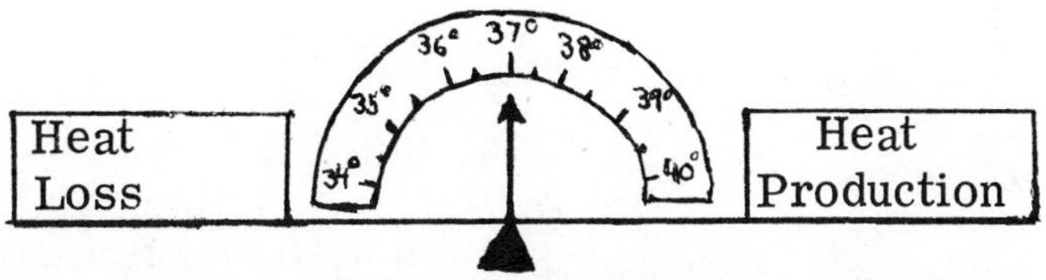

The delicate enzyme systems of the body function optimally only in the normal temperature range. Thus, normal body function depends on maintenance of relatively constant temperature. The thermoregulatory center in the hypothalamus controls the balance between heat production and heat loss to maintain normal body temperature at 37°C ± 1°C.

a) 

a decrease in body temperature can be caused by increased __________ and/or decreased __________.

b) 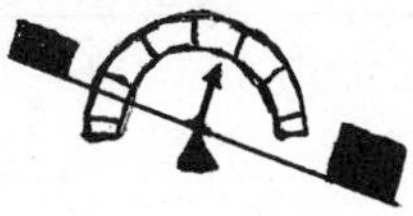

an increase in body temperature can be caused by increased __________ and/or decreased __________.

---

72. leukocytosis

---

73. A number of factors, apart from inflammation, may cause leukocytosis. Strenuous exercise, adrenalin injections, anxiety, and pain all can cause an elevated white count. Is a white count of 25,000/cu. mm. always caused by inflammation? ☐ no ☐ yes

56. nitrogen balance

---

57. When the body exhausts its carbohydrate supply and begins to use fatty acids, there is a great increase in the formation of ketones, a condition called __________.

---

119. 1. Mechanical Filter: reticular meshwork
2. Phagocytic Filter: phagocytic reticular cells and macrophages

---

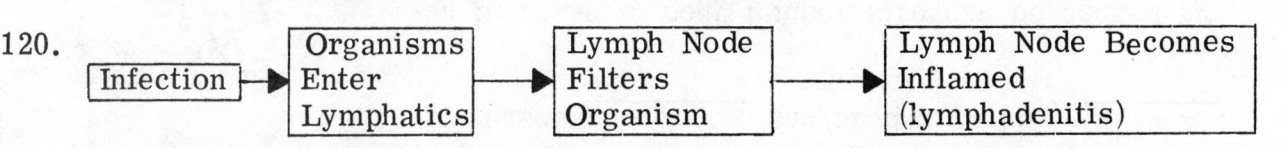

120. Infection → Organisms Enter Lymphatics → Lymph Node Filters Organism → Lymph Node Becomes Inflamed (lymphadenitis)

When a specific area of the body is infected, some of the organisms enter the lymphatics and are carried to the regional lymph nodes. Most bacteria are filtered and prevented from spreading farther, but the lymph nodes often become inflamed. Inflammation of the lymph nodes is called lymphadenitis. MATCH THE AREA OF PRIMARY INFECTION WITH THE MOST LIKELY AREA OF LYMPHADENITIS:

Area of Primary Infection	Lymphadenitis
___ infected knife wound in the left thigh	A. Inguinal Nodes
___ infected burn on the right arm	B. Axillary Nodes
___ infected tonsils	C. Cervical Nodes

9. a) increased heat loss   decreased heat production
   b) increased heat production   decreased heat loss

---

10. The normal body temperature averages ________ °C or ________ °F but often varies 0.5 to 0.7°C.

---

73. [✓] no

---

74. Normal white count ranges between ________ and ________ per cubic millimeter of blood.

55. a) fatty acids
    b) protein breakdown

---

56. The use of protein for fuel in large amounts causes metabolism of protein to exceed intake, which leads to negative _________ _________.

---

118. increased

119.

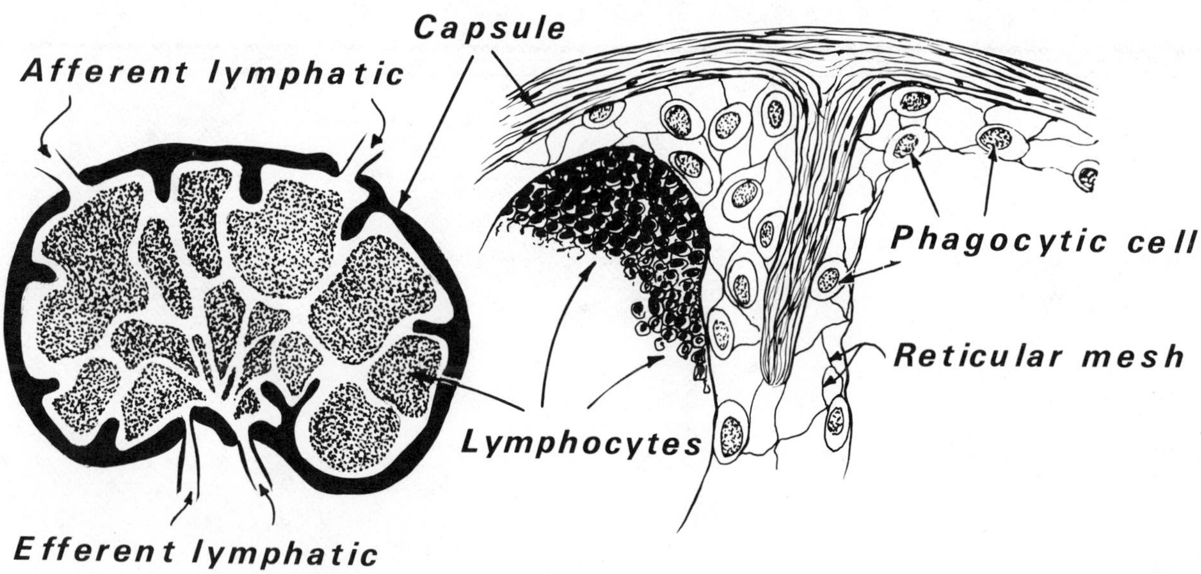

The reticular meshwork of the lymph sinuses may serve as a mechanical filter while the phagocytic activity of the reticular cells further improves the effectiveness of the lymph node. Lymph sinuses function as a filtering mechanism, preventing the dissemination of certain agents. What are the components of this filter?

1. ______________________________

2. ______________________________

10. The normal body temperature averages 37°C or 98.6°F but often varies 0.5 to 0.7°C.

---

11. Pyrexia is an abnormally __________ body temperature due to a __________ ____.

---

74. 5,000 (and) 10,000

---

75. For every neutrophil in circulation there are many mature cells held in the bone marrow reserve. Release of large numbers of these cells causes _____.

54. increase
increase

55.

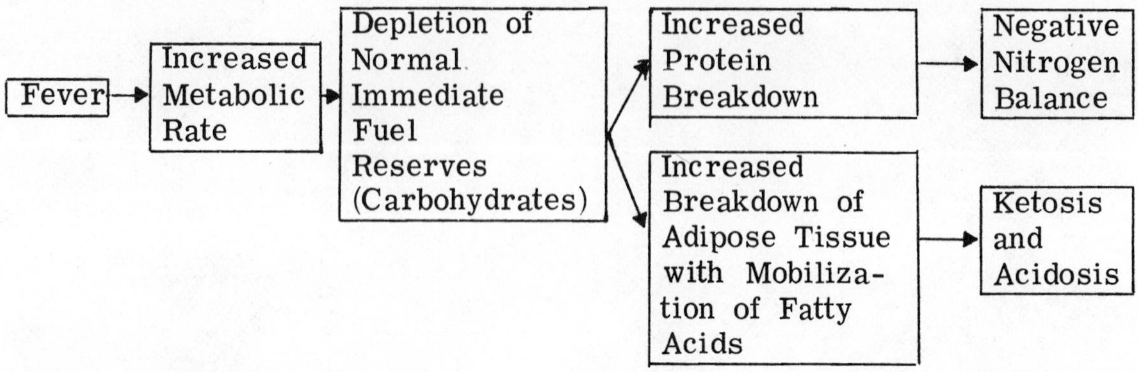

Loss of appetite is common in fever, and this, coupled with a high metabolic rate, leads to depletion of the normal fuel reserves, causing increased protein breakdown and mobilization of fatty acids.

In prolonged fevers:
a) loss of body adipose tissue is due to increased use of _________ _________ for metabolism,
b) wasting of muscles is due to increased _________ _________.

117. All are increased.

118. The substances which are taken up by the lymphatics are carried to the nearest lymph node, where the lymph fluid is filtered. During inflammation the filtration rate of the regional lymph nodes is greatly _________.

11. Pyrexia is an abnormally high body temperature due to a disturbance of the thermoregulatory center in the hypothalamus.

---

12. Heat production by the body depends on the __________ activity of the tissues.

---

75. leukocytosis

76.

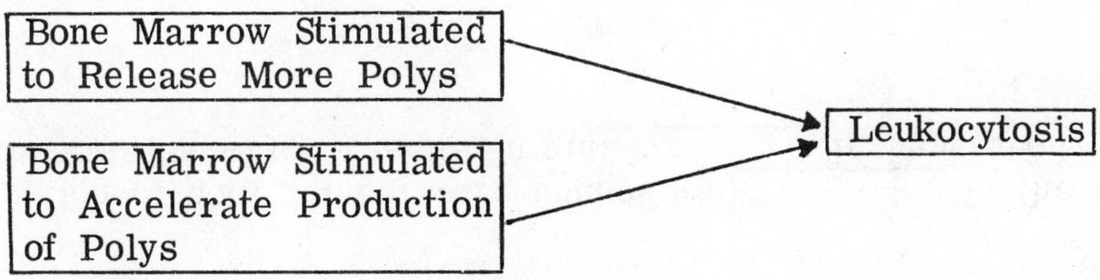

Leukocytosis is produced by two mechanisms:
1) release of more polys from reserves,
2) increased production of polys.

When the production of polys increases, the number of cells in the bone marrow increases. During leukocytosis the bone marrow undergoes ☐ hypertrophy ☐ hyperplasia .

53. systemic
systemic

54.

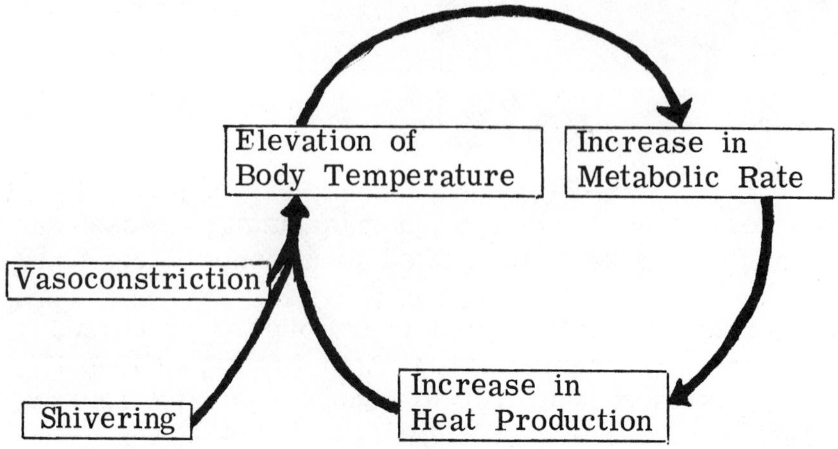

Elevation of body temperature causes a(n)__________ in the metabolic activity of the tissues, which results in a(n)__________ in heat production.

116. T
F
T
T

117. During inflammation, changes occur in the blood vessels and the lymphatics. INDICATE WHETHER THE FOLLOWING ARE INCREASED OR DECREASED OR REMAIN THE SAME DURING INFI AMMATION:

___ Blood Flow

___ Loss of Protein and Fluid from Vessels

___ Uptake of Fluid and Protein by Lymphatics

___ Lymph Flow

12. Heat production by the body depends on the metabolic activity of the tissues.

---

13. If the body is too cold, the regulatory center reduces heat loss and increases heat production by:
    1) Vasoconstriction, primarily of small superficial vessels,
    2) Shivering, if vasoconstriction is insufficient to raise body temperature.

    If you are outside on a cold day and your body temperature starts to drop, the vessels near the skin will __________; if body temperature is still too low, you will begin to __________.

---

76. [✓] hyperplasia

---

77. When release of polys is greatly increased, the normal reserves of cells are depleted and the rate of cell maturation cannot match the rate of cell release. Under these conditions the marrow releases immature cells. Prolonged stress on the marrow causes the release of increasing numbers of __________ cells.

52. A goose pimples
C drenching sweat
A chattering teeth
A sensation of cold
B, C sensation of heat
A shivering

53.

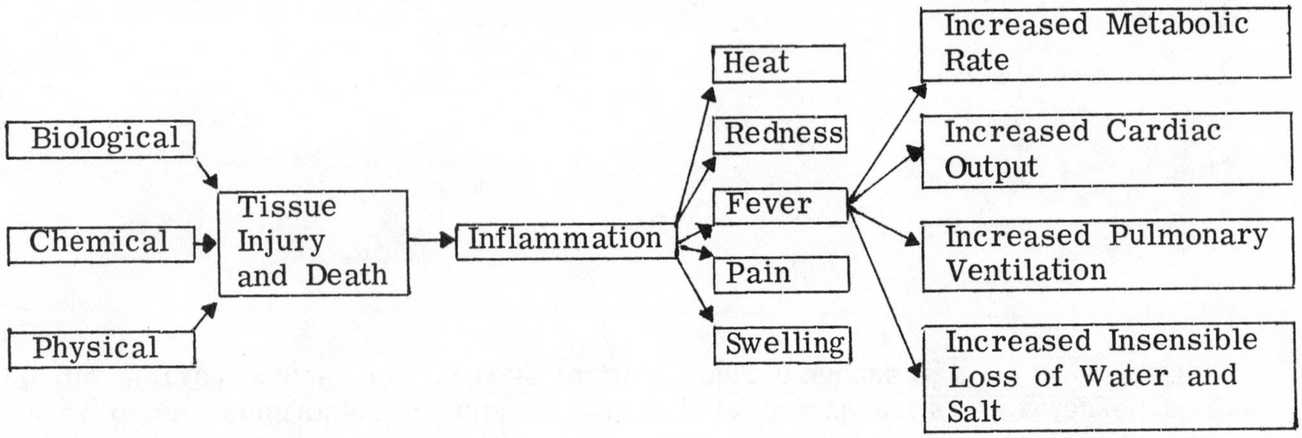

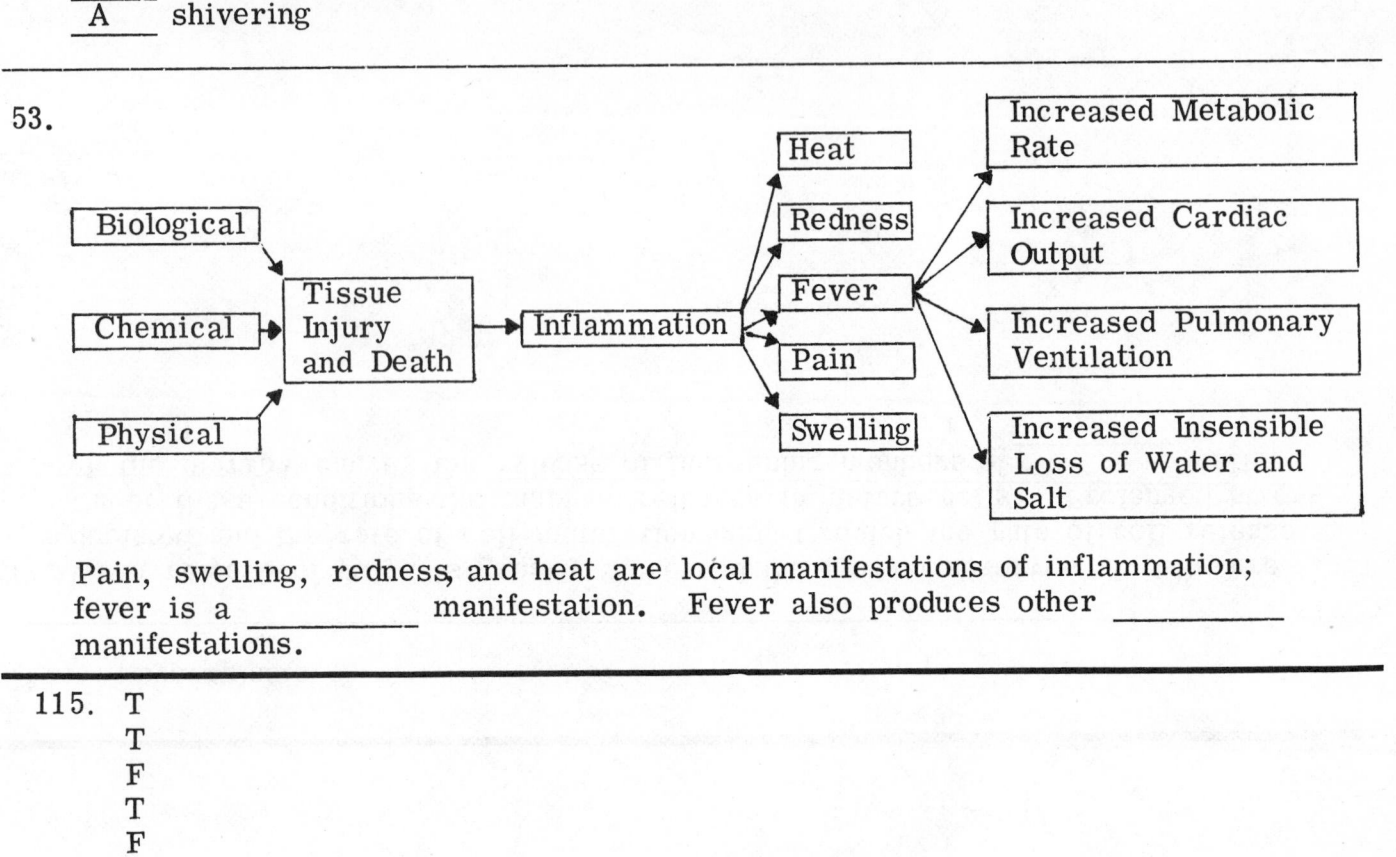

Pain, swelling, redness, and heat are local manifestations of inflammation; fever is a __________ manifestation. Fever also produces other __________ manifestations.

---

115. T
T
F
T
F
T

D. Lymphadenitis (11 frames)

When you complete this section, you will be able to select correct responses relating to the:

1. definition, mechanism, and manifestations of lymphadenitis.

116. Under normal conditions, the efflux of substances from the capillaries into interstitial space exceeds the influx from interstitial space into the capillaries. The excess fluid and molecules enter the lymphatics and return to the blood. During inflammation, the accelerated loss of fluid and protein from the blood vessels causes a great increase in the uptake of these substances by the lymphatics. INDICATE "T" TRUE OR "F" FALSE:

___ The increased blood flow to an inflamed area is associated with an increased lymph flow.
___ The lymphatics do not resorb proteins which leave the blood vessels under normal conditions.
___ Much of the protein lost from capillaries and venules during exudation is recovered by the lymphatics.
___ Obstruction of lymph flow under normal conditions can cause complications such as elephant scrotum.

13. If you are outside on a cold day and your body temperature starts to drop, the vessels near the skin will constrict; if body temperature is still too low, you will begin to shiver.

---

14. Shivering is involuntary twitching or quivering of the muscles. Shivering increases the __________ activity of the muscles and __________ heat production.

---

77. immature

---

78. As polys mature, their nuclei become increasingly segmented. The young neutrophil has a rod-like nucleus that is curved or bent. These are called stab or band neutrophils. Which neutrophil is the most immature?

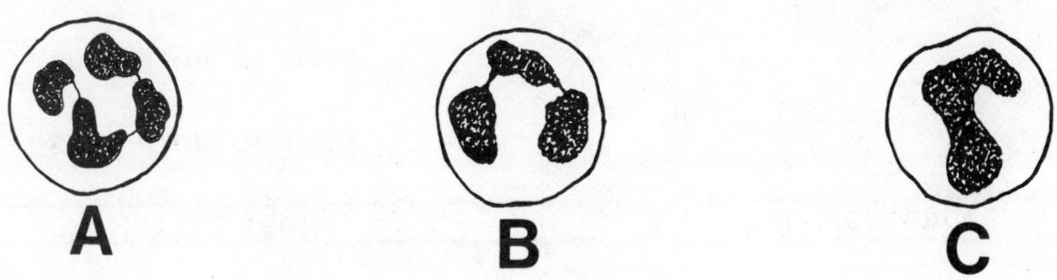

51. vasodilation

---

52. MATCH THE FOLLOWING (letters may be used more than once):

___ goose pimples	A. cold stage
___ drenching sweat	B. hot stage
___ chattering teeth	C. defervescence
___ sensation of cold	
___ sensation of heat	
___ shivering	

---

114. Lab. abnormality — Lab. abnormality
Lab. abnormality — Lab. abnormality
Symptom — Symptom

---

115. INDICATE "T" TRUE OR "F" FALSE:

	frame reference
___ Elevated fibrinogen and γ-globulin levels may be manifestations of inflammation.	100, 105
___ Increased antibody production is associated with elevated γ-globulin level.	100
___ ESR is a measure of the rate at which red cells form clots.	106
___ ESR is linearly related to fibrinogen concentration.	109
___ Fibrinogen levels are often used in diagnosis.	112
___ Leukocytosis and increased ESR often occur together.	114

14. Shivering is involuntary twitching or quivering of the muscles. Shivering increases the metabolic activity of the muscles and increases heat production.

15. Vasoconstriction of the superficial vessels reduces the volume of blood close to the surface of the body and thus __________ heat loss.

78.

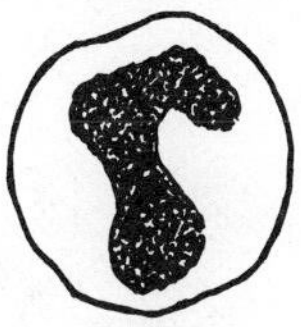

C

79. The age of a granulocyte can be roughly determined by the number and configuration of the nuclear lobes. The appearance of large numbers of immature polys indicates that:

a) an acute inflammation is beginning.

b) inflammation has been continuing for some time.

50. hot

---

51. When the drop in body temperature is abrupt, there is an intense subjective impression of heat and copious sweating. If the drop in temperature is more gradual, it is accomplished by __________ alone.

---

113. We suspect pregnancy.

---

114. INDICATE WHETHER THE FOLLOWING SYSTEMIC MANIFESTATIONS OF INFLAMMATION ARE SYMPTOMS, SIGNS, OR LAB ABNORMALITIES:

___ negative nitrogen balance

___ acidosis

___ malaise

___ increased ESR

___ leukocytosis

___ headache

15. reduces (decreases)

---

16. MATCH THE FOLLOWING:

____shivering	A. A physiologic mechanism to reduce heat loss
____vasoconstriction	B. A physiologic mechanism to increase heat production.

---

79. b)

80.

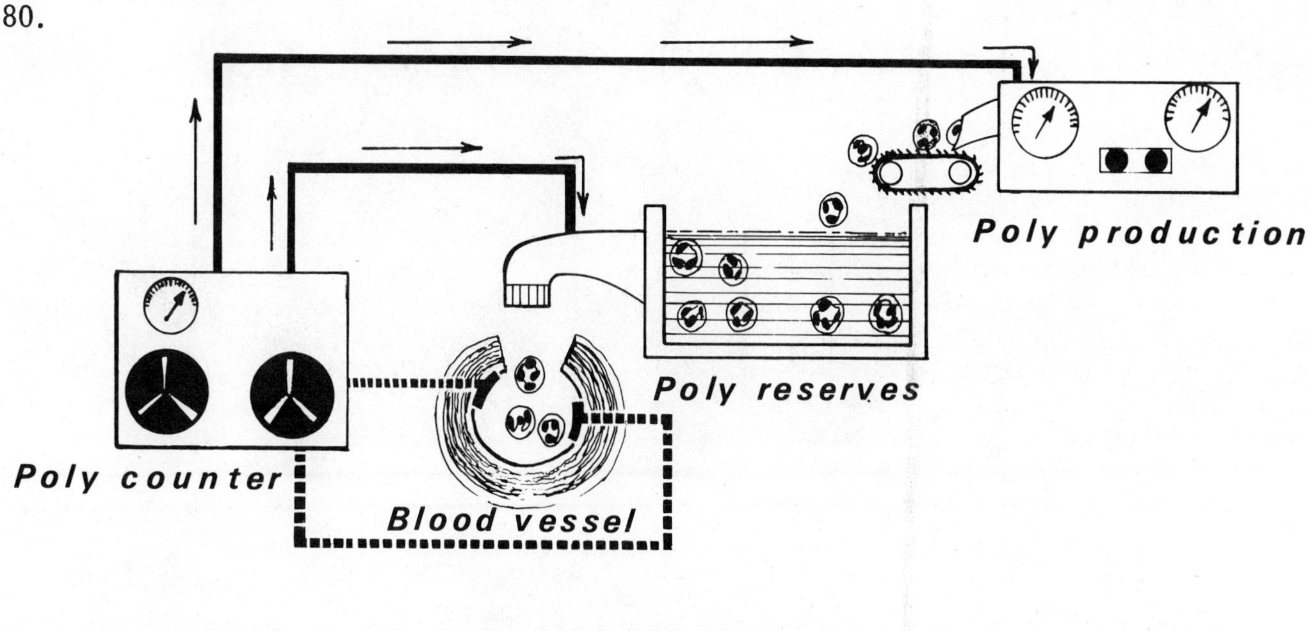

Two mechanisms are responsible for leukocytosis. They are:

1. ____.

2. ____.

49. vasodilation

---

50. Due to elevated body temperature and increased vasodilation, the individual feels __________ during fastigium.

---

112. ESR

---

113. An 18-year-old woman has an elevated ESR, normal white cell count, normal γ-globulin, normal temperature. She complains of "a tired feeling." WHICH DO YOU THINK IS MOST LIKELY?

___ She probably suffers from chronic infection.

___ She is probably pregnant.

16. B
A

---

17. If the body is too warm, the thermoregulatory center increases heat loss by:
1) vasodilation, primarily of small, superficial vessels;
2) sweating, if vasodilation is insufficient to lower body temperature.

Vigorous exercise raises central body temperature, which causes __________ of the superficial blood vessels. If this does not cool the body sufficiently, it is followed by __________.

---

80. 1. Release of more polys from reserves.
2. Increased production of polys.

---

81. The stimulus to leukocytosis in inflammation is poorly understood. At present there is evidence for two possible mechanisms:

1. A polypeptide, called leukocytosis-promoting factor (LPF), is present in inflammatory exudates and causes striking leukocytosis.

2. Disintegrating polys release a substance which stimulates the bone marrow.

It is very possible that these two mechanisms are the same and that the substance released from disintegrating polys is __________.

48. constant
    loss

---

49. In the hot phase, increased heat loss is not usually accomplished by sweating but by increased cutaneous __________.

---

111. No.

---

112. Fibrinogen levels are difficult to measure, so __________ is often measured instead.

17. Vigorous exercise raises central body temperature, which causes dilation of the superficial blood vessels. If this does not cool the body sufficiently, it is followed by sweating.

---

18. The manifestations of capillary dilation are:

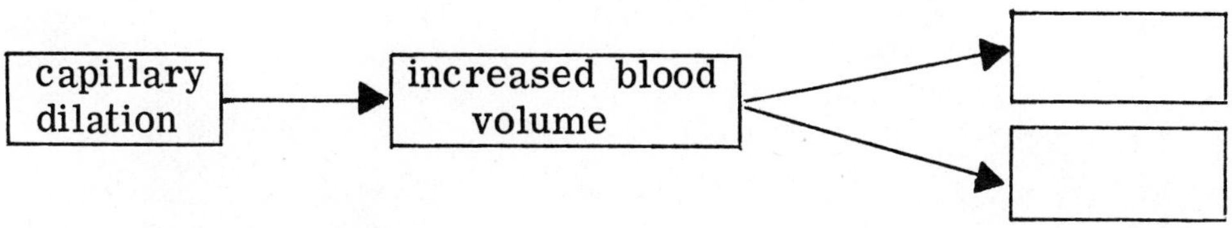

---

81. LPF (leukocytosis-promoting factor)

---

82. It has been demonstrated that injection of LPF will promote leukocytosis, but it is not certain that this is the primary mechanism. However, as soon as the number of circulating polys begins to drop, the bone marrow is stimulated. INDICATE THE DIRECT MECHANISMS OF LEUKOCYTOSIS BELOW:

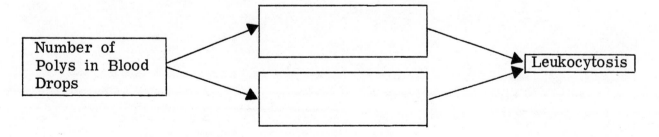

47. increases

---

48. Since body temperature remains __________ during fastigium, increased heat production must be balanced by increased heat __________.

---

110. Increased ESR in acute inflammation is primarily due to elevated fibrinogen. Increased ESR in chronic inflammation is primarily due to elevated γ-globulin.

---

111. ESR is increased with pregnancy, malignant tumors, rheumatic fever, and acute and chronic inflammation. Is an increase in ESR always associated with inflammation?

18. 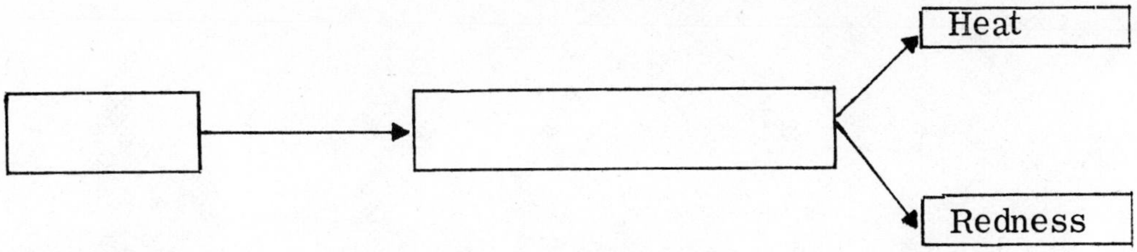

19. Vaporization of sweat from the body surface removes body heat. A certain amount of water is vaporized at all times. This insensible water loss normally contributes very little to body cooling; however, when vasodilation is insufficient to cool the body, sweating begins, increasing vaporization and heat ________.

82. 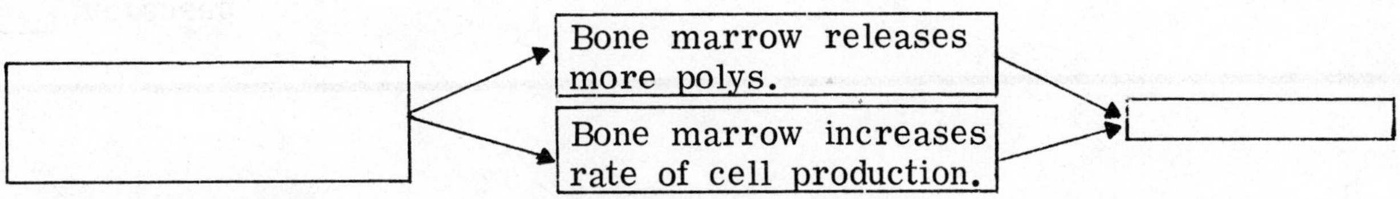

83. The number of polys in the blood drops temporarily in inflammations, especially infections, because they die in great numbers in the tissues. FILL IN THE DIAGRAM BELOW:

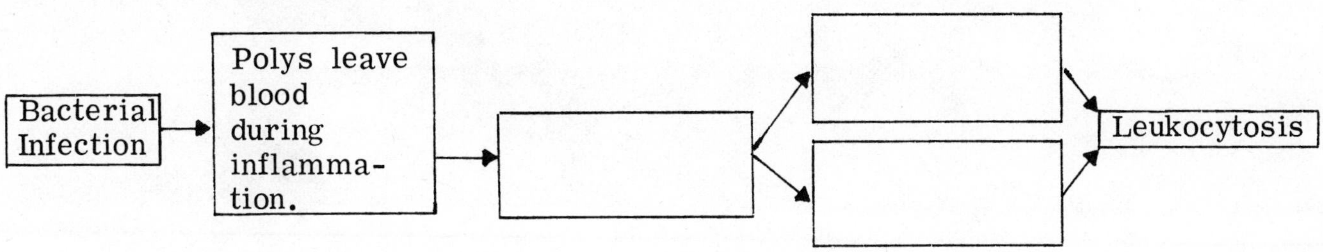

46. falls

---

47. During fastigium, or the hot stage, temperature is maintained at a high level. Heat production is increased over normal levels--not by shivering but by the acceleration of metabolism caused by increased body temperature. An increase in body temperature increases metabolic rate and an increase in metabolic rate further __________ body temperature.

---

109. ☑ increased

---

110. Increased ESR in acute inflammation is primarily due to elevated __________.

Increased ESR in chronic inflammation is primarily due to elevated __________.

19. loss

20. WHICH BOX(ES) INDICATE CORRECT RESPONSES?

	vessels increase in diameter	vessels decrease in diameter	heat loss increases	heat loss decreases
Vasoconstriction	☐	☐	☐	☐
Vasodilation	☐	☐	☐	☐

83.

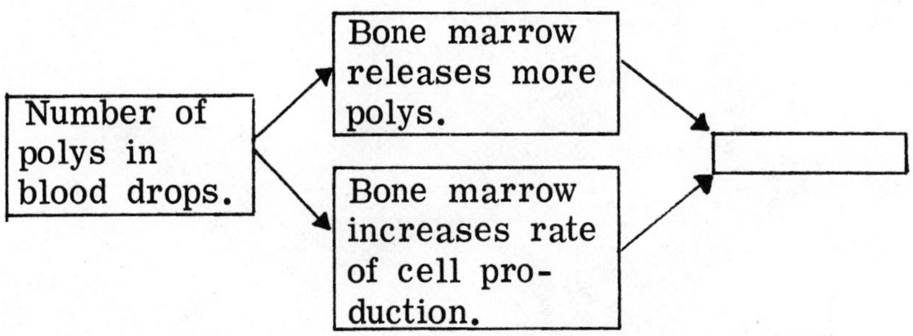
Number of polys in blood drops.
Bone marrow releases more polys.
Bone marrow increases rate of cell production.

84. Although leukocytosis commonly means an increase in the number of circulating __________, it may also mean an increase in number of the other types of white cells.

45. A faster temperature rise creates the sensation of cold. A very fast rise is the result of vasoconstriction and shivering.

---

46. During the cold stage, central body temperature rises while the temperature of the skin __________.

---

108. increased

---

109. Increased concentrations of fibrinogen and γ-globulin make the blood more viscous, which increases the tendency of red cells to clump together and therefore the cells settle faster.

ESR is most often ☐ increased ☐ normal ☐ decreased during inflammation.

20. ☐ ☒ ☐ ☒

☒ ☐ ☒ ☐

---

21. If the superficial blood vessels are constricted, ☐ less ☐ more blood is near the body surface and, therefore, ☐ less ☐ more heat is lost to the surroundings.

When the superficial vessels are dilated, ☐ less ☐ more blood is near the body surface and, thus, ☐ less ☐ more heat is lost.

---

84. neutrophils

---

85. A differential leukocyte count is the enumeration of the relative percentages of the various types of white blood cells as seen in stained films of peripheral blood. A differential count gives information about:

a) the number of white cells/cu. mm.

b) the relative proportions of the various types of white cells.

c) both a and b.

d) neither a nor b.

44. increases

---

45. When the temperature rises gradually, it is probably due to unnoticed vasoconstriction. A faster temperature rise creates the sensation of __________. A very fast rise is the result of __________ and __________.

---

107. b)

---

108. An increase in ESR means that erythrocytes settle out of the blood at an __________ rate.

21. If the superficial blood vessels are constricted, [✓] less blood is near the body surface and, therefore, [✓] less heat is lost to the surroundings.

When the superficial vessels are dilated, [✓] more blood is near the body surface and, thus, [✓] more heat is lost.

---

22. Alcohol causes vasodilation; therefore, someone who has been drinking will feel [ ] warm [ ] cold.

During a cold November football game, you have celebrated each touchdown scored from inside the 10-yard line with a straight shot of scotch and each touchdown scored from outside the 10 with two shots. After the fifth touchdown of the first quarter, you feel __________ because your skin temperature is [ ] increased [ ] decreased, which results in [ ] increased [ ] decreased body heat loss.

---

85. b)

86.

Normal Adult Leukocyte Values

	Minimum	Average	Maximum	Percentage
Total WBC	5,000	7,000 - 8,000	10,000	100%
Neutrophils	3,000	4,000 - 4,500	7,000	50-70%
Eosinophils	50	200	400	1-4%
Basophils	0	25	100	0-1%
Lymphocytes	1,500	2,000	3,000	25-40%
Monocytes	200	400	800	3-8%

Which cell is about ten times as common as eosinophils?
Which cell is about twice as common as eosinophils?
Which cell is about ten times as common as monocytes?
Which cell is about twice as common as lymphocytes?

43. reduced

---

44. In cases where the temperature rises very fast, as in malaria, shivering begins and __________ heat production.

---

106. b)

---

107. Anticoagulant is added to the whole blood in an ESR test to:

a) speed up sedimentation.

b) prevent clot formation.

22. [✓] warm

After the fifth touchdown of the first quarter, you feel warm because your skin temperature is [✓] increased, which results in [✓] increased body heat loss.

---

23. MATCH THE FOLLOWING:

___ vasoconstriction	A. produces heat
___ sweating	B. reduces heat loss
___ shivering	C. increases heat loss
___ vasodilation	
___ metabolic activity	

---

86. lymphocytes
monocytes
neutrophils
neutrophils

---

87. MATCH THE FOLLOWING:

% of normal total white count	Cell type
___ 3%	A. neutrophils
___ 6%	B. eosinophils
___ 30%	C. monocytes
___ 60%	D. lymphocytes

42. reduces
    raises

---

43. When the temperature rise is abrupt, there is a subjective sensation of cold as blood flow near the body surface is greatly ________.

---

105. inflammation

---

106. Erythrocyte sedimentation rate (ESR) is a measure of how rapidly red cells form a packed column in a tube of whole blood with an anticoagulant added. ESR is a measure of:

a) the density of the red cell precipitate.

b) the rate at which red cells settle out of the blood.

c) the rate at which red cells form a clot.

23. B vasoconstriction
C sweating
A shivering
C vasodilation
A metabolic activity

24.

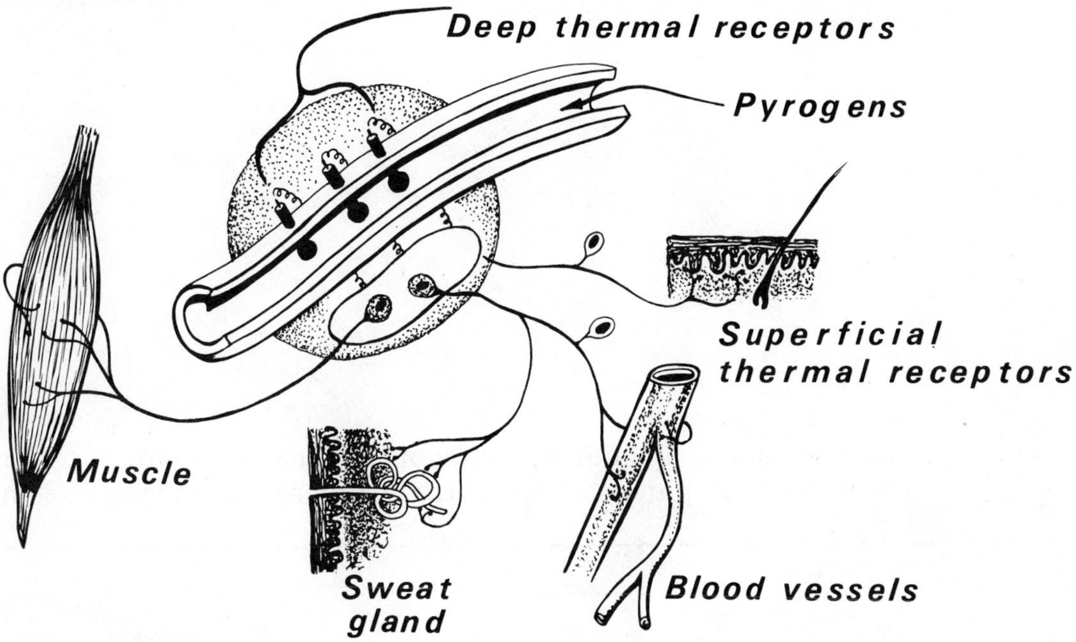

The thermoregulatory center responds to three different types of stimuli:

1) Blood temperature is monitored by deep thermal receptors in the hypothalamus.
2) Chemical agents called pyrogens from cells or bacteria affect the thermoregulatory center.
3) Surface body temperature is monitored by superficial thermal receptors.

When the body surface is cooled, superficial ________________ are stimulated and send afferent impulses to the ______________, which sends efferent impulses to blood vessels, causing ____________. If this is insufficient to maintain body temperature, muscles are stimulated, causing ____________________.

---

87. B. eosinophils 3%
C. monocytes 6%
D. lymphocytes 30%
A. neutrophils 60%

---

88. Some specific inflammatory states are associated with increased percentages of specific white cell types other than polys. Eosinophils often increase in number during parasitic infections and allergic states; a rise in the percentage of lymphocytes is associated with whooping cough and mononucleosis; and monocytes may increase up to 15% of the total during typhoid fever. In these cases, the ☐ white cell count ☐ differential count may be of diagnostic value.

41. C defervescence   A onset   B fastigium

---

42. The first sign of the onset of a fever is cutaneous vasoconstriction, which ________ heat loss and thus ________ body temperature.

---

104. fibrin

---

105. Fibrinogen levels in the blood are often elevated in inflammation. Increased amounts of fibrinogen and γ-globulins in the blood can be systemic manifestations of ________.

24. When the body surface is cooled, superficial thermal receptors are stimulated and send afferent impulses to the thermoregulatory center, which sends efferent impulses to blood vessels, causing vasoconstriction. If this is insufficient to maintain body temperature, muscles are stimulated, causing shivering.

---

25. A man with a complete transection of the spinal cord and sympathetic trunks at level T3 has complete anesthesia below T4. He immerses his body to the waist in a whirlpool bath with a temperature of 45°C. The vessels of his hands show:

a) vasoconstriction.

b) vasodilation.

c) no change.

EXPLAIN.

---

88. [✓] differential count

---

89. The significance of the systemic cellular response is that it makes available increased numbers of leukocytes and, in some cases, increased numbers of a specific type of leukocytes. Increased local need for a certain type of white cells is met by __________ release and production by the bone marrow.

40. B
A
C

41.

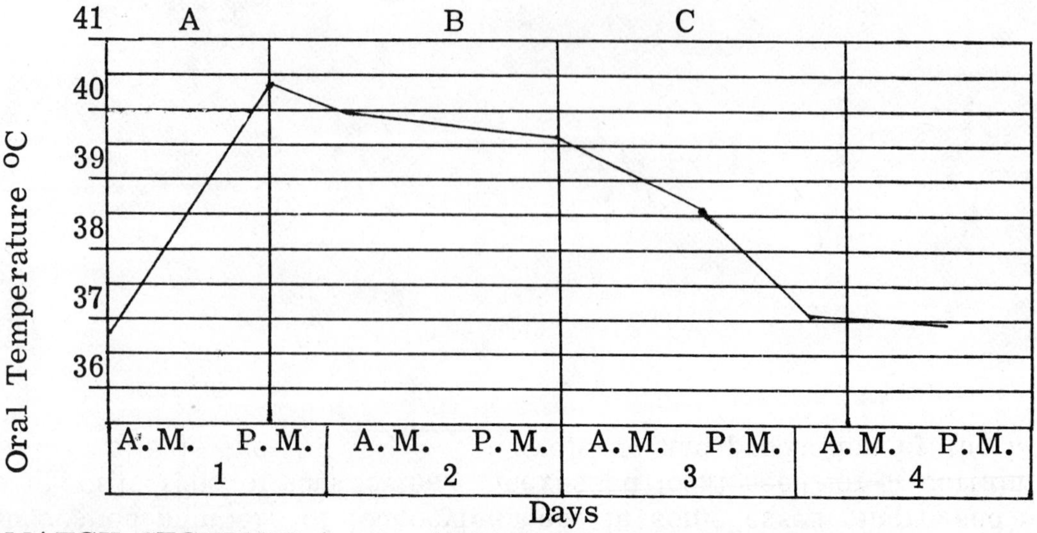

MATCH SECTIONS A, B, AND C OF THE CHART ABOVE WITH THE STAGE OF FEVER BELOW:

___ defervescence ___ onset ___ fastigium

---

103. proteins

---

104. Clot formation often plays an important part in inflammation and wound healing.

Clot Formation

Fibrinogen is the soluble precursor of the clot-forming protein __________.

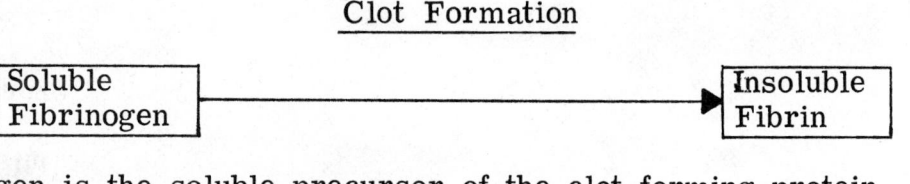

25. b) vasodilation.
The temperature of his blood is raised, stimulating the deep thermal receptors of the hypothalamus, which causes vasodilation.

---

26. Pyro- is a Greek root meaning "heat" and -gen means "producing," so the word pyrogen means __________ __________.

---

89. increased

---

90. Leukocytosis is an __________ in the number of circulating leukocytes, and leukopenia (leuko- in Greek refers to "white (cells)" and -penia to "poverty") is a __________ in the number of circulating leukocytes.

39. higher

---

40. There are three stages in fever. MATCH THE FOLLOWING:

___ onset: cold stage, when temperature is rising	A. heat production = heat loss
___ hot stage: fastigium (fas-tij´ee-um), when temperature is constant	B. heat production > heat loss
___ defervescence: when temperature is falling	C. heat production < heat loss

---

102. increased (elevated)

---

103. Fibrinogen and γ-globulins are both plasma __________.

26. heat-producing

---

27. A pyrogen is a fever-producing substance. The mechanism of pyrogen action is not entirely understood, but in some manner pyrogens affect the thermoregulatory center to reset the balance between heat production and heat loss. A pyrogen mimics the effect of ☐ heat ☐ cold on the hypothalamus.

---

90. increase

decrease

---

91. Leukopenia may develop in certain infections, such as typhoid, tularemia, and many viral infections. It may also be caused by an overwhelming prolonged infection. Conditions of prolonged stress are thought to make the bone marrow progressively less responsive. Can leukopenia be a manifestation of inflammation? Yes or no.

38. polymorphonuclear leukocytes

---

39. When an individual is febrile, his thermoregulatory mechanism behaves as if it were adjusted to maintain body temperature at a __________ than normal level.

---

101. F
T
F
T

---

102. An increase in antibody production is manifested by __________ plasma γ-globulin.

27. [✓] cold

---

28. Pyrogens produce __________ by resetting the body's thermostat at a higher level. When body temperature is rising, heat production [ ] exceeds [ ] equals heat loss.

---

91. Yes.

---

92. A white cell count of 2,000/cu. mm. is __________.

37. pyrogens (or fever)

---

38. Pyrogens are produced by __________ __________, but they may also be extracted from many other tissues, so at present it is difficult to be certain of the sequence of events in the production of fever.

---

100. b)
A certain period of time is necessary for the synthesis of a sufficient amount of antibody to elevate the gamma globulin level.

---

101. Normal Distribution of Plasma Proteins

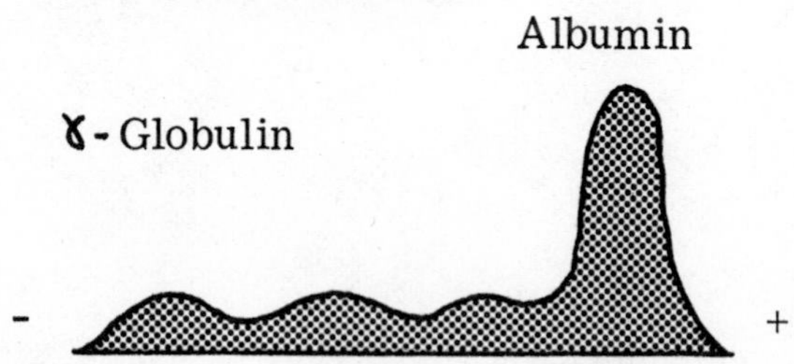

Patient's Distribution of Plasma Proteins

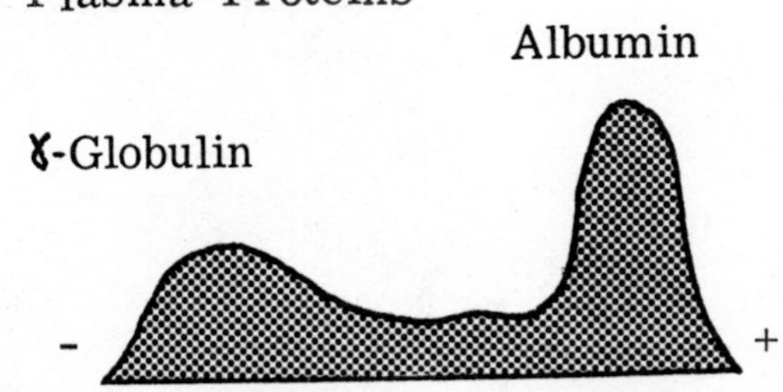

The patient with the plasma protein levels above had a white cell count of 25,000/cu.mm. and a number of immature polys. MARK THE FOLLOWING "T" TRUE OR "F" FALSE:

___ The patient probably has an acute inflammatory reaction to some biological agent.

___ The patient's antibody production is increased.

___ The patient's white cell production is probably normal.

___ The patient probably has an infection which has been continuing for at least several days.

28. fever
[✓] exceeds

---

29. If a patient has a fever which is constant at 39°C his heat production
[ ] is less than [ ] equals [ ] exceeds his heat loss.

---

92. leukopenia

---

93. MATCH THE FOLLOWING: (Of course it is not possible to make a diagnosis on the basis of white cells alone, but make the best choice on the basis of what you have learned.)

____depressed bone marrow due to toxic drugs

____pyogenic infection

____severe allergy

____prolonged severe infection

____parasitic infection of the liver

____acute appendicitis

A. neutrophils 90% of differential count

B. eosinophils 10% of differential count

C. leukopenia

36. [✓] yes

37.

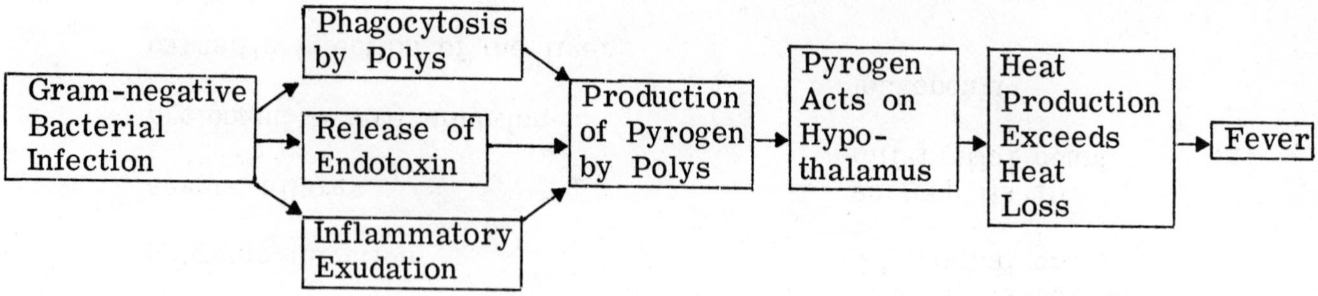

As can be seen in the diagram above, bacteria can cause the production of __________ in at least three ways.

---

99. systemic

---

100. Antibodies are part of the gamma (γ) globulin fraction of blood proteins. An elevation of plasma γ-globulin level is associated with:

a) early stages of inflammation.

b) late stages of, or continuing, inflammation.

EXPLAIN.

29. ☑ equals (If the temperature is constant, heat production must equal heat loss.)

---

30. The thermoregulatory center responds to stimuli from three sources:

1) superficial receptors which monitor the temperature of the __________;

2) deep receptors which monitor the temperature of the __________;

3) substances which cause fever, called __________.

---

93. C C
A B
B A

---

94. MATCH THE FOLLOWING:

___ fever	A. A systemic manifestation of inflammation which often has an important function.
___ leukocytosis	B. A systemic manifestation of inflammation which has no known function.

35. elevated body temperature
1. vasoconstriction
2. shivering

lowered body temperature
1. vasodilation
2. sweating

---

36. Considerable controversy exists over the sources of pyrogens in the various fever-producing states. It is possible that many different substances can act as pyrogens. However, it has been established that polymorphonuclear leukocytes generate pyrogen in response to specific stimuli; so far only gram-negative bacterial endotoxin, phagocytosis, and a factor in inflammatory peritoneal exudates have been proved to do this. Are most bacterial infections accompanied by fever? ☐ no ☐ yes

---

98. F
F
T
T
F
T

C. Increased Serum Gamma Globulin and Erythrocyte Sedimentation Rate (17 frames)

When you complete this section, you will be able to select correct responses relating to the:

1. significance of elevated gamma globulin and fibrinogen levels.
2. definition and mechanism of erythrocyte sedimentation rate.

99. Disturbances of leukocyte number and blood protein levels are __________ manifestations of inflammation.

30. 1) body surface (or skin)
2) blood
3) pyrogens

---

31. WHICH BOXES INDICATE CORRECT STIMULUS-RESPONSE RELATIONSHIPS?

Stimulus	Response: Raise Body Temperature	Response: Lower Body Temperature
Body surface too cold.		
Body surface too hot.		
Blood too cold.		
Blood too warm.		
Pyrogens in blood.		

---

94. B fever
A leukocytosis

---

95. WHICH OF THE FOLLOWING ARE POSSIBLE SYSTEMIC MANIFESTATIONS OF INFLAMMATION?

a) fever
b) alkalosis
c) decreased metabolic rate
d) leukocytosis
e) leukopenia
f) fall in body temperature
g) increased fluid loss
h) negative nitrogen balance

34. elevation of body temperature (not fever)

elevated (increased)

---

35. What mechanisms mediated by the thermoregulatory center cause:

elevated body temperature ?	lowered body temperature ?
1. ______	1. ______
2. ______	2. ______

---

97. T
T
F
T
T
T

---

98. INDICATE "T" TRUE OR "F" FALSE:

		frame reference
___	A large number of mature polys indicates a prolonged leukocytosis.	77
___	As polys mature, their nuclei become less segmented.	78
___	A differential count determines the relative proportions of the types of white blood cells.	85
___	An increase in the percentage of polys accompanies most infections.	88
___	Leukopenia is a white count of less than 10,000/cu.mm.	70, 90
___	The white cell count may drop just before leukocytosis begins.	82, 83

31.

	Raise Body Temperature	Lower Body Temperature
Body surface too cold.	✓	
Body surface too hot.		✓
Blood too cold.	✓	
Blood too warm.		✓
Pyrogens in blood.	✓	

32. An abnormally high body temperature due to a disturbance of the thermoregulatory center is a fever. WHICH ARE CAUSES OF FEVER?

___ body surface too cold ___ blood too cold ___ pyrogens

95. a, d, e, g, h

96.

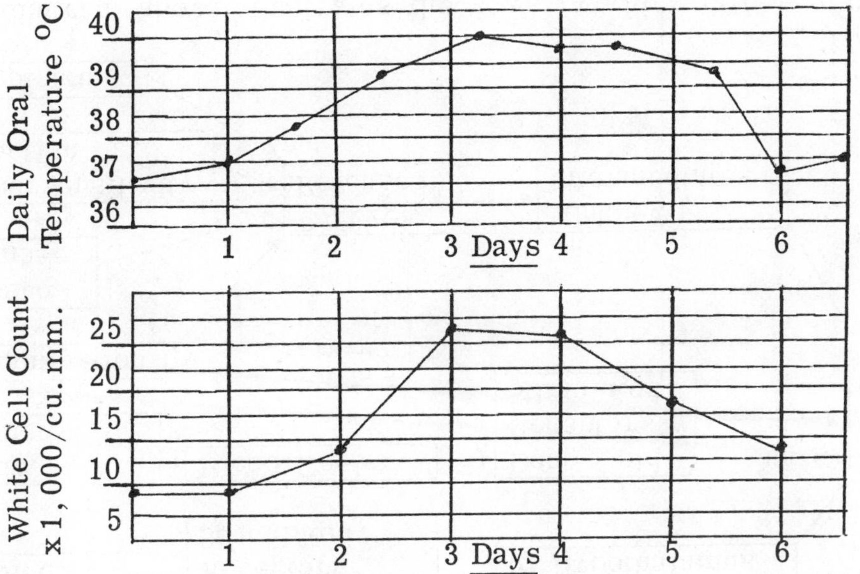

FRAME 96 CONTINUED ON NEXT PAGE

33. No. There are many possible causes of fever.

---

34. INDICATE THE PROPER RESPONSE TO THE BOX ON THE RIGHT AND IN THE BLANK BELOW:

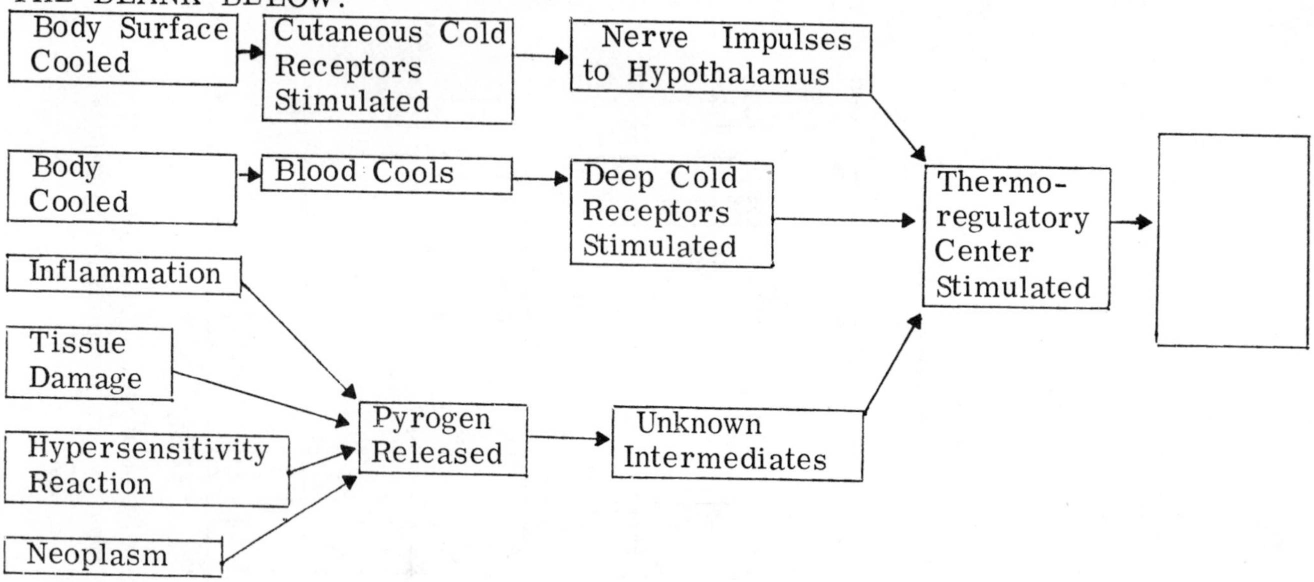

The diagram above illustrates the ways in which different types of stimuli cause the same response from the thermoregulatory center, __________ body temperature.

---

96. F
F
F
T

T
F
F

---

97. INDICATE "T" TRUE OR "F" FALSE:

		frame reference
___	Leukocytosis is a white cell count above 10,000/cu.mm.	70
___	Leukocytosis can be produced by inflammation or exercise.	72,73
___	For every poly in circulation there is about one in the bone marrow reserve.	75
___	Inflammation can stimulate increased release and production of leukocytes.	69,76
___	Leukocytosis is a systemic response which assists the local response.	89
___	In certain infections, leukopenia may develop.	91

32. ✓ pyrogens

---

33. Fever occurs in almost all inflammations lasting more than a few hours. By far the most common cause is infection, but fever may also occur after: 1) infarction (tissue death due to interruption of blood supply; 2) hemorrhage (bleeding); 3) some malignant neoplasms; 4) damage to the thermoregulatory center in the brain; and 5) hypersensitivity reactions such as serum sickness. Does the presence of a fever always indicate that inflammation is present?

TURN TEXT 180° AND CONTINUE.

---

96. (continued)

	Normal % of Leukocytes	% Leukocytes, Day 3
Neutrophils	50-70%	80%
Basophils	0-1%	0%
Eosinophils	1-4%	2%
Lymphocytes	25-40%	15%
Monocytes	3-8%	3%

INDICATE "T" TRUE OR "F" FALSE:

_____ The patient had a chronic infection.
_____ The data are within normal ranges.
_____ The patient had an allergic reaction.
_____ The patient had an inflammation, likely an infection.
_____ The patient had leukocytosis.
_____ The patient had lymphocytosis.
_____ The patient had neutropenia.

TURN TEXT 180° AND CONTINUE.

Unit 7. Necrosis

Unit 7. NECROSIS

OBJECTIVES

When you complete this unit, you will be able to select correct responses relating to the:

	starting page	frame numbers
A. Characteristics of Cell Death	7.3	1-17

1. definition of cell death.
2. structural and functional abnormalities used to identify dead cells and their specificity.

B. Classification of Cell Death	7.37	18-46

1. distinction between cell death due to fixation of tissue, necrosis, physiologic cell death, and somatic death in terms of definition and morphologic appearance.
2. definition of autolysis, situations in which it occurs, and morphologic differentiation from degeneration and necrosis.
3. effect of time and internal and external factors on the morphology of dead cells.

C. Mechanisms of Necrosis	7.28	47-68

1. relationship of the following causes of necrosis to the mechanisms by which they cause necrosis and distribution of the necrosis:

ischemia	systemic anoxia
caustic chemicals	osmotic changes
enzymes	infectious agents
allergic reactions	irradiation

2. definitions of ischemia, infarct, and ischemic atrophy.

D. Classification and Characteristics of Necrosis	7.27	69-110

1. distinguishing features of coagulation necrosis, liquefaction necrosis, caseous necrosis, enzymatic fat necrosis, and gangrenous necrosis on the basis of:
   a) defining characteristics
   b) gross and microscopic features
   c) causative agents and pathophysiologic mechanisms
   d) common sites of occurrence and relation to tissue modifications
2. differences among dry, wet, and gas gangrene.

PRETEST

UNIT 7. NECROSIS

SELECT THE SINGLE BEST RESPONSE.

1. Which indicate(s) irreversible cell damage?
   (A) pyknosis, karyolysis, karyorrhexis
   (B) permeability of the cell membrane to large molecules such as trypan blue
   (C) both
   (D) neither

2. A histologic examination of a section of tissue reveals swollen cells with cloudy cytoplasm, increased eosinophilia, and nuclei pushed peripherally. These changes are most characteristic of
   (A) degeneration
   (B) autolysis
   (C) coagulation necrosis
   (D) liquefaction necrosis

3. Which is LEAST helpful in distinguishing postmortem autolysis from necrosis?
   (A) polymorphonuclear leukocytic infiltrate
   (B) karyorrhexis, karyolysis, and pyknosis
   (C) a zone of congestion
   (D) a grossly wedge-shaped lesion

4. Choose the correct statement concerning a high-power view of the center of a renal infarct compared to a high-power view of a severely autolyzed kidney without necrosis:
   (A) The two views may look the same microscopically.
   (B) Cytoplasmic changes will be more striking in the autolyzed kidney without necrosis.
   (C) Nuclear changes will be more striking in the autolyzed kidney without necrosis.
   (D) The autolyzed kidney without necrosis will exhibit liquefaction.

5. X-rays cause necrosis by
   (A) producing DNA injury
   (B) precipitating cell proteins
   (C) both
   (D) neither

6. A localized slightly soft and slightly yellow lesion in a solid organ has red margins grossly. Microscopically it exhibits autolysis in the center and congestion and acute inflammation at the margins. Which type of necrosis is present?
   (A) coagulation
   (B) caseous
   (C) gangrenous
   (D) liquefaction

7. Macrophages, and epithelioid and giant cells are associated with
   (A) liquefaction necrosis
   (B) coagulation necrosis
   (C) caseous necrosis
   (D) gangrenous necrosis

8. Enzymatic fat necrosis is most closely associated with
   (A) pancreatic necrosis
   (B) fatty metamorphosis of the liver
   (C) dystrophic calcification
   (D) amyloidosis

GO ON TO NEXT PAGE AND BEGIN THE UNIT.

A. Characteristics of Cell Death (17 frames)

When you complete this section, you will be able to select correct responses relating to the:

1. definition of cell death.
2. structural and functional abnormalities used to identify dead cells and their specificity.

1. This unit begins the discussion of a second major category of basic structural and functional changes that occur in the body, namely cell degeneration and cell death. For convenience, the discussion of healing follows in Unit 8. Degenerative changes are discussed in Unit 9.

CLASSIFY THE FOLLOWING:

____ often a direct result of injury to the body

____ disturbances of cell maturation and proliferation, e.g., hyperplasia

____ the absence or malformation and/or malfunction of an organ or tissue due to genetic damage

____ complex cellular and vascular response of the body to injury

A. cell degeneration and cell death
B. inflammation and repair
C. disturbances of growth
D. developmental abnormality

---

1. A
   C
   D
   B

---

2. Cell death is the permanent cessation of the vital function of the cell (such as respiration, synthesis of enzymatic and structural protein, and maintenance of osmotic and chemical homeostasis).

   Cell degeneration refers to abnormal changes in cells which are potentially reversible.

   The distinction between cell degeneration and cell death is based on demonstrating whether or not the changes are ____________________.

---

57. b
c

---

58. Carbon monoxide produces systemic anoxia by competitively inhibiting the oxygen-carrying capacity of hemoglobin. Cyanide directly poisons the respiratory function of cells throughout the body. Both of the poisons kill people so fast that the morphologic changes of cell death do not have time to develop.

In contrast, aldehydes and caustic chemicals, such as strong acids and bases, produce immediate local effects by precipitating cell proteins.

MATCH THE FOLLOWING CASES WITH THE POSSIBLE CAUSES:

____ a child ingests a substance which produces severe patchy necrosis of lining of the esophagus and stomach

____ a child ingests a substance and dies almost immediately; no lesions are found at autopsy

A. cyanide

B. oven cleaner

TURN TEXT 180° AND CONTINUE.

2. reversible

---

3. Since reversibility is a function of change over a period of time, the ultimate distinction between cell death and cell degeneration requires observation over a period of time. Direct observation of individual cell function is rarely possible except in experimental situations. Morphologic observation of cells usually requires fixation, and, therefore, observation of an individual cell is limited to one point in time.

MATCH THE FOLLOWING:

____basis for ultimate distinction between cell degeneration and cell death, but not usually practical to measure at cellular level

____practical to observe at the cellular level, but may not be sufficient to distinguish cell degeneration and cell death

A. functional changes

B. morphologic changes

---

58. B
A

---

59. The cell membrane is primarily responsible for maintaining osmotic homeostasis. Three mechanisms which may disrupt this function include:

1. exposure to hypo- or hypertonic solutions, which may overcome the cell's ability to control water intake and the cell bursts or shrinks
2. physical trauma, which may disrupt the cell membrane and kill the cell
3. antigen-antibody reactions on the surface of the cell, which may activate, complement, and cause lysis of the cell membrane

MATCH THE FOLLOWING:

____direct exposure to hypo- or hypertonic solution

____occlusion of a coronary artery

____hammering your thumb instead of the nail

____swallowing of lye (strong base)

____lysis of red blood cells which follows administration of a certain drug

A. necrosis due primarily to anoxia

B. necrosis due primarily to protein precipitation

C. necrosis due primarily to rupture of cell membrane

56. A
B
A
A
B

---

57. Certain causes of anoxia which are systemic in nature may act to produce local anoxic effects. For example, shock, which produces systemic anoxia, may result in only selective local effects in the brain, kidney, and liver because of the great susceptibility of these tissues to anoxia.

WHICH IS/ARE TRUE ?

a. Systemic anoxia is likely to affect all organs equally.

b. Systemic anoxia is likely to affect susceptible cells within an organ diffusely.

c. Local anoxia due to occlusion of a vessel within an organ is likely to affect only a localized part of the organ.

3. A
   B

---

4. Certain cellular changes are always associated with irreversible loss of cell function, but a cell may be dead without exhibiting these changes. For example, destruction of the nucleus (except in red blood cells) is associated with permanent loss of cell function; whereas, a piece of fixed "normal" tissue will appear "normal" in microscopic sections but function cannot be restored.

CLASSIFY SOME ADDITIONAL EXAMPLES:

____ sections are taken immediately from various organs of a person who died from hanging

____ an area is observed microscopically in which cells have ruptured membranes and cytoplasmic content is extruding from the cells

A. morphologic change sufficient to establish cell death

B. cells dead but morphologic changes not sufficient to indicate cell death

---

59. C
    A
    C
    B
    C

---

60. Enzymatic digestion may be either the cause or the result of cell death.

MATCH THE FOLLOWING:

____ Enzymes released from clostridia in gas gangrene cause an advancing wave of cell lysis.

____ The center of an infarct gradually develops the cytoplasmic and nuclear changes of cell death.

____ Autolysis.

A. Enzymes causing cell death

B. Enzymatic digestion following cell death

55 B, C, E
A, D, F

---

56. Diffuse anoxia results from systemic lack of oxygen or blockage of oxygen transfer with systemic effects. For example, suffocation and anemia may produce systemic oxygen lack, and carbon monoxide poisoning produces systemic blockage of oxygen transfer.

MATCH THE FOLLOWING SPECIFIC CAUSES OF ANOXIA WITH THE EFFECTS THEY PRODUCE:

Causes	Effects
____suffocation	
____ischemia	A. diffuse effects
____CO poisoning	
____anemia	B. local or regional effects
____vascular occlusion	

---

110. T
T
T
F
T
F

THIS IS THE END OF UNIT 7. TAKE THE POSTTEST ON PAGE xxvi.

4. B
   A

---

5. Cell death is most often initiated by interference with cell function. Morphologic changes take time to develop after loss of function. Immediate fixation prevents the development of these morphologic changes.

   Sometimes cell death may be a direct result of physical injury, such as occurs with crushing.

   Which is/are true concerning the morphologic changes associated with cell death?

   a. They sometimes, but not always, are sufficient to establish that cell death has occurred.
   b. They often are not evident until sometime after the cell is dead.
   c. Fixation prevents development of these changes in cells that have died from anoxia (lack of oxygen).

---

60. A
    B
    B

---

61. Three sources of high concentration of enzymes which can cause necrosis are pancreas, polymorphonuclear leukocytes, and certain strains of clostridial organisms (anaerobic bacteria).

    Pancreatic digestive enzymes may be released locally, with injury to the pancreas and resultant digestion of pancreas and adjacent tissues.

    Polys may be called upon to digest tissue which is already dead, such as the edge of an infarct; on the other hand, when large numbers of polys are attracted by pyogenic bacteria, their enzymes may kill healthy tissue in the process of fighting the bacteria. In gas gangrene, the anaerobic clostridia grow only in dead tissue, but they liberate enzymes which spread into and kill surrounding healthy tissue.

    MATCH THE SITE OF ENZYMATIC NECROSIS WITH THE CAUSE:

    ____ adjacent to an injury contaminated by anaerobic bacteria
    ____ adjacent to the pancreas
    ____ in tissue invaded by Staphylococcus aureus (pyogenic coccus)

    A. pancreatic enzymes
    B. poly enzymes
    C. clostridial enzymes

54. B
A
C

---

55. MATCH THE FOLLOWING (LETTERS MAY BE USED MORE THAN ONCE AND MORE THAN ONE MAY BE USED):

____ An elderly man experiences pain in the foot and notices his toes have turned blue. Over the next ten days the toes turn blacker and are sharply demarcated from adjacent normal tissue.

____ An elderly man has noticed the gradual loss of hair on his feet and legs, thinning and scaling of his skin, and decrease in size of his leg muscles, with pain after walking several blocks.

A. Ischemic atrophy
B. Infarct
C. Acute ischemia
D. Chronic ischemia
E. Microscopic sections would reveal overt morphologic changes of necrosis
F. Microscopic sections would reveal imperceptible morphologic changes of necrosis

---

109. T
F
F
T
T
T

---

110. INDICATE TRUE (T) OR FALSE (F):

	frame reference
____ Caseous necrosis typically shows no cell detail or retention of cell outlines.	(84)
____ Caseous necrosis and enzymatic fat necrosis both are yellow and opaque and remain in the body for long periods.	(87, 97)
____ In dry gangrene, tissue is slowly invaded by putrefactive bacteria.	(104)
____ Gas gangrene is highly lethal because of the location of the lesion, whereas wet gangrene is highly lethal because of the self-perpetuating nature of the lesion.	(106)
____ Enzymatic fat necrosis is pathognomonic of pancreatic necrosis.	(97)
____ Gangrene is a spreading infection due to aerobic bacteria.	(100)

5. a, b, and c are true.

---

6. Cell death is defined ▱ functionally ▱ morphologically.

A pathologist most often identifies cell death ▱ functionally ▱ morphologically.

Cell death is ______________________________________.

---

61. C
A
B

---

62. Irradiation (and some anti-cancer drugs, such as nitrogen mustard) block DNA synthesis and thus have their greatest necrotizing effect on rapidly dividing cells such as some types of tumor cells, bone marrow cells, and the epithelial cells of the small intestine. Tissues which turn over at a slow rate, such as connective tissue, muscle, and brain, are not greatly affected except by very high doses of irradiation.

Which of the following are likely outcomes following exposure to x-rays in the appropriate area?

____ myocardial necrosis
____ mental retardation
____ anemia, leukopenia, and thrombocytopenia
____ diarrhea
____ necrosis of stromal tissue
____ necrosis within a malignant neoplasm

Irradiation ▱ does ▱ does not block cell proliferation.

53. Necrosis is the abnormal death of cells or groups of cells within the living body.
Ischemia is local or regional anoxia due to a functional and/or mechanical interference with blood flow.
An infarct is a localized area of ischemic necrosis.
Ischemic atrophy is the reduction in organ size due to ischemia but without overt evidence of necrosis.

---

54. CLASSIFY THE FOLLOWING EXAMPLES:

____The cytoplasm of most renal proximal tubule epithelial cells is eosinophilic, and nuclei are pyknotic or karyolytic. Gomeruli, distal tubules, connective tissue, and medulla appear normal. Grossly, the renal cortex is swollen and pale and the kidney is 25% heavier than normal.	A. infarct B. selective diffuse necrosis of one tissue component
____The upper pole of the kidney contains a wedge-shaped area with base at the renal capsule. Within this area, all cell detail is lost but cell outlines are retained. Other than this lesion, the kidney is grossly normal in appearance and the weight is normal.	C. ischemic atrophy
____The kidney tubules are all somewhat dilated, and the lining epithelium is thin. The amount of cortex appears reduced both grossly and microscopically. The kidney is one-half normal weight, and an atherosclerotic plaque occludes three-fourths of the lumen of the main renal artery.	

---

108. A, B, C
A
C
A

---

109. INDICATE TRUE (T) OR FALSE (F):

	frame reference
____An infarct is due to ischemia.	(52)
____All instances of ischemic necrosis are infarcts.	(52)
____Abscesses and enzymatic fat necrosis both are associated with a severe polymorphonuclear leukocytic reaction.	(97)
____Enzymatic fat necrosis always occurs in or near the pancreas.	(97)
____Coagulation necrosis is characterized by loss of cell detail with retention of cell outlines and coagulated intracellular protein.	(69)
____Brain infarcts are associated with liquefaction necrosis.	(82)

6. [✓] functionally
[✓] morphologically
Cell death is the permanent cessation of the vital functions of the cell. (or equivalent)

---

7. One can look at a microscopic section and determine which cells were undergoing irreversible changes and which were undergoing reversible changes before the time of fixation. With rare exceptions (e.g., red blood cells), the nucleus is a vital part of a cell, and, of course, the contents of the cell must be contained within an intact cell membrane.

Many changes in the cytoplasm of a cell can be repaired.

Which of the following are proof of cell death?

a. swelling of the cytoplasm
b. lysis of the nucleus
c. compacting of cytoplasm
d. rupture of cell membrane
e. granules in cytoplasm

---

62. _✓_ anemia, leukopenia, and thrombocytopenia
_✓_ necrosis within a malignant neoplasm
_✓_ diarrhea

Irradiation [✓] does block cell proliferation.

---

63. MATCH THE FOLLOWING:

Cause of Necrosis		Mechanism of Necrosis
____ ischemia	A.	injury to the pancreas
____ caustic chemicals	B.	protein precipitation
____ osmotic changes	C.	anoxia
____ enzymatic digestion	D.	rupture of cell membranes
____ irradiation	E.	blocking of DNA synthesis

52. 1. a. infarct

2. b. selective necrosis of most susceptible tissue element
Systemic anoxia does not directly produce infarcts.
Theoretically, systemic anoxia could produce atrophy, but this is not a common association.

---

53. DEFINE:

necrosis ______________________________

ischemia ______________________________

infarct ______________________________

ischemic atrophy ______________________________

---

107. C
A
B
C
A, B

---

108. MATCH THE FOLLOWING:

____anaerobic organisms	A. dry gangrene
____extremity with slow development of lesion	B. wet gangrene
____self-perpetuating due to toxin production	C gas gangrene
____not likely directly to kill the patient	

7. b. lysis of the nucleus
   d. rupture of cell membrane

---

8. The process of cell degeneration (reversible) to cell death (irreversible) is often a continuum. Since the cytoplasmic changes of degeneration often precede cell death, cytoplasmic changes ☐ would ☐ would not be present when changes of cell death develop and ☐ would ☐ would not be helpful in distinguishing cell death from cell degeneration. Nuclear changes ☐ would ☐ would not be helpful in distinguishing cell degeneration from cell death.

---

63. C
    B
    D
    A
    E

---

64. MATCH THE FOLLOWING:

Distribution of Necrosis	Cause of Necrosis
____ in or near the pancreas	A. ischemia
____ exposed areas composed of rapidly dividing cells	B. caustic chemicals
____ in locale of blood supply	C. x-irradiation
____ adjacent to a contaminated area of tissue necrosis	D. enzymatic digestion
____ on the skin or in upper digestive tract	E. systemic anoxia
____ in neurons and renal tubule cells	

51. A, B
B
C

---

52. Infarcts by definition are due to ischemia. A localized area of necrosis corresponding to the area supplied by an artery is unlikely to be due to another cause.

Selective necrosis of the most susceptible component of a tissue may be due to toxic injury or systemic anoxia as well as ischemia. For example, necrosis of proximal tubule epithelium might be due to shunting of blood from the renal cortex, mercury compounds, or severe systemic anoxia. Selective necrosis of neurons might be due to systemic anoxia or reduced blood flow to the brain or a combination of the two.

Atrophy may be caused by disease inherent within the tissue or disuse as well as by ischemia (usually more regional than local).

1. Which lesion(s) specifically indicate ischemia as the cause?
   a. infarct
   b. selective necrosis of most susceptible tissue element
   c. atrophy
2. Which lesion(s) commonly result from systemic anoxia?
   a. infarct
   b. selective necrosis of most susceptible tissue element
   c. atrophy

---

106. A, B, C
C
A, B
C
A

---

107. With gas gangrene, the dead tissue must be removed quickly to stop the disease. The disease can be prevented by removal of all dead tissue from wounds. During the Civil War, gas gangrene was extremely common in extremities with gunshot wounds, and amputation was used for prevention or treatment. In modern wars, gas gangrene has been prevented and limbs saved by careful surgical removal of dead tissue (called debridement). Gas gangrene can occur in internal organs but is more classically associated with wounds.

MATCH THE FOLLOWING:

____ a rapidly spreading necrosis of an extremity with bubbles in the tissue	A. dry gangrene
____ a sharply demarcated lesion of an extremity which turns black over a period of a few days	B. wet gangrene
____ a dark, boggy, friable, distended, foul-smelling segment of bowel	C. gas gangrene
____ most commonly associated with traumatic injuries	
____ most commonly associated with infarcts	

8. [✓] would
[✓] would not
[✓] would

---

9. The most common sequence of cell degeneration and death within the body is typified by the changes that follow anoxia.

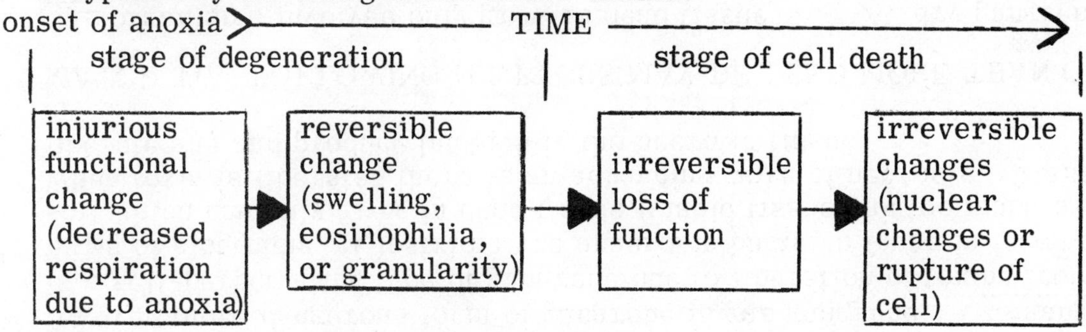

Which of the following is/are true?

a. The morphologic changes of degeneration will be present at the the time irreversible morphologic changes become apparent.
b. Cytoplasmic changes are often reversible.
c. Nuclear changes such as lysis of chromatin are irreversible.
d. Cytoplasmic changes will be present when nuclear changes develop.
e. Cell death and cell degeneration can usually be distinguished by changes in the cytoplasm.

---

64. D
C
A
D
B
E

---

65. Infectious agents (bacteria, fungi, viruses, protozoa, and metazoa) produce necrosis in a variety of ways. In many cases the exact cellular mechanisms are not known. See if you can discover the mechanism of necrosis in some typical examples.

MATCH THE FOLLOWING:

____ pyogenic bacteria attract polys
____ some viruses grow primarily within parenchymal cells of an organ
____ some viruses grow in small vessels and cause swelling and proliferation of endothelial cells
____ a few bacteria excrete highly potent toxins

A. local anoxia
B. compete with the host cell from within
C. cause host to release enzymes harmful to its own tissue
D. need more information to tell how cells are killed

50. B
A
C

---

51. When ischemia produces a localized area of complete tissue death, the lesion is called an infarct. An infarct is a localized area of ischemic necrosis.

There is no uniformly applied name for the selective necrosis of tissue elements due to regional ischemia. In the kidney this is referred to as acute tubular degeneration or necrosis.

Ischemic atrophy is the reduction in organ size due to ischemia without overt morphologic evidence of necrosis. This occurs with mild prolonged ischemia.

MATCH THE FOLLOWING (LETTERS MAY BE USED MORE THAN ONCE):

____infarct	A. localized area of necrosis
____selective ischemic tissue necrosis	B. overt necrosis
____ischemic atrophy	C. imperceptible necrosis

---

105. B
C
A (sometimes B)
B
A

---

106. Wet gangrene is particularly dangerous because the bacteria eat up the tissue, leading to perforation of organs and rapid spread of infection. An even more dangerous form of gangrene is gas gangrene. Gas gangrene is a self-perpetuating type of gangrene due to liberation of toxins from certain types of clostridia. Clostridia are anaerobic bacteria found in feces and soil which can only grow in dead tissue (viable tissue has too much oxygen). When toxin is liberated, there is an advancing wave of necrosis. These organisms liberate gas and produce bubbles in the necrotic tissue.

MATCH THE FOLLOWING (LETTERS MAY BE USED MORE THAN ONCE):

____organisms involved only grow in dead tissue	A. dry gangrene
____specific putrefactive organisms (clostridia)	
____non-specific putrefactive organisms involved	B. wet gangrene
____most rapidly spreading	
____spreads slowly if at all	C. gas gangrene

9. a
b
c
d

---

10. With the light microscope there are three types of nuclear changes that definitely indicate cell death: chromatin clumping, fragmentation of chromatin clumps within the nucleus, and digestion of stainable nuclear chromatin. From the following word derivations LIST THE NAMES WHICH CORRESPOND TO THE NUCLEAR CHANGES ABOVE:

pykno:	"condensation" - from the Greek
-osis:	"process of" - Greek suffix
karyon:	"nucleus" - from the Greek
-lysis:	"dissolution" - Greek suffix
-rhexis:	"breaking into smaller parts" - Greek suffix

chromatin clumping ______________________________
fragmentation of chromatin clumps ______________________
digestion of nuclear chromatin _________________________

---

65. C
B
A
D

---

66. Allergic reactions (altered responses due to previous exposure to various substances) may cause necrosis by damaging the cell membrane, by damaging vessels, by delayed reactions involving lymphocytes with loosening of cells from their neighbors and source of nutrition, and, in extreme cases, by release of histamine with swelling that compromises blood flow or oxygen transfer. MATCH THE MECHANISM OF NECROSIS WITH THE EXAMPLES OF THREE TYPES OF ALLERGIC REACTIONS:

____ Incompatible blood is transfused into a patient. The patient's blood contains antibodies which attach to antigenic sites on the donated red blood cells, activating an enzyme of the complement system, which eats a hole in the red cell.

____ Antigen-antibody complexes lodge in the basement membrane of a blood vessel and initiate an acute inflammatory reaction. Multiple small infarcts result.

____ An organ is transplanted to an incompatible recipient. After a few weeks, many lymphocytes, decreased numbers of parenchymal cells, and a few dead cells are seen in the organ on histologic examination.

A. Ischemia

B. Disruption of cell membrane

C. Delayed cellular hypersensitivity reaction

49. S emphysema
S anemia
I thrombus occluding a blood vessel
I shunting of blood away from the renal cortex
Ischemia [✓] is not always associated with physical blockage of blood vessels.

---

50. Ischemia may have three types of effects, depending on its severity and whether it is local or regional.

MATCH THE EFFECTS WITH THE EXAMPLES:

____shunting of blood away from renal cortex, with death and degeneration of the most susceptible cells (proximal tubule cells)

____occlusion of a coronary artery, causing an area of myocardial necrosis

____gradual loss of muscle mass, atrophy of skin, and loss of hair or lower extremities

A. localized area of complete tissue death
B. selective degeneration and/or necrosis of the most susceptible cells in an organ
C. death of a few cells at a time due to mild alteration of regional blood flow

---

104. [✓] slow, so slow that many authors do not consider this to be a form of gangrene
[✓] unlikely, although the dead tissue should be removed because of this possibility

---

105. Wet gangrene is characterized by a heavy, rapid secondary invasion by putrefactive organisms. It occurs in moist tissues which undergo necrosis and have access to entrance by putrefactive bacteria. The necrosis is often due to infarction but may be due to trauma or other causes. In general, dry gangrene is limited to the extremities. Wet gangrene may occur in the extremities but more commonly occurs in abdominal organs.

MATCH THE FOLLOWING:

____intestine
____brain
____legs
____rapid development and spread
____slow development and spread

A. dry gangrene
B. wet gangrene
C. neither A nor B

10. pyknosis (pik-no′ sis)
karyorrhexis (kar-ee-o-rek′ sis)
karyolysis (kar-ee-ol′ i-sis)

---

11. NAME THE NUCLEAR CHANGE IN EACH DRAWING:

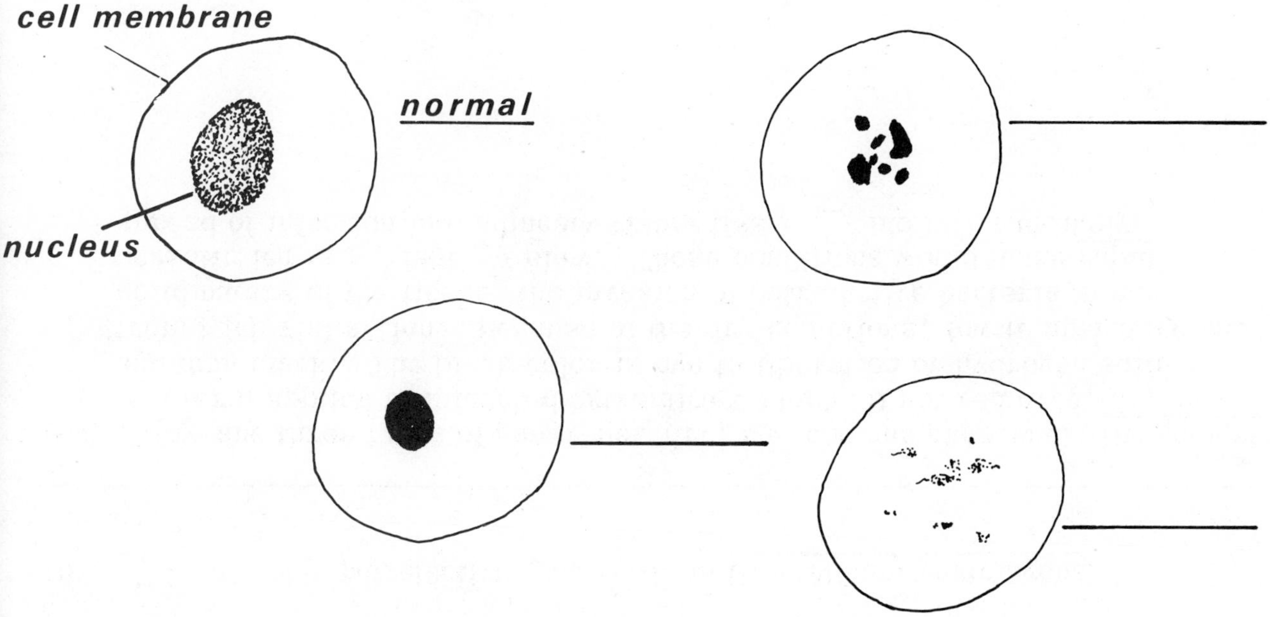

These changes are all ☐ reversible ☐ irreversible.

---

66. B
A
C

---

67. INDICATE TRUE (T) OR FALSE (F):

	frame ref.
____Ischemia is local or regional anoxia due to local or regional changes in blood flow.	(49)
____Ischemia always produces infarcts.	(50)
____Infarcts always are due to ischemia.	(52)
____Necrotic cells are prominent in ischemic atrophy.	(50,51)
____The presence of polys at the margin of myocardial infarct indicates that they are causing enzymatic necrosis.	(61)

48. A
A
B
A
B

---

49. Anoxia can also be classified according to whether it produces systemic (generalized) effects or local (or regional) effects.

Ischemia is local or regional anoxia due to a functional and/or mechanical interference with blood flow.

MATCH THE FOLLOWING:

Cause	Effect
____emphysema	S. systemic anoxia
____anemia	
____thrombus occluding a blood vessel	I. ischemia
____shunting of blood away from the renal cortex	

Ischemia ☐ is ☐ is not always associated with physical blockage of blood vessels.

---

103. ✓ anaerobic putrefactive rods such as Clostridium perfringens.

---

104. There are three types of gangrene: dry, wet and gas gangrene. Dry gangrene is a term applied to infarcted extremities which, if not removed, dry up and turn black. The black color is due to liberation of hydrogen sulfide from bacterial action. Because of the dry conditions, low temperature and solid nature of the tissue, the invasion of putrefactive bacteria into a necrotic leg is ☐ fast ☐ slow. These conditions would make rapid spread of infection into adjacent viable tissue ☐ likely ☐ unlikely.

11. pyknosis
karyorrhexis
karyolysis

These changes are all /✓/ irreversible.

---

12. When pyknosis, karyorrhexis, or karyolysis is seen by light microscopy, the cell is irreversibly damaged. Earlier reversible changes, such as margination of chromatin at the periphery of the nucleus, can be seen by electron microscopy and possibly by light microscopy.

Which is/are true?

a. Karyorrhexis and pyknosis are reversible changes that precede karyolysis.
b. Degenerative changes which precede cell death are easily detected in the nucleus by light microscopy.
c. Changes of cell death are easily detected in the nucleus by light microscopy.
d. Nuclear changes are associated with irreversible functional changes such as a decrease in DNA-dependent RNA synthesis.

---

67. T
F
T
F
F

---

68. INDICATE TRUE (T) OR FALSE (F):

		frame ref.
____	Suffocation, CO poisoning, and severe anemia often produce infarcts.	(52, 56)
____	Enzymatic necrosis is commonly associated with virus infections.	(61)
____	Allergic reactions may produce necrosis by selective damage to cell membranes, by producing ischemia, or by loosening of cells from their neighbors.	(66)
____	Irradiation kills cells by precipitating protein in cell membranes.	(62)

47. A
B
C
C and sometimes A or B

---

48. Lack of sufficient oxygen is the most common cause of necrosis. Anoxia may be caused by interference with any part of the respiratory pathway.
MATCH THE FOLLOWING INJURIES WITH THE OXYGEN TRANSFER PATHWAY THEY INTERRUPT:

Injuries	Oxygen Transfer
____emphysema (increased size and decreased number of pulmonary alveoli)	A. from air to blood
____asthma (contraction of smooth muscle of bronchi)	B. from blood to tissues
____arteriosclerosis	
____collapsed lung	
____thrombus occluding a blood vessel	

---

102. Gangrene is ☑ often secondary to ischemia.

Gangrene ☑ is not likely to develop in a sharp cut due to broken glass (little or no dead tissue would be present).

An infarct of the ☑ intestine will almost certainly develop into gangrene because of access to putrefactive organisms.

---

103. In gangrene the bacteria in the lesion are

____ordinary pyogenic cocci such as Staphylococcus aureus.

____anaerobic putrefactive rods such as Clostridium perfringens.

12. c
d

---

13. Following anoxic injury and degeneration, some cells recover, while others progress from degeneration to cell death. In examining tissue, cells which have obviously progressed to cell death can be identified by nuclear changes.

Some cells which exhibit only degenerative changes (cytoplasmic changes) may also be dead. Sometimes these cells can be detected by special techniques. Two such techniques of detecting early evidence of cell death include (1) the uptake of large colloidal particles such as the dye trypan blue (prior to fixation) due to irreversible damage to the cell membrane and (2) demonstration of severe loss of intracellular enzymes by enzyme histochemical techniques.

MATCH THE FOLLOWING:

____swelling of cytoplasm
____rupture of cell
____eosinophilia of cytoplasm
____leakage of large colloidal particles through cell membrane
____pyknosis, karyorrhexis, or karyolysis
____severe loss of cellular enzymes

A. occurs with cell death but may only represent reversible degenerative change

B. early evidence of cell death

C. late evidence of cell death

---

68. F
F
T
F

D. Classification and Characteristics of Necrosis (42 frames)

When you complete this section, you will be able to select correct responses relating to the:

1. distinguishing features of coagulation necrosis, liquefaction necrosis, caseous necrosis, enzymatic fat necrosis, and gangrenous necrosis on the basis of:
   a) defining characteristics
   b) gross and microscopic features
   c) causative agents and pathophysiologic mechanisms
   d) common sites of occurrence and relation to tissue modifications

2. differences among dry, wet, and gas gangrene.

GO ON TO THE NEXT PAGE

46. T
F
F
T
F

C. Mechanisms of Necrosis (22 frames)

When you complete this section, you will be able to select correct responses relating to the:

1. relationship of the following causes of necrosis to the mechanisms by which they cause necrosis and distribution of the necrosis:

ischemia	systemic anoxia
caustic chemicals	osmotic changes
enzymes	infectious agents
allergic reactions	irradiation

2. definitions of ischemia, infarct, and ischemic atrophy.

47. To some extent, the causes of necrosis can be grouped according to their specific modes of action and their relation to the general mechanisms by which necrosis is produced. MATCH THESE SPECIFIC MODES OF ACTION WITH THE GENERAL MECHANISMS BY WHICH NECROSIS OCCURS:

Specific Modes of Action	General Mechanisms
____ anoxia (lack of oxygen)	A. interference with respiration
____ protein precipitation	B. interference with synthesis or damage to cell proteins
____ osmotic injury	
____ accumulation of certain metabolic products	C. interference with osmotic or chemical hemostasis

101. ✓ infarcted leg
✓ severe traumatic crush wound of a limb
✓ gunshot wound
✓ criminal abortion
✓ infarct of the intestine
✓ necrotizing appendicitis

102. Gangrene is ☐ always ☐ often ☐ rarely secondary to ischemia.

Gangrene ☐ is ☐ is not likely to develop in a sharp cut due to broken glass.

An infarct of the ☐ lung ☐ intestine will almost certainly develop into gangrene because of access to putrefactive organisms.

13. A
C
A
B
C
B

---

14. Cytoplasmic swelling is the most common early degenerative change. It is due to cell membrane changes which allow K^+ to move out of the cell and Na^+ and H_2O to move into the cell. Cytoplasmic eosinophilia occurs later in the degenerative process and persists into the stage of cell death. It is due to movement of colloidal particles, electrolytes, and water out of the cell, with compacting of eosinophilic cytoplasmic membranes (mitochondria and endoplasmic reticulum).

ORDER THE FOLLOWING AS THEY OCCUR IN THE DEGENERATION-CELL DEATH PROCESS. WHICH IS/ARE DIAGNOSTIC OF CELL DEATH?

____ eosinophilia of the cytoplasm
____ pyknosis, karyorrhexis, or karyolysis
____ swelling of the cytoplasm

---

69. In the preceding section, common types of necrosis were considered in terms of causes and mechanisms. This section deals with well-known morphologic types of necrosis which help us to ascertain causes. Many types of necrosis are non-specific morphologically, but the types to be discussed here can be closely related to causes.

Coagulation necrosis is a solid type of necrosis due to coagulation of proteins and is associated with loss of cell detail but retention of cell outlines. The changes within the necrotic area are often predominantly due to autolysis with resultant gradual nuclear disintegration and cytoplasmic eosinophilia.

Coagulation necrosis is associated with ☐ rapid ☐ slow disintegration of tissue.

Outline of the tissue framework ☐ can ☐ cannot be identified in the coagulated area.

45. T
T
T
F

---

46. INDICATE TRUE (T) OR FALSE (F):

	frame ref.
____Enzymes, bile, salt solutions, mechanical damages, and temperature are all factors which affect the rate at which dead cells decompose.	(43, 44)
____Intracellular digestive enzymes produce nearly the same affect on the rate of autolysis in all tissues.	(41)
____Cardiac muscle and connective tissue tend to undergo postmortem autolysis more rapidly than the brain and liver.	(41)
____With normal tissue, autolysis is dependent on the time from removal or somatic death to fixation; whereas, with necrosis, it is dependent on the time from cell injury to fixation.	(36, 37)
____Necrosis and autolysis are easily distinguished by nuclear and cytoplasmic changes.	(35, 36)

---

100. coagulation necrosis
a
e

---

101. Gangrene does not occur spontaneously. The putrefactive bacteria will not invade live tissue because they require anaerobic conditions. Gangrene occurs in areas of necrosis where there is access to contamination from intestinal or soil putrefactive bacteria.

INDICATE THE SITUATIONS IN WHICH GANGRENE IS LIKELY:

____infarcted leg
____the stump of a cleanly severed limb
____severe traumatic crush wound of a limb
____gunshot wound
____criminal abortion
____myocardial infarct
____infarct of the intestine
____necrotizing appendicitis

14. 2 eosinophilia of the cytoplasm (may be present with either degeneration or cell death)
  3 pyknosis, karyorrhexis, or karyolysis (indicates cell death)
  1 swelling of the cytoplasm

---

15. Supplemental frame -- No response required.

Ultrastructural studies of chemical and anoxic injury to cells have provided additional explanation of the classic light microscopic findings in the cytoplasm associated with cell degeneration and cell death.

The early changes which are characterized under the light microscope by enlargement, pallor, and vacuolation of the cell are largely accounted for by swelling of mitochondria and endoplasmic reticulum.

The later shrinkage and eosinophilia result from collapse and denaturation of the eosinophilic membranes that make up mitochondria and endoplasmic reticulum. The dissolution of the basophilic ribosomes contributes to the relative eosinophilia.

Granules may appear at various stages due to intracellular phagocytosis of degenerating cell elements with resultant formation of lysosomal bodies (phagosomes). The ultimate dissolution of the cell may be due to release of lysosomal enzymes into the cell sap and self-digestion of the cell.

Rupture is probably a result of cell death rather than a cause of it.

GO ON TO NEXT PAGE

---

69. Coagulation necrosis is associated with ☐ slow disintegration of tissue. (Autolysis is a relatively slow process; if the process were rapid, cell outline would be lost.)
Outline of the tissue framework ☐ can be identified in the coagulated area (except in very late stages of the process).

---

70. Ischemia is the most common cause of coagulation necrosis. Other forms of anoxia and chemical poisons such as mercury compounds and carbon tetrachloride also produce coagulation necrosis. Heat and caustic substances will coagulate tissue, but in larger amounts they will cause complete disintegration of the tissue (a burn).

Coagulation necrosis is ☐ usually ☐ sometimes ☐ rarely due to ischemia.

Coagulation necrosis can be caused by ☐ ischemia ☐ severe systemic anoxia ☐ toxins and can be ☐ localized ☐ diffuse involving the most susceptible cells in an organ, such as neurons or renal tubule cells.

44. [✓] cells for tissue culture
[✓] mechanical movement [✓] bile [✓] endogenous enzymes
[✓] exogenous enzymes (fixatives will act on live or dead cells equally)

---

45. INDICATE TRUE (T) OR FALSE (F):

	frame ref.
____ Fixation is treatment of tissue with a solution which stops decomposition by finely precipitating tissue protein.	(34)
____ Cell death is an integral part of necrosis, physiologic cell death, somatic death, and fixation of normal tissue.	(18, 19, 20, 21)
____ Autolysis is a factor in determining the morphologic appearance of necrosis, physiologic cell death, and somatic death.	(35, 36)
____ Necrosis is characterized by irreversible changes in the injured cell without surrounding tissue changes.	(29)

---

99. pancreas

---

100. Gangrene is necrosis with secondary tissue invasion by putrefactive bacteria. Putrefactive bacteria are a variety of anaerobes which will not grow in living tissue. They digest the dead tissue, liberating foul-smelling, volatile compounds associated with decomposing tissue. Gangrene is generally, but not always, caused by ischemia and thus appears microscopically in the early stages as tissue with cell outlines but no cell detail in which bacteria are growing.

Gangrenous necrosis is often a subtype of ____________ necrosis.

Which is/are examples of gangrene?

a. an infarcted leg which has turned black and is beginning to smell
b. a septic (infected) infarct of the kidney causes a thrombus containing Staphylococcus aureus (an aerobic bacteria)
c. myocardial infarct
d. acute appendicitis
e. acute appendicitis with thrombosis of appendiceal artery and secondary invasion by anaerobes

16. INDICATE TRUE (T) OR FALSE (F):

		frame ref.
____	Cell death is defined by structural changes.	(2, 3)
____	Functional changes of cell death are easily measured.	(3)
____	The uptake of some colloidal dyes such as trypan blue by an intact cell indicates cell death.	(13)
____	Structural changes of cell death usually precede functional changes that indicate cell death.	(5)

---

70. Coagulation necrosis is [✓] usually due to ischemia.

Coagulation necrosis can be caused by [✓] ischemia [✓] severe systemic anoxia [✓] toxins and can be [✓] localized [✓] diffuse.

---

71. Coagulation necrosis appears as an area of tissue that has lost cell detail but retained cell outlines. MATCH THE FOLLOWING DRAWINGS OF CARDIAC MUSCLE:

A. coagulation necrosis B. normal C. liquefaction of tissue

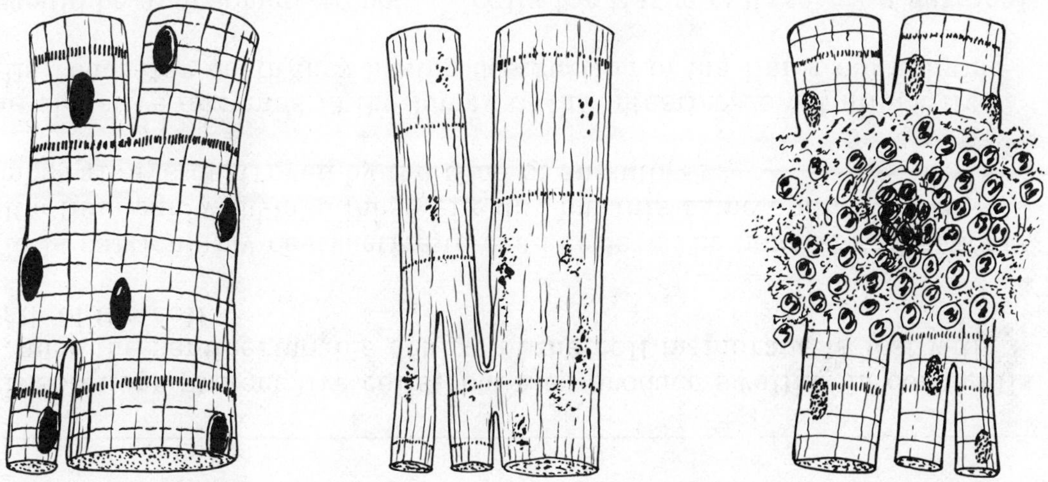

______ ______ ______

43. a
    b

---

44. Salt solutions protect live cells, but they produce swelling in dead cells because the semipermeable quality of the cell membrane is lost with death of the cell.

Bile is particularly destructive to dead cells. The normal gallbladder epithelium can withstand these effects, but this same epithelium is almost always destroyed by the time of an autopsy.

The digestive enzymes in the lumen of the intestine do not attack live cells, but after death they hasten destruction of the lining epithelium.

It would be appropriate to put ☐ cells for tissue culture ☐ a surgical pathology biopsy specimen in balanced salt solution.

In general, live cells as compared to dead cells are amazingly resistant to the action of ☐ mechanical movement ☐ bile ☐ endogenous enzymes ☐ exogenous enzymes ☐ fixatives.

---

98. B
    A
    C

---

99. Enzymatic fat necrosis is generally considered to be pathognomonic of injury or inflammation of the ______________.

16. F
F
T
F

---

17. INDICATE TRUE (T) OR FALSE (F):

frame ref.

____By light microscopy, structural changes diagnostic of cell death are most easily detected in the cytoplasm. (7, 8)

____Structural changes occur first in the cytoplasm of cells that are destined to die. (8)

____All dead cells seen in paraffin-embedded specimens as seen by light microscopy will exhibit "changes of cell death." (4)

____Eosinophilia of cytoplasm indicates cell death. (9, 14)

____Eosinophilia of dead cells is due to loss of water, denaturation of protein, and loss of ribosomes. (14,15)

---

71. B, A, C

---

72. The microscopic changes of coagulation necrosis are the classic microscopic changes of cell death. The rate of the changes varies with the type of tissue, but the sequence of the changes is the same for most tissues. The early changes resemble those of degeneration; late in the process, nuclei may be completely gone and some cells may rupture, with eventual blurring of cell outlines.

CLASSIFY THE FOLLOWING MICROSCOPIC CHANGES OF COAGULATION NECROSIS AS EARLY (E) OR LATE (L):

____swelling and/or eosinophilia of cytoplasm

____complete karyolysis

____pyknosis and karyorrhexis

____some loss of cell outlines

INDICATE WHETHER THE DEVELOPMENT OF COAGULATION NECROSIS WOULD BE RAPID (R) OR SLOW (S) IN INFARCTS OF THE FOLLOWING ORGANS:

____heart

____kidney

____intestine

____lower extremity

42. ✓ a three-day-old area of necrosis in myocardium
✓ a kidney removed and fixed at the end of an autopsy
✓ uncooked sweetbreads (pancreas)
✓ an epithelial tumor of the colon examined one day after removal

---

43. The most common factors affecting the disintegration of dead cells are relative content of enzymes in the tissue and time.

Warm temperature and moist environment promote postmortem changes by increasing rates of enzymatic reactions and providing a good environment for putrefactive bacteria.

Dead tissue which is undergoing autolysis is much more susceptible to damage from mechanical handling than live tissue or fixed tissue. This is much more true for flexible complex tissue such as intestine than for solid, slowly autolyzing tissue such as connective tissue or muscle. Careful handling and rapid fixation markedly reduce postmortem artifacts in intestinal and similar tissues.

Which of the following procedures would reduce postmortem changes?
a. refrigeration of the body
b. embalming of the body
c. humid atmospheric conditions
d. washing the bowel prior to fixation

---

97. A
B
A
C
B
A
C

---

98. Enzymatic fat necrosis should be distinguished from necrosis of adipose tissue (coagulation or non-specific type). Adipose tissue can undergo infarction like any other tissue, but perhaps more commonly it undergoes a non-specific type of necrosis due to traumatic injury. When breast, subcutaneous tissue, or other adipose tissue is injured, neutral fat is released and a reaction of macrophages and giant cells (which engulf the lipid) is commonly found.

MATCH THE FOLLOWING:

A. enzymatic fat necrosis
B. necrosis of adipose tissue, non-specific type
C. infarct

____ A pendulous breast is injured by a mop handle. Sections reveal a focus of necrotic cells, foamy histocytes, and giant cells.
____ The omentum is studded with 3- to 8-mm-size, yellow, opaque nodules.
____ An appendix epiploica (globule of adipose tissue attached to the colon) twists, the resultant necrosis causes the globule to be detached, and it falls into the peritoneal cavity. The peripheral part that is bathed in peritoneal fluid appears normal; the central portion has lost cell nuclei but retains outlines of fat cells.

17. F
T
F
F
T

B. Classification of Cell Death (29 frames)

When you complete this section, you will be able to select correct responses relating to the:

1. distinction between cell death due to fixation of tissue, necrosis, physiologic cell death, and somatic death in terms of definition and morphologic appearance.
2. definition of autolysis, situations in which it occurs, and morphologic differentiation from degeneration and necrosis.
3. effect of time and internal and external factors on the morphology of dead cells.

18. The morphologic study of human tissue is performed on surgically removed tissues or tissue removed at autopsy. In both of these situations all or most of the cells are dead by the time they are examined grossly and microscopically. If left at room temperature, all such tissue will develop morphologic changes of cell death. Fixation prevents these changes. WHICH IS/ARE TRUE?
a. All dead cells exhibit the morphologic changes of cell death.
b. All dead cells will exhibit the morphologic changes of cell death if left unfixed for a period of time.

---

72. E swelling and/or eosinophilia
L complete karyolysis
E pyknosis and karyorrhexis
L some loss of cell outlines

S heart
R kidney
R intestine
S lower extremity

(Remember, muscle and connective tissue autolyze slowly.)

---

73. Coagulation necrosis has which of following characteristics?

____ retention of cell detail
____ loss of cell detail

____ retention of cell outlines
____ loss of cell outlines

____ grossly liquid
____ grossly solid

41. S cardiac muscle
R brain
R kidney tubules

R pancreas
S skeletal muscle
S blood vessel walls
R small intestine

---

42. Another very important factor affecting the appearance of dead cells is time. The most important effect of time is on the degree of autolysis. In attempting to determine the age of a necrotic area, the degree of autolytic changes and the stage of the inflammatory-repair response are evaluated. Postmortem autolysis superimposed on the autolysis associated with necrosis makes this evaluation more difficult.

FOR EACH OF THE FOLLOWING PAIRS, INDICATE WHICH WOULD EXHIBIT THE MOST STRIKING NUCLEAR AND CYTOPLASMIC CHANGES OF AUTOLYSIS:

____ a one-day-old area of necrosis in myocardium
____ a three-day-old area of necrosis in myocardium

____ uncooked T-bone steak
____ uncooked sweetbreads (pancreas)

____ a kidney removed and fixed at the beginning of an autopsy
____ a kidney removed and fixed at the end of an autopsy

____ a fibroblastic tumor examined one day after removal from the body
____ an epithelial tumor of the colon examined one day after removal

---

96. B
A
A
B
A
B

---

97. Enzymatic fat necrosis is a specific type of necrosis occurring in and about the pancreas as a result of release of pancreatic enzymes due to inflammation or trauma. The enzymes digest tissue, converting lipids to free fatty acids, which combine with calcium ions to form soaps. Grossly, this process produces white to yellow, opaque, chalky nodules in the pancreas, retroperitoneal adipose tissue, and omentum. Microscopically, the necrotic area is amorphous and more hematoxaphilic (blue) than other types of necrosis because of the high calcium content. Early lesions have a mild polymorphonuclear leukocytic reaction at the margin, but older lesions have surprisingly little reaction and remain for a long time.
MATCH THE FOLLOWING:

____ solid
____ liquid
____ small nodules in and about the pancreas
____ necrosis due to enzymatic digestion
____ large numbers of polys
____ relatively inert necrotic material with little purulent reaction
____ tissue outline gone

A. enzymatic fat necrosis

B. abscess

C. both A and B

18. b

---

19. In the practice of medicine we are concerned with identifying when cells are dying abnormally within the living body. The term necrosis is used to identify this situation. Necrosis is the abnormal death of cells or groups of cells within the living body. Necrosis does not include death of cells due to aging or death of cells due to removal of tissue from the body.

WHICH IS/ARE TRUE ?

a. All cells dying within the living body are said to be undergoing necrosis.
b. Necrosis cannot occur after a patient has died.

---

73. ✓ loss of cell detail
✓ retention of cell outlines
✓ grossly solid

---

74. Coagulation necrosis by definition is solid, but it is generally softer than surrounding normal tissue, due to some disintegration of the cells. In the early stages an area of coagulation necrosis may be slightly swollen due to swelling of the cells, but in later stages there is usually some shrinkage due to loss of cellular substances. Hemorrhage may be superimposed, making the lesion red; otherwise the coagulated area will become progressively more yellow due to lipid accumulation.

INDICATE WHICH FEATURES MAY CHARACTERIZE COAGULATION NECROSIS GROSSLY:

___ yellow color	___ soft	___ slightly swollen	___ liquid
___ red color	___ hard	___ somewhat shrunken	___ solid

40. Autolysis is the self-destruction of cells (or equivalent).

Autolysis occurs after somatic death, after surgical removal of tissue, with necrosis, with physiologic cell death. (or equivalent)

---

41. The rate at which a tissue autolyzes is affected by various factors, but the most important is the amount of intracellular digestive enzymes the tissue contains. The brain, kidney tubule epithelium, glands that secrete digestive enzymes, and mucosal linings of the small intestine and stomach contain large amounts of digestive enzymes. Muscle and connective tissue contain small amounts of digestive enzymes.

MATCH THE FOLLOWING TISSUES TO THE RATE AT WHICH YOU WOULD EXPECT THEM TO UNDERGO AUTOLYSIS:

Tissue		Rate Autolyzed
____cardiac muscle	____pancreas	R. rapidly
____brain	____skeletal muscle	
____kidney tubules	____blood vessel walls	S. slowly
	____small intestine	

---

95. A
B
B
A
A
B

---

96. MATCH THE FOLLOWING ITEMS WITH THE BASIC TYPE OF NECROSIS WITH WHICH THEY ARE MOST CLOSELY ASSOCIATED:

____abscess	A. caseous necrosis
____granuloma	
____chronic inflammation	B. liquefaction necrosis
____acute inflammation	
____incomplete digestion of dead cells and debris	
____total digestion of dead cells and debris	

19. b

---

20. Physiologic cell death (also called necrobiosis) is the "normal" death of cells within the living body due to aging and "normal" wear and tear of cells. For example, cells of the epidermis as they move outward undergo changes in their cytoplasm followed by pyknosis and lysis of their nuclei, leaving an eosinophilic mass (keratin).

INDICATE WHETHER THE FOLLOWING ARE ATTRIBUTES OF PHYSIOLOGIC CELL DEATH (P), NECROSIS (N), BOTH (B), OR NEITHER (O):

____ occur within the living body
____ may develop after death of the whole organism
____ will exhibit the morphologic changes of cell death
____ morphologic changes of degeneration are likely to precede those of cell death
____ dead cells are likely to occur in predictable locations and predictable numbers
____ dead cells are likely to occur in variable locations and variable numbers, depending on extent and nature of injury

---

74. ✓ yellow
✓ red
✓ soft
✓ slightly swollen
✓ somewhat shrunken
✓ solid

---

75. The site and distribution of coagulation necrosis are dependent on its cause; conversely, the site and distribution often help identify the cause.

Infarction is the most common, important, and distinctive cause of coagulation necrosis. The distribution of infarcts is clearly related to distribution of blood vessels.

Other examples of localized areas of coagulation necrosis include the effects of heat or caustic agents and necrosis in the center of tumors that outgrow their blood supply.

More diffuse types of coagulation necrosis result from selective vulnerability of cells to regional or systemic anoxia or to chemicals which selectively kill certain types of cells. Neurons, renal tubule epithelial cells, and centrilobular hepatocytes appear to be most vulnerable to anoxia. Examples of selective chemical injury include the effects of mercury compounds on renal tubule cells and carbon tetrachloride on centrilobular hepatocytes.

MATCH THE FOLLOWING:

Lesion	Distribution of Lesion
____ centrilobular necrosis of liver due to carbon tetrachloride	A. local in distribution of an artery
____ centrilobular necrosis of liver due to anoxia	B. local at site of injury
____ infarct	C. diffuse, susceptible cells involved
____ burn by caustic agent	

39. Any of the following:

pyknosis
karyorrhexis
karyolysis

swelling
increased eosinophilia
disruption of cell membrane

---

40. Autolysis is ______________________________.

NAME THREE SITUATIONS IN WHICH AUTOLYSIS CAN OCCUR.

____

____

____

---

94. B
A
B
A
B
A
B
A
B

---

95. MATCH THE FOLLOWING ITEMS WITH THE BASIC TYPE OF NECROSIS WITH WHICH THEY ARE ASSOCIATED:

____macrophages and giant cells
____neutrophils and macrophages
____pyogenic bacteria
____M. tuberculosis, fungi
____lung, lymph nodes, bone
____brain

A. caseous necrosis

B. liquefaction necrosis

20. B occur within the living body
O may develop after death of the whole organism
B will exhibit the morphologic changes of cell death
B morphologic changes of degeneration are likely to precede those of cell death
P dead cells are likely to occur in predictable locations and predictable numbers
N dead cells are likely to occur in variable locations and variable numbers, depending on extent and nature of injury

---

21. Somatic death is the death of an individual. It is associated with lack of heartbeat lack of breathing, and failure in brain function. The time of somatic death is legally defined, the time being based on previous observations of circumstances in which recovery is not possible. Usually it is easy to recognize a dead person as one who does not respond to stimuli, is not breathing, and has no heartbeat.

WHICH IS/ARE TRUE?

a. At the time of somatic death all cells in the body are dead.
b. A patient with a heartbeat but no spontaneous breathing, or vice versa, is dead.
c. At some time following somatic death, all cells in the body will die.

---

75. C
C
A
B

---

76. Infarcts are most commonly caused by (1) atherosclerosis, a disease which often causes obstruction of medium-sized systemic arteries, especially those in the heart and brain, but also in arteries of the legs, mesentery, and kidney, or by (2) thrombi (blood clots in vessels) that arise in the legs or pelvic veins and are carried through the inferior vena cava to the right heart and pulmonary arteries, where they lodge and obstruct blood flow. Thrombi may also arise in the left side of the heart and be carried widely to lodge in arteries of the brain, kidneys, spleen, intestine, and legs. (There are many other causes of infarcts, such as accidental surgical ligation of an artery and specific diseases of the vessels.)

Atherosclerosis most commonly produces infarcts of clinical importance in which two organs? ______________________

Infarcts in the lung are most commonly due to ▱ atherosclerosis ▱ thrombi arising in the leg veins.

When infarcts occur in multiple organs, one should look for the source of thrombi in the ▱ leg veins ▱ heart.

38.

	pure postmortem autolysis	necrosis	degeneration
cytoplasmic changes	✓	✓	✓
nuclear changes	✓	✓	
surrounding tissue reaction		✓	

39. LIST TWO NUCLEAR AND TWO CYTOPLASMIC CHANGES YOU MIGHT EXPECT TO SEE WITH AUTOLYSIS:

________________ ________________

________________ ________________

93. C
A
B

94. MATCH THE FOLLOWING ITEMS WITH THE BASIC TYPE OF NECROSIS WITH WHICH THEY ARE MOST CLOSELY ASSOCIATED:

____granuloma
____infarct
____Mycobacterium tuberculosis
____ischemia
____no cell detail or cell outline
____no cell detail but retention of cell outline
____epithelioid and giant cells
____autolysis
____allergic reaction

A. coagulation necrosis

B. caseous necrosis

21. c

---

22. DEFINE:

necrosis ____________________

physiologic cell death (necrobiosis) ____________________

____

somatic death ____________________

---

76. heart, brain
Infarcts in the lung are most commonly due to ☑ thrombi arising in leg veins.
When infarcts occur in multiple organs, one should look for the source of thrombi in the ☑ heart.

---

77. The most common cause of coagulation necrosis is ____________________

Other causes of coagulation necrosis include: ____________________

____

Causes of localized coagulation necrosis include: ____________________

____

Causes of selective coagulation necrosis of tissue elements include:

____________________ ____________________

37. B
A
B
A

---

38. INDICATE THE TYPES OF CHANGES SEEN WITH EACH OF THE FOLLOWING:

	pure postmortem autolysis	necrosis	degeneration
cytoplasmic changes			
nuclear changes			
surrounding tissue reaction			

---

92. C
A
C
B,C
A

---

93. Coagulation necrosis is usually due to anoxia and rarely due directly to a biological agent.

Abscesses are almost always due to biological agents, **most often pyogenic** bacteria. Pyogenic agents are small and difficult to see in tissue sections but are easily and quickly cultured.

Caseous necrosis is caused by microorganisms that can often be seen in tissue sections with special stains, thus permitting early presumptive diagnosis. However, culture is required to prove the identity of the specific organism, but this may take days to weeks.

MATCH THE FOLLOWING:

____caseous necrosis
____coagulation necrosis
____liquefaction necrosis (abscess)

A. no causative microorganisms present
B. causative organism usually identified by culture only
C. causative organism usually identified by special stains and culture

22. Necrosis is the abnormal death of cells or groups of cells within the living body.
Physiologic cell death (necrobiosis) is the normal death of cells within the living body.
Somatic death is the death of an individual.

---

23. MATCH THE FOLLOWING SPECIFIC EXAMPLES WITH THE GENERAL PROCESSES:

____sloughing of stratum corneum of skin
____cessation of cardiac function
____a small myocardial infarct
____a liver biopsy specimen with no abnormal findings
____red blood cells die after 120 days
____small-intestine crypt cells divide and migrate to the top of the villi and are sloughed

A. necrosis
B. somatic death
C. physiologic cell death
D. fixation of normal tissue

---

77. The most common cause of coagulation necrosis is ischemia (or infarction)

Other causes of coagulation necrosis include:
moderate injury due to heat or caustic agents
regional or systemic anoxia, certain chemicals

Causes of localized coagulation necrosis include:
ischemia (or infarction)
heat or caustic agents or tumor outgrowing blood supply

Causes of selective coagulation necrosis of tissue elements include:
regional or systemic anoxia
certain chemicals

---

78. In organs with dual supply, such as lung and liver, or with extensive collateral circulation, such as intestine, blood continues to flow into the necrotic area, producing a hemorrhagic (red) infarct.

In other organs, infarcts take on the yellow color of necrotic tissue except for a zone of inflammatory congestion at the margin.

MATCH THE FOLLOWING:

____heart
____lung
____liver

____kidney
____spleen
____intestine
____leg

R. red (hemorrhagic) infarct
Y. yellow infarct

36. a
c

---

37. In some types of necrosis, autolysis (self-digestion) is responsible for the nuclear and cytoplasmic changes of cell death in the necrotic lesion.

MATCH THE FOLLOWING:

____helpful in identifying some types of necrosis	A. postmortem autolysis
____tends to obscure morphologic evidence of necrosis as well as other processes	B. antemortem autolysis
____associated with necrosis and physiologic cell death	
____associated with somatic death	

---

91. The most important organ involved by caseous necrosis is lung.

The two most important organs involved by infarcts are heart and brain.

The purulent type of liquefaction necrosis occurs in many organs, while the nonpurulent type of liquefaction necrosis occurs in the brain.

---

92. MATCH THE FOLLOWING (LETTERS MAY BE USED MORE THAN ONCE):

____high content of digestive enzymes	A. caseous necrosis
____caused by organisms that are difficult to kill even after phagocytosis	B. coagulation necrosis
____caused by organisms that promote chemotaxis	C. liquefaction necrosis
____may be caused by ischemia	
____allergic reaction involved	

23. C
B
A
D
C
C

---

24. Physiologic cell death is a low-grade continuous process and, therefore, one could expect to see evidence of it ☐ grossly ☐ microscopically in specimens removed ☐ from a living patient ☐ immediately after death.

Necrosis may or may not be visible grossly, depending on the size of the lesion and whether there has been time for development of the cellular changes of cell death. By definition, necrosis ☐ can ☐ cannot develop after somatic death. Somatic death is a gross finding and ☐ can ☐ cannot also be associated with necrotic lesions in individual organs.

---

78. Y heart
R lung
R liver
Y kidney
Y spleen
R intestine
Y leg

---

79. In organs with a tree-like arterial system, such as kidney, spleen, liver, and lung, the infarct will be wedge- or pie-shaped with widest part at the periphery. In the heart, the distribution follows the muscle bundles. The intestine has a segmental arterial distribution, and the leg has a longitudinal distribution.

MATCH THE SHAPE OF INFARCTS WITH THE VARIOUS ORGANS:

____ heart
____ lung
____ liver
____ kidney
____ spleen
____ intestine
____ leg

W. wedge-shaped

N. not wedge-shaped

35. The morphologic changes of autolysis ☑ would be the same as the nuclear and cytoplasmic changes of cell death.

a
b   Autolysis would contribute to the changes of cell death
c   in all of these situations.
d

---

36. Autolysis is the destruction of cells by the enzymes contained within their own lysosomes. When it occurs after somatic death (or after surgical removal of tissue), it is called postmortem autolysis.

Postmortem autolysis, if not stopped early by fixation, can obscure the identification of both normal tissue and lesions.

WHICH IS/ARE TRUE?

a. Autolysis affects diseased as well as normal tissue.
b. Autolysis does not occur in the living body.
c. Postmortem autolysis may obscure the changes of necrosis.

---

90. B
A

---

91. Caseous necrosis is most frequently seen in the lung in association with tuberculosis and systemic fungal infections. In the initial infection there usually is spread of the infection to pulmonary hilar lymph nodes, with development of similar caseous lesions. Less commonly, these infections spread to involve other organs. The organs most commonly involved in secondary spread are organs of the reticuloendothelial system (lymph nodes, spleen, liver, bone marrow), bone, kidney, and meninges. Abscess may involve any organ but is most commonly seen in the skin, head and neck region, lung, and areas adjacent to the gastrointestinal tract and kidney.

The most important organ involved by caseous necrosis is ____________.

The two most important organs involved by infarcts are ____________ and ____________.

The purulent type of liquefaction necrosis occurs in many organs, while the nonpurulent type of liquefaction necrosis occurs in the ____________.

24. [✓] microscopically
[✓] from a living patient [✓] immediately after death
[✓] cannot
[✓] can

---

25. A healthy young person dies immediately from a cardiac arrhythmia (failure in the heart's electrical conduction system) due to an electric shock. If an autopsy were done immediately and appropriate tissue fixed for preparation of microscopic sections, one would find

[ ] gross [ ] microscopic evidence of physiologic cell death
[ ] gross [ ] microscopic evidence of necrosis
[ ] gross [ ] microscopic evidence of somatic death

79.

N	heart	W	kidney
W	lung	W	spleen
W	liver	N	intestine
		N	leg

---

80. A localized area of coagulation necrosis due to ischemia is likely to be red if ______________________________.

A localized area of coagulation necrosis due to ischemia is likely to be wedge-shaped if ______________________________.

34. Fixation [✓] preserves cell structure and [✓] destroys cell function.

---

35. In the absence of fixation, dead cells undergo autolysis even in the living body. Autolysis, which literally means "self-lysis," is the self-destruction of cells. After a cell's function fails, its own hydrolytic enzymes begin to digest it. The morphologic changes of autolysis are the same as those in cells killed by lack of oxygen.

The morphologic changes of autolysis [ ] would [ ] would not be the same as the nuclear and cytoplasmic changes of cell death.

In which of the following situations would self-destruction of cells occur due to lack of fixation?

a. in tissues after somatic death when the autopsy was delayed
b. in surgically removed tissues in which pathologic examination was delayed
c. in tissue which has died in the body from inadequate blood supply
d. in physiologic cell death

---

89. C
B, D
A

---

90. MATCH THE FOLLOWING DIAGRAMS TO THE TYPE OF NECROSIS WITH WHICH THEY ARE MOST COMMONLY ASSOCIATED:

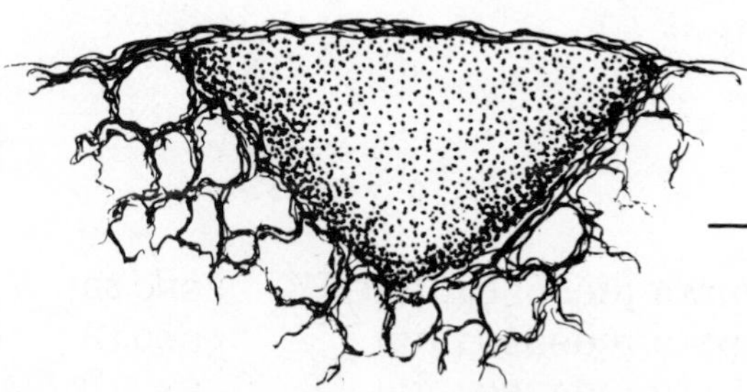

______

A. caseous necrosis

B. coagulation necrosis

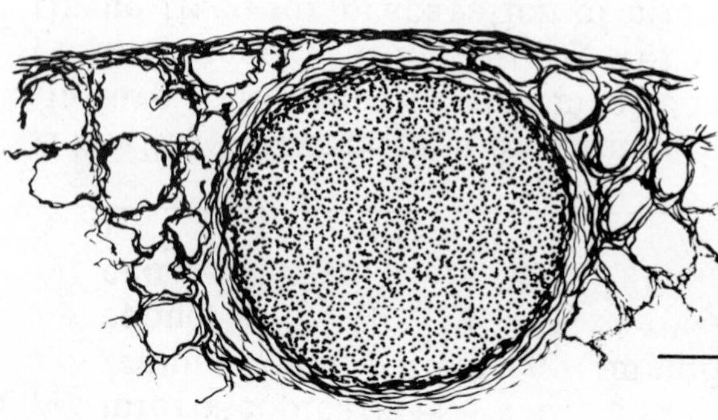

______

25. ☑ microscopic evidence of physiologic cell death
☑ gross evidence of somatic death
Necrosis (localized area of cell death) would not be present, and if it were, it would not have had time to develop so that the changes could be seen.

---

26. The lesions of necrosis are usually localized or multifocal whereas the changes that follow somatic death are diffuse but vary somewhat among tissues. The morphologic changes of cell death in necrosis and following somatic death may be quite similar and are greatly dependent on time before fixation.

Which is most helpful in distinguishing necrosis from changes following somatic death?

____ distribution of the changes ____ microscopic changes in the dead cells

---

80. red if the organ has a dual blood supply or extensive collateral circulation.

wedge-shaped if the organ has a tree-like arterial system.

---

81. WHICH ARE FEATURES OF COAGULATION NECROSIS?

a. rapid liquefaction of tissue
b. commonly associated with yellow, wedge-shaped lesions at the periphery of solid organs such as kidney and spleen
c. may diffusely affect an organ, e.g., selective damage to renal tubules due to poor renal perfusion or poisons selective for renal tubules such as mercury
d. cell membranes are especially affected, resulting in rupture and loss of tissue outlines
e. within an area of coagulation necrosis, connective tissue and parenchymal elements are likely to undergo changes at a different rate because autolysis occurs at different rates in these cells

33. congestion
inflammatory cell response
healing response

---

34. Adequate fixation or the lack of it is one of the most important factors affecting the appearance of tissue visualized under the microscope. Most fixatives act primarily by precipitating and denaturing protein. Thus, they preserve the protein framework of the cell but destroy the semipermeability of the membranes and most of the intracellular chemical functions.

Fixation ☐ preserves ☐ destroys cell structure and
☐ preserves ☐ destroys cell function.

88.

COAGULATION NECROSIS

	Caseous Necrosis	Early	Well Developed	Late
Cell detail maintained		X		
Cell or tissue outlines retained		X	X	"(X)"

---

89. Grossly, a typical initial caseous lesion of tuberculosis or systemic fungus infection occurs as a spherical mass at the periphery of the lung. If the lesion heals (is surrounded or replaced by fibrous tissue), it becomes calcified and remains for years. If it spreads initially or later breaks down and spreads, it becomes a larger, irregular mass with more extensive caseation.

MATCH THE GROSS APPEARANCE OF THE FOLLOWING LUNG LESIONS WITH THEIR POSSIBLE CAUSE (USE EACH LETTER ONCE):

____wedge-shaped peripheral hemorrhagic soft lesion
____spherical hard calcified mass with central soft friable yellow material
____spherical mass filled with thick yellow material that runs out when mass is cut

A. infection due to Staphylococcus aureus (a pyogenic coccus)
B. tuberculosis
C. ischemia due to thrombus in pulmonary artery
D. histoplasmosis (a fungus infection)

26. ✓ distribution of the changes

---

27. In order to identify a lesion as necrotic, three questions must be answered affirmatively:
    A. Are the cells dead?
    B. Did they die while the patient was alive?
    C. Are there more dead cells than might be expected from normal physiologic cell death?

MATCH THE FOLLOWING STATEMENTS WITH THE LETTERS OF THE QUESTIONS THEY HELP ANSWER:

____There is morphologic evidence of irreversible nuclear change.
____The dead cells are not localized to surfaces where cell turnover is normally rapid.
____There is a distinct inflammatory or healing response to the dead cells.

---

81. b
c
e

---

82. Liquefaction necrosis is simply defined as necrosis in which dead tissue is liquefied. For practical purposes, this occurs in two situations: in brain infarcts and in abscesses or phlegmons.

Abscesses (localized) and phlegmons (ramifying areas of liquefaction of tissue) are produced by enzymes liberated from the large numbers of polymorphonuclear leukocytes. These lesions are caused by pyogenic cocci or other types of bacteria such as those originating from the intestinal tract. Brain infarcts are peculiar in that they initially start to undergo coagulation necrosis, but then this tissue, with high lipid content, begins to break down and the lipid is phagocytized by macrophages. Later the debris is carried away, leaving a hole filled with clear fluid.

MATCH THE FOLLOWING:

____caused by bacteria
____caused by ischemia
____contains clear fluid
____contains pus
____promoted by chemostatic agents which attract polys

A. brain infarct

B. abscess

32. a
b
d

---

33. FROM THE PRECEDING FRAME, NAME THREE MORPHOLOGIC FEATURES THAT HELPED PROVE THAT THE DEAD CELLS WERE DUE TO NECROSIS:

____

____

____

---

87. Caseous necrosis ☑ is a destructive lesion which ☑ does leave permanent tissue damage.
The dead cells ☑ do exhibit the morphologic changes of cell death.
The main histologic difference from coagulation necrosis is that cell outlines disappear.

---

88. Caseous necrosis and infarcts are both sharply demarcated, and with time the central portion of a large infarct may resemble the center of a caseous mass.

INDICATE APPROPRIATE CHARACTERISTICS IN THE FOLLOWING CHART:

	Caseous Necrosis	Coagulation Necrosis: Early	Coagulation Necrosis: Well Developed	Coagulation Necrosis: Late
Cell detail maintained				
Cell or tissue outlines retained				

27. A
C
B

---

28. The morphologic changes of cell death occur with or following

___necrosis
___physiologic cell death
___somatic death
___immediate fixation of normal tissue

The term necrosis /_/ is /_/ is not synonymous with the term cell death.

---

82. B
A
A
B
B

---

83. Liquefaction necrosis is ______________________________.

LIST TWO TYPES OF LIQUEFACTION NECROSIS AND THEIR CAUSES:

Types	Causes
______________	______________
______________	______________

31. A
D
C
B

---

32. Necrotic tissue provides a mild to moderate stimulus to the vascular and cellular inflammatory response and a strong stimulus to the repair response.

An area of myocardium dies because of insufficient blood supply. Which of the following are likely reactions to the dead tissue?

a. a zone of congestion around the dead tissue
b. moderate numbers of polys at the margin of the dead tissue
c. many polys throughout the dead tissue with enzymatic liquefaction of all the dead tissue
d. prominent ingrowth of new connective tissue into the dead tissue after several days

---

86. Caseous necrosis occurs with [✓] some granulomatous inflammations.
Caseous necrosis [✓] does not occur in the absence of a granulomatous type process.
Caseous necrosis is probably due to a [✓] host allergic reaction to the causative agent.

---

87. The lesion preceding the development of caseous necrosis is a hard tubercle consisting of masses of plump macrophages (epithelioid cells), often surrounded by a rim of lymphocytes. As the lesion enlarges, the center becomes caseous, i.e., it undergoes necrosis, with disruption of nuclei and cytoplasm to form an amorphous eosinophilic mass. In the early stages, remnants of pyknotic and karyorrhectic nuclei (nuclear dust) are present. The necrotic material is very resistant to digestion and is the site of calcium deposition. Small lesions (1 to 2 cm.) may be completely replaced by fibrous tissue, but in larger lesions the necrotic material is surrounded by a wall of fibrous tissue and remains for years, often with viable organisms in the center.

Caseous necrosis [ ] is [ ] is not a destructive lesion which [ ] does [ ] does not leave permanent tissue damage.
The dead cells [ ] do [ ] do not exhibit the morphologic changes of cell death.
The main histologic difference from coagulation necrosis is that ____________ ____________ disappear.

28. ✓ necrosis
✓ physiologic cell death
✓ somatic death (if tissue not fixed)
The term necrosis [✓] is not synonymous with the term cell death.

EXPLANATORY NOTE: The term necrosis is used in two different ways: (1) It may be used to describe the process of cell death within the body from the time of initial injury; in this case there may be no morphologic changes until some time after the injury; or (2) it may be used to describe the morphologic changes of abnormal cell death that occurred in the living body. The meaning should be clear from the context.

---

29. The best indication that tissue died before it was removed from the patient is reaction to the dead tissue, such as inflammation or healing. In the early stages of necrosis, host reaction may be minimal, and the distribution of the lesion provides the only clue to the fact that the damage occurred in vivo.

The morphologic presence of dead cells is [ ] necessary to identify [ ] diagnostic of necrosis in tissue sections.

Helpful features in distinguishing necrosis from postmortem disintegration include [ ] host reaction to dead cells [ ] localized lesions.

---

83. Liquefaction necrosis is necrosis in which the dead tissue is liquefied.

Types	Causes
brain infarct	ischemia (or infarct)
abscess	bacteria (or more directly, enzymes from polys)

---

84. Caseous necrosis is so named because it has the appearance of crumbly (friable) cheese. Caseous necrosis is a solid type of necrosis which grossly resembles crumbly cheese and microscopically is characterized by loss of cell detail and cell outlines. It is important because its presence immediately suggests the presence of tuberculosis or systemic fungal infection (it is occasionally mimicked by necrotic tumor and may occur to a minor extent in leprosy).

COMPARE THE ATTRIBUTES OF COAGULATION, LIQUEFACTION, AND CASEOUS NECROSIS (LETTERS MAY BE USED MORE THAN ONCE):

____ grossly solid
____ cell outlines maintained
____ frequently caused by ischemia
____ frequently caused by pyogenic bacteria
____ frequently caused by tuberculosis and fungi

A. coagulation necrosis
B. liquefaction necrosis
C. caseous necrosis

30. The morphologic changes of cell death occur with ✓ necrosis ✓ physiologic cell death ✓ somatic death.
A reaction to dead cells occurs with ✓ necrosis (and to a minimal extent with physiologic cell death).

---

31. When a localized portion of the body dies as a result of injury (necrosis), the body reacts to the dead tissue. The first reaction is often simple congestion. This is followed by an inflammatory cell reaction to the dead tissue. Healing may begin in a few hours or a few days, depending on the extent and duration of the injury. A myocardial infarct is a localized lesion of heart muscle due to loss of blood supply to that area. The progression of congestion, inflammatory cell response, and healing is rather slow with a myocardial infarct, because there are no exogenous agents to speed up decomposition and muscle deteriorates slowly.

MATCH THE TIME WITH THE PREDOMINANT SURROUNDING TISSUE REACTION (USE EACH LETTER ONLY ONCE):

Time	Predominant Reaction
____ 0-18 hours	A. no reaction
____ 18 hours to 1 day	B. healing
____ 1-5 days	C. inflammatory cells
____ more than 5 days	D. congestion

---

85. Caseous necrosis is a ☑ solid type of necrosis which grossly resembles crumbly cheese and microscopically is characterized by loss of ☑ cell detail and ☑ cell outlines.

It is usually caused by tuberculosis or systemic fungus infection.

---

86. Caseous necrosis is almost invariably associated with granulomatous inflammation, but not all types of granulomatous inflammation progress to caseous necrosis. (The best example of this is sarcoidosis.) A delayed hypersensitivity reaction (allergic reaction mediated by lymphocytes rather than antibodies) is probably involved, since caseous necrosis will not develop for about 2 weeks after first exposure to tubercle bacilli but occurs within a few days on reexposure to the organism.

Caseous necrosis occurs with ☐ some ☐ all granulomatous inflammations.
Caseous necrosis ☐ does ☐ does not occur in the absence of a granulomatous type process.
Caseous necrosis is probably due to a ☐ direct action of a causative agent ☐ host allergic reaction to the causative agent.

29. The morphologic presence of dead cells is /✓/ necessary to identify necrosis in tissue sections.
Helpful features in distinguishing necrosis from postmortem disintegration include /✓/ host reaction to dead cells /✓/ localized lesions.

---

30. The distinction between necrosis and physiologic cell death rarely presents problems. In fact, physiologic cell death is so slow in most tissues and the dead cells removed so rapidly by macrophages or by sloughing that they are rarely seen in sections except in tissues with rapid turnover, such as epidermis and endometrium.

The morphologic changes of cell death occur with
____necrosis ____physiologic cell death ____somatic death

A reaction to dead cells occurs with
____necrosis ____physiologic cell death ____somatic death

TURN TEXT 180° AND CONTINUE.

---

84. A, C
A
A, B
B
C

---

85. Caseous necrosis is a / / solid / / liquid type of necrosis which grossly resembles crumbly cheese and microscopically is characterized by loss of / / cell detail / / cell outlines.

It is usually caused by ____________________________ or

____________________________.

TURN TEXT 180° AND CONTINUE.

Unit 8. Healing

Unit 8. HEALING

OBJECTIVES

When you have completed this unit, you will be able to select correct responses relating to the:

	starting page	frame numbers
A. Healing: Resolution and Repair	8.3	1-23
B. Repair: Parenchymal and Connective Tissue Proliferation	8.49	24-42
C. Healing: Classification	8.62	43-115
D. Healing: Agent and Host Factors	8.54	116-137

A. Healing: Resolution and Repair — 8.3 — 1-23

1. definition of healing, resolution, sloughing, repair, and physiologic replacement.
2. recognition of examples and non-examples of healing.

B. Repair: Parenchymal and Connective Tissue Proliferation — 8.49 — 24-42

1. definition of labile, stable, and permanent cells.
2. classification of the following as labile, stable, or permanent:
   hematopoietic tissue
   glandular parenchymal tissue
   surface epithelia
   muscle (smooth, striated, and cardiac)
   nerve cells
   bone and cartilage
   connective tissue

C. Healing: Classification — 8.62 — 43-115

1. distinction between resolution, orderly regeneration, disorderly regeneration, and organization in terms of:
   a) definitions
   b) type of preceding injury
   c) organs involved
   d) time course and resulting structural and functional changes
   e) common examples

D. Healing: Agent and Host Factors — 8.54 — 116-137

1. definition and differentiation of healing by first intention and healing by second intention in terms of time, sequence of events, outcome, and factors determining which course will be followed.
2. local and systemic factors likely to produce rapid or slow healing, increased susceptibility to infection, excessive scarring, or failure of the healing process.

PRETEST

UNIT 8. HEALING

SELECT THE SINGLE BEST RESPONSE:

1. Repair and physiologic replacement are by definition
   (A) basic pathologic processes
   (B) both involved in healing
   (C) both involved with cell proliferation
   (D) primarily connective tissue processes

2. Which is the correct order from greatest to least regenerative capacity?
   (A) nerve, smooth muscle, cardiac muscle
   (B) smooth muscle, nerve, cardiac muscle
   (C) cardiac muscle, smooth muscle, nerve
   (D) cardiac muscle, nerve, smooth muscle

3. In which of the following are both tissues composed of stable cells?
   (A) glandular parenchyma and bone marrow
   (B) nerve tissue and myocardium
   (C) bone and adipose tissue
   (D) glial cells and surface epithelium

4. Anoxic damage to proximal kidney tubules due to shock heals by
   (A) resolution alone
   (B) orderly regeneration
   (C) disorderly regeneration
   (D) organization

5. Two weeks after an abdominal operation, histologically the scar would appear
   (A) acellular, avascular, disorderly fibrous
   (B) acellular, avascular, orderly fibrous
   (C) cellular, vascular, orderly fibrous
   (D) cellular, vascular, disorderly fibrous

6. A 4-centimeter nodule found periphery of the lung consists of central amorphous, eosinophilic material surrounded by a layer of dense, relatively acellular, fibrous tissue containing a few lymphocytes. The age of this lesion is most likely
   (A) 1 day
   (B) 1 week
   (C) 1 month
   (D) 1 year

7. After treatment with a cancer chemotherapeutic agent, a patient's white blood count drops to 2,000 cells/mm^3. After discontinuing the agent, the bone marrow is likely to undergo
   (A) resolution only
   (B) orderly regeneration
   (C) disorderly regeneration
   (D) organization

8. Which is most likely to produce significant delay in healing?
   (A) presence of necrotic tissue
   (B) moderate protein deficiency
   (C) diabetes mellitus
   (D) vitamin B_{12} deficiency

GO ON TO THE NEXT PAGE AND BEGIN THE UNIT

A. Healing: Resolution and Repair (23 frames)

This is an introduction to the subject of healing. When you complete this section, you will be able to select correct responses relating to the:

1. definition of healing, resolution, sloughing, repair, and physiological replacement.

2. recognition of examples and non-examples of healing.

1. Healing is the sequence of events directed toward restoring normal structure and function of the body after injury. The body cannot always completely restore normal structure and function, but the attempt is still a form of healing. Processes involved include removal of exudates, replacement of the original tissue by regrowth, and replacement by new connective tissue.

   WHICH OF THE FOLLOWING ARE EXAMPLES OF HEALING?

   a. replacement of burned skin by new squamous epithelium
   b. replacement of burned skin by masses of scar tissue
   c. scar formation around a liver abscess
   d. formation of serous exudate following a burn
   e. response of polys to bacterial invasion

---

1. a
   b
   c

---

2. WHICH OF THE BASIC RESPONSES OF THE BODY TO INJURY ARE COMMONLY FOLLOWED BY HEALING?

   a. inflammation
   b. cell degeneration and cell death
   c. abnormal development
   d. disturbances of growth

---

70. COMPLETE THE FOLLOWING DIAGRAM:

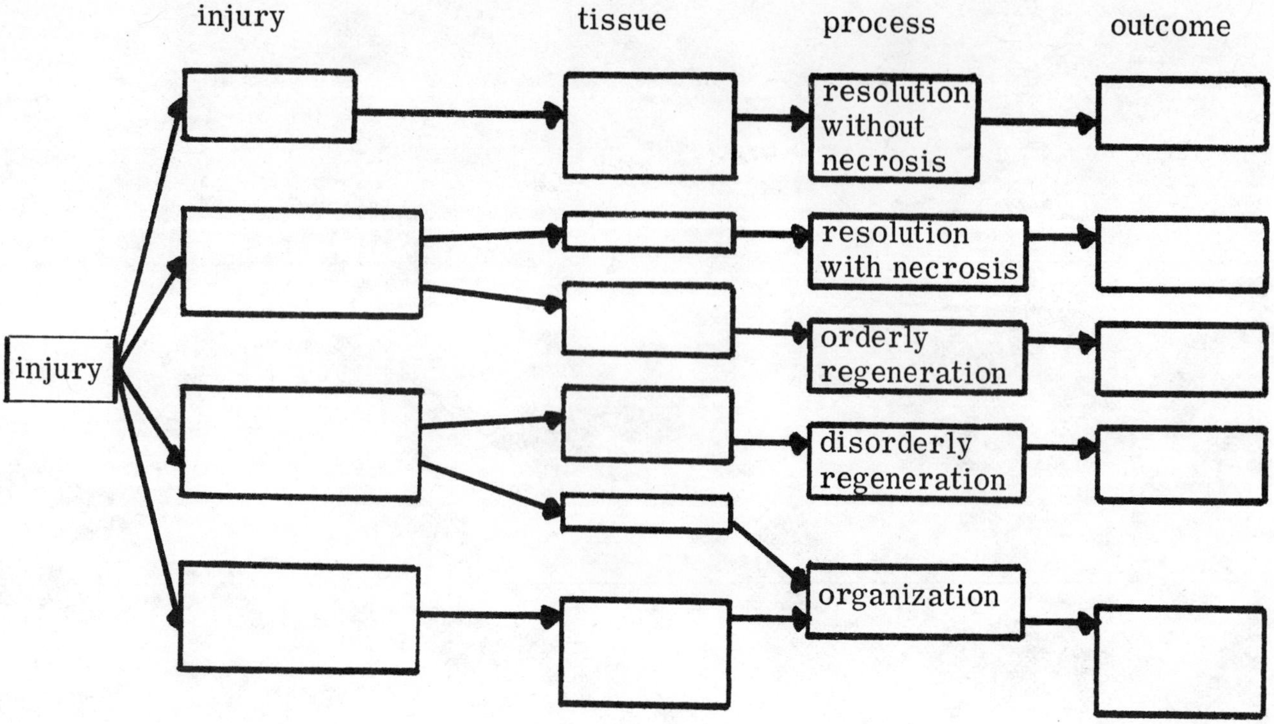

TURN TEXT 180° AND CONTINUE.

2. a
   b

3. FILL IN THE EMPTY BOX:

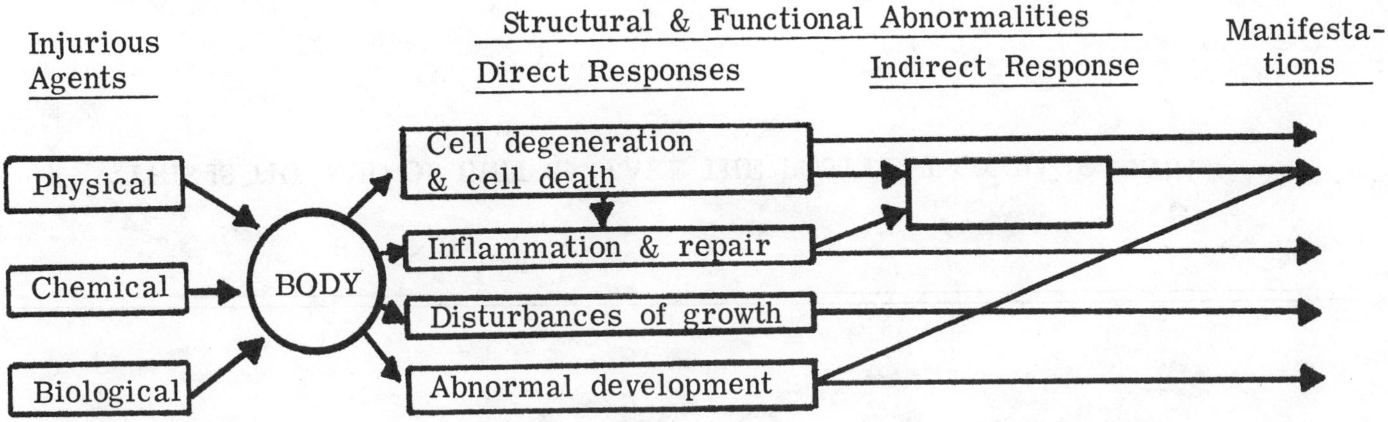

70.

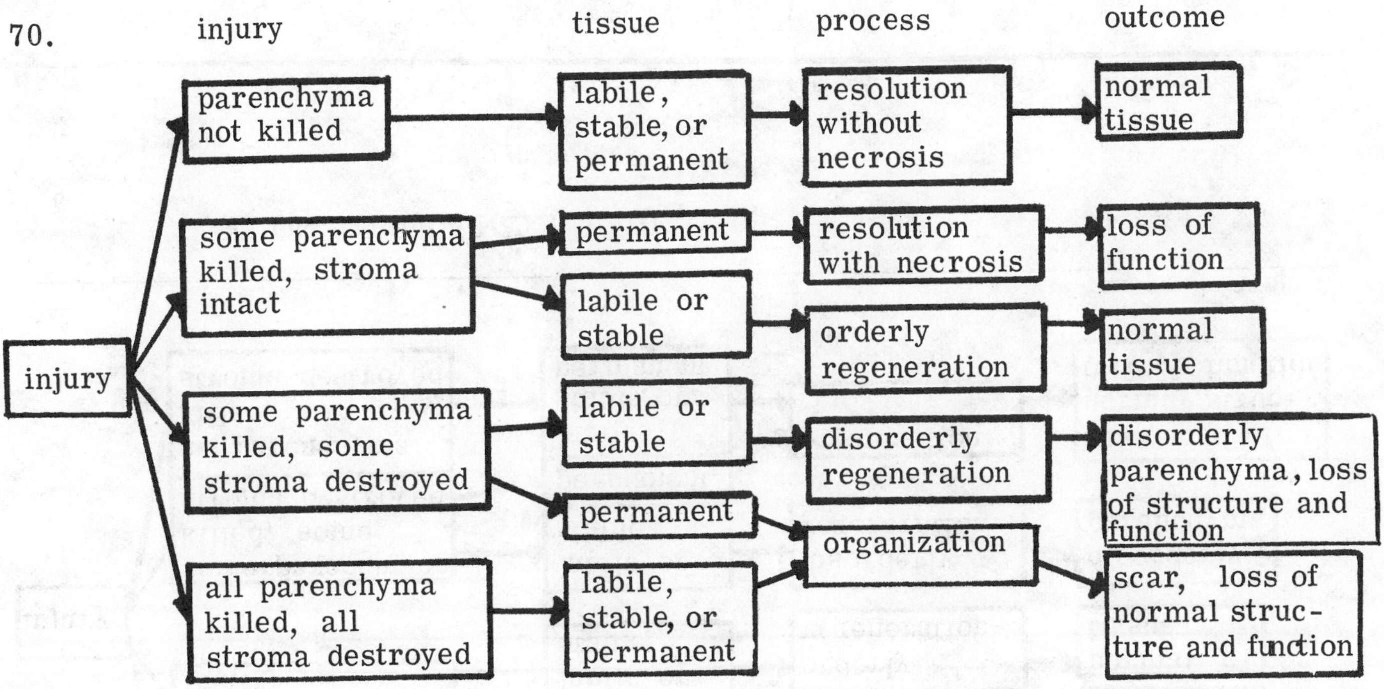

71. Resolution is commonly the only process that acts on an inflammatory exudate. If resolution is slow to occur (as it is in 10 to 20% of untreated pneumococcal pneumonias), organization occurs. What outcome would this lead to?

69.

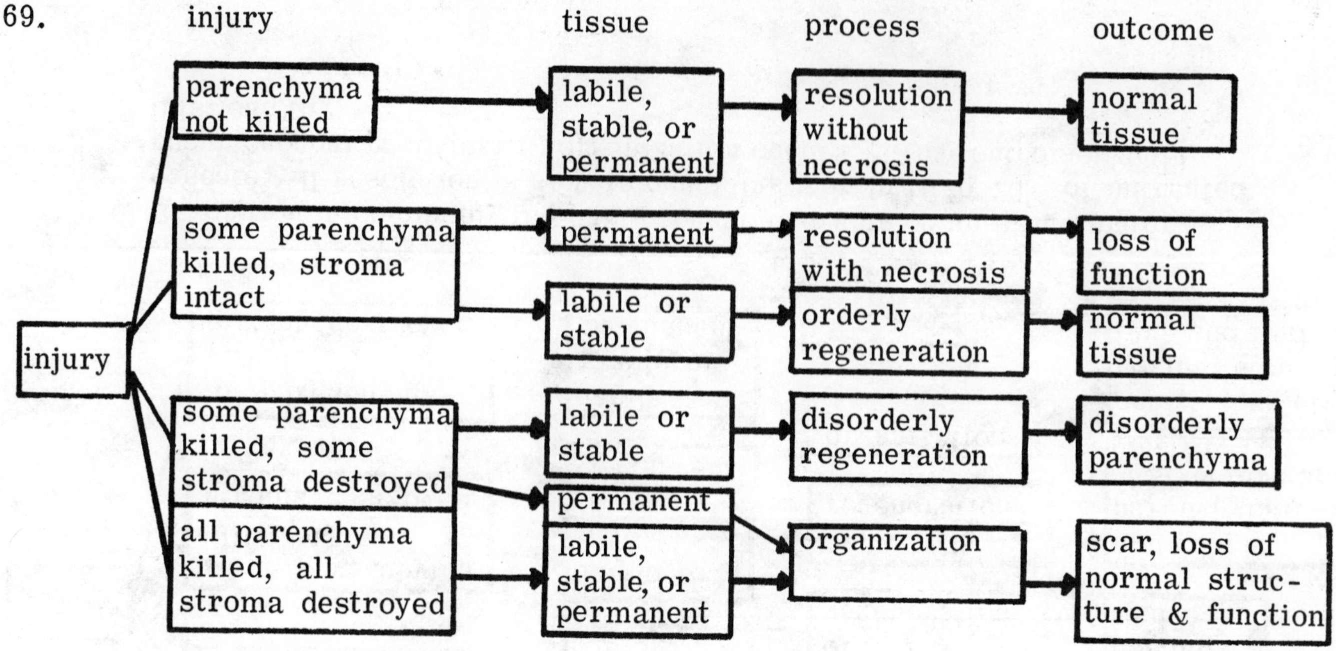

GO ON TO THE NEXT PAGE.

137. F
F
F
T
T
F

THIS IS THE END OF UNIT 8. TAKE THE POSTTEST ON PAGE xxviii.

3. Healing

---

4. Three different processes may be involved in healing.

1) resolution: the resorption of transudate, exudate, or liquefied debris
2) sloughing (sluf' ing): the separation of dead tissue or exudate from an external or internal body surface.
3) repair: the replacement of dead or injured tissues by new cells of parenchymal or stromatic origin.

MATCH THE FOLLOWING:

____ liquefaction and resorption of a fibrinous exudate	A. repair
____ the shedding of a fibrinous exudate from a mucosal surface	B. resolution
____ ingrowth of fibroblasts into fibrinous exudate with later scar formation	C. sloughing

---

71. scar, with loss of normal structure and function

---

72. INDICATE WHICH CONDITION CAUSES EACH OUTCOME IN THE LUNG:

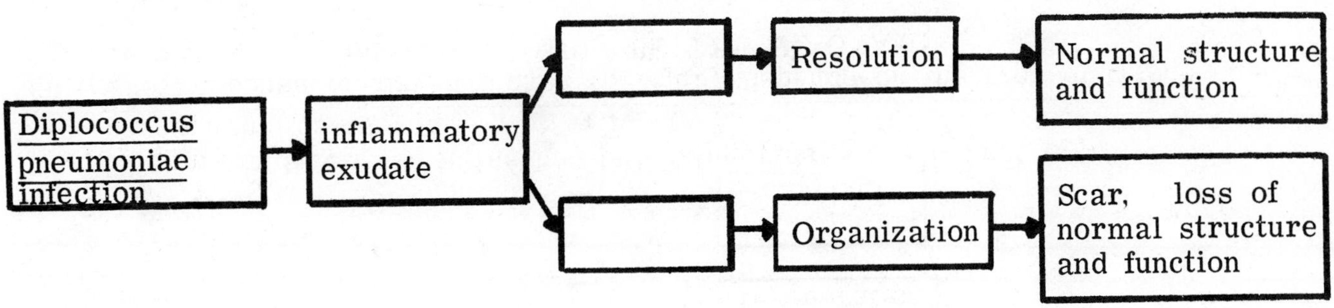

68.

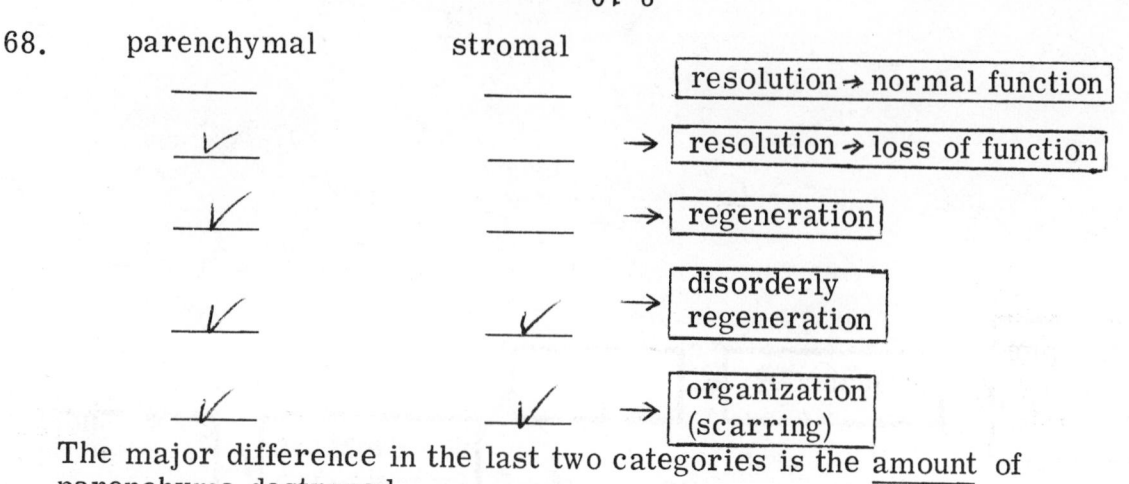

parenchymal	stromal	
___	___	resolution → normal function
✓	___	→ resolution → loss of function
✓	___	→ regeneration
✓	✓	→ disorderly regeneration
✓	✓	→ organization (scarring)

The major difference in the last two categories is the <u>amount</u> of parenchyma destroyed.

69. The response an organ makes to injury depends on the type of tissue as well as the injury. COMPLETE THE DIAGRAM:

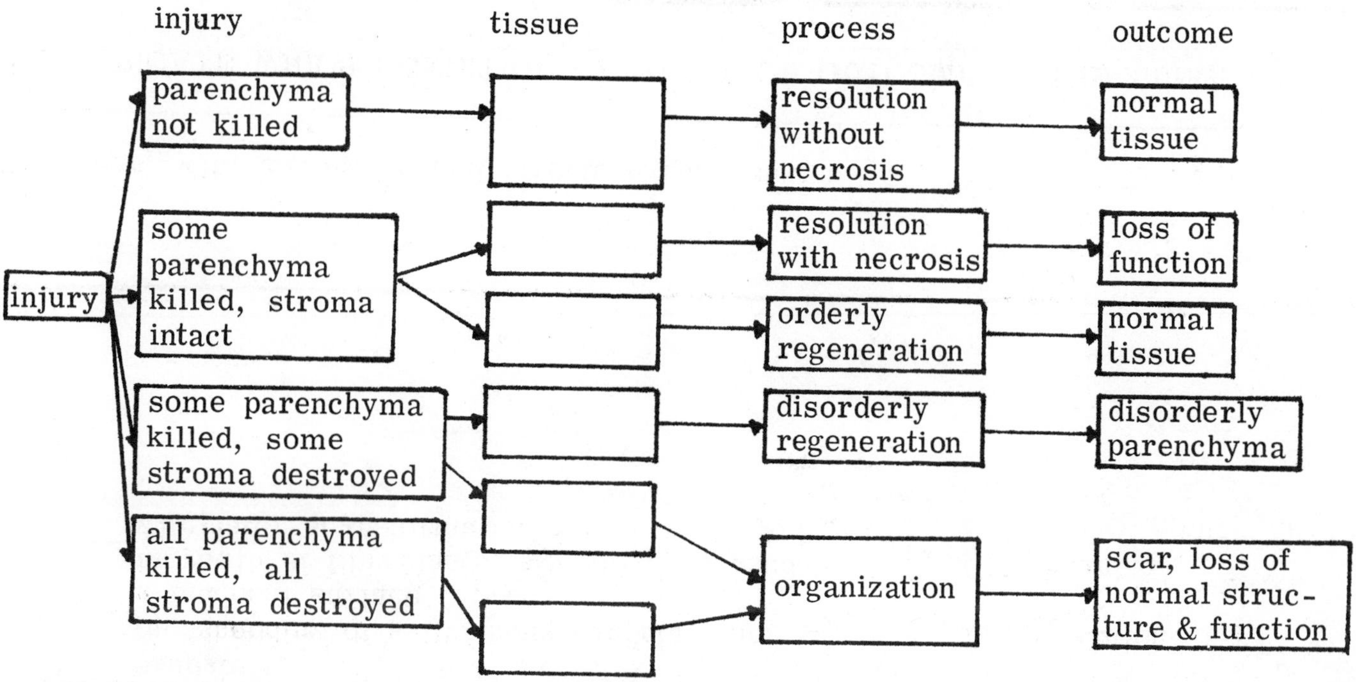

136. youth
growth hormone

137. INDICATE "T" TRUE OR "F" FALSE:

frame ref.

____If poor apposition, necrosis, or infection is present, a wound will heal by first intention. (116)

____A surgeon should remove stitches sooner after surgery if the patient is receiving corticosteroids. (133, 134)

____Mild protein deficiency will slow the healing of an injury. (131)

____An injury in an old man in good health will heal more slowly than one in a young man. (132)

____Foreign bodies may predispose to abscess formation. (125)

____Systemic factors have more dramatic effects on wound healing than local factors. (130)

4. B
C
A

---

5. Healing is directed toward restoring __________ __________ and __________ by removal of debris or exudate and/or replacement of dead or injured cells.

MATCH THE FOLLOWING:

____resolution
____repair
____sloughing

A. replacement of dead or injured cells
B. removal of exudate or debris from interstitial space
C. removal of exudate and debris from a body surface

72.

rapid removal of injurious agent (or equivalent)

slow removal of injurious agent

---

73. Organization is a process which occurs in every organ in the body. Its useful function is to provide strength in permanently injured organs. When exudates are organized, the result is almost always deleterious, an unnecessary loss of normal structure and function. CHOOSE WHETHER EACH EXAMPLE OF ORGANIZATION IS "U" USEFUL OR "H" HARMFUL:

____organization of exudate in the pericardium
____organization of a myocardial infarct
____organization occurring after a cut
____organization in an arthritic joint
____fibrous adhesions between visceral and parietal pleura or between loops of bowel

67. A
C
E
B
D

---

68. INDICATE TYPES OF TISSUE INJURED, IF ANY, TO PRODUCE THE FOLLOWING OUTCOMES:

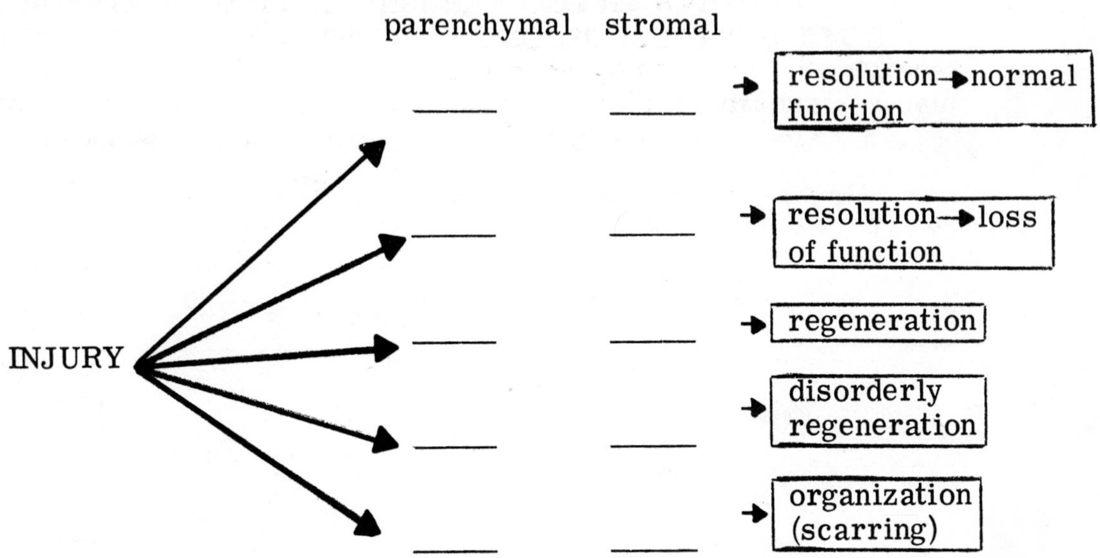

The major difference in the last two categories is the ______________ of parenchyma destroyed.

---

135. extreme protein deficiency
debilitating disease
old age
corticosteroid treatment
vitamin C deficiency

---

136. GIVE TWO SYSTEMIC FACTORS WHICH WILL INCREASE THE RATE OF REPAIR.

5. normal structure and function

B
A
C

---

6. Resolution commonly follows inflammation and necrosis. It may consist simply of resorption of exudate or may involve liquefication of dead tissue and debris followed by resorption.

FOR THE FOLLOWING SITUATIONS, INDICATE WHICH PROCESS(ES) WOULD OCCUR DURING RESOLUTION:

____necrotic heart muscle
____dense fibrinous exudate
____transudate
____serous exudate

A. liquefaction
B. resorption
C. liquefaction and resorption

---

73. H
U
U
H
H

---

74. When organization occurs, the invading reparative tissue is called granulation tissue. It consists primarily of two types of cells, fibroblasts and endothelial cells.

MATCH THE FOLLOWING:

____fibroblasts
____endothelial cells

A. produce new blood vessels
B. produce collagen

66. A
A
C
B

---

67. SELECT THE PROCESS(ES) MOST LIKELY TO OCCUR:

____selective anoxic damage to neurons
____cirrhosis of the liver (nodules of hepatocytes surrounded by fibrous tissue)
____brain infarct
____mild carbon tetrachloride injury to liver
____replacement of infarcted myocardium by fibrous tissue

A. resolution only
B. orderly regeneration
C. disorderly regeneration
D. organization
E. gliosis

---

134. twice

---

135. GIVE 4 SYSTEMIC FACTORS WHICH WILL DECREASE THE RATE OF REPAIR.

6. C
C (Fibrin is a solid protein which must be lysed before resorption can occur.)
B
B

---

7. Resolution is a form of healing and therefore is directed toward ____.

In a case of swelling with very little necrosis followed by resolution, what would you expect the outcome to be? ☐ loss of normal structure and function ☐ restoration of normal structure and function

---

74. B
A

---

75. In rheumatoid arthritis, a mild inflammation of the joints stimulates the growth of granulation tissue into the joint space and into the articular cartilage. What do you think is a frequent result of this granulation tissue proliferation? Is this useful or harmful organization?

65. injury tissue process outcome

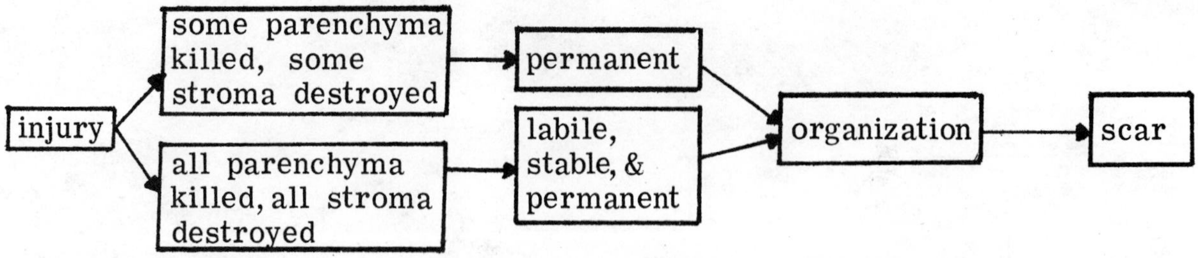

---

66. Brain injury illustrates the processes that can occur in a tissue containing permanent-type parenchymal cells (neurons).

With mild injury, swelling (edema) may occur and be resolved.

With diffuse anoxic damage, neurons are often selectively killed; other components are not affected as the dead cells and associated edema are removed, but neuronal function is lost in proportion to the number of dead cells.

Most localized necrotizing lesions, such as infarcts, produce complete loss of cells in an area,with some proliferation of glial cells at the margin of the area. Abscesses are an exception; they cause fibroblastic proliferation in the brain,leading to scarring around the abscess.

MATCH THE FOLLOWING:

____brain edema	A. resolution only
____anoxic neuronal damage	B. organization
____brain infarct	C. gliosis
____brain abscess	

---

133. B
B
B
A
A
B
B

---

134. A surgeon operates on a patient receiving cortisone treatments for rheumatoid arthritis. He will wait (half/twice) as long before he removes the stitches.

7. restoration of normal structure and function.

[✓] restoration of normal structure and function

---

8. A common cause of pneumonia is Diplococcus pneumoniae. In pneumococcal pneumonia, lobar consolidation of the lung occurs due to filling of alveolar spaces with inflammatory exudate. Shortly after removal of the injurious agent, resolution occurs. Since there is usually no necrosis of lung tissue in this infection, what would you expect the outcome to be?

---

75. scarred, useless (immovable) joints, harmful

---

76. The outcome of organization is a scar. Thus, you would expect the granulation tissue to gradually become (more/less) vascular, (more/less) cellular, and (more/less) fibrous.

64. tissue

permanent

labile, stable, or permanent

65. WHAT CONDITIONS FREQUENTLY RESULT IN ORGANIZATION ?

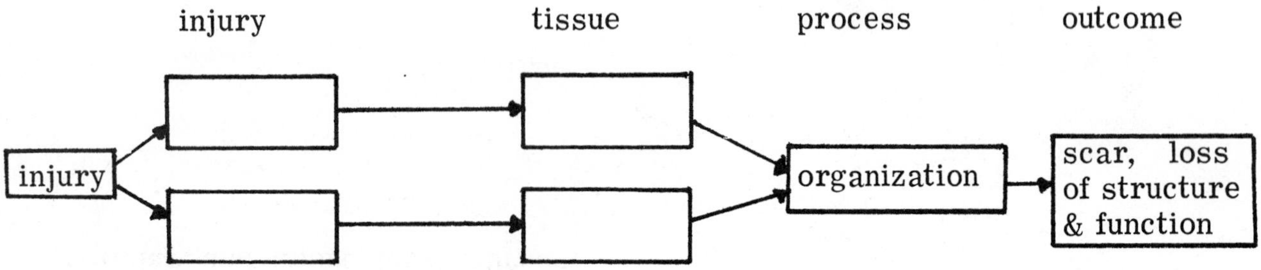

132. B
B
A
B
B

133. Increased levels of growth hormone, produced by the anterior pituitary, increase the rate of granulation tissue growth and repair. Corticosteroids, which are widely used therapeutically to depress the inflammatory reaction also reduce greatly the rate of granulation tissue growth and of repair.
CHOOSE THE CORRECT EFFECT:

____debilitating disease
____old age
____corticosteroids
____youth
____growth hormone
____extreme vitamin C deficiency (scurvy)
____extreme protein deficiency

A. increased rate of healing

B. decreased rate of healing

8. normal structure and function (or equivalent)

---

9. When resolution is the only form of healing involved, restoration of normal structure and function can occur rapidly. How rapidly it occurs depends on the amount and nature of the material to be resolved. Small lesions may be resolved in a few hours, whereas large ones may take a number of days.

MATCH THE FOLLOWING:

Lesion		Time for resolution
____swelling after bee sting	A.	hours
____lung consolidation	B.	3-5 days

---

76. You would expect the granulation tissue gradually to become less vascular, less cellular, and more fibrous.

---

77. We will now consider in greater detail the process of organization as it proceeds in a small, uncomplicated injury.

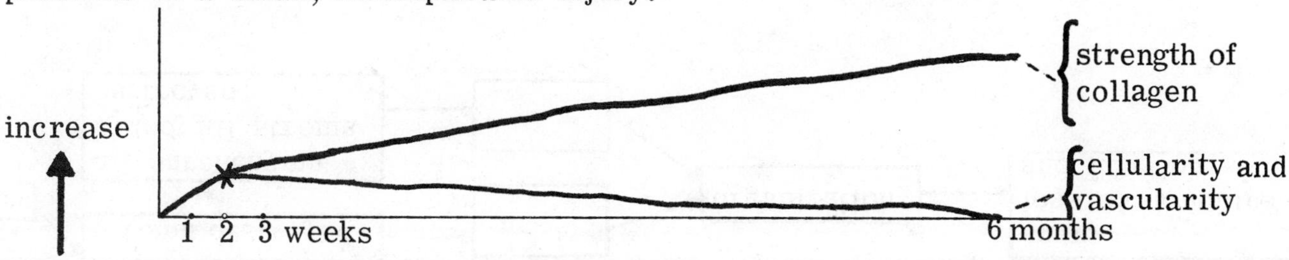

At the end of two weeks, a cellular vascular scar is present, some collagen has been laid down in a disorderly fashion, and the scar has attained some strength. What happens to the cellularity and vascularity of the scar during the next several months?

63. organization

64. INDICATE THE APPROPRIATE TISSUE TYPES:

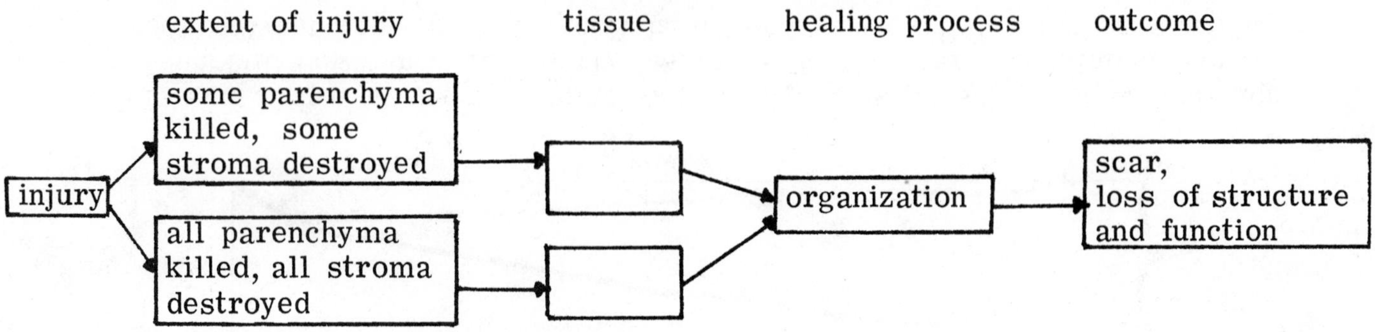

131. b
c

132. Other systemic factors also modify the rate of repair. Those correlated with good physical condition increase the rate, while those correlated with poor physical condition decrease the rate of repair.

CHOOSE THE CORRECT EFFECT:

____vitamin C deficiency
____extreme protein deficiency
____youth
____old age
____debilitating disease

A. increased rate of healing

B. decreased rate of healing

9. A
   B

---

10. The term resolution is often used in a broad sense. When corrective measures are taken for congestive heart failure, and the accompanying edema (swelling) of the legs is alleviated, the edema is said to be __________________. Did cell injury or inflammation precede healing? / / yes / / no

---

77. They decrease slowly.

---

78. During the next six months, collagen is laid down and rearranged, and the wound becomes contracted, that is, smaller. In addition, most of the blood vessels are pinched off. This in turn causes a decreased cellularity in the scar. The end result of these processes is a mature scar. Given this information and the chart in the previous frame, what histological attributes do you think the scar would have?

62. orderly regeneration - orderly replacement of lost cells by proliferation of remaining parenchymal cells

organization - ingrowth of fibroblasts and endothelial cells into an injured area, with later formation of fibrous tissue

gliosis - growth of glial tissue into an injured area of the brain or spinal cord

adiposity - replacement of atrophied tissue by adipose tissue

---

63. WHICH PROCESS WILL MOST COMMONLY OCCUR UNDER THESE CONDITIONS TO PRODUCE THIS OUTCOME?

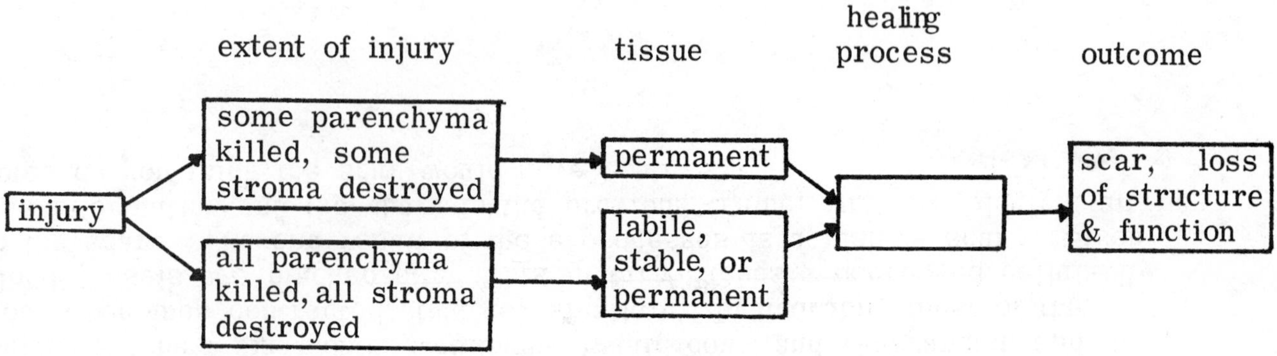

---

130. Thus, it is unable to produce collagen, and wound strength does not increase.

---

131. Protein deficiency slows repair only if the deficiency is extreme. This is because the body breaks down proteins elsewhere to supply the amino acids needed for the repair.

INDICATE THE CONDITION(S) WHICH WILL RESULT IN SLOW REPAIR:

a. 2 days of fasting
b. being lost at sea for 3 weeks with nothing but water and some limes
c. advanced cancer with severe weight loss

10. resolved

☑ no

---

11. Most organs have two distinct types of tissue components. One component maintains the structure of the organ and the other performs the functions peculiar to the organ. The structural tissue is called stroma, and the cells responsible for the main function of the organ are called parenchyma.

FOR EACH OF THE FOLLOWING PAIRS, IDENTIFY STROMA (S) AND PARENCHYMA (P)

____bile-producing cells of the liver	____fibrovascular connective tissue
____reticulin fibers and connective tissue cells of portal triad	____cardiac muscle fibers
____neurons	____villus epithelial cells
____glial cells	____lamina propria

---

78. acellular,
avascular, (or equivalent)
orderly fibrous

---

79. The three processes causing the production of an acellular, avascular, orderly fibrous scar are:

1) the contraction deposition and rearrangement of ____________

2) a decrease in ____________

3) a decrease in ____________

61. orderly regeneration
disorderly regeneration
organization
gliosis
adiposity

---

62. DEFINE THE FOLLOWING:

orderly regeneration:

organization:

gliosis:

adiposity (associated with atrophy):

---

129. b
d

---

130. Systemic factors are also important in determining how a wound heals, but they affect the outcome less frequently and to a lesser extent than do local factors. Extreme vitamin C deficiency (scurvy) is rarely seen now. When it occurs, the body is unable to hydroxylate the proline in procollagen fibrils. Thus, it is unable to produce ______________, and wound strength (does/does not) increase.

11. P bile-producing cells of the liver
S reticulin fibers and connective tissue cells of portal triad

S fibrovascular tissue
P cardiac muscle fibers

P neurons
S glial cells

P villus epithelial cells
S lamina propria

---

12. In tissues containing both connective tissue and epithelium, the epithelium is the more specialized and therefore is the parenchymal element. All epithelial tissues have a stroma, even though it may be slight. It is difficult to make a distinction between stroma and parenchyma in highly specialized connective tissues such as bone and cartilage.

FOR EACH OF THE FOLLOWING TISSUE OR TISSUE COMPONENTS, INDICATE STROMA (S) OR PARENCHYMA (P) OR BOTH (B):

___ epidermis and its appendages
___ dermis

___ renal tubule cells
___ vascular renal connective tissue

___ bone
___ cartilage

---

79. collagen
vascularity
cellularity

---

80. During the first two weeks after the injury, granulation tissue proliferates to produce the young scar. What two cell types play the primary role in organization? ______________________

____

Cellularity reaches a maximum at about ______________.

60. regeneration
C
A
B

---

61. NAME THE PROCESS:

Process		Outcome	
regrowth of parenchyma	→	return to normal	________
regrowth of parenchyma	→	disorderly structure	________
ingrowth of fibrous connective tissue	→	scarring	________
ingrowth of glial cells	→	dense glial tissue	________
replacement of atrophic tissue by fat cells	→	adipose tissue	________

---

128. B
A
B
A

---

129. The healing of a cut on the scalp proceeds rapidly, with little likelihood of bacterial infection. Fibroblasts proliferate rapidly and begin to lay down collagen in a day or two. In contrast, a myocardial infarct heals slowly, with little collagen formation for a week.

WHICH OF THE FOLLOWING FACTORS ACCOUNT FOR THE SLOWER HEALING OF THE MYOCARDIAL INFARCT?

a. presence of bacteria in the lesion
b. large amount of necrotic tissue
c. higher temperature than skin
d. decreased blood supply
e. presence of foreign-body material

12. P epidermis and its appendages
S dermis

P renal tubule cells
S vascular renal connective tissue

B bone
B cartilage

---

13. In general, parenchymal cells are much more susceptible to injury than stroma. In particular, stromal cells are much less likely to be killed by anoxia.

FOR THE FOLLOWING PAIRS, INDICATE WHICH IS MOST LIKELY TO BE DAMAGED BY ISCHEMIA (ANOXIA RESULTING FROM REDUCED BLOOD SUPPLY):

____ bile-producing cells of liver
____ sinusoidal lining cells of liver

____ renal tubule epithelial cells
____ endothelial and mesangial cells of glomeruli

____ glial cells
____ neurons

____ mucosa of small intestine
____ submucosa of small intestine

---

80. fibroblasts
endothelial cells (from blood vessels)
Cellularity reaches a maximum at about 2 weeks.

---

81. The first day after the injury, the mature fibroblasts in the vicinity take on additional cytoplasm and assume immature star and bipolar forms. They then divide and migrate into the injured area. What would you expect them to do next?

59. 1. 3-5 days
    2. 1-2 days
    3. 7-14 days

---

60. Replacement of lost cells by proliferation of new parenchymal cells is ____________________.

Connective tissue repair is the invasion and replacement of dead tissue or exudate by new cells derived from the structural framework of the organ. In most instances the connective tissue growth initially consists of capillaries and fibroblasts, with later formation of fibrous tissue. This process is called organization. Sometimes with slow death of tissue, the old tissue is replaced by adipose tissue. This is called adiposity. In the brain the connective tissue proliferation usually consists of glial elements and is called gliosis.

MATCH THE FOLLOWING:

____proliferation of astrocytes around an area of brain injury
____proliferation of fibroblasts and capillaries around an infarct
____ingrowth of adipose tissue in an organ undergoing atrophy

A. organization
B. adiposity
C. gliosis

---

127. b d
     c e
       f

---

128. The presence of necrotic tissue, with its lack of blood supply, is probably the most important factor in bacteria overcoming the host's defenses in an injured area. Since necrotic tissue must be resolved in healing, the amount of it which is present is also an important factor in determining how fast an injury will heal.

MATCH THE FOLLOWING:

____slow healing
____little scar formed
____greatest likelihood of bacterial infection
____heals mainly by resolution

A. small amount of necrotic material in lesion
B. large amount of necrotic material in lesion

13. ✓ bile-producing cells of the liver
✓ neurons
✓ renal tubule epithelial cells
✓ mucosa of small intestine

---

14. With anoxic brain damage, frequently neurons are destroyed without damage to the much hardier glial cells. The necrotic neurons are liquefied and resorbed.

Which healing process has occurred? What is the outcome?

---

81. produce collagen

---

82. FILL IN THE EMPTY BOX:

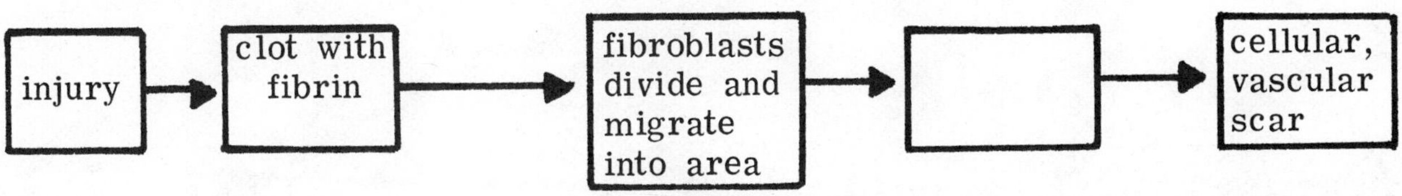

58. b
c
a

---

59. GIVE THE APPROXIMATE TIME NEEDED TO REGENERATE THE FOLLOWING TISSUES AFTER INJURY:

1. liver parenchyma
2. intestinal mucosa
3. kidney tubules

---

126. The new, larger wound he has created will not heal and will go through the same process, and he will have to amputate again, because there was not sufficient blood supply to permit healing. (or equivalent)

---

127. Let us review some of the interrelations between local factors which may greatly affect healing. Pyogenic bacteria such as Staphylococcus aureus or coliform bacteria from the intestines can turn a clean wound into a necrotic purulent mess which greatly sets back the healing process. Most open wounds are contaminated by small numbers of these bacteria, but they are easily handled by the body's defense mechanism if they are close to a viable capillary bed.

INDICATE WHICH FACTORS, IF PRESENT IN A WOUND, WOULD FAVOR BACTERIAL GROWTH:

a. high oxygen tension
b. decreased blood flow
c. necrotic tissue
d. a surgical sponge (gauze)
e. hematoma (localized collection of blood)
f. a dead space filled with serous fluid

14. resolution
loss of function (or equivalent)

---

15. The outcome of resolution is partially determined by the nature of the injury. FILL IN THE EMPTY BOXES:

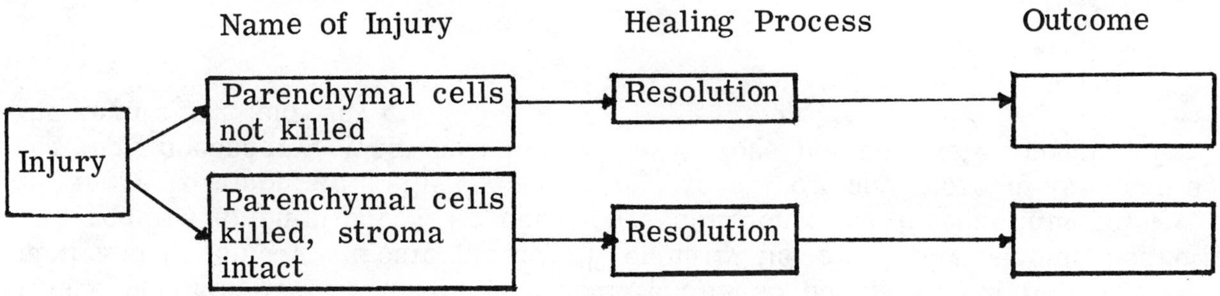

---

82. collagen laid down

---

83. FILL IN THE EMPTY BOX:

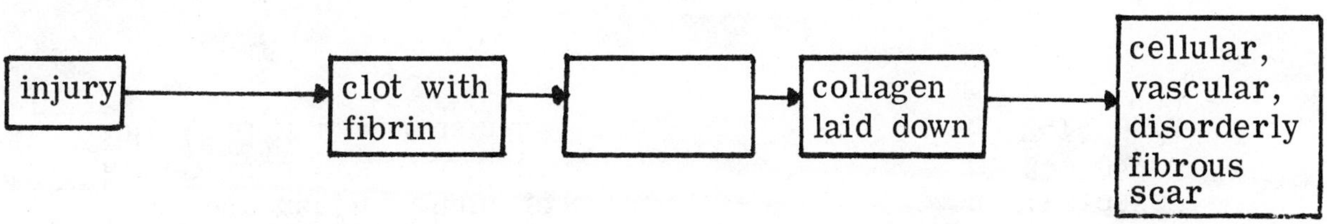

57. Regeneration of comparable size injuries is generally slower than resolution.

shortest = small intestine (a)
longest = kidney tubules (c)

---

58. MATCH THE FOLLOWING INJURIES WITH THE TIME NEEDED TO REGENERATE THE TISSUES:

____liver parenchyma damage	a. 1-2 days
____kidney tubule damage	b. 3-5 days
____intestinal mucosa damage	c. 7-14 days

---

125. Granulomatous reaction or infection may occur because suture may invoke a foreign-body response and may harbor bacteria.

---

126. Repair rate of tissue increases with the blood supply and temperature of the tissue. An extreme example of the problems caused by poor blood supply is an older diabetic patient who clips his toenail too short and cuts the tissue beneath it. Because his circulation is so poor, the cut may fail to heal and become a chronic ulcer. Eventually the area may become necrotic and require amputation. The question a surgeon must face at this point is where to amputate. He does not want to cut off any more of the man's leg than necessary. What will happen if he does not amputate enough of the man's leg and why?

15. normal structure and function

loss of structure and function

---

16. FILL IN THE EMPTY BOXES:

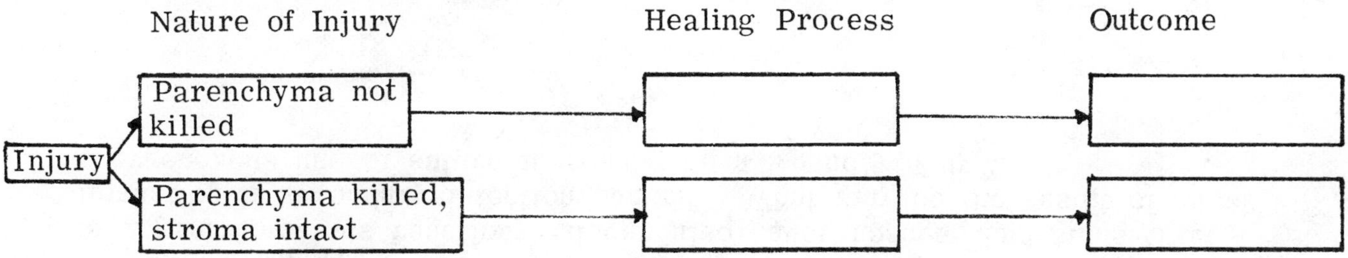

---

83. fibroblasts divide and migrate into area

---

84. The second day after the injury, endothelial cells from the blood vessels in the surrounding healthy tissue divide and migrate into the area, forming solid cords. These cords are soon canalized and blood flow commences.

Healthy young granulation tissue would appear ☐ cloudy gray-yellow ☐ pink; whereas, infected granulation tissue with fibrinopurulent exudate would appear ☐ cloudy gray-yellow ☐ pink.

In healthy granulation tissue, maximum vascularity occurs at about ______________.

56. B
A

---

57. The speed of regeneration varies from organ to organ. The gut is capable of regenerating mucosa in 1 to 2 days. The liver is capable of regenerating parenchyma in 3 to 5 days. The kidney tubules are somewhat slower, requiring 7 to 14 days to regenerate. Is regeneration of comparable size injuries faster or slower than resolution?

Which would probably occur in the shortest time following mild injury?

a. reepithelialization of small intestine
b. restoration of liver parenchyma
c. recovery of kidney tubules

Which would take the longest?

---

124. b
d
f
regeneration and organization

---

125. Necrotic tissue, poor apposition, and infection are three of the most important factors in delaying healing. In addition, several other local and systemic factors must be considered in relation to the healing process in general.
When a foreign body causes a lesion, it is most commonly in the form of a granulomatous reaction. It can also cause abscess and sinus tract formation if secondary infection occurs. What may be the result of an overgenerous use of suture in sewing up a wound? Why?

16. Healing Process — Outcome

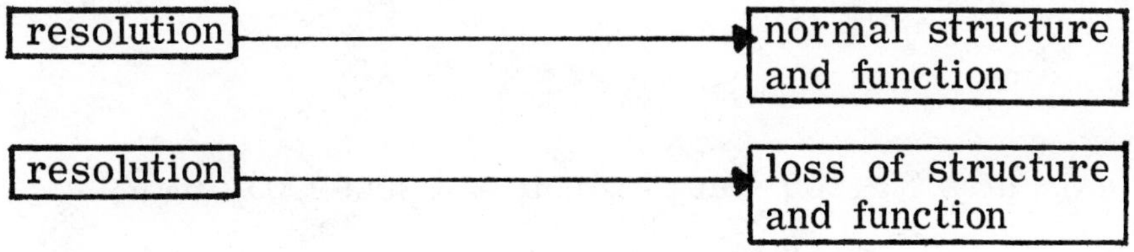

---

17. What determines the outcome of an injury which heals by resolution?

---

84. [✓] pink
[✓] cloudy gray-yellow
2 weeks

---

85. FILL IN THE EMPTY BOX:

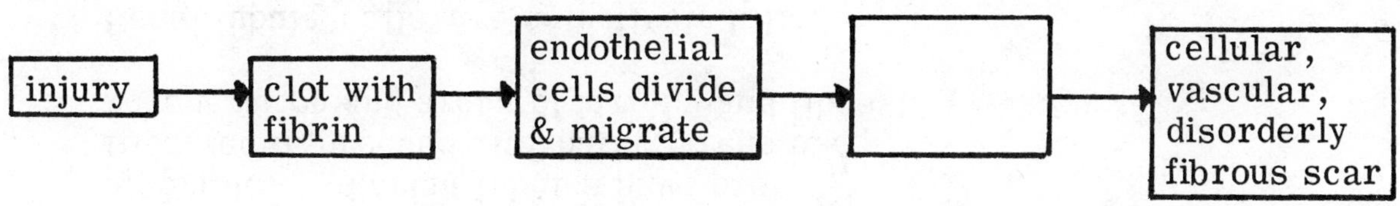

55. A. Because the new cells are parenchymal in origin, this is an example of regeneration.

---

56. MATCH THE FOLLOWING:

Kidney Changes	Type of Healing
____Scattered afferent glomerular arterioles are occluded, causing injury and fibrous replacement of glomeruli and ischemic atrophy of tubules supplied by the efferent arteriole. Adjacent tubules have proliferated to produce alternating areas of regeneration and areas of atrophy and fibrosis.	A. orderly regeneration
____Renal tubule cells are selectively killed by shunting of blood away from the renal cortex. Restoration of blood flow results in complete replacement of the cells in a few weeks.	B. disorderly regeneration

---

123. A
B
B

---

124. The sequence of events in healing by first and second intention is the same: injury → inflammation → formation of granulation tissue and ingrowth of epithelium from the margins. The major differences occur because the wound margins are spread apart in healing by second intention.

Which of the following distinguish between healing by first and second intention?

a. presence of acute inflammation
b. degree of acute inflammation
c. presence of granulation tissue
d. presence of exposed granulation tissue
e. epithelial regeneration
f. extent of epithelial regeneration

What two processes are involved in a healing skin wound?

17. whether parenchymal cells have been killed or not (or equivalent)

---

18. MATCH THE FOLLOWING:

____	replacement of dead or injured cells by new cells of parenchymal or stromal origin	A. Sloughing
____	separation of dead tissue or exudate from a body surface	B. Resolution
____	removal of a transudate, exudate, or liquefied debris	C. Repair

---

85. **canalization of cords** (or equivalent)

---

86. After an injury, inflammation occurs. Within a few hours, polys and macrophages are attracted to the area. They phagocytose and digest the injured tissue, working from the edges toward the middle. While resolution may take weeks if the injured area is large, organization commences behind the macrophages, within 24-36 hours of the injury. Hence, there usually are three processes occurring in an injured area for some time after the injury. What are they?

54. normal structure & function

---

55. When the kidney glomeruli are damaged, the epithelial cells frequently are stimulated to proliferate. The structure is so complex, however, that normal structure is often not regained.
WHICH IS/ARE CORRECT?

A. Because the new cells are parenchymal in origin, this is an example of regeneration.

B. Because normal structure and function are not regained, this is orderly regeneration.

---

122. regeneration

---

123. Which will heal by first intention? ____
Which will heal by second intention? ____
Which will heal with exposed granulation tissue? ____

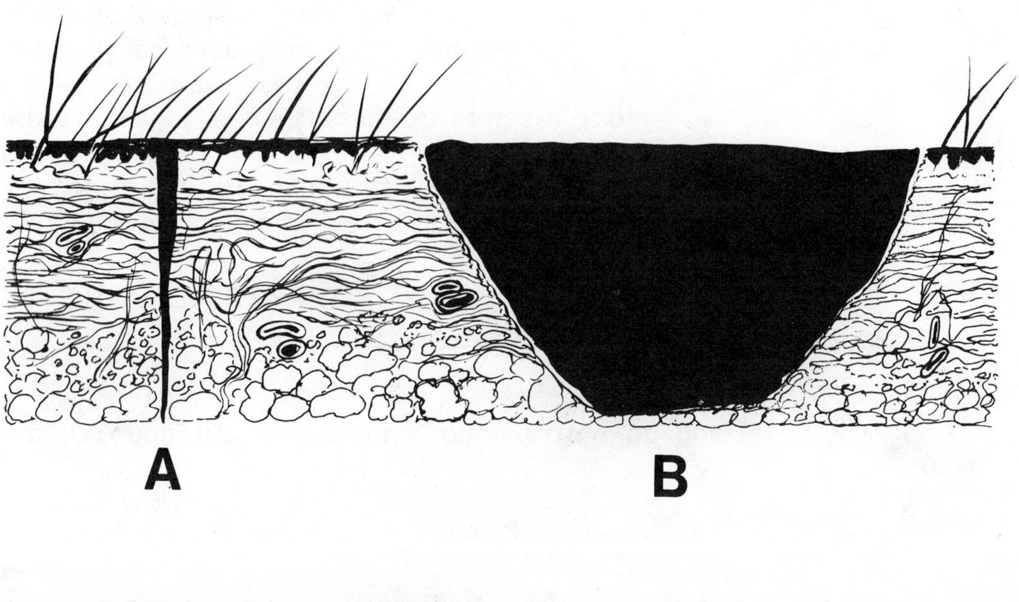

A B

18. C
A
B

---

19. WHICH ARE EXAMPLES OF SLOUGHING?

a. a scab coming off the skin
b. removal of dead neurons
c. the shedding of a pseudomembrane into the lumen of the gut
d. resorption of an exudate in the lungs
e. coughing up of necrotic lung tissue

---

86. inflammation
resolution
organization

---

87. Fibroblasts appear to have some phagocytic ability, especially in the immature, active form. Thus, for example, in myocardial infarcts they may be seen growing directly into the necrotic muscle.

Which is/are correct?

A. Fibroblasts may take part in both resolution and organization.

B. Resolution may be accomplished by fibroblasts and/or macrophages.

53. orderly regeneration of tubule epithelium

---

54. FILL IN THE EMPTY BOX:

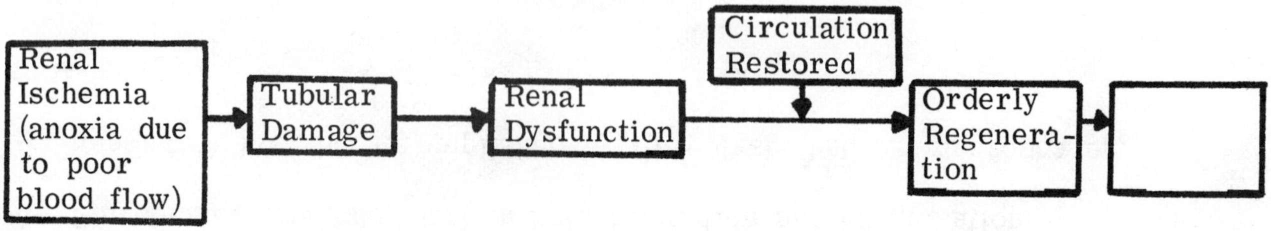

---

121. less, less, less, faster
a, b, c

---

122. The epithelium must regain continuity in wounds of the skin. In healing by first intention this occurs rapidly, in about two days. The epithelial cells divide and migrate over the defect. This part of the healing is an example of which reparative process?

19. a
c
e

---

20. <u>Repair</u> is the replacement of dead or injured tissues by new cells of parenchymal or stromal origin. It is the body's primary response to inflammation and necrosis.
<u>Physiologic replacement</u> is the continuous proliferation of cells in tissue in which physiologic cell death is occurring.

Repair, physiologic replacement, and disturbances of growth have some similar characteristics, but they are usually considered to be distinct processes. MATCH THE FOLLOWING:

___continuous proliferation of osteoblasts and remodeling of bone
___proliferation of osteoblasts, producing new bone after a fracture
___proliferation of crypt cells of the small intestine with formation of new villus cells
___proliferation of cells in a neoplasm
___hyperplasia of squamous epithelium after years of exposure to the sun

A. Repair
B. Physiologic replacement
C. Disturbance of growth

---

87. Both A and B

---

88. The next series of frames will consider specific common examples of healing relating to myocardial infarction, bone, skin, peripheral nerve, brain, abscesses, granulomas, liver, and kidney.

A patient has had a small (3-4 mm. diameter) myocardial infarct. With an infarct of this size, most of the necrotic tissue should have been removed by the end of the second week.

DESCRIBE THE ARRANGEMENT OF THE COLLAGEN AT THIS TIME.

How strong will the area be?

52.

	composed of labile or stable parenchyma	supporting stroma undamaged	orderly regeneration
1. brain infarct			
2. anoxic damage to neurons		✓	
3. partial-thickness burn to dermis	✓	✓	✓
4. burn damaging epidermis and full thickness of dermis	✓		
5. kidney infarct	✓		
6. ischemic kidney tubule necrosis	✓	✓	✓
7. myocardial infarct			

---

53. A person who has been in an auto accident is admitted to the hospital emergency room. He is bleeding profusely. The bleeding is stopped and he is treated for shock. The following day his urine output is observed to be far below normal. The patient is given proper supportive treatment and after 10 to 14 days his urinary output rapidly rises toward normal.

What repair process has occurred in the renal tubules ?

---

120. poor apposition
necrotic tissue
infection

---

121. In healing by first intention, the amount of necrotic tissue is small and the space which must be filled is also small. Thus, as compared with healing by second intention, you would expect (more/less) inflammation, (more/less) granulation tissue, (more/less) scarring, and that the whole process would be (faster/slower).

Which of the following sequences are possible explanations for the increased scarring from healing by second intention ?

a. poor apposition → increased exudate → increased granulation tissue

b. necrotic tissue → infection → poor apposition
(necrotic tissue, infection, poor apposition) → increased exudate → increased granulation tissue

c. infection → necrotic tissue → poor apposition
(infection, necrotic tissue, poor apposition) → increased exudate → increased granulation tissue

20. B
A
B
C
C

---

21. MATCH THE FOLLOWING:

____follows inflammation or necrosis	A. Physiologic replacement
____occurs in a tissue continuously throughout life	B. Repair
____involves proliferation of cells	

---

88. Disorganized loose collagen will be present.
It will have regained some strength.

---

89. Assuming there are no complications, how long would you wait before allowing the patient to return to normal activity (i.e., until the tissue strength has returned to normal)?

51.

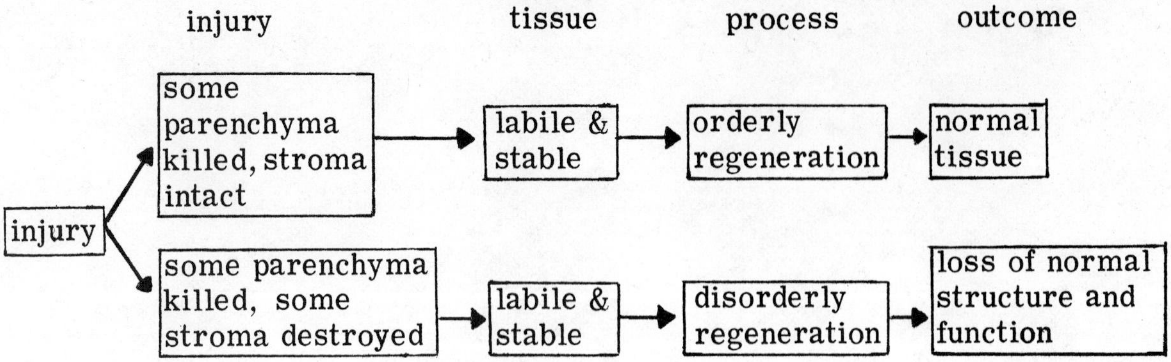

52. INDICATE WHICH CONDITIONS ARE PRESENT AND WHETHER ORDERLY REGENERATION WILL OCCUR:

	composed of labile or stable parenchyma	supporting stroma undamaged	orderly regeneration
1. brain infarct			
2. anoxic damage to neurons			
3. partial-thickness burn to dermis			
4. burn damaging epidermis and full thickness of dermis			
5. kidney infarct			
6. ischemic kidney tubule necrosis			
7. myocardial infarct			

119. A
B
A
B

120. GIVE THREE FACTORS, ANY OF WHICH IS SUFFICIENT TO CAUSE A WOUND TO HEAL BY SECOND INTENTION RATHER THAN FIRST INTENTION.

21. B
A
A, B

---

22. MATCH THE FOLLOWING WORDS AND DEFINITIONS:

____the death of cells and tissues within the living body
____the replacement of dead cells and tissues by new ones of parenchymal or stromal origin in response to injury
____the vascular and cellular response to injury
____the replacement of dead cells by new ones of the same type in response to normal physiologic cell death

A. inflammation
B. necrosis
C. repair
D. physiologic replacement

---

89. several months (or equivalent)

---

90. The healing of a broken bone involves granulation tissue, but it also involves other connective tissue elements, namely, cartilage and bone. Granulation tissue grows into the blood clot produced by the fracture and is gradually replaced by new bone and some cartilage. The cartilage serves as a framework for endochondral bone formation and eventually is completely replaced as the site is remodeled into mature bone.

The reparative elements of a fractured bone include ____________, ____________, and ____________. Of these components, the one that is temporarily present in the middle phase of the process is ____________.

50.

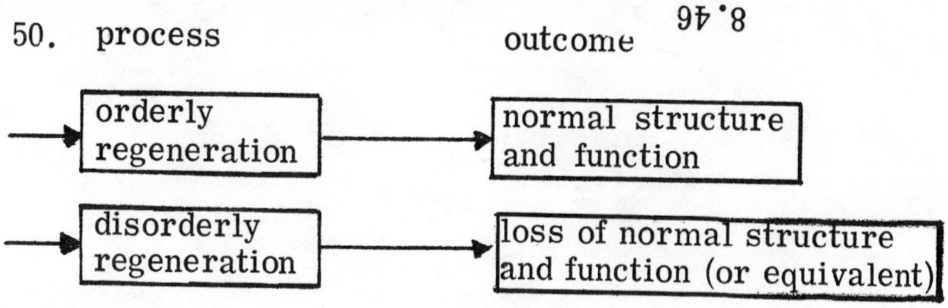

51. INDICATE THE CONDITIONS FOR EACH PROCESS:

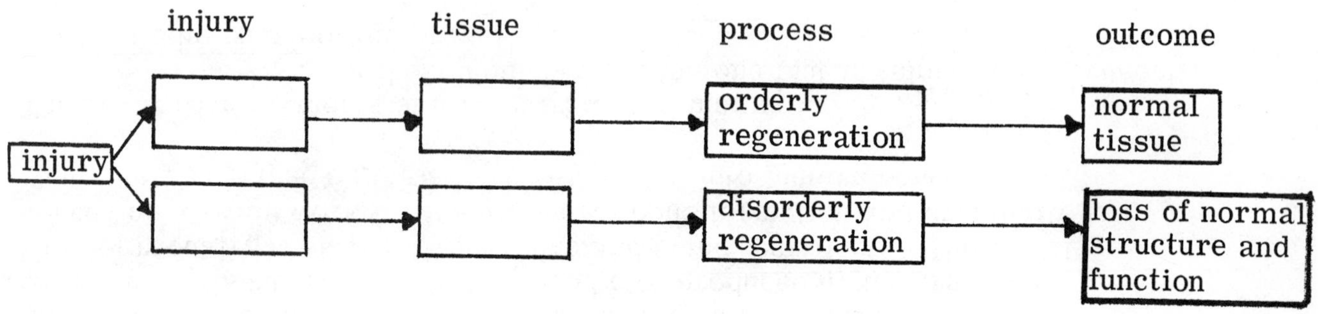

118. b

119. INDICATE WHETHER THE FOLLOWING EXAMPLES WOULD HEAL BY (A) FIRST INTENTION OR (B) SECOND INTENTION:

____ a cut by a sickle, cleaned and stitched up one hour after the accident

____ a dirty cut by a sickle, not cleaned and stitched until ten hours after the accident

____ a clean surgical incision

____ a surgical incision which after two days became infected

22. B
C
A
D

---

23. INDICATE "T" TRUE OR "F" FALSE:

	frame ref.
____The universal outcome of healing is restoration of normal structure and function.	(1)
____Necrosis and/or inflammation usually precede healing.	(2, 3)
____Resolution and sloughing involve the replacement of dead or injured cells.	(4)
____Resolution may consist of liquefaction of debris and resorption of exudate and liquefied debris.	(6)
____The amount of exudate determines whether the outcome of resolution will be restoration of normal structure and function.	(8, 9,15)
____Physiologic replacement occurs only after injury.	(20)

---

90. granulation tissue, cartilage, and bone
cartilage

---

91. When the break occurs, periosteum may be elevated from either side. The periosteal cells start multiplying and form a collar around each end. Then they migrate toward each other and reestablish continuity if the bone is immobilized. The fibroblasts in the new granulation tissue soon differentiate into chondroblasts and osteoblasts and begin producing ______________ and ______________.

MATCH THE LABELS WITH THE PICTURE OF THE BONE AS IT WOULD APPEAR AFTER 2 to 3 WEEKS:

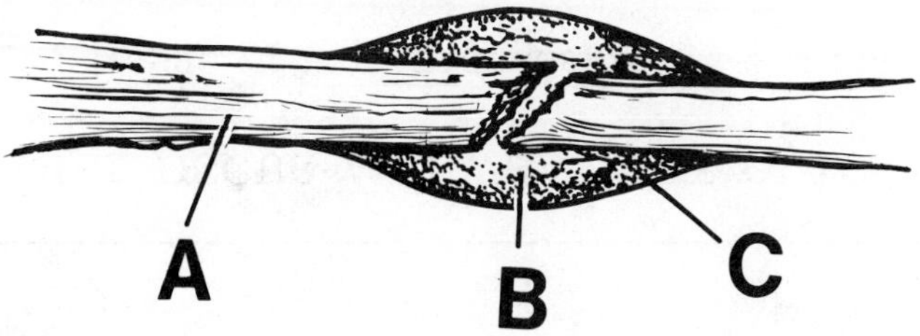

____old bone fragment
____proliferating periosteum
____mixture of fibrous tissue, disorganized bone, and cartilage

49. 1) The tissue parenchyma must be labile or stable (or the tissue parenchyma must be capable of proliferation).
2) Some viable parenchyma must remain.
3) The stroma must be intact.

---

50. INDICATE WHICH PROCESS WILL OCCUR AND WHAT THE OUTCOME WILL BE:

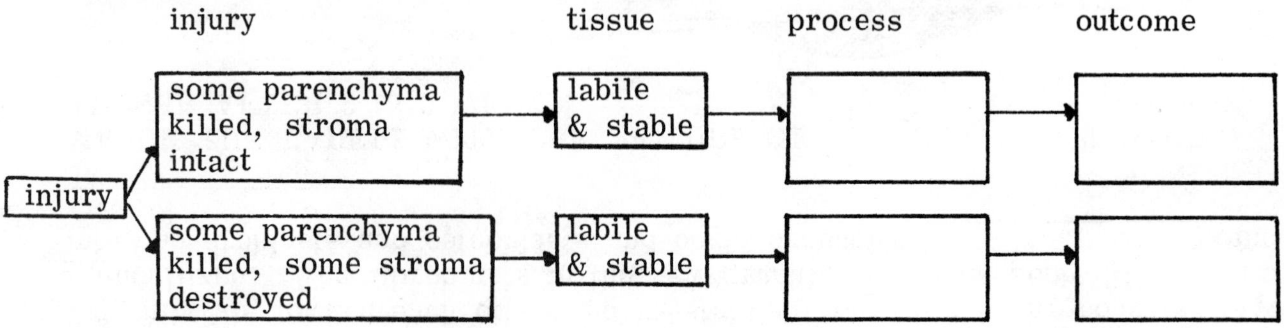

---

117. 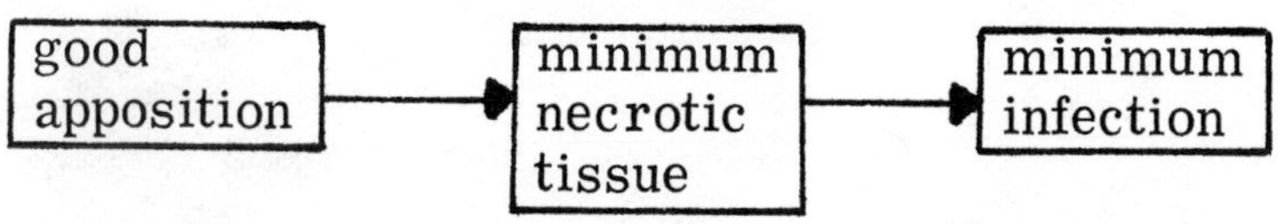

(in any order)

---

118. It is known from experience that wounds of less than six hours duration which have been cleaned of dead tissue and foreign material will heal in spite of the presence of small numbers of bacteria. If a wound has remained open for longer than six hours or so, bacterial infection is likely to have become established and the wound is not likely to heal by first intention in spite of cleansing.

WHICH IS/ARE TRUE?

a. The presence of bacteria in a 2-hour-old wound indicates infection.
b. If a 2-hour-old wound is sutured without removal of all dead tissue, bacterial infection is likely.

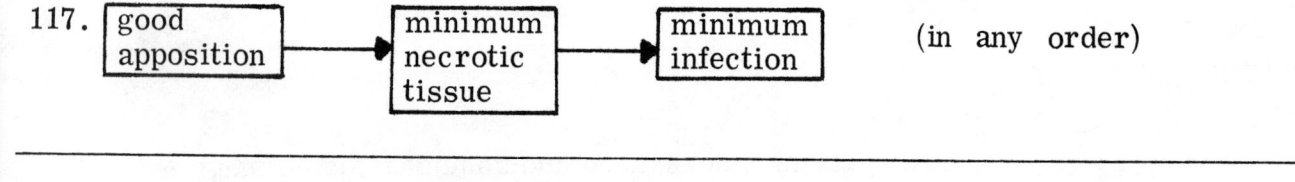

23. F
T
F
T
F
F

B. Repair: Parenchymal and Connective Tissue Proliferation (19 frames)

When you complete this section, you will be able to select correct responses relating to the:

1. definition of labile, stable, and permanent cells.

2. classification of the following as labile, stable, or permanent.

   hematopoietic tissue
   glandular parenchymal tissue
   surface epithelia
   muscle (smooth, striated, cardiac)
   nerve cells
   bone and cartilage
   connective tissue

GO ON TO NEXT PAGE

---

91. cartilage and bone

A
C
B

---

92. Over a period of months, most scar tissue rearranges along lines of stress. In a healing fracture, fibrous tissue can differentiate into bone. Since normal bone is structured along lines of stress, the ultimate outcome of this repair is usually ________________.

48. O
D
O

49. In the last two frames, three factors were given as being necessary for extensive orderly regeneration. One concerned the nature of the tissue at the location of the injury and the other two concerned the type of injury.

What are the three factors necessary for extensive orderly regeneration?

116.

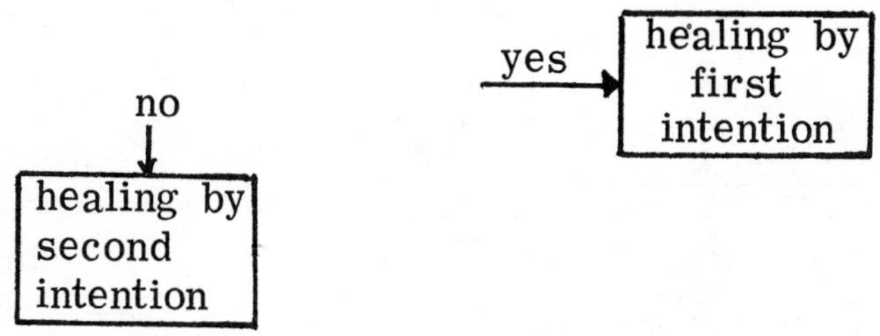

117. FILL IN THE EMPTY BOXES:

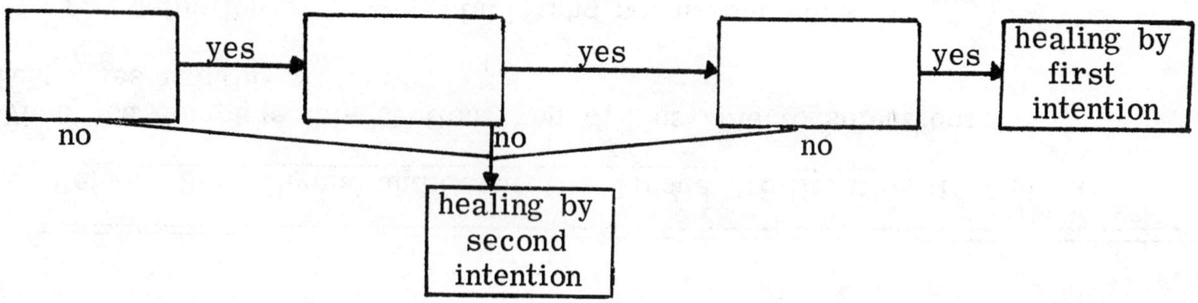

24. The proliferative capability of a cell is one of the primary determinants of the type of repair which will occur.

Most tissues can be classified by the proliferative capacity of the constituent cells as:

1) labile: proliferate continuously throughout life
2) stable: proliferate to a minimal extent in adult life except when stimulated to proliferate by certain factors such as tissue injury
3) permanent: do not undergo mitosis in postnatal life

MATCH THE FOLLOWING:

____mitosis occurs normally	L. labile cells
____mitosis occurs in response to injury	S. stable cells
____mitosis does not occur	P. permanent cells

---

92. normal bone. (or equivalent)

---

93. INDICATE WHICH OF THE FOLLOWING ARE, IN GENERAL, TYPICAL OF ORGANIZATION:

____formation of granulation tissue
____an outcome of normal structure and function
____proliferation of fibroblasts and endothelial cells
____the formation of a new scar after a couple of weeks
____deposition of bone and cartilage
____differentiation of fibroblasts into specialized cells

47. _✓_ labile _✓_ stable

_✓_ skin
___ brain
_✓_ liver
___ heart

_✓_ intestinal mucosa
_✓_ kidney tubule
_✓_ bone
_✓_ bone marrow

---

48. The type of injury is an important factor in determining whether regeneration will occur and if so, which type. If regeneration is to occur, there must be some parenchymal tissue left to proliferate. If the stroma is intact, orderly regeneration will occur; if not, disorderly regeneration is more likely.

INDICATE ORDERLY REGENERATION (O) OR DISORDERLY REGENERATION (D) FOR THE FOLLOWING EXAMPLES:

____ centrilobular damage to hepatocytes (mild carbon tetrachloride injury)
____ submassive hepatic necrosis with islands of uninjured cells remaining in a collapsed, disorganized stroma
____ diffuse anoxic injury to many proximal renal tubule cells, without collapse or disorganization of renal architecture

---

116. Surgeons noted years ago that some incisions and sutured wounds healed "by first intention," while others started to heal, broke down, and eventually healed "by second intention." We now know that three factors are important in producing healing by first intention:
1) good apposition of wound margins
2) minimum necrotic tissue
3) minimum bacterial infection

FILL IN THE BLANKS:

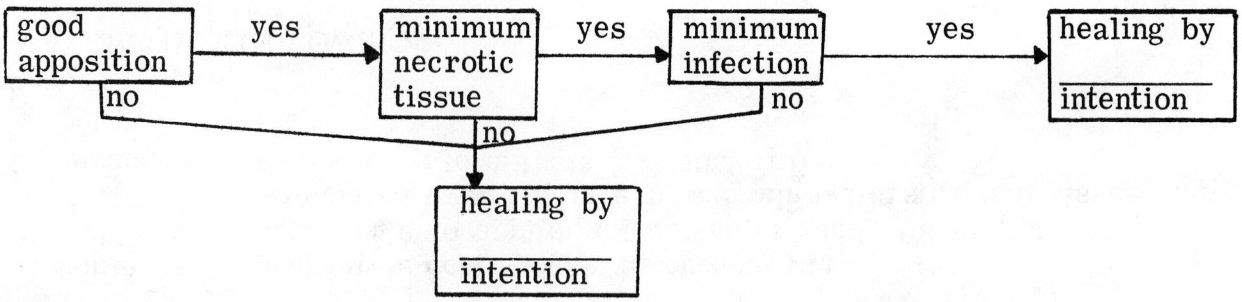

24. _L_ mitosis occurs normally
_S_ mitosis occurs in response to injury
_P_ mitosis does not occur

---

25. Stable cells are so named because

☐ they are stable under all circumstances.

☐ they are stable in the "normal" state.

---

93. _✓_ formation of granulation tissue
_✓_ proliferation of fibroblasts and endothelial cells
_✓_ the formation of new scar after a couple of weeks

---

94. INDICATE WHICH OF THE FOLLOWING OCCUR WITH A TYPICAL HEALING FRACTURE:

___ formation of granulation tissue
___ an outcome of normal structure and function
___ proliferation of fibroblasts and endothelial cells
___ the formation of new scar after a couple of weeks
___ deposition of bone and cartilage
___ differentiation of fibroblasts into specialized cells

46. B
A (normal function restored)

---

47. Regeneration can only occur in tissues in which the parenchymal cells are capable of proliferation.

INDICATE WHICH TYPE(S) OF TISSUE ARE CAPABLE OF REGENERATION:

____labile ____stable ____permanent

INDICATE TISSUES WHERE EXTENSIVE REGENERATION MAY OCCUR:

____skin	____intestinal mucosa
____brain	____kidney tubule
____liver	____bone
____heart	____bone marrow

---

115. F
T
T
F
T

D. Healing: Agent and Host Factors (22 frames)

When you complete this section, you will be able to select correct responses relating to the:

1. definition and differentiation of healing by first intention and healing by second intention in terms of time, sequence of events, outcome, and factors determining which course will be followed.

2. local and systemic factors likely to produce rapid or slow repair, increased susceptibility to infection, excessive scarring, or failure .of the repair process.

GO ON TO THE NEXT PAGE

25. Stable cells are so named because

[√] they are stable in the "normal" state.

---

26. Epithelial surfaces and hematopoietic (myeloid and lymphoid) tissues proliferate continuously and therefore are classified as labile tissues.

INDICATE THE LABILE TISSUES OR CELLS:

____lymphocytes
____epidermis
____bone marrow
____smooth muscle
____liver parenchymal cells
____nerve cells

---

94. all of them

---

95. The skin will regenerate with little scarring if less than full thickness injury occurs. The skin appendages (hair follicles, sebaceous glands, and sweat glands) will regenerate if a part of them is uninjured.
MATCH THE INJURIES AND OUTCOMES:

Level of Injury

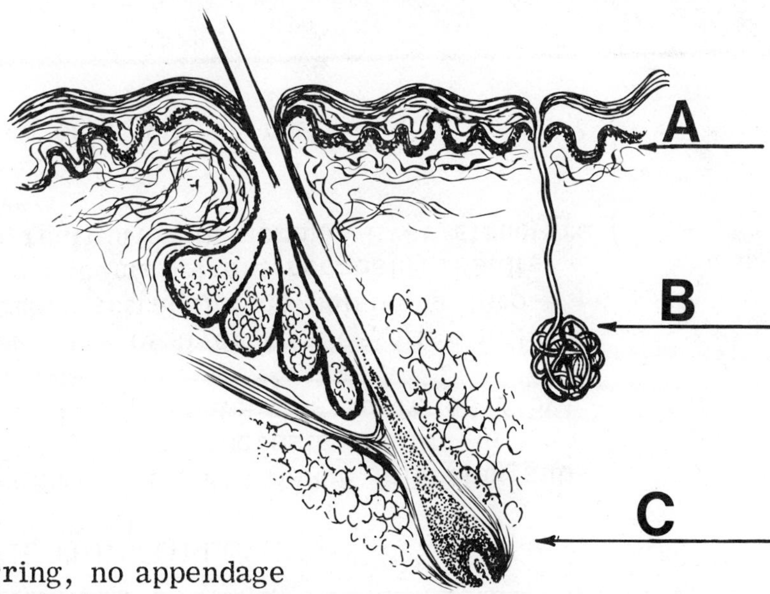

A scrape

B partial thickness

C full thickness

Outcome

____scarring, no appendage regeneration
____little or no scarring, rapid regeneration of injured tissue
____little or no scarring, all injured tissues eventually regenerate

45. A
B
B
A

---

46. MATCH THE FOLLOWING:

____regrowth of liver tissue following submassive liver necrosis results in nodules of hepatocytes surrounded by fibrous tissue	A. orderly regeneration
____regrowth of liver lobules after mild carbon tetrachloride poisoning (produces centrilobular necrosis) results in restitution of normal liver structure	B. disorderly regeneration

In which case will normal function return?

---

114. T
F
T
T
F

---

115. INDICATE "T" TRUE OR "F" FALSE:

	frame ref.
____The cells primarily involved in regeneration are the stroma of the injured organ.	(44)
____The liver will heal by orderly regeneration if only the parenchymal cells are damaged or by disorderly regeneration and scarring if large areas of parenchymal and stromal tissue are damaged.	(107, 111)
____If repair occurs in organs where the functional tissue is permanent, it will be by organization or gliosis.	(66, 69)
____Repair should be completed in about one week if it is by regeneration, regardless of which organ it is occurring in.	(57)
____The outcome of orderly regeneration is normal structure and function.	(45)

26. _✓_ lymphocytes
_✓_ epidermis
_✓_ bone marrow

---

27. The continuous proliferation of labile cells is called physiologic replacement. You would expect that the tissues involved would be ☐ the same as ☐ different from those undergoing physiologic cell death.

Physiologic replacement is particularly prominent for which of the following cells or tissues?

____ blood cells

____ endometrium

____ cells lining the surface of the intestinal tract

____ neurons

---

95. C
A
B

---

96. GIVE THE OUTCOME OF THE FOLLOWING SKIN INJURIES:

a scrape

a partial-thickness burn

a full-thickness burn

44. R
C
R
C

---

45. Regeneration can be orderly, restoring normal structure and function, or disorderly, resulting in disorganized structure and consequent loss of function. Disorderly regeneration is a combination of parenchymal regeneration and connective tissue repair.

MATCH THE FOLLOWING:

____parenchymal regrowth to produce normal histology	A. orderly regeneration
____scarring or other connective tissue repair process prevents orderly parenchymal regrowth, resulting in disorganized parenchymal regrowth	B. disorderly regeneration
____involves scarring	
____does not involve scarring	

---

113. B
A
C

---

114. INDICATE "T" TRUE OR "F" FALSE:

	frame reference
____The liver and kidney are two organs where disorderly regeneration is commonly observed.	(106-112)
____The cells primarily involved in organization are macrophages and endothelial cells.	(74)
____Regeneration occurs if the supporting stroma is uninjured and if the functional parenchymal cells are labile or stable.	(47, 48)
____As it matures, granulation tissue becomes less vascular, less cellular, and more fibrous, forming a mature scar after several months.	(77,78)
____The outcome of disorderly regeneration is normal structure and function.	(45)

27. [✓] the same
✓ blood cells
✓ endometrium
✓ cells lining the surface of the intestinal tract

---

28. Stable cells, which comprise the majority of cell types, reproduce minimally or not at all in normal situations but can proliferate in response to injury.

Stable cells, however, vary greatly in their capacity to proliferate in response to injury.

MATCH THE FOLLOWING:

____ The epithelial, endothelial, and mesangial cells of a renal glomerulus can proliferate but will not form new glomeruli.

____ Removal of a lobe of liver will be followed by formation of new liver lobules to replace the lost volume.

A. extensive replacement capacity

B. limited replacement capacity

---

96. little or no scarring, rapid regeneration of injured tissue
little or no scarring, all injured tissues eventually regenerate
scarring, no appendage regeneration

---

97. While the nervous system response to injury may at first appear to be unusual, it can be predicted by application of the principles learned in the earlier parts of this program.

MATCH THE NERVE INJURY TO THE OUTCOME:

Injury

a. radial nerve cut and ends reapproximated
b. radial nerve cut and ends not reapproximated

Outcome

____ tangle of fibrous tissue, Schwann cells (from nerve sheath), and axons, resulting in a neuroma

____ neurons grow back down the sheaths and near-normal function eventually returns

43. A
Yes, the necrotic tissue must be removed before repair can occur.

---

44. Regeneration is the replacement of lost cells by proliferation of the remaining parenchymal cells.

Connective tissue repair is the replacement of lost cells by proliferation of the stroma (connective tissue) of an organ. Scarring, the most common form of connective tissue repair, is the process of replacement by dense fibrous (collagenous) tissue.

INDICATE WHETHER EACH OF THE FOLLOWING IS AN EXAMPLE OF REGENERATION (R) OR CONNECTIVE TISSUE REPAIR (C):

____replacement of a burned area of skin by new squamous cells
____replacement of a burned area of skin by fibrous scar tissue
____replacement of damaged kidney tubules by new tubule cells
____replacement of a damaged kidney glomerulus by fibrous tissue

---

112. We would call it disorderly regeneration, because there is both scarring and regeneration without restitution of normal structure.

---

113. Kidney lesions provide a nice contrast in repair responses. If one tissue element which is capable of replacing itself is selectively damaged, return to normal may be expected. Complete necrosis of a localized area can only heal by scarring. Patchy damage involving several tissue components will involve some that can regenerate and others that will scar or atrophy.

MATCH THE TYPES OF REPAIR WITH THE TYPES OF KIDNEY DAMAGE:

____ischemic tubular necrosis	A. organization
____infarct	B. orderly regeneration
____nephron vascular damage	C. disorderly regeneration and organization

28. B
A

---

29. In general, the parenchyma of glandular organs and most mesenchymal tissues are composed of stable cells.

Examples of gland parenchyma include kidney tubules, gastric secretory glands, and thyroid acini.

Examples of cells of mesenchymal origin include fibrovascular stroma (connective tissue) and more specialized tissue such as bone, cartilage, adipose tissue, and the glial connective tissue cells of the central nervous system.

INDICATE THE STABLE TISSUES OR CELLS:

____hepatocytes
____fibrocytes
____Brunner's glands of duodenum
____capillaries

____epidermis
____dermis
____bone marrow
____bone

____neurons
____glial cells
____subcutaneous fatty tissue

---

97. b
a

---

98. GIVE THE OUTCOME OF THE FOLLOWING INJURIES:

1. a cut radial nerve with ends reapproximated closely

2. a cut radial nerve with ends not reapproximated

42. F
F
T
T
F

C. Healing: Classification (73 frames)

This section discusses the various types of repair. When you have completed this section, you will be able to select correct responses relating to the:

1. distinction between resolution, orderly regeneration, disorderly regeneration, and organization in terms of:
   a. definitions
   b. type of preceding injury
   c. organs involved
   d. time course and resulting structural and functional changes
   e. common examples

43. Repair is the replacement of dead or injured tissue with new, viable tissue. Resolution may precede or occur with repair. Resolution can occur alone, but repair seldom does, since repair, by definition, does not include the removal of debris (which may block the process of replacement of injured tissue by new cells).

WHICH IS/ARE TRUE ?

A. Resolution frequently occurs without repair.
B. Repair frequently occurs without resolution.

If an area of heart muscle undergoes necrosis, will resolution begin before the scar begins to form ? Explain.

---

111. C
C
A
B
B
B

---

112. The kidney's architecture is such that vascular damage may cause necrosis of individual nephrons. When the afferent arteriole or glomerulus becomes occluded, most of the nephron unit dies and some granulation tissue grows into the area and later becomes a small scar. However, some tubules may survive, proliferate, and become cystically dilated. Adjacent nephron units with intact vessels may undergo hyperplasia. When many nephrons are involved, the process is one of alternating small scars with dilated tubules and normal-appearing tubules. This process is called arterionephrosclerosis.

What type of repair process is occurring in these kidneys ?

29. ✓ hepatocytes
✓ fibrocytes
✓ Brunner's glands of duodenum
✓ capillaries
✓ dermis
✓ bone
✓ glial cells
✓ subcutaneous fatty tissue

---

30. Osteoblasts and cartilage cells present an interesting contrast in regenerative capacity of stable cells. Both types of cells can proliferate from pre-existing tissue or can be derived from other connective tissue cells such as fibroblasts. Osteocytes can form bone and can remodel the bone to normal. Cartilage cells form disorganized cartilage which may be replaced by bone, but it cannot be remodeled into normal cartilaginous structures.

Which of the following cannot be repaired to normal?

a. a football injury producing a fracture of the tibia
b. a football injury with disruption of cartilage in the knee
c. rheumatoid arthritis with fibroblastic tissue replacing articular cartilage
d. a fracture site in which some cartilage is formed during the remodeling process

---

98. 1. neurons grow back down the sheaths, and near-normal function eventually returns
2. tangle of fibrous tissue, Schwann cells, and axons, forming a neuroma

---

99. The brain is unusual in its reactions to injury. After simple edema, resolution without necrosis usually occurs. Anoxic brain damage causes necrosis of neurons, which is also usually followed by resolution. Infarction leads to necrosis of neurons and glia, with proliferation of new glial cells around the area (gliosis).
Infection with abscess formation may provoke organization. In the brain abscesses frequently spread and are difficult to wall off. If treated, these result in scarring, and if untreated, usually result in death. The usual response to brain abscess, in contrast to other types of brain injury, is organization rather than gliosis.

MATCH THE MOST CHARACTERISTIC RESPONSE WITH THE TYPE OF BRAIN INJURY:

____ anoxic neuronal damage
____ infarct
____ abscess
____ edema

A. resolution
B. regeneration
C. organization
D. gliosis

41. T
T
F
F
F

---

42. INDICATE "T" TRUE OR "F" FALSE:

	frame reference
____All epithelial cells are classified as stable.	(26, 29, 40)
____Glial cells and neurons of the central nervous system are both permanent cell types.	(29, 35)
____Bone and cartilage cells are stable cells.	(29, 30)
____Renal glomeruli, even though composed of stable cells, may not regenerate to normal with severe injury.	(28)
____Adipose tissue is classified as labile.	(29)

---

110. ☑ yes

---

111. Several repair responses are possible in the liver, depending on the injury. Regenerative nodules occur when there is collapse of many lobules with remaining liver cells in between. MATCH THE INJURY WITH THE RESPONSE:

____a whole lobe is surgically removed
____necrosis of individual cells or groups of cells within lobules
____necrosis of groups of cells involving several lobules at one time and multiple areas of the liver
____abscess
____infarct
____caseous granuloma

A. disorderly regeneration
B. scarring
C. orderly regeneration

30. b
c

---

31. There is also variability in replacement capacity of parenchymal epithelial cells. Epithelial cells of major organs, such as kidney and liver, which are most susceptible to damage by anoxia and poisons, are most capable of rapid proliferation in response to injury. Glands which serve as supporting secretory appendages, such as salivary glands and Brunner's glands, have less replacement capacity.

MATCH THE FOLLOWING:

____damaged selectively by systemic causes	A. hepatocytes and renal tubule cells
____damaged by local injury or disease	B. lacrimal glands and submucosal esophageal glands
____complete replacement of injured cells likely	
____complete replacement of injured cells unlikely	

---

99. anoxic neuronal damage ——→ A. resolution (with loss of function)
infarct ——→ D. gliosis
abscess ——→ C. organization
edema ——→ A. resolution (without loss of function)

---

100. A lesion that usually produces scarring rather than gliosis in the central nervous system is a(an) ________________.

An infarct in the brain will produce loss of function of neurons which are ☐ localized to one area ☐ diffusely scattered.

Anoxic damage in the brain will produce loss of function of neurons which are ☐ localized to one area ☐ diffusely scattered.

40. S
L
P

Labile:	surface epithelium hematopoietic tissue	Permanent:	muscle neurons
Stable:	gland parenchyma mesenchymal connective tissue		

Epithelial cells are either labile or stable.

---

41. INDICATE "T" TRUE OR "F" FALSE:

	frame ref.
____Stable cells undergo mitosis in postnatal life.	(24)
____Gland parenchyma and cells of mesenchymal origin are classified as stable cells.	(29)
____Neurons and skeletal muscle cells can multiply if they have intact nuclei and sheaths.	(36)
____Smooth muscle is incapable of proliferation after birth.	(37)
____Following damage to less than half the cell, cardiac muscle fibers will undergo intracellular regeneration.	(36)

---

109. disorderly regeneration

---

110. Because Prometheus stole fire from the gods, he was punished by being chained to a rock. Periodically a vulture would fly down and eat a lobe of his liver. The liver is unusual; if an entire lobe is removed surgically and empty space is left, it may regenerate perfectly in a few weeks. On the basis of this information, is it possible that the ancient gods knew more than they were letting on to mortal men?

☐ yes ☐ no

31. A
B
A
B

---

32. MATCH THE FOLLOWING:

____epithelial surfaces — L. labile

____parenchyma of glandular organs — S. stable

____hematopoietic tissue (lymphoid and myeloid)

____mesenchymal connective tissues

---

100. abscess
☑ localized to one area
☑ diffusely scattered

---

101. GIVEN THE TYPE OF BRAIN INJURY, PREDICT WHICH REPARATIVE PROCESS WILL OCCUR AND THE OUTCOME:

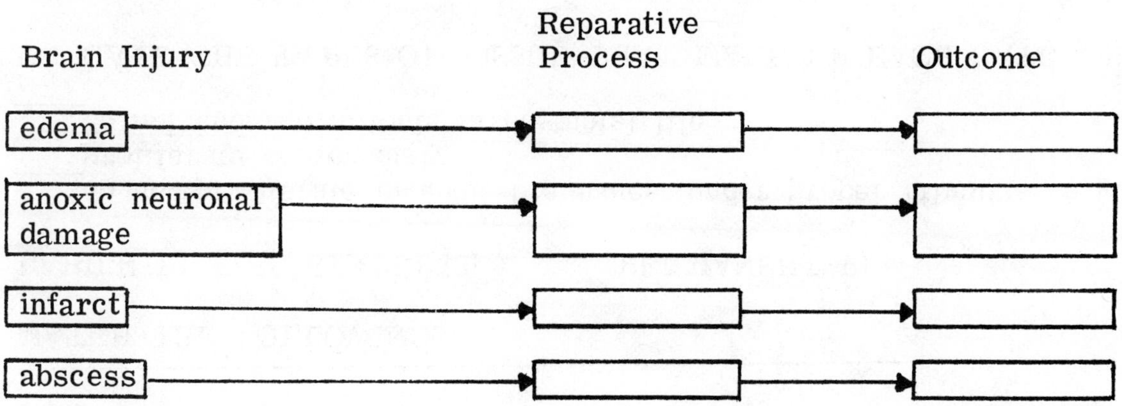

39. L epithelial surfaces
S mesenchymal connective tissues
L hematopoietic tissues
P nerve cells
S gland parenchyma
P muscle cells

---

40. MATCH THE FOLLOWING:

LABILE (L) STABLE (S) PERMANENT (P)

____ do not proliferate in adult life except under proper stimulus, e.g., injury
____ proliferate continuously
____ do not undergo mitosis in postnatal life

INDICATE THE TYPES OF TISSUE THAT MAKE UP EACH CATEGORY :

Labile ____________ Permanent ____________
____________ ____________

Stable ____________
____

Epithelial cells are either ______________ or ______________.

---

108. A
B

---

109. Chronic alcoholic damage to the liver leads to cirrhosis. In cirrhosis both destructive and reparative processes continue for long periods of time. The repair process is chronic ____________ ____________.

32. L
S
L
S

---

33. What two types of tissue are labile? What two types of tissue are stable?

CLASSIFY THE FOLLOWING AS LABILE (L) OR STABLE (S):

____ mature fibroblasts
____ bone marrow
____ hepatocytes
____ kidney tubule cells

____ kidney glomerulus cells
____ lymphocytes
____ blood vessel endothelium
____ adipose tissue

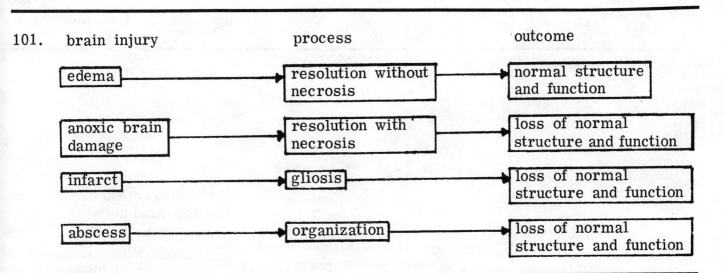

101.

brain injury	process	outcome
edema →	resolution without necrosis →	normal structure and function
anoxic brain damage →	resolution with necrosis →	loss of normal structure and function
infarct →	gliosis →	loss of normal structure and function
abscess →	organization →	loss of normal structure and function

---

102. Infarcts, abscesses, and caseous granulomatous nodules are all localized necrotic lesions which, in general, provoke a fibroblastic healing reponse. Small lesions will be completely replaced by granulation tissue, which will evolve into a dense scar. Large lesions will be walled off by formation of a fibrous rim.

Infarcts, abscesses, and caseous granulomas heal by the process of __________.

The necrotic material may be completely replaced by scar if the lesions are ________________.

38. S P (or S)
S P
L S

Most smooth muscle is classified as <u>permanent</u> tissue, but vascular smooth muscle and the muscularis mucosae of the gut could be classified as <u>stable</u> tissue.

---

39. CLASSIFY THE FOLLOWING TISSUE TYPES AS LABILE (L), STABLE (S), OR PERMANENT (P):

____ epithelial surfaces
____ mesenchymal connective tissues
____ hematopoietic tissues
____ nerve cells
____ gland parenchyma
____ muscle cells

---

107. disorderly regeneration

108.

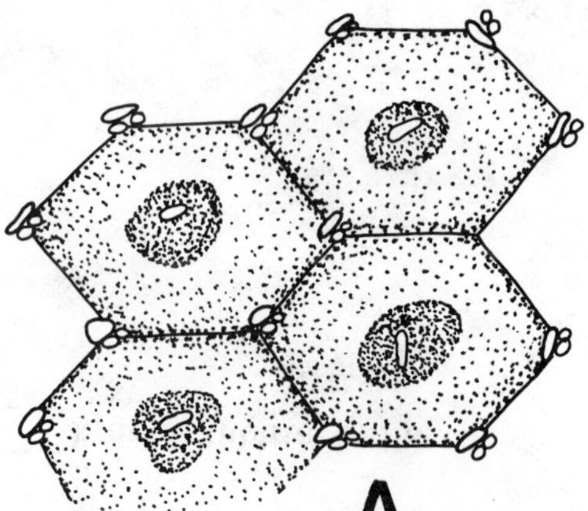

A

centrilobular necrosis

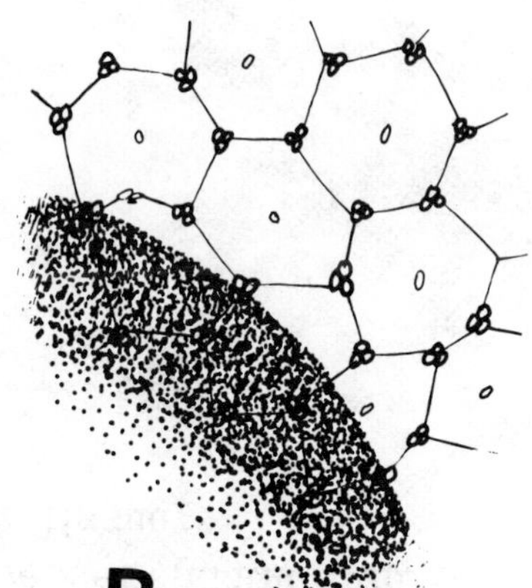

B

panlobular necrosis

Which will lead to orderly regeneration? ______

Which will lead to disorderly regeneration? ______

33. Labile: hematopoietic, surface epithelium
Stable: gland parenchyma

S	mature fibroblasts	S	kidney glomerulus cells
L	bone marrow	L	lymphocytes
S	hepatocytes	S	blood vessel endothelium
S	kidney tubule cells	S	adipose tissue

---

34. CLASSIFY THESE TISSUES AS LABILE (L) OR STABLE (S):

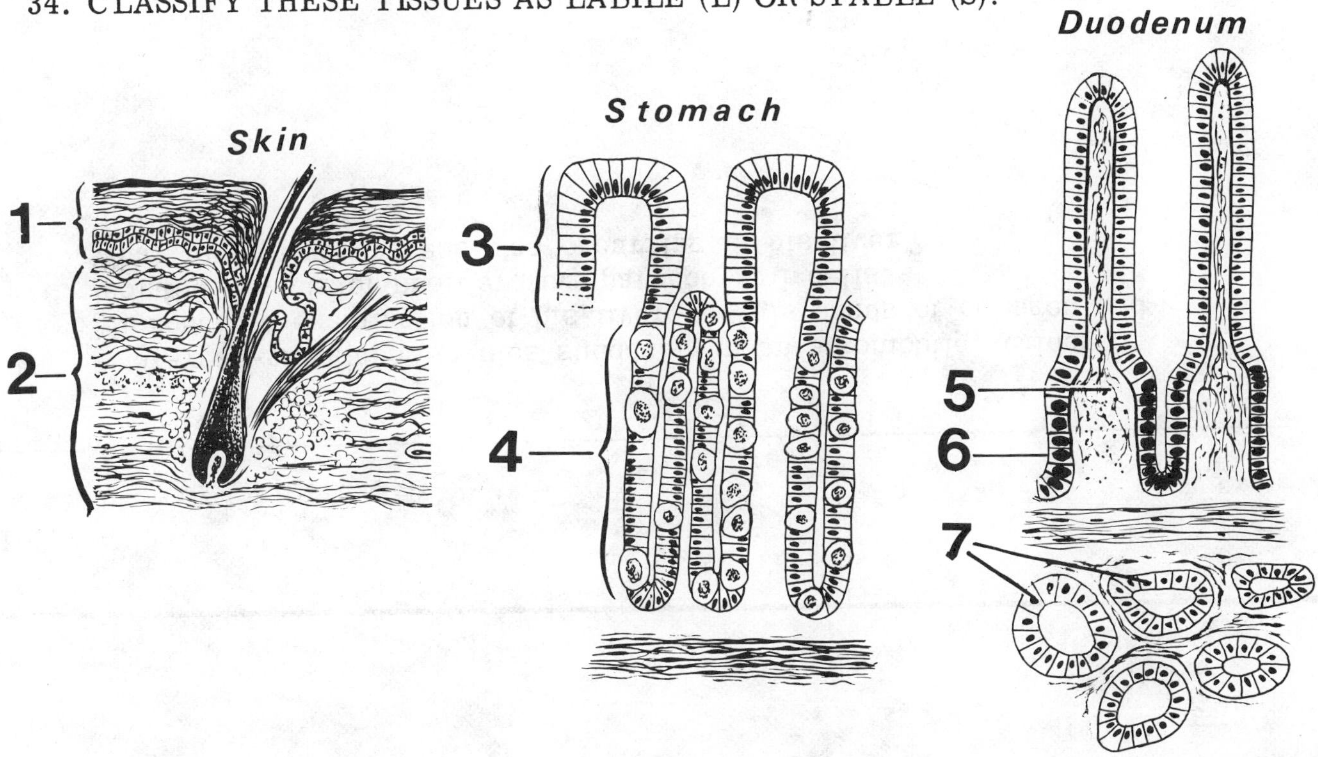

---

102. Infarcts, abscesses, and caseous granulomas heal by the process of organization.

The necrotic material may be completely replaced by scar if the lesions are small.

---

103. An abscess contains the injurious agent and large numbers of polys in the central area. Thus, a large amount of lytic enzyme is present in the central area.

If the abscess is small, once the injurious agent is removed and the content is liquefied by enzymes, resolution will be the predominant healing process. If the abscess is large, it cannot resolve, and organization will occur, resulting in scar formation. Large abscesses may rupture and collapse, producing irregular scars.

MATCH THE FOLLOWING:

____ 2-cm diameter abscess in liver	A. organization predominant
____ 2-mm diameter abscess in liver	B. resolution predominant

37. C
A
B
A

---

38. CLASSIFY THE FOLLOWING TISSUES AS LABILE (L), STABLE (S), OR PERMANENT (P):

____chondrocytes
____glial cells
____transitional epithelium of the urinary tract
____smooth muscle of the gut
____nerve cells of the brain
____stomach glands

Most smooth muscle is classified as ______________ tissue, but vascular smooth muscle and the muscularis mucosae of the gut could be classified as ______________ tissue.

---

106. a
b
c

---

107. A 57-year-old alcoholic dies suddenly in an automobile accident. Microscopic examination of his liver reveals bands of collagen and isolated islands of proliferating parenchymal cells. What reparative process was occurring in his liver?

34. 1. epidermis - L
2. dermis - S
3. surface epithelium - L
4. gastric glands - S
5. lamina propria - S
6. crypt epithelium - L
7. Brunner's glands - S

Note: The proliferative zone in the stomach is in the superficially placed pits and in the small intestine it is in the deep-lying crypts.

---

35. Nerve cells and muscle cells seldom if ever undergo mitosis in postnatal life, and, therefore, are classified as _______________ tissues.

CLASSIFY THE FOLLOWING TISSUES AS LABILE (L), STABLE (S), OR PERMANENT (P):

____bone marrow
____cardiac muscle
____osteocytes
____glial cells
____nerve cells
____sweat glands
____kidney (tubule cells)

---

103. A
B

---

104. Granulomas contain the injurious agent and epithelioid macrophages in the central areas. They are formed around agents which are difficult for the body to remove. Because of this and the fact that there is little lytic enzyme, it may take many years to organize a caseous granuloma. Both old abscesses and old granulomas have a tendency to undergo calcification, but this seems to occur more frequently in old granulomas.

CHOOSE WHETHER EACH FEATURE IS CHARACTERISTIC OF ABSCESSES (A) OR GRANULOMAS (G) OR BOTH (B):

____provoke formation of a fibrous wall
____greater tendency to calcify
____take longer to heal
____little lytic enzyme in central area
____healing by organization
____occasional healing primarily by resolution

36. A and B
They have intact nuclei and cell membranes.

---

37. Regenerating smooth muscle can be observed in two specific situations:

1) When new blood vessels are formed after an injury, new smooth muscle can be found in the media.

2) When the mucosa of a small area of the gut is lost, the entire muscosa, including the muscularis mucosae, is regenerated.

MATCH THE FOLLOWING:

____cardiac muscle	A. capable of intracellular regeneration
____neurons	B. capable of limited proliferation
____smooth muscle	C. no observable regenerative capability
____skeletal muscle	

---

105. A, B, C
A
B
C
A
C

---

106. Examples of disorderly regeneration are not as clear-cut because disorderly regeneration is not a "pure" process—it is a combination of organization and proliferation of parenchyma.

WHICH IS/ARE TRUE ?

a. Disorderly regeneration is a response to injury where both the parenchyma and stroma proliferate.

b. Because there is no longer an orderly framework, the proliferating parenchyma will lack order.

c. Scarring is likely to be a component of disorderly regeneration.

35. L bone marrow
P cardiac muscle
S osteocytes

S glial cells
P nerve cells
S sweat glands
S kidney (tubule cells)

---

36. Most permanent tissues are only relatively so. Smooth muscle is capable of some regeneration, though large areas cannot be replaced. Striated muscle and nerves are capable of intracellular regeneration. As long as the sarcolemma or neurolemma is intact and there is an intact nucleus present, the cell can regenerate an injured part. Cardiac muscle possesses virtually no regenerative capability.

WHICH OF THE CELLS MIGHT BE CAPABLE OF INTRACELLULAR REGENERATION? WHY?

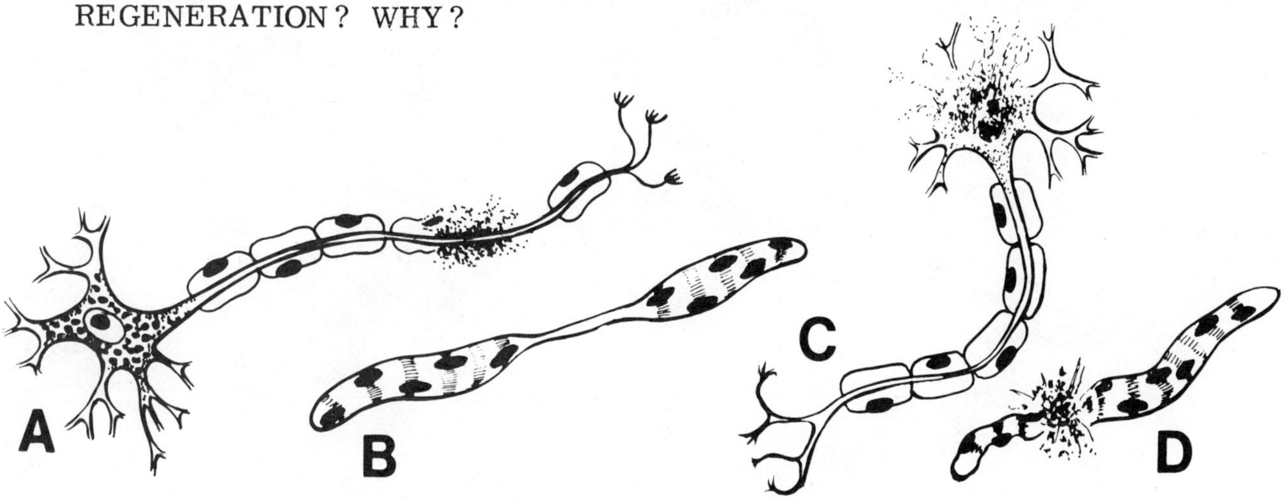

TURN TEXT 180° AND CONTINUE.

---

104. B
G
G
G
B
A

---

105. Except in the brain, where liquefaction occurs, infarcts produce coagulation necrosis, which provides a strong stimulus and good framework for ingrowth of granulation tissue. Infarcts up to several centimeters in diameter will be completely replaced by scar, which, with time, will contract to reduce the size of the lesion.

MATCH THE FOLLOWING:

____ heals with scar tissue
____ most likely to be completely replaced by scar
____ most likely to have solid, amorphous necrotic material in center which does not become organized
____ most likely to rupture, producing irregular scar
____ produces liquefaction and gliosis in brain
____ produces liquefaction and fibrosis in brain

A. infarct
B. caseous granuloma
C. abscess

TURN TEXT 180° AND CONTINUE.

Unit 9. Degeneration

Unit 9. DEGENERATION

OBJECTIVES

When you complete this unit, you will be able to select correct responses relating to the:

	starting page	frame numbers
A. Characteristics of degenerations	9.3	1-28

1. major differences among necrosis and acute and chronic degenerations in terms of morphologic appearance, causative mechanisms, and likelihood of reversibility.

	starting page	frame numbers
B. Classification of degenerations	9.59	29-149
(B1) Introduction	9.63	29-33
(B2) Degeneration involving water	9.73	34-45
(B3) Degeneration involving carbohydrate	9.62	46-65
(B4) Degeneration involving lipid	9.22	66-108
(B5) Degeneration involving protein	9.71	109-139
(B6) Degeneration involving calcium	9.26	140-149

1. Definition and proper use of: accumulation, storage, deposit, infiltration, hyaline, hyalin.
2. Information and procedures used to identify water, carbohydrate, fat, protein, and calcium in tissue.
3. Comparison of degenerations involving mainly
   water: cloudy swelling, hydropic degeneration
   carbohydrate: glycogen storage, mucoid change
   lipid: fatty metamorphosis, adiposity, mineral oil, granuloma, lipidoses, xanthoma, atheroma, lipofuscin
   protein: hyalinization of collagen, amyloidosis, fibrinoid change, Mallory body, Zenker's hyaline change
   calcium: dystrophic calcification, metastatic calcification

   in terms of
   definition
   type of material deposited
   morphologic appearance
   common sites and disease associations
   pathogenesis
   clinical significance

PRETEST

UNIT 9. DEGENERATION

SELECT THE SINGLE BEST RESPONSE:

1. Acute cell degeneration is characterized by dysfunction of the cell
   (A) cytoplasm
   (B) nucleus
   (C) both
   (D) neither

2. Which of the following is suggested when the morphologic features of chronic degeneration are associated with a fibrous reaction?
   (A) a specific lysosomal defect
   (B) a relative degree of anoxia
   (C) imperceptible necrosis
   (D) bacterial infection

3. Which type of degeneration is characterized by extracellular lipid deposits?
   (A) fatty metamorphosis
   (B) adiposity
   (C) mineral oil granuloma
   (D) xanthoma

4. Which is/are characteristically deposited intracellularly?
   (A) amyloid
   (B) glycogen
   (C) both
   (D) neither

5. Which occur(s) in the liver?
   (A) adiposity
   (B) fatty metamorphosis
   (C) both
   (D) neither

6. Which is/are usually reversible?
   (A) hydropic change
   (B) amyloid deposition
   (C) both
   (D) neither

7. Dystrophic calcification is defined by
   (A) elevated serum calcium levels
   (B) occurrence at sites of injury
   (C) both
   (D) neither

8. Reduced protein synthesis is likely to produce
   (A) atherosclerosis
   (B) fatty metamorphosis
   (C) both
   (D) neither

GO ON TO NEXT PAGE AND BEGIN THE UNIT

A. <u>Characteristics of Degeneration</u> (28 frames)

When you complete this section, you will be able to select correct responses relating to the:

1. major differences among necrosis and acute and chronic degenerations in terms of morphologic appearance, causative mechanisms, and likelihood of reversibility.

1. INDICATE THE FOURTH MAJOR RESPONSE OF THE BODY TO INJURY:

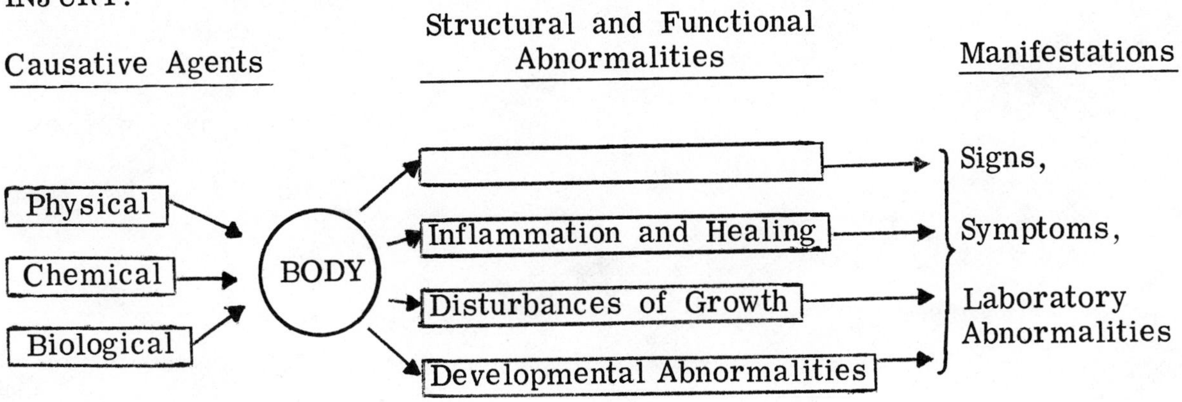

74. A
C
B
D

---

75. Lipid stains such as oil red O or Sudan black act by dissolving the colored oily stain in the non-colored oily tissue lipid.

Triglyceride droplets stain brightly with oil red O in frozen sections and are represented by clear holes in paraffin sections.

INDICATE WHICH HEPATOCYTE IS FROM A FROZEN SECTION STAINED WITH OIL RED O:

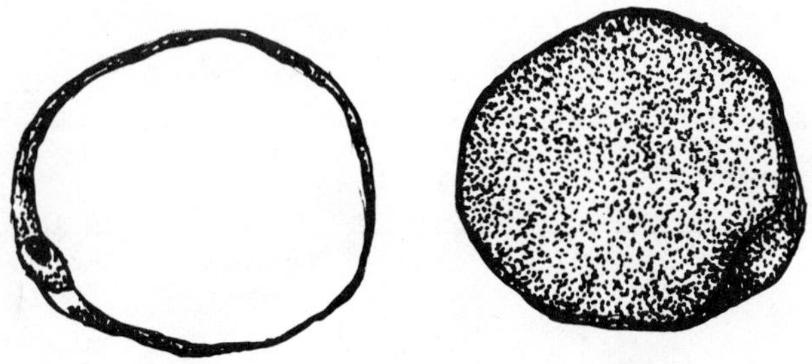

A B

TURN TEXT 180° AND CONTINUE.

1. | Cell Degeneration and Cell Death | or | Degeneration and Necrosis |

---

2. Degeneration refers to cellular and/or interstitial changes in which cells are not killed.

Acute degenerations are characterized by cytoplasmic injury and occur with injury not severe enough to produce necrosis (localized cell death within the living body).

Chronic degenerations are characterized by accumulations of a variety of substances either intra- or extracellularly and are caused by a variety of mechanisms.

MATCH THE FOLLOWING:

____cell death involved	A. necrosis
____reversible cytoplasmic injury	B. acute degeneration
____deposits within cells or interstitium	C. chronic degeneration

---

75. B

---

76. Intracellular lipoprotein accumulations also stain brightly for lipid in frozen sections and may stain faintly for lipid in pariffin sections because all of the lipoprotein may not be extracted by the tissue processing.

Cholesterol crystals do not stain in frozen sections because they are solids; in routine sections they are represented by cleft-shaped holes.

WHICH OF THE FOLLOWING STAIN STRONGLY (+), PARTIALLY (+/-), OR NOT AT ALL (0) WITH OIL RED O?

Triglyceride globules in hepatocytes in ___frozen sections___paraffin sections

Cholesterol crystals in an aortic intimal plaque in ___frozen sections ___paraffin sections

Lipoprotein complexes in macrophages in lipid storage diseases in ___frozen sections ___paraffin sections

73. B
A
B
A
A

---

74. Lipids appear as holes in tissue sections unless the sections are cut directly from frozen tissue (either fresh or fixed).

MATCH THE FOLLOWING (use each response only once):

____never seen directly in tissue sections	A. water
____seen in ordinary formalin-fixed H & E sections	B. glycogen
	C. mucus
____remains in tissue after direct fixation in alcohol	D. lipid
____removed from tissue except in frozen sections	

---

149. T
T
F
F
T

THIS IS THE END OF UNIT 9. TAKE THE POSTTEST ON PAGE xxx.

2. A
B
C

---

3. INDICATE THE PROCESS OCCURRING IN THE LIVER CELLS BELOW:

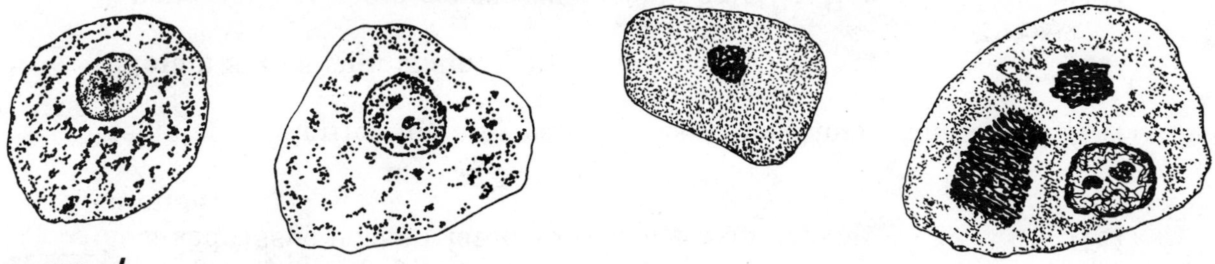

normal ______ ______ ______

A. necrosis (nuclear and cytoplasmic changes of cell death)
B. acute degeneration (non-specific swelling of cytoplasm, normal nucleus)
C. chronic degeneration (deposits in cytoplasm, normal or displaced nucleus)

---

76. Triglyceride globules in hepatocytes in _+_ frozen sections _0_ paraffin sections
Cholesterol crystals in an aortic intimal plaque in _0_ frozen sections
_0_ paraffin sections
Lipoprotein complexes in macrophages in lipid storage diseases in
_+_ frozen sections _+/-_ paraffin sections.

---

77. Considerable information can be gained from looking at ordinary H & E sections without resorting to special stains and fixatives.

Triglycerides form a droplet which displaces cytoplasm and nucleus and leaves a hole after being dissolved out.

Mucus often forms a globule in an epithelial cell but is not removed and stains faintly. It may or may not displace the nucleus.

Water, glycogen, and lipoproteins are finely dispersed without displacement of the nucleus, and all are removed in processing to produce a pale or vacuolated cytoplasm.
MATCH THE FOLLOWING CELLS WITH THE MATERIAL IN THEM:

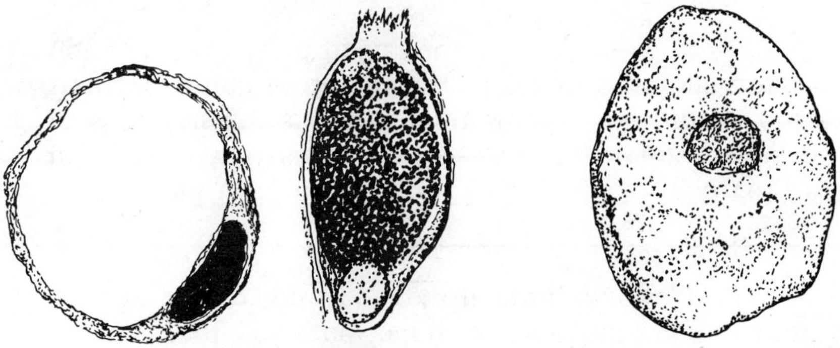

A **B** **C**

___mucus

___water, glycogen, or lipoprotein

___triglyceride

72. A strictly exogenous lipid is mineral oil.
Lipid droplets are most likely to contain triglyceride or mineral oil.
Dispersed intracellular lipid is in the form of lipoprotein complexes.
Cholesterol may be found extracellularly as crystals and intracellularly as dispersed lipoprotein complexes.

---

73. Lipids and lipid complexes, including cholesterol crystals, are removed prior to paraffin infiltration by the solvents used in routine tissue processing (xylene and chloroform). Lipids are not removed by watery fixatives such as formalin. Frozen sections must be used to directly demonstrate lipid in tissue.

MATCH THE FOLLOWING:

____water-soluble, removed by formalin	A. lipid
____not water-soluble, not removed by formalin	B. glycogen
____if fixed in alcohol, not removed during paraffin embedding	
____always removed by paraffin embedding process	
____may be demonstrated by frozen section after formalin fixation	

---

148. C
A
D
B

---

149. INDICATE "T" TRUE OR "F" FALSE:

	frame reference
____Dystrophic calcification is the deposition of calcium in diseased tissue unassociated with changes in serum calcium.	(141)
____Metastatic calcification may cause kidney stone formation.	(147)
____Calcium stains with eosin.	(144)
____Hyperparathyroidism causes dystrophic calcification.	(141, 147)
____Atherosclerosis may cause dystrophic calcification.	(141, 147)

3. B A C

4. COMPARE:	necrosis	acute degeneration	chronic degeneration
intact nucleus			
altered cytoplasm			
likely to be immediate reaction to injury			
deposits present in cells or between cells			
cells dead			

77. C
A
B

78. COMPLETE THE FOLLOWING TABLE BY INDICATING APPROPRIATE BOXES:

	water	glycogen	mucin	triglyceride	lipoprotein	cholesterol crystals
material removed in tissue processing, producing holes in H & E sections						
some residual material may be bound to cells and can be stained						
PAS-positive						
PAS-positive after amylase digestion						
characteristic needle-shaped clefts in H & E sections						
oil red O-positive in frozen sections						

71. B
A
C

---

72. A strictly exogenous lipid is ____________________.

Lipid droplets are most likely to contain __________ or ______________.

Dispersed intracellular lipid is in the form of ______________ complexes.

Cholesterol may be found extracellularly as ________________ and intracellularly as dispersed ______________ complexes.

---

147. A
B
A
B

---

148. MATCH THE DEGENERATIVE PROCESSES THAT MAY BE INVOLVED IN A SEVERE ATHEROSCLEROTIC LESION OF THE AORTA WITH THE DESCRIPTIONS:

____dense, eosinophilic, acellular areas

____foamy macrophages

____masses of hematoxaphilic granules

____needle-shaped empty spaces

A. intracellular cholesterol deposits
B. extracellular cholesterol deposits
C. hyalinization of collagen
D. dystrophic calcification

4.

	necrosis	acute degeneration	chronic degeneration
intact nucleus		✓	✓
altered cytoplasm	✓	✓	✓
likely to be immediate reaction to injury	✓	✓	
deposits present in cells or between cells			✓
cells dead	✓		

5. Immediate types of injury usually produce both degeneration and necrosis. The transition from early cytoplasmic swelling to later shrunken eosinophilic cytoplasm to the nuclear changes that establish cell death can be analyzed to judge the severity and time of injury.

ASSUMING THE SEVERITY OF INJURY TO BE THE SAME, RANK THE FOLLOWING FROM EARLIEST (1) TO LATEST (3) STAGE OF THE INJURY:

____ Many cells have eosinophilic cytoplasm and pyknotic nuclei, and there is congestion and infiltration of leukocytes.

____ The tissue is swollen due to cells with enlarged, vacuolated cytoplasm.

____ Some cells have vacuolated cytoplasm, while others have more eosinophilic cytoplasm; some cells exhibit pyknosis, karyorrhexis, and karyolysis.

---

78. material removed in tissue processing: water, glycogen, triglyceride, lipoprotein, cholesterol crystals

some residual material may be bound to cells and can be stained: glycogen, lipoprotein

PAS-positive: glycogen, mucin

PAS-positive after amylase digestion: mucin

characteristic needle-shaped clefts in H & E sections: cholesterol crystals

oil red O-positive in frozen sections: triglyceride, lipoprotein

---

79. Degenerations involving triglyceride accumulation involve the two types of cells that store triglyceride: adipose tissue cells and hepatocytes.

The adipose tissue cell is designed to store triglyceride as a spherical droplet in its cytoplasm and to release it when needed by the body for energy.

The hepatocyte does not normally contain enough triglyceride to form a droplet, but in many disease situations, triglyceride accumulates in hepatocytes, forming a droplet which displaces cytoplasm and nucleus.

Triglyceride accumulates ☐ intracellularly ☐ interstitially.

Cells accumulating droplets of triglyceride which push cytoplasm and nucleus to the periphery include:

____ hepatocytes ____ adipose tissue cells ____ macrophages

70. B
A

---

71. Cholesterol complexed to lipoprotein often accumulates in macrophages, especially when serum cholesterol is high. In areas of cholesterol deposition, there is often a mixture of extracellular crystals and foamy macrophages containing the complexed cholesterol.

MATCH THE FOLLOWING:

____quickly ingested and removed by macrophages when spilled extracellularly	A. cholesterol
____partially ingested by macrophages, partially stored as crystals	B. triglyceride
____remains extracellular, cannot be removed by macrophages	C. mineral oil

---

146. basophilic (hematoxaphilic, blue) granules

---

147. Dystrophic calcification can frequently be seen in roentgenograms and, therefore, is helpful in locating degenerative or necrotic lesions which have calcified.

Metastatic calcification may result in primary injury, especially in the kidney where it may damage renal parenchyma or may result in kidney stone formation.

MATCH THE FOLLOWING:

____indicates site of previous injury	A. dystrophic calcification
____may initiate injury	
____a spherical, calcified, granulomatous lesion in the periphery of the lung	B. metastatic calcification
____kidney stones associated with hypercalcemia	

5. 3
1
2

---

6. ASSUMING THE TIME FROM INJURY TO BE THE SAME, RANK THE FOLLOWING FROM LEAST (1) TO MOST SEVERE (3) DEGREE OF INJURY:

____Only cytoplasmic changes are evident.

____All cells in an area exhibit cytoplasmic and nuclear changes.

____Some cells exhibit only cytoplasmic changes while others have both nuclear and cytoplasmic changes.

In distinguishing acute degenerative changes from necrosis, one should be most concerned about the presence or absence of ☐ cytoplasmic ☐ nuclear changes.

---

79. ☑ intracellularly
_✓_hepatocytes _✓_adipose tissue cells

---

80. Adiposity may refer to
   1) a generalized increase in body adipose tissue (called obesity),
   2) replacement of parenchymal organs by normal-appearing adipose tissue (adiposity associated with parenchymal atrophy).

MATCH THE FOLLOWING:

____adiposity of subcutaneous tissue and some organs associated with overeating

____adiposity of the heart and pancreas commonly found with aging

____foamy macrophages accumulate locally in subcutaneous adipose tissue

A. adiposity with parenchymal atrophy

B. obesity

C. injury to adipose tissue

69. ✓ yes
✓ foreign-body granuloma

---

70. A transient form of extracellular lipid occurs when adipose tissue is injured, with liquid triglyceride escaping from the ruptured adipocytes. Macrophages quickly accumulate and phagocytose the triglyceride. They apparently convert the triglyceride to a complex which is evenly dispersed in the cytoplasm of the macrophage.

MATCH THE FOLLOWING:

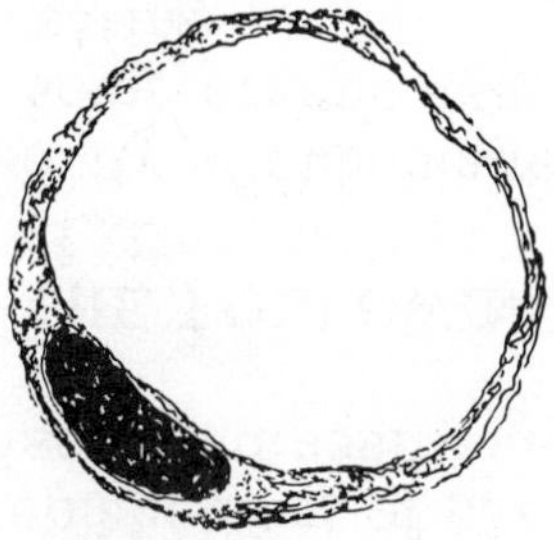
____

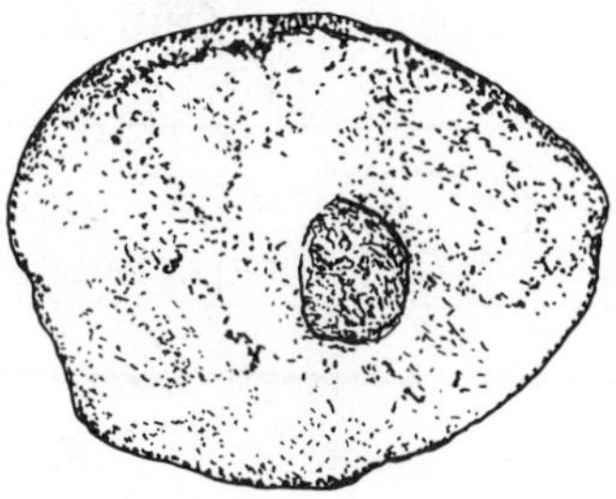
____

A. macrophage with ingested lipid

B. adipocyte with liquid triglyceride droplet

---

145. dystrophic calcification

---

146. Morphologically, dystrophic calcification appears in areas of old injury as small ________ ________.

6. 1
   3
   2

In distinguishing acute degenerative changes from necrosis, one should be most concerned about the presence or absence of

☑ nuclear changes.

---

7. The causes of acute degeneration are generally the same as those for necrosis. Anoxia is the most frequent cause.

The causes of chronic degeneration are diverse and often are not capable of producing overt necrosis (if they did produce much necrosis, they would kill the patient and therefore would not be chronic).

MATCH THE FOLLOWING:

____often a non-specific reaction to injury associated with necrosis	A. acute degeneration
____often a specific reaction associated with mechanism that does not produce overt necrosis	B. chronic degeneration

---

80. B
    A
    C

---

81. Aging and atrophy are frequently associated with innocuous adiposity of the myocardium and pancreas. Adipose tissue cells are not found in the parenchyma of liver, kidney, spleen, lung, or brain.

Adiposity might account for

A. liver enlargement
B. heart failure
C. both
D. neither

68. C
D
D
B
A

---

69. The body reacts to extracellular lipid. Macrophages (either singly or as foreign-body giant cells) are the principal reacting cell. If the macrophages cannot ingest and remove the extracellular lipid, fibrous tissue is formed to wall off the area.

Would you expect cholesterol crystals and mineral oil to be associated with permanent tissue damage?

____yes
____no

The reaction to cholesterol crystals and mineral oil would be best classified as

____acute inflammation
____non-specific chronic inflammation
____foreign-body granuloma

---

144. B,C
A
B,C
A

---

145. Granular deposits of calcium in areas of old injury are called ____________ ____________________.

7. A
B

---

8. Chronic degenerative processes are sometimes referred to as "infiltrations" because they are characterized by deposition of mineral, carbohydrate, lipid, or protein.

These substances accumulate because 1) they are difficult to remove, and 2) they do not kill cells.

MATCH THE FOLLOWING:

____quite variable in appearance, depending on substance involved	A. acute degeneration
____more likely to be reversed	
____frequently caused by the same mechanism that produces overt necrosis	B. chronic degeneration
____frequently caused by processes which are not capable of producing overt necrosis	

---

81. D. neither (parenchymal adiposity is innocuous)

---

82. Fatty metamorphosis of the liver is the accumulation of globules of neutral lipid (predominantly triglyceride) within hepatocytes. The swollen hepatocytes individually resemble adipose tissue cells, with their peripheral rim of cytoplasm and displaced, flattened nucleus, even though they are of radically different origin (endodermal vs. mesodermal) and differences between fatty liver and adipose tissue are easily recognized at low power or grossly. The liver responds to obesity by fatty metamorphosis and not adiposity.

MATCH THE FOLLOWING:

____large vacuoles in cells with displaced nuclei and cytoplasm	A. fatty metamorphosis
____abnormal storage of triglyceride	
____occurs in liver	B. adiposity
____does not occur in liver	
____involves epithelial cells	
____involves specialized connective tissue cells	

67. B
A
C
☑ specific

---

68. With the exception of cholesterol crystals and exogenous oils (such as mineral oil which is accidently inhaled when used as a laxative), lipids are found intracellularly.

MATCH THE FOLLOWING:

____triglyceride	A. extracellular lipid droplets
____lipoproteins	B. extracellular lipid crystals
____cholesterol bound by lipoprotein	C. intracellular lipid droplets
____cholesterol crystals	D. intracellular dispersed lipid
____mineral oil	

---

143. Dystrophic calcification is calcification at sites of degeneration or necrosis not associated with disorders of calcium metabolism (or equivalent). Metastatic calcification is calcification due to elevated serum calcium (or equivalent).

---

144. Calcium deposited in tissue appears as granular basophilic (hematoxaphilic) material.

MATCH THE FOLLOWING (more than one letter may apply):

____blue in H & E sections	A. hyaline degeneration
____red in H & E sections	B. dystrophic calcification
____particulate	C. metastatic calcification
____homogeneous	

8. B
A
A
B

---

9. In chronic degeneration, cellular homeostasis is set at an altered level over a long period of time. By definition this means the cells are neither returning to normal nor progressing to cell death, even though they are potentially able to do so.

INDICATE THE BOXES WHICH REPRESENT ACUTE AND CHRONIC DEGENERATION:

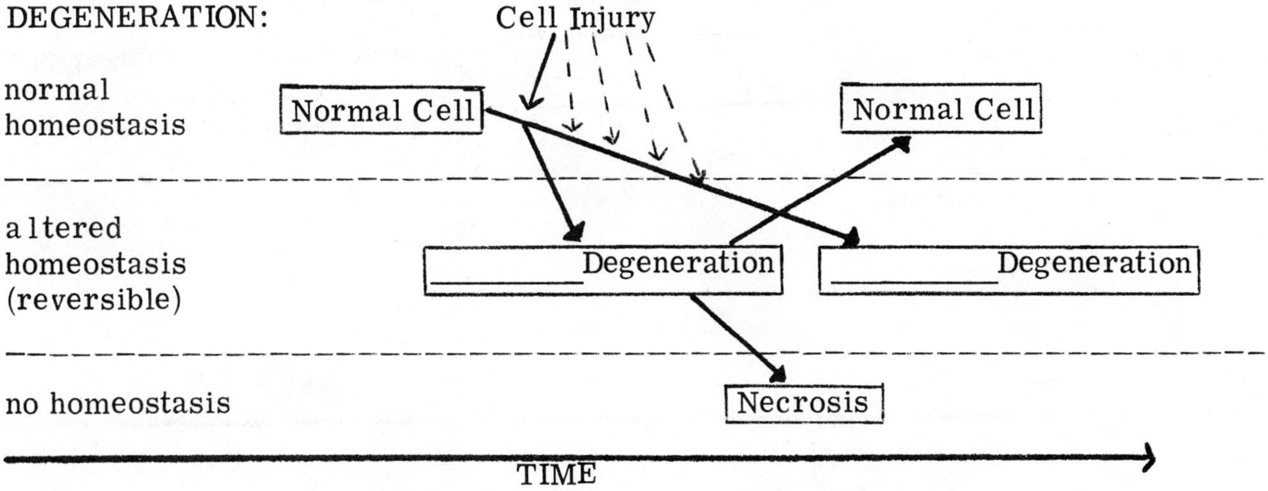

---

82. A, B
A, B
A
B
A (i.e., hepatocytes)
B

---

83. To help understand the pathogenesis of fatty metamorphosis, recall a few broad generalizations about lipid metabolism:

1) Triglyceride globules, the main dietary fat, are split in the intestinal lumen, absorbed, and reform into triglyceride globules in intestinal epithelial cells.
2) Intestinal epithelial cells add a lipoprotein coat which allows triglyceride to be transported into lymphatics and thus to the blood in the form of fine droplets (chylomicrons).
3) Chylomicrons are taken up by hepatocytes and adipose tissue cells (and other cells to a lesser extent).
4) The adipose tissue stores triglyceride, whereas the liver may store it, use it for energy, or add a lipoprotein coat and export it.

MATCH THE FOLLOWING:

____ major dietary input of lipid to liver
____ major dietary input to adipose tissue
____ metabolic product of liver which facilitates lipid transport
____ metabolic product of intestinal epithelial cells which facilitates transport of lipid droplets

A. triglyceride in form of chylomicrons
B. lipoprotein

66. A
A
B
C

67. MATCH THE FOLLOWING:

 ______

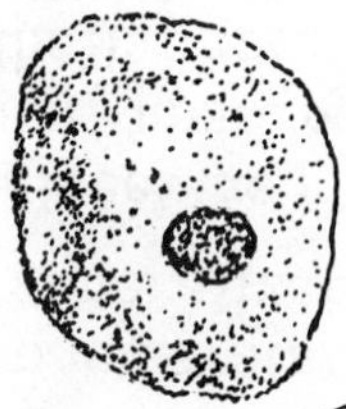 ______

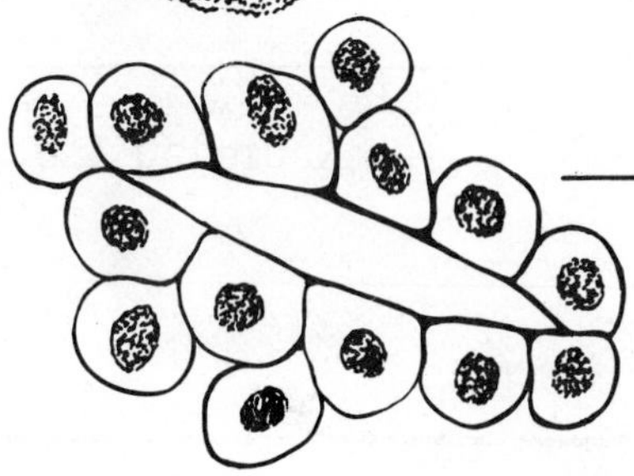 ______

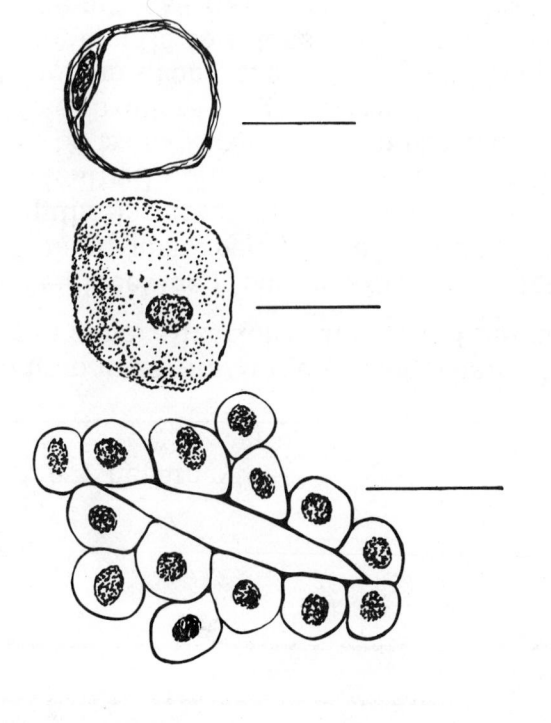

A. finely dispersed lipid complexes or small droplets, nucleus not displaced
B. droplets of neutral fat (triglyceride) in liver cell or adipose tissue cell displacing cell nucleus and cytoplasm
C. cholesterol crystal surrounded by macrophages containing dispersed lipid complexes.

The spaces caused by cholesterol crystals are ▱ specific
▱ not specific for cholesterol.

142. B
A
B
A

143. Dystrophic calcification is ______________________________.

Metastatic calcification is ______________________________.

9. acute degeneration | chronic degeneration

---

10. LABEL THE BOXES:

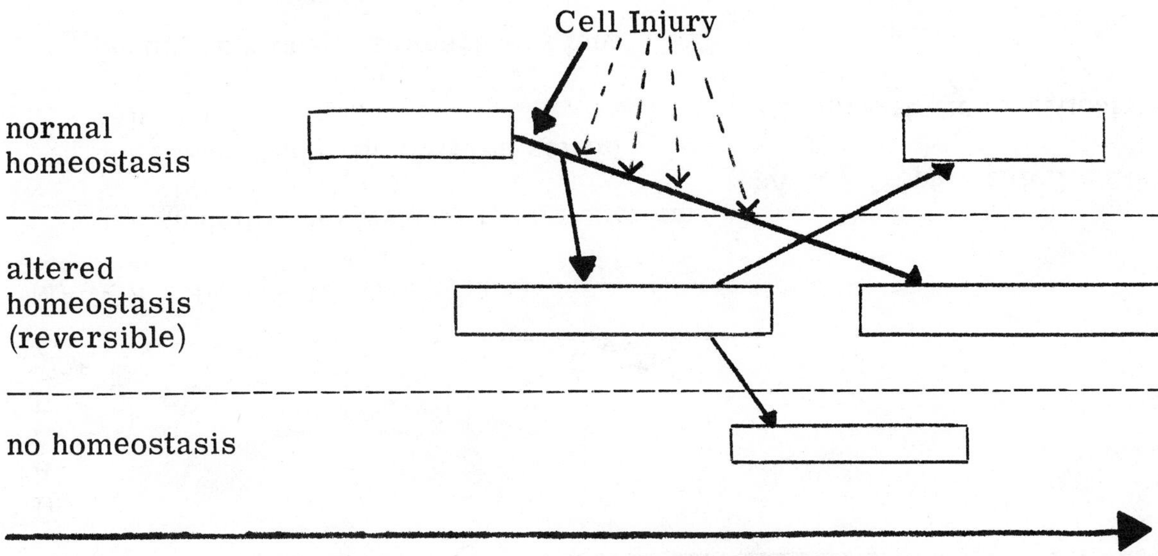

---

83. A
A
B
B

---

84. Adipose tissue is a simpleminded tissue: its job is to store triglyceride and, when needed, to break down triglyceride to free fatty acids to be used by the body cells for energy.

The triglyceride comes to the adipose tissue from either the intestine or the liver, since these are the organs capable of supplying the lipoprotein coat needed for transport in the blood. When more storage capacity is needed, more adipose tissue cells are formed and when not needed, they disappear.

Adipose tissue ☐ is ☐ is not capable of undergoing hyperplasia.
Adipose tissue ☐ is ☐ is not heavily involved in storage of glycogen.

The two principal functions of adipose tissue are:

____

____

65. T
T
T
F
F

<u>Degeneration Primarily Involving Lipid</u> (43 frames)

66. Lipids in tissue take one of three forms: liquid droplets, protein-bound complexes, or crystals (specifically cholesterol).

MATCH THE FOLLOWING:

A. lipid droplets
B. lipid-protein complexes
C. lipid crystals

____Triglycerides are stored in liver or adipose tissue cells, producing a spherical droplet.

____Mineral oil, an indigestible, exogenous oil, produces a spherical defect in tissue walled off by inflammatory cells and fibrous tissue.

____Lipoproteins, including lipoprotein-cholesterol complexes, are bipolar molecules that can be dispersed in cell cytoplasm.

____In high concentration, cholesterol may crystallize to form diagnostic needle-shaped crystals.

---

141. B
A
A
B

---

142. MATCH THE FOLLOWING:

A. dystrophic calcification
B. metastatic calcification

____associated with elevated serum calcium

____not associated with elevated serum calcium

____occurs in kidney, stomach, and lung

____occurs at sites of degeneration and necrosis

10.

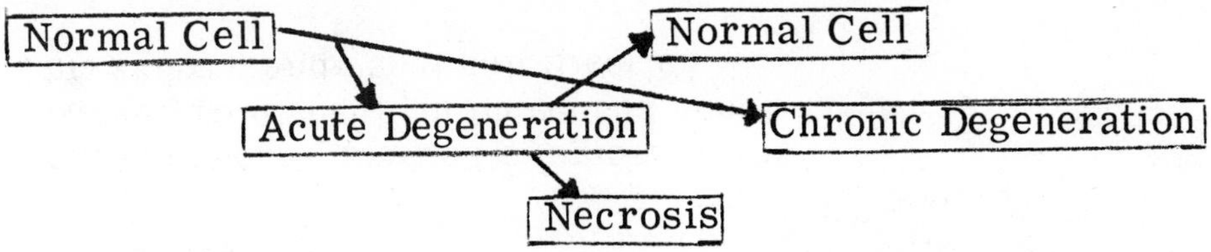

---

11. Acute degenerative changes are similar to those of necrosis up to the point of irreversible damage.

Subacute and chronic degenerative changes are characterized by accumulation of a variety of substances within cells or interstitial areas due to non-lethal changes in cell function.

MATCH THE FOLLOWING:

____ frequently due to interference with vital cell functions (such as cell respiration, synthesis of enzymatic and structural protein, and osmotic and chemical homeostasis)	A. acute degeneration
____ frequently due to interference with specific non-lethal cellular metabolic pathways	B. chronic degeneration
____ all types tend to be similar in appearance	
____ wide variety of types	
____ involves cells predominantly	
____ involves either cells or interstitium	

---

84. Adipose tissue [✓] is capable of undergoing hyperplasia.
Adipose tissue [✓] is not heavily involved in storage of glycogen.
The two principal functions of adipose tissue are:

storage of triglyceride

breakdown of triglyceride to free fatty acids as needed by the body for energy (or equivalent)

---

85. The liver's involvement in lipid metabolism is very complex. The liver may receive lipid in the form of chylomicrons and medium-chain fatty acids from the intestine and free fatty acid from plasma.

The liver can manufacture lipid from carbohydrate or protein.

The liver exports lipid in the form of various lipoproteins and as triglyceride coated with lipoprotein. The main export is to adipose tissue for storage.

MATCH THE FOLLOWING (more than one letter may apply):

____ synthesizes triglyceride and provides lipoprotein coat for transport	A. liver
____ site of lipid storage in obese people	B. adipose tissue
____ major direct provider of lipid as a fuel	
____ major factory for manufacture of lipid from other substances	C. intestine

64. F
T
T
F
F
T

---

65. INDICATE "T" TRUE OR "F" FALSE:

		frame reference
____	Mucus in or outside of epithelial cells is pale and faintly staining in H & E sections and strongly PAS-positive even after amylase treatment.	(57)
____	Glycogen storage diseases are progressive disorders associated with enlargement of various organs such as liver, skeletal muscle, and heart, depending on the type.	(54, 55)
____	Mucinous change is a descriptive term rather than a specific disease.	(59)
____	Mucinous changes are confined to the cytoplasm of cells since glycoproteins are produced in cells.	(58, 59)
____	Glycogen is frequently found in extracellular locations.	(52)

---

140. minerals

---

141. Calcification is the most common degeneration involving minerals. Dystrophic calcification occurs at sites of tissue degeneration or necrosis and does not involve any disorder of calcium metabolism. Metastatic calcification is the result of elevated (or saturated) serum calcium levels with metastasis of calcium to specific sites, namely kidney, gastric mucosa, and lung. These organs all excrete acid. Precipitation of calcium at these sites has been attributed to the relative alkaline state of the tissue due to acid excretion.

MATCH THE FOLLOWING EXAMPLES WITH THE TYPE OF CALCIFICATION:

____ rapid breakdown of bone calcium due to extensive involvement with cancer

____ old tuberculous foci usually are densely radiopaque on chest films

____ old atherosclerotic plaques often are brittle

____ parahormone- producing tumors of the parathyroid result in increased bone breakdown and renal calcification

A. dystrophic calcification

B. metastatic calcification

11. A
B
A
B
A
B

---

12. Necrosis liberates substances which provoke an acute inflammatory reaction. Acute degeneration without necrosis generally does not result in a significant inflammatory reaction.

MATCH THE FOLLOWING:

____ liver cells contain focal glossy, homogeneous, eosinophilic deposits in their cytoplasm	A. necrosis
____ glossy, homogeneous, eosinophilic material is seen between muscle cells in the myocardium, muscularis of the intestine, and muscularis of small arterioles and tongue	B. acute degeneration
____ kidney tubule cells have a diffuse swelling of their cytoplasm but nuclei are intact	C. chronic intracellular degeneration
____ anterior horn cells of the spinal cord have eosinophilic cytoplasm associated with some cells without nuclei and some infiltration of polys in the area	D. chronic interstitial degeneration

---

85. A, C
A, B
B
A

---

86. Factors which favor the development of fatty metamorphosis of the liver include:
    1) increased input of lipid to liver
    2) decreased utilization of lipid by the liver for energy
    3) inability to export triglyceride due to defective synthesis of lipoproteins

MATCH THE FOLLOWING:

____ prolonged, excessive overeating	A. increased input of lipid to liver
____ decreased metabolism due to anoxia	B. decreased utilization of lipid by the liver for energy
____ injury by poisons which block protein synthesis (CCl_4, alcohol, phosphorus)	C. inability to export lipid

63. a
b
c

---

64. INDICATE "T" TRUE OR "F" FALSE:

	frame reference
____Cloudy swelling is a synonym for accumulation of infiltration.	(32, 35)
____Hydropic degeneration is an acute degeneration that either leads to necrosis or leads to complete recovery.	(34, 41)
____Hydropic degeneration and glycogen storage disease both produce enlarged cells having pale, vacuolated cytoplasm.	(38, 51)
____Hydropic degeneration affects the nucleus, whereas glycogen storage does not.	(38, 53)
____Diabetes mellitus and glycogen storage disease are both caused by increased rates of glycogen formation.	(47)
____The PAS reaction following amylase treatment of sections will detect glycoprotein but not glycogen.	(50, 57)

---

139. F
T
F
T
T

Degeneration Primarily Involving Calcium (10 frames)

140. Deposits of calcium, phosphorus, iron, and inorganic crystalline deposits, the exact composition of which is unknown, are commonly seen as degeneration. These materials may be classified as ______________.

12. C
D
B
A

---

13. A mild but distinct acute inflammatory cell response suggests:

____necrosis

____acute degeneration

____chronic degeneration

---

86. A
B
C

---

87. Increased input of lipid to the liver may result from dietary excess or from excessively rapid liberation of lipid from adipose tissue as occurs in acute starvation or insulin deficiency (diabetes mellitus). Insulin promotes uptake of lipid by adipose tissue; the lack of insulin activity favors lipolysis in adipose tissue.

Which of the following favor the development of fatty metamorphosis due to excessive input of lipid to the liver?

____insulin therapy
____untreated diabetes mellitus
____obesity
____poisons
____being lost in the woods for two days

62. mucoprotein
glycogen
water

---

63. The gross recognition of mucin may help identify the underlying disease process. Grossly, mucin is gray and translucent. Connective tissue mucins have the consistency of firm gelatin; epithelial mucins are more fluid and sticky.

The gross recognition of mucin might be helpful in which of the following circumstances?

a. classifying a connective tissue tumor of the thigh as myxomatous

b. indicating duct obstruction in a mucus-secreting organ

c. classifying an epithelial neoplasm as mucinous

d. identifying specific metabolic defects causing mucinous degeneration

---

138. F
F
T
F
F

---

139. INDICATE "T" TRUE OR "F" FALSE:

	frame reference
____Extracellular hyaline deposits are easily removed during healing.	(113, 118, 120)
____Fibrinoid change is found in subcutaneous nodules associated with rheumatoid arthritis and in vessels with vasculitis.	(124, 126, 128)
____A fibrinous material may be fibrin or some other material.	(124)
____Aging collagen is a common cause of hyalinization.	(118)
____Special stains are useful in distinguishing types of protein deposits.	(114)

13. _✓_ necrosis

---

14. Imperceptible necrosis means that neither necrotic cells nor acute inflammatory cell reaction to necrotic cells can be seen in histologic sections, but the slow death of many cells can be inferred from other observations.

MATCH THE FOLLOWING:

____ changes of cell death associated with acute inflammatory reaction	A. overt necrosis
____ an organ is reduced to half its normal weight; remaining cells are of normal size	B. imperceptible necrosis
____ the parenchymal cells of an organ are half replaced by fibrous or adipose tissue	

---

87. _✓_ untreated diabetes mellitus
_✓_ obesity
_✓_ being lost in the woods for two days

---

88. Decreased utilization of lipid by the liver may result from carbohydrate deprivation (carbohydrate is needed to feed the carboxylic acid cycle) or anything that interferes with oxidative function.

MATCH THE FOLLOWING CAUSES OF FATTY METAMORPHOSIS WITH THEIR MECHANISM:

____ increased lysis of lipid stores in adipose tissue	A. increased input of lipid to liver
____ impairment of mitochondrial oxidative function	B. decreased utilization of lipid by the liver for energy
____ relative lack of carbohydrate in liver cells	

61. A C
B D
B C D
A C

---

62. Below are descriptions of cells with pale or vacuolated cytoplasm.

INDICATE WHETHER THEY CONTAIN WATER, GLYCOGEN, OR MUCOPROTEIN:

____The cytoplasm is strongly PAS-positive after formalin or alcohol fixation, with or without amylase digestion.

____The cytoplasm is weakly PAS-positive after formalin fixation, strongly PAS-positive after alcohol fixation, and PAS-negative in sections treated with amylase.

____The cytoplasm is PAS-negative after either formalin or alcohol fixation.

---

137. ✓ gray
✓ amyloidosis of liver
✓ hyalinized scar

---

138. INDICATE "T" TRUE OR "F" FALSE:

	frame reference
____Hyalin is a specific substance which can be identified by special staining reactions.	(110, 114)
____Mallory bodies are acutely degenerating hepatocytes with diffusely eosinophilic cytoplasm.	(133, 134)
____Amyloid is a substance with a distinctive staining reaction.	(114, 115)
____Amyloid is deposited at the site of chronic inflammation.	(120)
____Amyloid is a denser, tougher material than collagen.	(137)

14. A
B
B

---

15. Chronic degeneration is sometimes associated with slow death of cells, which may produce fibrosis and/or a mild infiltration of chronic inflammatory cells.

Acute degeneration is sometimes associated with ☐ overt necrosis ☐ imperceptible necrosis.

Chronic degeneration is sometimes associated with ☐ overt necrosis ☐ imperceptible necrosis.

---

88. A
B
B

---

89. Inability to export triglyceride is due to defective synthesis of lipoproteins to coat the triglyceride for transport in the blood. Lipoprotein synthesis is impaired with protein deficiencies, choline deficiency, and a variety of poisons such as carbon tetrachloride, alcohol, and phosphorus.

MATCH THE FOLLOWING:

cause	mechanism of lipid accumulation
____insufficient carbohydrate to feed carboxylic acid cycle	A. decreased utilization of lipid by liver
____substances interfere with protein production	B. decreased export of lipid by liver
____impaired oxidation	
____caused by several types of poisons	

60. hydropic degeneration: ___ nucleus ✓ cytoplasm ___ interstitium
glycogen degeneration: ✓ nucleus ✓ cytoplasm ___ interstitium
mucoid degeneration: ___ nucleus ✓ cytoplasm ✓ interstitium

---

61. MATCH THE FOLLOWING WITH THE INDICATED NUMBER OF RESPONSES:

___ ___ readily reversible

___ ___ not readily reversible

___ ___ ___ PAS-positive

___ ___ due to acutely increased cellular uptake of substance involved

A. hydropic degeneration

B. glycogen storage disease

C. glycogen in renal tubule cells associated with severe glycosuria

D. mucus production by cancer cells

---

136. 0 hydropic degeneration
+/- glycogen storage disease
0 fatty metamorphosis
0 adiposity
+/- lipidoses
\+ amyloid
\+ Mallory bodies

---

137. Proteinaceous deposits may be seen grossly only if they are large masses. Old hyalinized scar is tough, glistening, and gray-white. Amyloid deposits in organ parenchyma may produce large, pale, gray, soft organs. Fibrin deposits are gray-white and stringy when fresh, friable when old (if they have not been replaced by fibrous tissue). Masses of protein are grossly ___ red ___ yellow ___ gray.

Which of the following would you expect to see grossly?

___ amyloidosis of liver
___ amyloidosis in vessels of rectal submucosa
___ Mallory bodies
___ hyalinized scar

15. [✓] overt necrosis
[✓] imperceptible necrosis

---

16. MATCH THE FOLLOWING:

____ large droplets of lipid are seen in most hepatocytes	A. degeneration only
____ large droplets of lipid are seen in most hepatocytes; the hepatocytes are separated into lobules by bands of fibrous tissue	B. degeneration with active necrosis
____ large droplets of lipid are seen in many hepatocytes; other hepatocytes contain eosinophilic cytoplasmic deposits; and some polys are seen in the stroma	C. degeneration with slow imperceptible necrosis

---

89. A
B
A
B

---

90. Starvation has two effects which promote fatty metamorphosis: one has relatively more effect acutely and the other chronically.

In the early phase of starvation, more lipid is brought to the liver from adipose tissue stores than can be exported. In late or prolonged starvation, protein deficiency results in inability to produce enough lipoprotein for export.

MATCH THE FOLLOWING:

____ import of lipid by liver greater than export	A. acute starvation
____ import of lipid by liver equals export but export mechanism deficient	B. chronic starvation

59. B
A
C

---

60. INDICATE WHERE YOU WOULD LOOK FOR CHANGES IN EACH OF THE FOLLOWING TYPES OF DEGENERATIONS:

hydropic degeneration: ____nucleus ____cytoplasm ____interstitium

glycogen degeneration: ____nucleus ____cytoplasm ____interstitium

mucoid degeneration: ____nucleus ____cytoplasm ____interstitium

---

135. C cloudy swelling
C glycogen storage disease
A fatty metamorphosis
D atheroma
D xanthoma
A Mallory bodies
B Zenker's hyaline change

---

136. INDICATE WHICH CONTAIN MATERIALS REMAINING (+), PARTIALLY REMAINING (+/-), OR REMOVED (0) AFTER ROUTINE TISSUE PROCESSING:

____hydropic degeneration

____glycogen storage disease

____fatty metamorphosis

____adiposity

____lipidoses

____amyloid

____Mallory bodies

16. A
C
B

---

17. MATCH THE FOLLOWING:

____decrease in tissue mass due to gradual loss of cells	A. overt necrosis
____rapidly reversible cytoplasmic changes	B. imperceptible necrosis
____intracellular or extracellular deposits	C. acute degeneration
____nuclear and cytoplasmic changes with associated acute inflammation	D. chronic degeneration

---

90. A
B

---

91. MATCH THE FOLLOWING CAUSES OF FATTY METAMORPHOSIS OF THE LIVER WITH THEIR MAJOR CAUSATIVE MECHANISM:

____prolonged, excessive overeating	A. input overload of lipid
____acute starvation	
____anoxia	B. decreased utilization of lipid by liver cells
____deficiency in factors such as choline involved in phospholipid synthesis	
____prolonged severe protein deficiency	C. failure to manufacture soluble lipid products for export
____injury by poisons which block protein synthesis (CCl_4, alcohol, phosphorus)	

In each of these situations, what is the type of lipid that accumulates?

58. A A C B

---

59. There are no distinct mucinous degenerations, although the term is loosely applied to situations where mucin content of tissue is increased, such as the following:

1) in uncommon connective tissue tumors which produce ground substance (myxomas)

2) in atrophy of connective tissue where there is a relative increase in ground substance

3) in mucin-producing cancers which may spill pools of mucin into connective tissue

4) in plugged excretory ducts where mucin cannot be removed

MATCH THE FOLLOWING:

____subacute or chronic degeneration with deposits in cytoplasm or nucleus

____acute degeneration involving cytoplasm

____a descriptive term for increase of material in cytoplasm or interstitium

A. hydropic degeneration

B. glycogen degeneration

C. mucinous degeneration

---

134. B
A
A
B
A
B
A, B

---

135. MATCH THE FOLLOWING:

____cloudy swelling
____glycogen storage disease
____fatty metamorphosis
____atheroma
____xanthoma
____Mallory bodies
____Zenker's hyaline change

A. may occur within hepatocytes

B. may occur within skeletal muscle cells

C. both A and B

D. neither A and B

17. B
C
D
A

---

18. At the cellular level acute degeneration is characterized by morphologic changes in the cell cytoplasm only, whereas necrosis is characterized by cytoplasmic, nuclear, and surrounding tissue changes.

MATCH THE FOLLOWING:

____cells with swollen, granular cytoplasm with normal nucleus, but without congestion, inflammation, or healing in surrounding tissue

____cells without nuclei, but some membranes and membrane debris visible, circumscribed by cellular inflammatory response

A. necrosis

B. degeneration

---

91. A
A
B
C
C
C
triglyceride (fatty acids are quickly transformed into triglyceride if not used)

---

92. The normal liver shows no evidence of fatty metamorphosis histologically. Mild to moderate fatty metamorphosis may be transient or prolonged and usually is not associated with clinically detectable change in liver function.

Severe fatty metamorphosis is more likely to be prolonged (although reversible with treatment) and may be associated with a greatly enlarged soft liver, abnormalities in liver function tests, and occasionally jaundice.

MATCH THE FOLLOWING:

____acute or chronic degeneration
____chronic degeneration
____often an incidental morphologic finding
____often a clinically significant finding

A. mild to moderate fatty metamorphosis

B. severe fatty metamorphosis

57.

	water	glycogen	mucin
leave vacuoles after formalin fixation	✓	✓	
PAS-positive		✓	✓
PAS-positive after amylase digestion			✓

58. Mucins are normally found in extracellular ground substance of connective tissue and in mucus-secreting epithelial cells. In epithelial cells mucus either forms a globule in the cytoplasm, which displaces the nucleus (goblet cell), or is diffusely located in apical cytoplasm with a basally placed undistorted nucleus.

IDENTIFY THE CONTENT OF THE FOLLOWING CELLS:

A. mucin B. glycogen C. glycogen or water

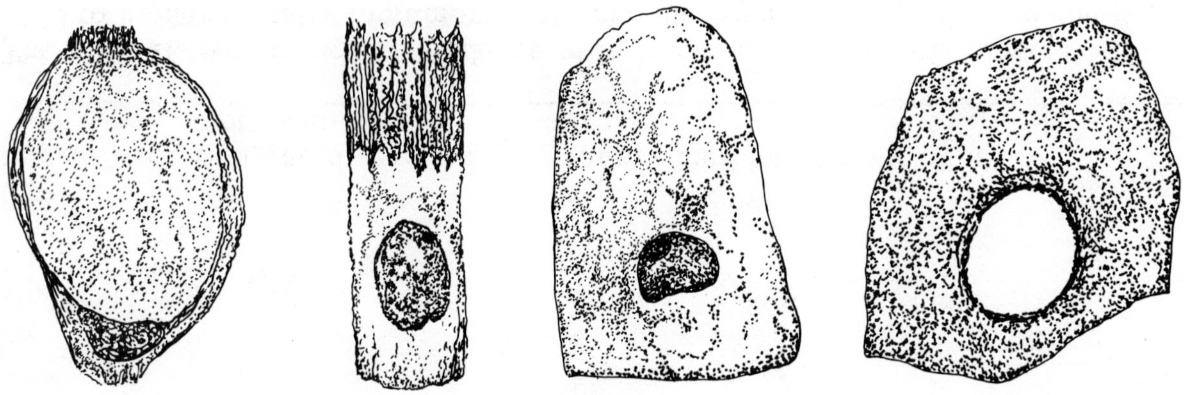

133. B
A

134. Mallory bodies are found in some alcoholics, particularly after a prolonged bout with the bottle. They may gradually disappear over weeks to months during periods of reduced alcohol intake.

MATCH THE FOLLOWING:

A. Mallory bodies

B. Zenker's hyaline change

____acute

____chronic

____focal cytoplasmic change

____diffuse cytoplasmic change

____associated with alcoholism

____found in people dying of typhoid fever

____term(s) related to only one type of tissue

18. B
A

---

19. RECALL WHETHER THE FOLLOWING MORPHOLOGIC CHANGES ARE (R) REVERSIBLE OR (I) IRREVERSIBLE:

____swollen cytoplasm

____pyknosis and karyorrhexis

____irregular cell margins

____phagocytic vacuoles

____increased granularity of cytoplasm

____rupture of cell membrane with debris

____karyolysis

____cloudiness

---

92. A
B
A
B

---

93. Severe fatty metamorphosis is likely to be caused by severe prolonged alcoholism or severe prolonged protein deficiency, such as is seen in children in various parts of the world with the dietary protein deficiency known as kwashiorkor.

Moderate fatty metamorphosis is likely to be caused by many less prolonged or less severe disturbances, such as fasting of a few day's duration, poorly controlled diabetes mellitus, moderate or episodic alcoholism, obesity, and various wasting diseases.

Fatty metamorphosis is very common and is usually ☐ symptomatic ☐ asymptomatic.
Clinically significant fatty metamorphosis is most often associated with ____________ and ____________
Fatty metamorphosis ☐ is ☐ is not present in a normal liver.

56. B
B
A
B

57. Like other proteins, mucins are solidified by fixatives and not removed during tissue processing. They stain faintly with eosin or hematoxylin, depending on their chemical composition. They stain strongly PAS-positive and cannot be removed by amylase digestion.

COMPARE THE FOLLOWING:

	water	glycogen	mucin
leave vacuoles after formalin fixation			
PAS-positive			
PAS-positive after amylase digestion			

132. ☑ acute
protein

133. Mallory bodies are fluffy, localized eosinophilic deposits within hepatocytes. Individual dead hepatocytes are sometimes called Councilman bodies.

MATCH THE FOLLOWING:

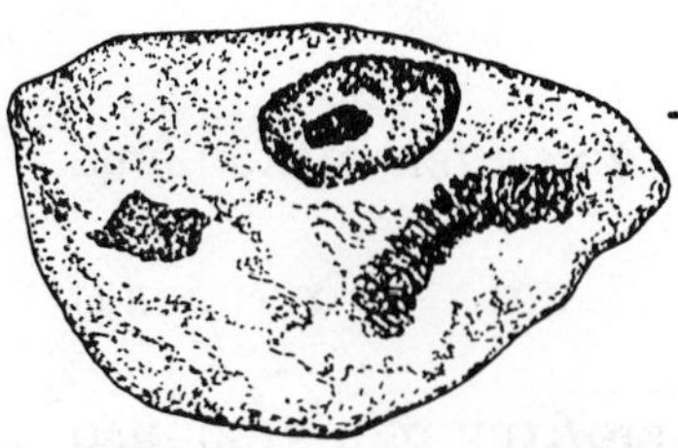 ______

A. Mallory body

B. Councilman body

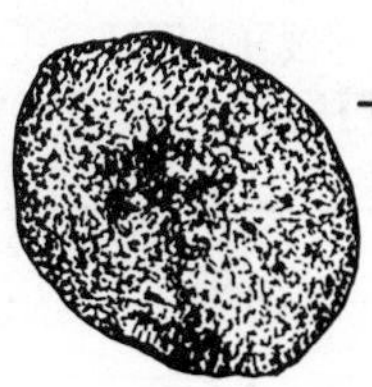 ______

19. R R
I I
R I
R R

---

20. Acute degeneration is usually caused by the same agents that cause necrosis. The degree of injury depends on the pathogenicity of the agent, the amount of the agent, the duration of exposure, and tissue susceptibility.

For example, carbon tetrachloride when inhaled or swallowed is absorbed readily and produces injury to the liver and kidney which either is fatal or is followed by complete recovery.

CLASSIFY THE FACTOR WHICH WILL DETERMINE WHETHER DEGENERATION AND/OR NECROSIS WILL OCCUR IN THE FOLLOWING SITUATIONS:

____ The length of time a person uses to put out a fire with a fire extinguisher containing CCl_4

____ The degree to which ventilation prevents accumulation of CCl_4 while he is extinguishing the fire

____ Whether the fire extinguisher contains CO_2 or CCl_4

____ Whether the injury at the fire is due to CCl_4 fumes or carbon monoxide (which produces death due to brain injury via anoxia)

A. pathogenicity of the agent
B. amount of the agent
C. duration of exposure
D. tissue susceptibility

---

93. [✓] asymptomatic
alcoholism and severe protein deficiency (or equivalent)
[✓] is not

---

94. MATCH THE FOLLOWING CAUSES OF FATTY METAMORPHOSIS WITH THE PREDOMINANT MECHANISM:

____ protein deficiency
____ obesity
____ acute fasting
____ diabetes mellitus (increased lipolysis)
____ alcoholism

A. increased lipid uptake by liver
B. decreased lipid mobilization by the liver

55. A
B
B
A

---

56. The second form of carbohydrate frequently observed in tissues is a heterogeneous group of carbohydrate-protein compounds variously referred to as:

glycoprotein - emphasizes chemical composition
mucopolysaccharide - emphasizes carbohydrate component
mucoprotein - emphasizes protein component
mucin - refers to connective tissue and epithelial glycoproteins
mucus - refers to epithelial mucin

MATCH THE FOLLOWING:

____variable chemical structure — A. glycogen

____many synonyms — B. glycoproteins

____located intracellularly

____located in cells or connective tissue ground substance

---

131. ✓ carbohydrate ✓ lipid ✓ protein
protein

---

132. Two examples of intracellular protein degeneration will be contrasted. You will encounter other examples later in the course.

Zenker's hyaline degeneration is the name given to the diffuse change commonly seen in skeletal muscle fibers of the rectus abdominis muscle and diaphragm of people dying of severe febrile illnesses, such as typhoid fever, and in anaphylactic shock. The entire cytoplasm appears eosinophilic, and often the changes proceed to frank coagulation necrosis.

Zenker's hyaline degeneration is a part of the degeneration-necrosis process and, therefore, is ☐ acute ☐ chronic.

The reason this change is so striking and was given a special name by early pathologists is probably related to the fact that skeletal muscle has abundant cytoplasm with high ____________ content.

20. C
B
A
D

---

21. The most common cause of acute degenerative changes is anoxia. One cause of anoxia is shock, a condition characterized by inadequate perfusion of blood to the tissues.

MATCH THE STATEMENTS WITH THE FACTOR INVOLVED (use each response only once):

____ Shock resulting from pooling of blood in veins is mild compared to shock from extensive blood loss.
____ If shock from blood loss is not corrected rapidly, permanent brain damage results.
____ Neurons, renal tubule cells, and centrilobular hepatocytes are most likely to be affected by shock.
____ Anoxia is potentially capable of affecting all cells.

A. pathogenicity of the agent
B. amount of the agent
C. duration of exposure
D. tissue susceptibility

---

94. B
A
A (The increased lipid mobilized by adipose tissue cannot be fully utilized or exported by the liver.)
A
B

---

95. LIST FOUR CAUSES OF FATTY METAMORPHOSIS:

____

____

____

____

54. B
A
B

---

55. The site of glycogen accumulation in glycogen storage diseases is variable, depending upon which enzyme is deficient. For example, in von Gierke's disease (Type I), the liver and kidney are most prominently involved. In Pompe's disease (Type II), the heart and skeletal muscles are involved.

MATCH THE FOLLOWING:

____enlarged abdomen	A. von Gierke's disease
____progressive weakness	B. Pompe's disease
____heart failure	
____convulsions due to low blood sugar (the liver regulates blood sugar)	

---

130. chronic
acute

---

131. Chronic intracellular degenerative processes may involve the accumulation of ____water ____carbohydrate ____lipid ____protein.

Of these materials, the only one that is always retained in the cell during tissue processing by routine techniques is ________________.

21. B
C
D
A

---

22. LIST FOUR FACTORS THAT INFLUENCE WHETHER AN AGENT WILL CAUSE DEGENERATION OR NECROSIS:

____

____

____

____

---

95. Any of the following: alcoholism
protein deficiency
starvation
diabetes mellitus
obesity

---

96. Mild fatty metamorphosis is a common histologic finding in association with a variety of diseases, but it is not evidenced clinically by significant liver enlargement or alteration in function.
Moderate to severe fatty metamorphosis is associated with varying degrees of liver enlargement and sometimes significant abnormalities in function. The liver is soft and yellow.

MATCH THE FOLLOWING:

____ normal to slightly enlarged liver with scattered cells containing large clear cytoplasmic vacuoles displacing the nucleus
____ large pale liver with diffusely vacuolated cells without nuclear displacement
____ large flabby yellow liver with single cytoplasmic vacuoles in most cells
____ liver with multiple large firm nodules which exude gelatinous material when cut

A. glycogen storage disease
B. mild fatty metamorphosis
C. severe fatty metamorphosis
D. mucus-secreting cancer which has spread to the liver

53. A
D
D
D

---

54. In contrast to diabetes, the several types of glycogen storage disease are 1) rare, 2) are more uniformly serious, leading to death in childhood from malnutrition or infections, and 3) cause prominent organ enlargement and malfunction. Diagnosis may be suspected from clinical and morphologic findings but is proved by demonstration of the specific tissue enzyme deficiency.

MATCH THE FOLLOWING:

____fatal disturbance of glycogen metabolism	A. diabetes mellitus
____common	B. glycogen storage disease
____may produce greatly enlarged liver due to glycogen accumulation	

---

129. C B A

---

130. Intracellular degenerations involving proteins also produce hyaline changes.

In acute degenerations the entire cytoplasm may become more compact and eosinophilic due to changes in proteins.

Chronic intracellular protein changes may be associated with formation of discrete hyaline masses in the cytoplasm.

Focal cytoplasmic changes suggest that the degeneration is ________________, while diffuse cytoplasmic changes suggest ________________ degeneration and/or necrosis.

22. pathogenicity of agent
amount of agent
duration of exposure
tissue susceptibility

---

23. All agents capable of causing necrosis can cause degeneration, but not all agents capable of causing degeneration can cause necrosis. For example, the glycogen storage diseases may produce an imbalance between glycogenesis and glycogenolysis, which often results in glycogen deposition, a chronic degeneration recognizable by the appearance of glycogen within the cytoplasm and nuclei of affected cells. Such an imbalance between glycogenesis and glycogenolysis will not result in overt necrosis.

MATCH THE FOLLOWING CAUSES WITH USUAL OUTCOMES:

____anoxic injury	A. degeneration only
____imbalance between glycogenolysis and glycogenesis	B. both necrosis and degeneration

---

96. B
A
C
D

---

97. Fatty metamorphosis may develop rapidly, as with starvation for a few days or injury with a poison such as CCl_4. With alcoholism, prolonged protein deficiency, or uncontrolled diabetes, for example, fatty metamorphosis is often chronic.

Adipose tissue increases and decreases slowly. Adiposity associated with atrophy might better be termed a metaplasia than a degeneration. Adiposity is commonly encountered at autopsy in the pancreas and heart and is of no clinical importance.

MATCH THE FOLLOWING:

____hydropic degeneration	A. an acute condition
____glycogen storage disease	B. a chronic condition
____adiposity	C. may be either acute or chronic
____fatty metamorphosis	

52. [✓] intracellular
[✓] increased uptake of glucose [✓] decreased breakdown of glycogen

---

53. The intracellular glycogen accumulations in diabetes are of little clinical significance: They are reversible with good control of the diabetes, and they do not produce significant organomegaly or organ malfunction.

Nuclear glycogen in hepatocytes is a common finding and is suggestive of diabetes, but the diagnosis is evident clinically.

Renal tubular glycogen deposits associated with severe glycosuria (glucose in urine) are specific for diabetes but are seen only at autopsy.

MATCH THE FOLLOWING:

____pathognomonic of diabetes	A. renal tubular glycogen deposits
____useful in detection of new diabetics	B. hepatic nuclear glycogen
____significant physiologic effects	C. both
____cause of clinically evident organ enlargement	D. neither

---

128. B
A
C

---

129. Amyloid in small arteries tends to be very homogeneous, with disappearance of smooth muscle nuclei.

Collagen in arteriolar sclerosis is more laminated, with some nuclei present.

Fibrinoid necrosis of arterioles shows patchy hyalinization, with nuclear debris and perivascular inflammation.

MATCH THE FOLLOWING SMALL ARTERIES WITH THE MATERIAL DEPOSITED:

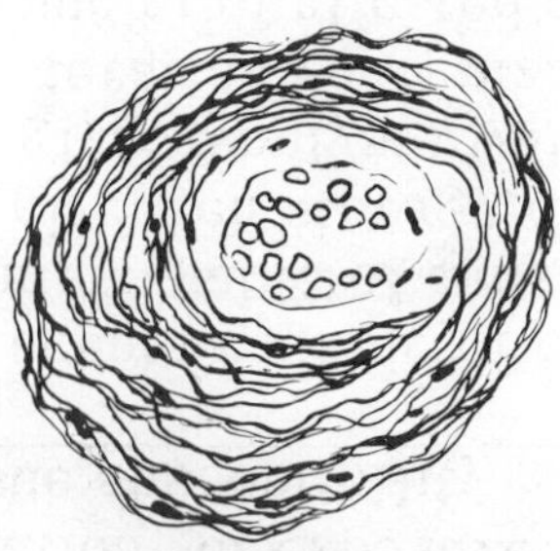

A

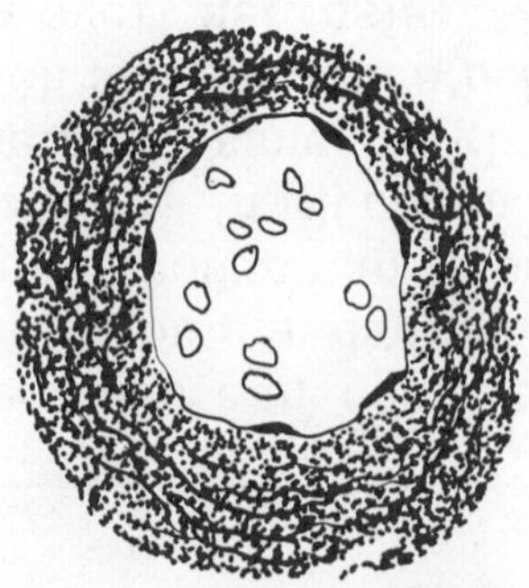

B

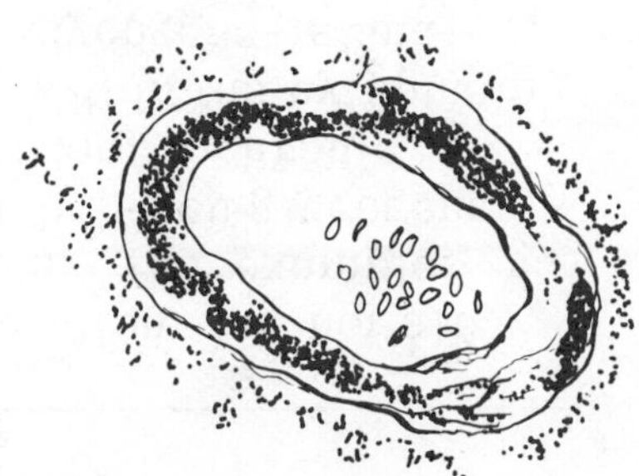

C

____fibrinoid ____amyloid ____collagen

23. B
A

---

24. Which is/are true?

a. Agents causing acute degeneration are usually capable of causing overt necrosis.

b. Agents causing chronic degeneration are usually capable of causing overt necrosis.

---

97. A
B
B
C

---

98. Mineral oil granulomas are an example of a foreign-body reaction to exogenous oils (hydrocarbons). The indigestible extracellular lipid is surrounded by giant cells and histiocytes; later, fibrosis occurs around the pools of lipid. This occurs most significantly in chronic users of mineral oil as a laxative who inhale the mineral oil in small amounts over a long period of time. Often there are surprisingly few symptoms, even when the lung becomes very fibrotic in areas and grossly exudes lipid droplets.

Mineral oil granulomas are ☐ acute ☐ chronic
are characterized by ☐ intracellular ☐ extracellular lipid
are characterized by ☐ dispersed ☐ globular lipid
produce ☐ pronounced ☐ little, if any, systemic reaction
☐ can ☐ cannot eventually produce severe destruction of lung.

51. A
B
C

---

52. Glycogen is a normal constituent of all cells but is most abundant in liver and muscle.

In glycogen storage diseases, there is a quantitative increase in glycogen in the cytoplasm and nuclei of various cells.

In poorly controlled diabetes mellitus, with high blood and urine sugar levels, glycogen is formed and accumulates in two sites: hepatic cell nuclei and renal tubule epithelial cells.

Glycogen accumulations are ☐ intracellular ☐ extracellular and are caused by ☐ increased uptake of glucose ☐ decreased breakdown of glycogen.

---

127. B
A
D
C

---

128. Hyalinization of small blood vessels may be due to several types of material and has important clinical implications.

In long-standing hypertension, the renal arterioles become thick-walled and rigid, with narrowing of the lumen due to replacement of their walls by dense collagen.

In acute or malignant hypertension and some inflammatory diseases of vessels, the walls of small and medium-size arteries in the kidney and other organs take on the appearance of fibrin due to necrosis of the vessel wall and/or fibrin deposition.

In amyloidosis, small arterioles are characteristically thick and homogeneously eosinophilic. Rectal submucosa and gingiva are common sites biopsied to demonstrate this change, but the lesions may be very widespread.

MATCH THE FOLLOWING:

____ Congo red-positive hyalinization of small vessels	A. collagen
____ thickening of small renal arterioles in hypertension	B. amyloid
____ a more granular and patchy eosinophilia seen with vasculitis	C. fibrinoid

24. a

---

25. The cellular changes in acute degenerations are characterized by injury to basic cell structures resulting in diffuse cytoplasmic changes such as swelling or eosinophilia.

The cellular changes of chronic degenerations are characterized by accumulations which may result from uptake of substances or metabolic blocks allowing buildup of substances from within.

MATCH THE FOLLOWING:

____ Lipid complexes (lipofuscin) accumulate as brown pigment granules at the poles of myocardial nuclei as a result of focal cellular damage associated with aging.

____ Myocardial muscle fibers are swollen due to changes in mitochondria and endoplasmic reticulum.

____ Glycogen accumulates in cardiac muscle fibers due to a genetic biochemical defect.

A. acute degeneration

B. chronic degeneration

---

98. ☑ chronic
☑ extracellular lipid
☑ globular lipid
☑ little, if any, systemic reaction
☑ can eventually produce severe destruction of lung

---

99. MATCH THE FOLLOWING:

____ a degeneration

____ an inflammatory reaction

____ liver

____ lung

____ intracellular lipid

____ extracellular lipid

____ endogenous lipid

____ exogenous lipid

A. mineral oil granuloma

B. fatty metamorphosis

50. <u>+/-</u> routine formalin-fixed sections
<u>+</u> tissue fixed in alcohol prior to routine processing
<u>-</u> alcohol and/or formalin-fixed sections incubated with salivary amylase

---

51. In von Gierke's type glycogen storage disease, large amounts of glycogen accumulate in hepatocytes because of deficiency of the glycogen-splitting enzyme glucose 6-phosphatase.

The glycogen stains faintly in eosin-stained sections, but is strongly PAS-positive. The cells are highly vacuolated when fixed primarily in a watery fixative.

MATCH THE HEPATOCYTES IN VON GIERKE'S DISEASE WITH THE FIXATIVE AND STAIN:

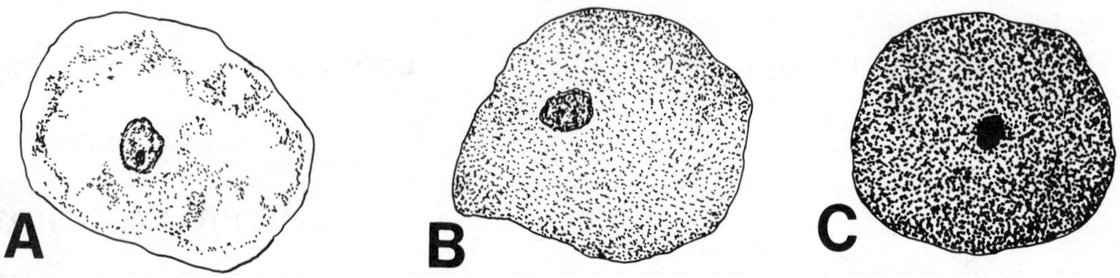

____formalin, hematoxylin, and eosin
____alcohol, hematoxylin, and eosin
____alcohol, PAS

---

126. In the early stage of the disease, a compacted fibrinous exudate may form on the synovial surface.
Organization of this exudate leads to formation of fibrous tissue, which is responsible for limiting mobility of the joint.
In old, relatively inactive joint lesions, homogenization and eosinophilia due to hyalinized collagen become prominent.
In the active stages of the disease, subcutaneous nodules may develop a peculiar central hyalinization called fibrinoid degeneration (or necrosis).
Prolonged active disease over many years may lead to amyloid deposits in other organs, such as liver, spleen, kidney, and adrenals.

---

127. MATCH THE FOLLOWING WITH THEIR IMPLIED MECHANISMS:

____a distinctive abnormal protein

____a result of aging of reparative tissue

____a descriptive term that does not imply a mechanism of formation

____material resulting from fibrin formation

A. hyalinized collagen

B. amyloid

C. fibrinous

D. fibrinoid

25. B
A
B

---

26. Chronic degenerations may involve interstitial deposits or alteration of existing interstitial material. The materials involved usually are relatively inert; otherwise, they would provoke overt necrosis and inflammation. Sometimes normal cells may be crowded out and undergo atrophy.

Some chronic degenerations involve crystalline deposits, such as cholesterol and uric acid, which provoke a foreign-body giant cell response.

Chronic interstitial degenerations are sometimes associated with:

a. deposits of abnormal material only

b. acute inflammation

c. foreign-body response

d. overt necrosis

e. imperceptible necrosis

---

99. B
A
B
A
B
A
B
A

---

100. Xanthomas are localized collections of histiocytes containing cholesterol which are usually found in the skin and are often associated with elevated serum cholesterol.

Lipidoses are any of several rare genetic metabolic defects associated with storage of lipoprotein complexes in reticuloendothelial or other type cells.

MATCH THE FOLLOWING:

____cholesterol deposited	A. xanthomas
____various lipoproteins accumulate	B. lipidoses
____intracellular lipid	C. both
____various cells involved, depending on defect	D. neither
____can be seen on physical examination	

49. C
B
A

50. Glycogen is water-soluble, so it is removed by watery fixatives such as formalin. Glycogen is incompletely removed by formalin because some of the glycogen sticks to cell proteins.

Alcohol renders glycogen insoluble in water; therefore, alcohol fixation followed by the routine formalin fixation will preserve glycogen.

INDICATE THE PAS-POSITIVITY (+, +/-, -) OF THE NORMAL GLYCOGEN IN HEPATOCYTES UNDER THE FOLLOWING CONDITIONS:

____routine formalin-fixed sections

____tissue fixed in alcohol prior to routine processing

____alcohol and/or formalin-fixed sections incubated with salivary amylase

---

125. B
A

126. Many aspects of rheumatoid arthritis, a chronic destructive disease of joints, can be described in terms of descriptors of degeneration.

USE THE WORDS ON THE RIGHT TO FILL IN THE BLANKS:

In the early stage of the disease, a compacted ________________ exudate may form on the synovial surface.	hyalinized collagen
Organization of this exudate leads to formation of ____________ tissue, which is responsible for limiting mobility of the joint.	fibrinoid
In old, relatively inactive joint lesions, homogenization and eosinophilia due to ________________ become prominent.	fibrinous
In the active stages of the disease, subcutaneous nodules may develop a peculiar central hyalinization called ______________ degeneration (or necrosis).	fibrous
Prolonged active disease over many years may lead to ________________ deposits in other organs, such as liver, spleen, kidney, and adrenals.	amyloid

26. a
c
e

27. INDICATE FEATURES WHICH CHARACTERIZE ACUTE AND CHRONIC DEGENERATIONS:

	Pure Acute Degeneration	Pure Chronic Degeneration
May be characterized as an intracellular process		
May be characterized as an interstitial process		
Agents often same as cause necrosis		
Agents often different than cause necrosis		
Reversible injury		
Often does not revert to normal		

100. A
B
C
B
A

101. Histiocytes containing lipid are often called foamy histiocytes, or xanthoma cells. They have a clear cytoplasm with sparse cytoplasmic components and a centrally placed nucleus. Grossly, localized collections of lipid-containing histiocytes are yellow lesions.

MATCH THE FOLLOWING (MORE THAN ONE LETTER MAY APPLY):

____grossly yellow

____nucleus displaced by a material accumulated

____characteristically found in skin

____characteristically found in liver

____contains cholesterol

____characteristically occurs in childhood

A. hydropic degeneration

B. glycogen storage disease

C. fatty metamorphosis

D. xanthoma

48. B
A
A

---

49. In the preparation of routine paraffin-embedded histologic sections, there are three major factors in determining the appearance of deposited materials:

A. the effect of the fixative on the material

B. specific steps used to remove a material selectively

C. the type of stain used

MATCH THE FACTORS ABOVE WITH THE EXAMPLES BELOW:

____Glycogen is PAS-positive.

____Glycogen can be digested out of the sections using amylase.

____Glycogen is mostly removed by watery fixatives such as formalin, leaving a vacuolated appearance to the cell.

---

124. fibrin-like
fibrinous
fibrinoid
fibrinoid
fibrinous

---

125. One should be particularly careful not to confuse the terms fibrinous and fibrous in referring to the presence of fibrin and collagen respectively.

MATCH THE FOLLOWING:

____tissue that develops as part of the repair process (organization)	A. fibrinous
____does not refer to a type of tissue but rather to a type of exudate or component of coagulated blood	B. fibrous

27.

	Acute Degeneration	Chronic Degeneration
may be characterized as intracellular	✓	✓
may be characterized as interstitial		✓
agents often same as cause necrosis	✓	
agents often different than cause necrosis		✓
reversible injury	✓	
often does not revert to normal		✓

28. INDICATE "T" TRUE OR "F" FALSE:

	frame reference
____ Degeneration is a non-lethal change in cell structure characterized by an alteration or accumulation of material within cells or interstitial tissue.	(2)
____ Anything which causes degeneration can cause necrosis but not everything that can cause necrosis can also cause degeneration.	(23)
____ Factors in determining whether injury will result in degeneration or necrosis are: pathogenicity of agent, amount of agent, duration of exposure, and tissue susceptibility.	(20)
____ Certain nuclear changes, such as pyknosis, are characteristic of either degeneration or necrosis.	(18)
____ Morphologically, degeneration is characterized by cytoplasmic changes in the cell without nuclear or surrounding tissue changes or by stromatic accumulations of material without acute inflammatory reaction.	(3, 18, 26)

---

101. C, D
C
D
B, C
D
B

---

102. Atherosclerosis is a complex disease characterized by deposits of lipids, especially cholesterol, in the intima of large and medium-size arteries. The lesions, particularly the early isolated and uncomplicated lesions, are often referred to as atheromas. Grossly, they first appear as yellow streaks in the intima of arteries.

MATCH THE FOLLOWING (more than one response may apply):

____ occur(s) in arteries	A. atheromas
____ yellow	
____ predominantly cholesterol	B. xanthomas
____ may be focal lesions	
	C. fatty metamorphosis

47. A
B

---

48. NOTE: An understanding of the histochemistry of materials deposited in degenerations is useful in understanding the morphology and pathogenesis of the diseases involving these substances. Therefore, in this section and the ones following, we will begin by comparing the histochemistry of the substances involved.

Carbohydrates are characterized in tissue sections by their strongly positive periodic acid-Schiff reaction (PAS-positive).

MATCH THE FOLLOWING:

____water	A. PAS-positive
____glycogen	B. PAS-negative
____mucoid substances (glycoprotein)	

---

123. D
A
C
B

---

124. Compacted fibrin may become hyaline in appearance. This occurs most commonly in thrombi due to compacting of coagulated blood within blood vessels and on inflamed serosal surfaces, such as pleura and joint surfaces. Material with an appearance similar to compacted fibrin occurs in the center of subcutaneous inflammatory nodules associated with rheumatoid arthritis and in the walls of small arteries and arterioles in certain inflammatory vascular diseases and with severe hypertension. Because it is difficult to prove that this material is fibrin, it was called fibrinoid, which means fibrin ____________________.

INDICATE WHETHER "Fibrinous" OR "Fibrinoid" IS MOST APPROPRIATE:

____pericarditis is commonly seen in patients with long-standing renal failure

____change was noted in the wall of many small arteries in this patient with multisystem disease due to vasculitis

____is a descriptive term used to mean hyaline or slightly granular eosinophilic desposits

____implies that the observer is sure of the chemical nature of the material he is looking at

28. T
F
T
F
T

B. Classification of Degenerations (121 frames)

When you complete this section, you will be able to select correct responses relating to the:

1. Definition and proper use of:
   accumulation, storage, deposit, infiltration, hyaline, hyalin
2. Information and procedures used to identify water, carbohydrate, fat, protein, and calcium in tissue
3. Comparison of degenerations involving mainly
   water: cloudy swelling, hydropic degeneration
   carbohydrate: glycogen storage, mucoid change
   lipid: fatty metamorphosis, adiposity, mineral oil, granuloma, lipidoses, xanthoma, atheroma, lipofuscin
   protein: hyalinization of collagen, amyloidosis, fibrinoid change, Mallory body, Zenker's hyaline change
   calcium: dystrophic calcification, metastatic calcification

in terms of
definition
type of material deposited
morphologic appearance
common sites and disease associations
pathogenesis
clinical significance

GO ON TO THE NEXT PAGE

---

102. A
A, B, C
A, B
A, B

---

103. In the earliest stages of atheroma formation, foamy cells containing much bound cholesterol predominate. Later these cells break down, with liberation of lipid, resulting in formation of cholesterol crystals.

Atheromas:

occur in the ___ ________________ of ________________.

have a ________________ color.

contain ________________ ▱ intracellularly ▱ extracellularly.

46. A
B
A
B

---

47. Storage of glycogen occurs in the two situations with opposite pathogenic mechanisms.

Glycogen storage diseases are a group of rare metabolic defects in which enzymes involved in the breakdown of glycogen are deficient, resulting intracellular accumulation of glycogen and poor mobilization of glucose.

Diabetes mellitus is a defect of glucose utilization with high blood and urine levels of glucose leading to uptake and conversion of glucose to glycogen in renal tubule cells and hepatic nuclei.

MATCH THE FOLLOWING:

____defective breakdown and export of glycogen	A. glycogen storage disease
____increased uptake of glucose and storage as glycogen	B. glycogen in renal tubules in diabetes

---

122. B A

---

123. The mechanism of amyloid formation is not precisely known. Amyloid is thought to be produced by plasma cells. This may explain the association of amyloid with long-standing inflammation and with malignant tumors of plasma cells (multiple myeloma).

MATCH THE FOLLOWING MECHANISMS WITH THE TYPE OF DEGENERATION WITH WHICH THEY MAY BE ASSOCIATED:

____change in membrane permeability	A. amyloidosis
____production of an abnormal protein by plasma cells	B. hyalinized collagen
____altered rate of metabolism	C. fatty metamorphosis
____compacting of reparative tissue	D. cloudy swelling

EXPLANATORY NOTE: This is a long complex section which lays the groundwork for understanding many different diseases. You will be asked to define and compare many conditions associated with tissue accumulation of water, carbohydrate, lipid, protein, and minerals. It is suggested that you not try to complete this section in one sitting.

The subsections of the remainder of this unit are:

Introduction (5 frames)
Degeneration primarily involving water (12 frames)
Degeneration primarily involving carbohydrate (20 frames)
Degeneration primarily involving lipid (42 frames)
Degeneration primarily involving protein (32 frames)
Degeneration primarily involving calcium (10 frames)

GO ON TO NEXT PAGE

---

103. occur in the intima of arteries
have a yellow color
contain cholesterol [✓] intracellularly [✓] extracellularly

---

104. Lipofuscin (lip o-fus' sin) is an insoluble, granular brown pigment composed of complexes of lipid with protein and/or carbohydrate which represents the indigestible residue of intracellular lysosomal digestion.

MATCH THE FOLLOWING:

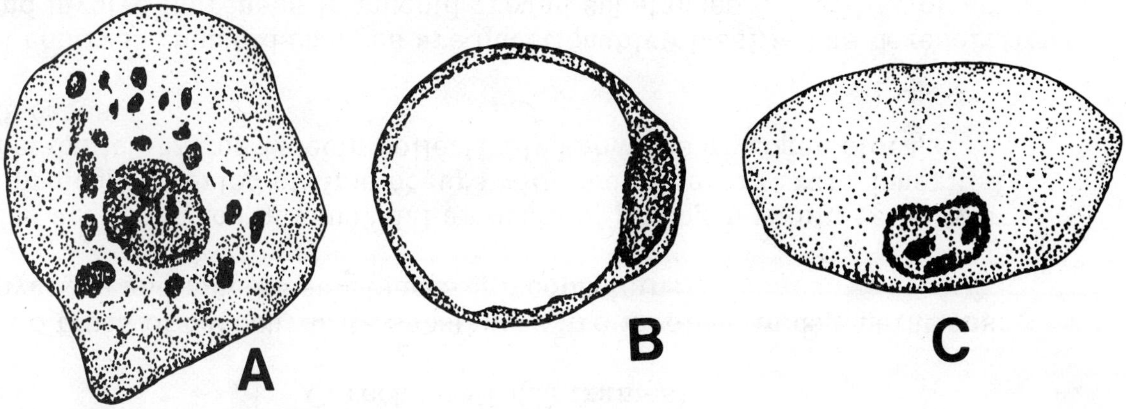

____hepatocyte containing triglyceride
____hepatocyte containing lipofuscin
____Kupffer cell containing lipoprotein complexes in lipidosis

45. F
T
T
F
T

Degeneration Primarily Involving Carbohydrate (20 frames)

46. Two types of carbohydrate substances are involved in degenerations: glycogen and mucoid substances (glycoproteins).

The accumulation of abnormal amounts of glycogen within cells over a prolonged period of time occurs with one of several rare inherited metabolic enzyme defects collectively known as glycogen storage diseases.

In contrast, mucoid changes are questionably classified as degenerations and involve increases in mucoid ground substances or spilling of epithelial mucins into connective tissues.

MATCH THE FOLLOWING:

____intracellular	A. glycogen storage disease
____extracellular	
____specific chemical defect	B. mucoid change
____descriptive term	

---

121. B
A
C

---

122. MATCH THE FOLLOWING:

A. replacement of arteriolar smooth muscle, characteristic of primary type amyloidosis
B. replacement of liver parenchyma with pressure atrophy of hepatocytes, characteristic of secondary type amyloidosis

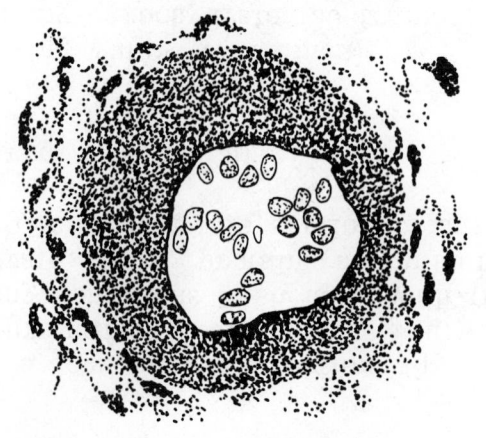

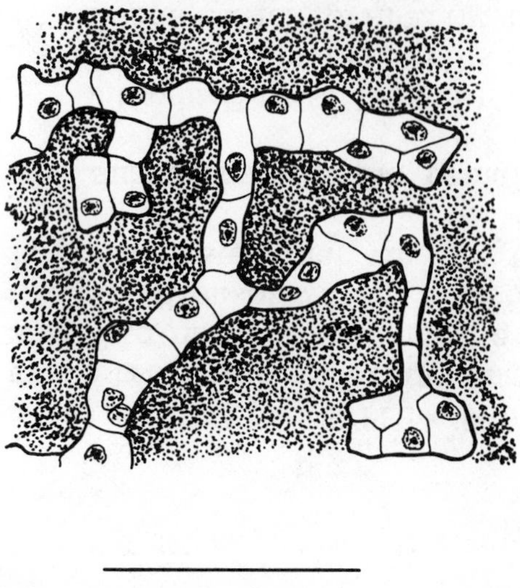

____

____

Introduction (5 frames)

29. Recall the definition of degeneration: ____________________

____

---

104. B
A
C

---

105. Lipofuscin is most commonly seen in the heart and liver with aging. The process is referred to as brown atrophy (brown color grossly due to lipofuscin; atrophy refers to slow, prolonged degeneration in this case). Brown atrophy is an insignificant autopsy finding.

MATCH THE FOLLOWING:

____grossly brown liver	A. fatty metamorphosis
____grossly yellow liver	B. atheroma
____focal yellow intimal lesions	C. brown atrophy
____granular intracellular pigment microscopically	
____large intracellular vacuole microscopically	
____foamy histiocytes and specific extracellular cleft-like spaces microscopically	

44. F
F
T
F

---

45. INDICATE "T" TRUE OR "F" FALSE:

	frame reference
____Cloudy swelling is seen in most organs at autopsy, since anoxia is an inevitable precursor of death.	(41,42)
____Increased organ weight is a useful, although not always specific, indicator of cloudy swelling.	(36)
____Edema is usually used to refer to extracellular water accumulation and is not classified as a degenerative disorder.	(34)
____Water produces discrete vacuoles in cells.	(35, 38)
____Osmotic injury to cells may produce hydropic degeneration.	(42,43)

---

120. B
A
A
B

---

121. Primary (= no antecedent cause known) amyloidosis is associated with hyaline deposits in muscle, particularly cardiac muscle, smooth muscle of small blood vessels and the gastrointestinal tract, and skeletal muscle of the tongue.

Amyloid tumors are rare solitary masses in the region of the upper respiratory tract.

MATCH THE FOLLOWING:

____deposits in abdominal organs associated with very long-standing chronic inflammations	A. primary amyloidosis
____possible explanation for large tongue and large heart	B. secondary amyloidosis
____might be confused clinically with a cancer of larynx or trachea	C. amyloid tumor

29. Degeneration is cellular and/or interstitial change in which cells are not killed.

---

30. Degenerations may be classified according to the type of chemical material altered or accumulated.

NAME FIVE CHEMICAL CLASSES OF MATERIAL THAT CAN ACCUMULATE IN DEGENERATION.

____

____

____

____

____

---

105. C
A
B
C
A
B

---

106. Lipofuscin accumulation within cells does not appear to interfere with the cells' function. The brown cytoplasmic lipofuscin granules can be differentiated from other pigments by their faint acid-fast staining, mild PAS-positivity, and failure to stain for iron. A similar pigment, called ceroid, accumulates in smooth muscle cells in vitamin E deficiency and may produce a brown color in the bowel wall.

MATCH THE FOLLOWING:

____specific lipoproteins	A. brown atrophy
____lipofuscin	
____ceroid	B. vitamin E deficiency
____granular brown intracellular pigment not dissolved in tissue processing	C. lipidoses
____enlarged pale cells with central nucleus	

43. a
b
c

---

44. INDICATE "T" TRUE OR "F" FALSE:

	frame reference
____Cloudy swelling is a chronic form of degeneration.	(35)
____Cloudy swelling involves extracellular accumulation of water.	(35)
____Cloudy swelling and hydropic degeneration are sometimes used as synonyms.	(35)
____Hydropic degeneration, in contrast to cloudy swelling, produces nuclear changes.	(35)

---

119. ☑ specifically
☑ extracellular
☑ irreversible

---

120. Secondary amyloidosis is secondary to long-standing inflammation (tuberculosis, osteomyelitis, rheumatoid arthritis, etc.) The amyloid is deposited at sites remote from the inflammatory process, most commonly in the liver, spleen, kidneys, and adrenals.

MATCH THE FOLLOWING:

____hyaline type material associated with chronic inflammation but deposited at sites remote from the inflammation (abdominal organs)

____hyaline type material which may occur at the site of long-standing chronic inflammation

____retention of some structure, and its location often allows for its identification

____very homogeneous deposits which can be positively identified by special histologic techniques

A. hyalinized collagen

B. amyloid deposits in secondary amyloidosis

30. water
mineral
carbohydrate [or equivalent]
lipid
protein

---

31. In this text we are using the word degeneration as a generic term to indicate (CHOOSE THE APPROPRIATE RESPONSES):

____that an abnormal amount of water, mineral, carbohydrate, lipid, or protein is present in some tissue

____that the morphologic change is associated with cell death

____that the change is at least potentially reversible

____that the change is intracellular and chronic

---

106. C
A
B
A, B
C

---

107. INDICATE "T" TRUE OR "F" FALSE:

	frame reference
____Triglyceride accumulation with formation of a globule displacing the nucleus is characteristically found in normal adipose tissue cells and in hepatocytes in fatty metamorphosis.	(66, 67, 75, 79)
____Adiposity and fatty metamorphosis are synonyms.	(80, 81, 82)
____Fatty metamorphosis is commonly caused by vitamin E deficiency and certain lipidoses.	(86)
____Atheromas are characterized by both intra- and extracellular lipid deposits.	(102, 103)
____Lipidoses are rare metabolic disorders often involving the reticuloendothelial organs.	(100)

42. A
B

---

43. Which of the following are pathogenic mechanisms for hydropic degeneration and/or cloudy swelling?

a. mild local injury

b. systemic infections, anoxemias, and toxemias

c. osmotic effects on certain specialized cells

---

118. hyalinized
scar (fibrous, connective) tissue

---

119. Amyloidosis refers to a group of rare, slowly progressive, chronic conditions in which a rather specific proteinaceous material composed of alpha and gamma globulins and glycoprotein is deposited in tissues.

It may occur as primary amyloidosis, secondary amyloidosis, or (rarely) amyloid tumors.

You would expect the proteinaceous deposits seen with amyloidosis to stain ▱ specifically ▱ non-specifically, to be ▱ intracellular ▱ extracellular, and to be ▱ reversible ▱ irreversible.

31. ✓ that an abnormal amount of water, mineral, carbohydrate, lipid, or protein is present in some tissue

✓ that the change is at least potentially reversible

---

32. Early pathologists gave various names to processes which we now classify as degenerations. These names tended to imply whether the material was produced locally or brought into the tissue.

TRY TO MATCH THE SYNONYM FOR DEGENERATION WITH THE IMPLIED ORIGIN OF THE MATERIAL PRESENT IN EXCESS:

____accumulation	A. increased local production or decreased export
____storage	
____deposit	B. excess material brought into tissue
____infiltration	

---

107. T
F
F
T
T

---

108. INDICATE "T" TRUE OR "F" FALSE:

	frame reference
____Brown atrophy frequently results in prolonged heart failure.	(105)
____Mineral oil granulomas occur most commonly in the colon and are innocuous lesions.	(98)
____Fatty metamorphosis is very common but usually is not the direct cause of symptoms.	(92, 93)
____Depletion of carbohydrate stores may lead to lipid accumulation in the liver.	(88)
____Deficient protein production may lead to lipid accumulation in the liver.	(89)

41. B
A
[✓] tissue susceptibility

---

42. Clinically, cloudy swelling of the liver, kidneys, and heart are classically associated with various severe acute infections, anoxemias, toxins or poisons, and severe burns.

The best examples of hydropic degeneration are seen in the renal tubules as a result of intravenous administration of hypertonic sugar solutions, diethylene glycol poisoning, or severe depletion of body potassium.

MATCH THE FOLLOWING:

____ more likely to occur as a mild change in several organs as result of severe systemic disease

____ more likely to appear in special tissue types with selected types of injury such as changes in osmotic pressure

A. cloudy swelling

B. hydropic degeneration

---

117. Hyaline is a descriptive term meaning "homogeneous and translucent" (or, more narrowly, a homogeneous, eosinophilic microscopic appearance).
collagen, fibrin, amyloid--also edema fluid, certain foreign bodies, or platelet masses
Special stains [✓] are helpful in distinguishing these materials.

---

118. Hyalinization of collagen is very common and is part of the process of aging of scar tissue as it becomes acellular and avascular. This not only occurs in surgical scars and healing lesions such as old granulomas, it also occurs in certain degenerative conditions such as atherosclerosis.

In the early stages of atherosclerosis, lipids are deposited and take the form of foamy histiocytes (lipid dispersed in histiocytes). As the atherosclerotic plaque enlarges, it also begins to scar. Older plaques become compact, homogeneous, and eosinophilic and, therefore, are referred to as ________________ized intimal plaques. Degeneration of collagen is really part of the process of aging of ________________ tissue.

32. A
A
B
B

---

33. Some degenerations are called changes because it is questionable whether they fit the definition of degeneration. Others have the suffix -oma because they resemble tumors or -osis simply to indicate a non-specific condition.

MATCH THE FOLLOWING:

Type of Degeneration	Implication of Name
____xanthoma	A. does not exactly fit with degenerations
____fibrinoid change	B. tumor-like
____amyloidosis	C. nature of condition not specified

---

108. F
F
T
T
T

Degeneration Primarily Involving Protein (31 frames)

109. Degenerations characterized by accumulations of protein or protein-like material can be classified according to whether they are extracellular or intracellular. Microscopically, protein deposits typically have a glistening, homogeneous, eosinophilic appearance.

MATCH THE FOLLOWING CHARACTERISTICS OF DEGENERATION WITH THE SUBSTANCES INVOLVED (more than one letter may apply):

____produce(s) empty spaces in H & E sections	A. water
____eosinophilic	B. fat
____considered a degeneration only when it accumulates intracellularly	C. protein
____may be intracellular or extracellular form of degeneration	

40. necrosis

---

41. Cloudy swelling is a common non-specific degeneration which occurs in most tissues following mild injury. However, when due to agents which act systemically, it is most often observed in specialized tissues such as epithelium of renal tubules, hepatocytes, myocardium, and neurons.

MATCH THE FOLLOWING:

____cloudy swelling in area of injury	A. toxemia or anoxia
____cloudy swelling in specialized tissues	B. mild local injury

The commonness of cloudy swelling in kidneys, liver, and heart can be accounted for on the basis of ▱ duration of injury ▱ tissue susceptibility ▱ intensity of injurious agent.

---

116. B
A
C

---

117. Hyaline is ____________________.

Extracellular hyaline deposits are likely to be composed of

____

____

____

Special stains ▱ are ▱ are not helpful in distinguishing these materials.

33. B
A
C

Degeneration Primarily Involving Water (12 frames)

34. Acute degenerations involving increases in cell size due to increases in water content are called cloudy swelling or hydropic degeneration.

A chronic increase in intracellular water is not a recognized entity.

Acute or chronic increase in water between cells (interstitially) is called edema and is classified as a hemodynamic disorder rather than a degeneration.

MATCH THE FOLLOWING:

____acute	A. cloudy swelling or hydropic degeneration
____chronic	B. edema
____intracellular	
____extracellular	

---

109. A, B
C
A
B, C Increased extracellular water (edema) is not usually considered a degeneration.

---

110. The term hyaline is frequently used to describe proteinaceous deposits. Hyaline is a descriptive adjective which means homogeneous and translucent and can be used to describe either gross or microscopic findings. The material deposited may be called hyalin even though this refers to appearance rather than chemical structure. Hyaline is often used in a more narrow sense by microscopists to mean homogeneous and eosinophilic.
Hyalin is a ☐ noun ☐ adjective which refers to a ☐ chemical ☐ morphologic substance characterized by which of the following:

____fibrillary structure
____ground glass (cloudy) appearance
____uniform structure
____deep blue color

39. increased cell size (distended)
vacuolated cytoplasm [or equivalent]
intact, nondisplaced nucleus

---

40. If some of the cells in an area of hydropic degeneration have indistinct, pale, or fragmented nuclei, this indicates that ________________ is present.

---

115. C
A
B
C

---

116. In addition to the differences in physical appearance, fibrin, collagen, and amyloid can usually be distinguished by the context in which they occur.

Fibrin masses are associated with inflammatory lesions where the fibrin has a chance to accumulate.

Collagen, of course, is a normal connective tissue constituent. It is only considered a degeneration when dense masses of old acellular scar tissue accumulate.

Amyloid occurs in the rare condition amyloidosis and accumulates in the walls of small blood vessels, between muscle fibers (smooth, skeletal, and cardiac), and between cells of parenchymal organs such as liver, spleen, kidney, and adrenal gland.

MATCH THE FOLLOWING:

____associated with old injury — A. fibrin

____associated with acute inflammation — B. collagen

____distributed in muscle, small vessels, and organ parenchyma — C. amyloid

34. A, B acute
B chronic
A intracellular
B extracellular

---

35. Cloudy swelling and hydropic degeneration are acute degenerations characterized by increase in water in the cell cytoplasm; they may be used as synonyms, or cloudy swelling may be used to indicate the milder form characterized microscopically by cloudy cytoplasm and hydropic degeneration for the more severe form with vacuolated (hydropic) cytoplasm. The vacuoles are not discrete and the distinction between the two processes is one of interpretation.

Cloudy swelling and hydropic degeneration involve changes in
☐ interstitium ☐ cytoplasm ☐ nucleus.

Cloudy swelling is generally considered to be a ☐ more ☐ less severe change than hydropic degeneration.

---

110. Hyalin is a ☑ noun which refers to a ☑ morphologic substance characterized by
✓ ground glass (cloudy) appearance, i.e., translucent
✓ uniform structure, i.e., homogeneous

---

111. Hyaline is a commonly used term because many materials seen histologically have an eosinophilic, homogeneous appearance. Most substances that have a hyaline appearance are compacted protein, but this is not always the case.

A hyaline microscopic appearance is ☐ always ☐ usually ☐ sometimes associated with protein deposits and usually is associated with a ☐ red ☐ blue color in H & E stained sections.

38. B

---

39. LIST THE MICROSCOPIC FINDINGS OF HYDROPIC DEGENERATION.

____

____

____

---

114. A, B, C
C
B
A, B, C

---

115. In H & E sections, amyloid is very homogeneous. The amyloid fibers are birefringent (optically rotate light) and when stained with Congo red give a green birefringence.

Collagen often appears wavy in H & E sections and may exhibit slight birefringence, but this is not green. Fibrin masses tend to be slightly granular in H & E sections and are not birefringent; in looser areas, fibrin strands can be seen.

MATCH THE FOLLOWING:

____most homogeneous	A. fibrin
____least homogeneous	B. collagen
____wavy bundles	C. amyloid
____specific birefringence	

35. ☑ cytoplasm
☑ less

---

36. The gross changes of cloudy swelling or hydropic degeneration are:
1) increased organ weight in proportion to increased water in cells
2) increased opaqueness or cloudiness of organ, often with pallor
3) tension on the organ capsule in organs such as liver and kidney

FOR EACH PAIR, INDICATE WHICH GROSS FINDING IS MOST LIKELY WITH CLOUDY SWELLING:

____150-gm kidney

____180-gm kidney

____kidney cortex pale and translucent

____kidney cortex congested

____kidney tissue bulges outward when capsule is cut

____kidney tissue retracts when capsule is cut

---

111. ☑ usually associated with protein deposits
☑ red in H & E sections

---

112. In the broad sense, hyaline is a descriptive term which indicates that a material is ______________________ and ______________________.

Most hyaline deposits are composed of ____________________, which ☐ is ☐ is not removed in tissue processing.

37. increased organ weight
cloudy (opaque, translucent, pale) appearance [or equivalent]
tension on capsule

---

38. Microscopically, the increased cell water of hydropic degeneration or cloudy swelling is identified by inference (since water cannot be seen in sections).

1) Cell size is increased due to distention of the cell membrane.
2) Cell constituents are more widely spaced, producing the so-called vacuolated appearance. Vacuoles are not distinct.
3) The nucleus is intact and not displaced.

Which cell is undergoing hydropic degeneration?

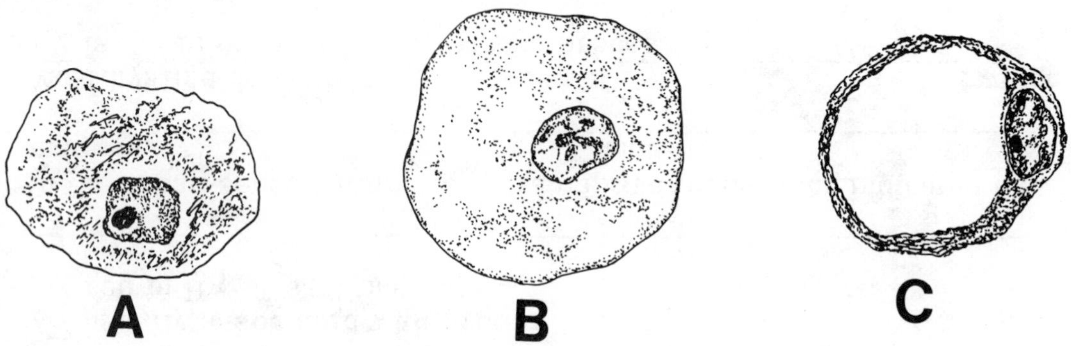

---

113. C
B
A

---

114. Extracellular, hyaline, proteinaceous deposits of fibrin, collagen, and amyloid (an abnormal protein which slowly accumulates is a condition known as amyloidosis) can be distinguished by their appearance in H & E sections, staining reactions, location, associated conditions, and by electron microscopy.

Electron microscopy is the least practical but most distinctive, since all three substances are long proteins with distinctively different fibrillar structures.

In routine paraffin sections, amyloid stains with Congo red and metachromatically with azo dyes such as crystal violet. Collagen can be stained with trichrome stains (blue or green, depending on type used).

MATCH THE FOLLOWING:

____hyaline	A. fibrin
____Congo red positive	B. collagen
____stains with trichrome stain	C. amyloid
____specific structure by electron microscopy	

36. ✓ 180-gm kidney ✓ kidney cortex pale and translucent
✓ kidney tissue bulges outward when capsule is cut

---

37. LIST THE GROSS FINDINGS OF CLOUDY SWELLING OR HYDROPIC DEGENERATION:

____

____

____

TURN TEXT 180° AND CONTINUE.

---

112. homogeneous and translucent (or equivalent)
protein
☑ is not removed in tissue processing

---

113. Most extracellular hyaline deposits are composed of collagen, fibrin, amyloid, edema fluid with high protein content, and certain foreign bodies. Masses of compacted platelets will also appear to be extracellular, although they are themselves cellular.

MATCH THE FOLLOWING EXAMPLES WITH THE NATURE OF THE HYALINIZED MATERIAL:

____ an old atheroma gradually is replaced by fibrous tissue, and the fibrous tissue becomes compact and acellular

____ the rough surface of an old atheroma in the aorta is covered by masses of small cellular fragments derived from the bloodstream

____ upon exposure to certain noxious gases the pulmonary alveoli fill with rather acellular inflammatory exudate

A. edema fluid
B. platelet thrombi
C. collagen

TURN TEXT 180° AND CONTINUE.

Unit 10. Developmental Abnormalities: Embryonic and Fetal, Genetic and Chromosomal

Unit 10. DEVELOPMENTAL ABNORMALITIES: EMBRYONIC AND FETAL, GENETIC AND CHROMOSOMAL

OBJECTIVES

When you complete this unit, you will be able to select correct responses relating to the:

		starting page	frame numbers
A.	Definition of Terms	10.5	1-13

1. definition of the following terms:

developmental abnormality	fetal period
genetic disease	cell growth
congenital disease	cell differentiation
familial disease	involution
embryonic period	

		starting page	frame numbers
B.	Classification of Developmental Abnormalities	10.31	14-27

1. classification of developmental abnormalities by
   a. cause: physical, chemical, biologic, or unknown
   b. pathogenic mechanism: intrauterine injury, genetic, or chromosomal
   c. onset of manifestations: congenital or noncongenital
   d. general type of structural and functional abnormalities: gross body deformities, gross organ deformities, diffuse or focal tissue reactions, or physiologic and/or biochemical defects only

		starting page	frame numbers
C.	Embryonic and Fetal Abnormalities	10.61	28-52

1. embryonic and fetal abnormalities: pathogenesis, common features, causes, and examples

		starting page	frame numbers
D.	Genetic Abnormalities	10.20	53-81

1. genetic abnormalities: pathogenesis, common features, classification, and examples

		starting page	frame numbers
E.	Chromosomal Abnormalities	10.49	82-106

1. chromosomal abnormalities: pathogenesis, classification, and features of common examples

		starting page	frame numbers
F.	Additional Data	10.32	none

PREREQUISITES
BASIC GENETICS, CYTOGENETICS, AND MOLECULAR GENETICS

A basic knowledge of genetics is a prerequisite to this unit on developmental abnormalities. If you cannot meet the following prerequisite objectives, we suggest that you study the appropriate material in one of the following references before beginning the unit.

OBJECTIVES

1. Recognize examples of the following types of inheritance and predict genotypes and phenotypes of parents or offspring: autosomal dominant, autosomal recessive, sex-linked dominant, sex-linked recessive.

2. Predict the likelihood of occurrence of traits which follow classic Mendelian patterns.

3. Define and recognize examples of and significance of penetrance, expressivity, linkage, balanced polymorphism, simple (autosomal) inheritance, multifactor inheritance.

4. Given a photograph of a karyotype, determine the sex and whether there is an abnormality in sex or autosomal chromosomes.

5. Indicate the significance of Barr bodies and drumstick appendages on nuclei of polys.

6. Given a pedigree, indicate the most likely type of inheritance.

7. Describe how the genetic message gets from the DNA to expression and how DNA, rRNA, tRNA, mRNA, and proteins are involved.

REFERENCES

Wintrobe MM, et al, Harrison's Principles of Internal Medicine, 7th edition, McGraw-Hill Co., New York, 1974, Chapter 62.

McKusick VA, Human Genetics, 2nd edition, Prentice-Hall, Englewood Cliffs, New Jersey, 1969.

Thompson JS, Genetics in Medicine, W. B. Sanders, Philadelphia, 1973.

PRETEST

UNIT 10: DEVELOPMENTAL ABNORMALITIES: EMBRYONIC AND FETAL, GENETIC AND CHROMOSOMAL

SELECT THE SINGLE BEST RESPONSE:

1. Familial disorders are
   (A) the same as genetic disorders
   (B) usually congenital
   (C) commonly associated with chromosomal abnormalities
   (D) sometimes caused by infectious agents

2. Involution is
   (A) the cause of aplasia and hypoplasia
   (B) due to a genetic abnormality
   (C) the most common cause of congenital abnormalities
   (D) controlled by the phenomenon of induction

3. Congenital heart disease and other gross organ defects are produced by injury during
   (A) gametogenesis
   (B) the fetal period
   (C) both
   (D) neither

4. Which may be detected on preparations of dividing cells (karyotyping)?
   (A) genetic disorders
   (B) embryonic injuries
   (C) both
   (D) neither

5. Abortion because of a possible embryonic defect might be considered if the mother had rubella
   (A) 2 weeks after the last menstrual period
   (B) 8 weeks after the last menstrual period
   (C) 16 weeks after the last menstrual period
   (D) 32 weeks after the last menstrual period

6. Injuries during the fetal period are most likely to interfere with which of the following?
   (A) involution
   (B) cell differentiation
   (C) cell growth
   (D) organogenesis

7. Genetic diseases rarely are the cause of
   (A) storage diseases
   (B) metabolic deficiencies
   (C) tissue damage from toxic metabolites
   (D) gross organ deformities

8. Of the following, which probably accounts for the greatest percentage of abortions?
   (A) genetic abnormalities
   (B) chromosomal abnormalities
   (C) embryonic injuries
   (D) fetal injuries

GO ON TO NEXT PAGE AND BEGIN THE UNIT

A. Definition of Terms (13 frames)

When you complete this section, you will be able to select correct responses to the:

1. definition of the following terms:

developmental abnormality
genetic disease
congenital disease
familial disease
embryonic period
fetal period
cell growth
cell differentiation
involution

1. Developmental abnormalities are structural and functional abnormalities which result from the application of an injurious agent before birth. Injuries occurring at the time of birth are not included in this group of disorders.

MATCH THE FOLLOWING:

____ injury to previous generations transmitted by genes

____ injury to the embryo

____ injury at birth

____ abnormal growth after birth

A. developmental abnormality

B. inflammation and repair, or degeneration and necrosis, or disturbance of growth

---

59. A
B

---

60. Below is a diagram of a series of enzymatic steps operating on a substance A:

$$A \xrightarrow{a} B \xrightarrow{b} C \xrightarrow{c} D$$

The capital letters represent substrates and the small letters enzymes.

If enzyme b is lacking, you would expect an excess of substance ________________ or perhaps substance ________________. Also, there would probably be a deficiency of substance ________________ and ________________.

Which of these four abnormalities could possibly cause observable disease?

TURN TEXT 180° AND CONTINUE.

1. A
A
B
B

---

2. This definition of developmental abnormalities is based primarily on the time of application of the injurious agent, i.e., before birth. The injury may be in the form of abnormal genes, abnormal chromosomes, or a variety of reactions to agents acting during in utero development.

Developmental abnormalities are often not classifiable as inflammation, degeneration, necrosis, or disturbance of growth. A few, however, can logically be classified as developmental abnormalities and by the type of tissue reaction.
MATCH THE FOLLOWING:

____ disease resulting from a genetic defect

____ an in utero infection which causes gross structural malformation

____ an in utero infection which causes chronic inflammation

A. developmental abnormality

B. inflammation and healing, or degeneration and necrosis, or disturbance of growth

C. both A and B

---

60. B or A
C and D
any of them

---

61. Phenylketonuria is a genetic disease due to absence or inactivity of phenylalanine hydroxylase.

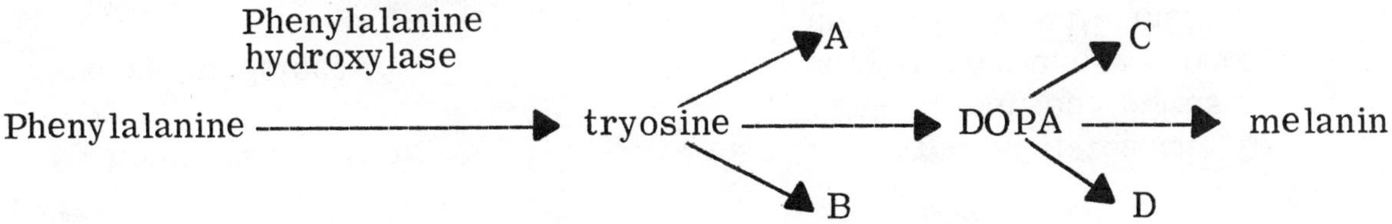

The excess phenylalanine is disposed of in two ways:

1) When the blood level rises above a certain point, it is excreted by the kidney. This gives the lab abnormality, phenylketon______.
2) Some of it is degraded via alternate pathways.

INDICATE WHICH OF THE FOLLOWING BIOCHEMICAL ABNORMALITIES WOULD BE PRESENT IN PHENYLKETONURIA (PKU):

____ ↑ serum melanin
____ ↑ urine phenylalanine
____ ↓ serum phenylalanine

58. ✓ dominant ✓ autosomal (A sex-linked gene is carried on the X chromosome and cannot be passed from father to son.)
✓ no

---

59. In theory, inherited (genetic) abnormalities produce logical defects. Each gene corresponds to one protein. If the protein is a structural protein, defects will be seen wherever that protein is. If it is an enzyme, the defects will be in some way related to the substrate and products of the enzyme.

MATCH THE FOLLOWING:

____structural protein defect A. abnormal skeleton due to weak epiphyseal plates

____enzyme defect B. decreased glucose 6-phosphatase in the liver, with increased storage of glycogen

---

f. SYMPTOMATIC CARE
- Down's syndrome
- non-correctable disfiguring embryonic anomalies
- brain damage secondary to fetal diseases
- genetic diseases
  - Friedreich's ataxia
  - lipid storage diseases
  - glycogen storage disease
  - (and many others)

THIS IS THE END OF UNIT 10. TAKE THE POSTTEST ON PAGE xxxii.

2. A
A
C

---

3. Abnormal genes, abnormal chromosomes, and intrauterine injury may be manifest before birth, at birth, after birth, or not at all.
INDICATE TRUE (T) OR FALSE (F):

____ Injurious agents acting after birth sometimes cause developmental abnormalities.

____ Developmental abnormalities may not be apparent until years after birth.

Developmental abnormalities are ______________________.

---

61. This gives the lab abnormality phenylketon<u>uria</u>.
__✓__ urine phenylalanine

---

62. During the fetal period, the mother's liver metabolizes the excess phenylalanine produced by the fetus. Thus, at birth the baby presents initially a normal biochemical picture.

INDICATE WHICH CURVE SHOWS THE CHILD'S SERUM LEVELS OF PHENYLALANINE:

A. level
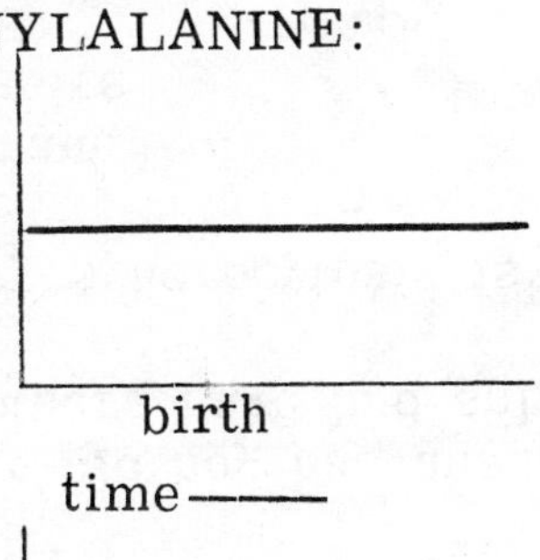

C. level
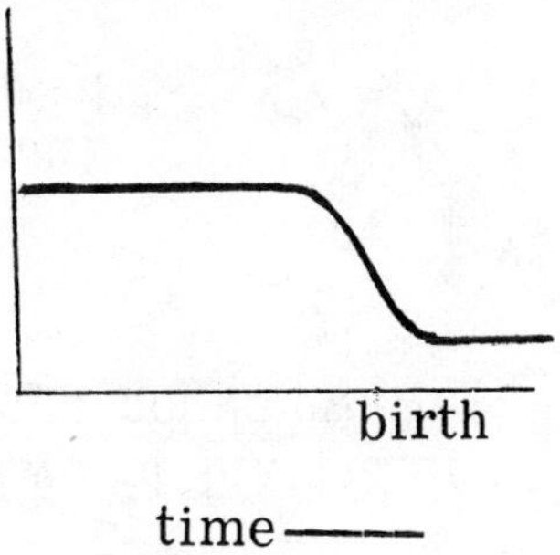

B. level
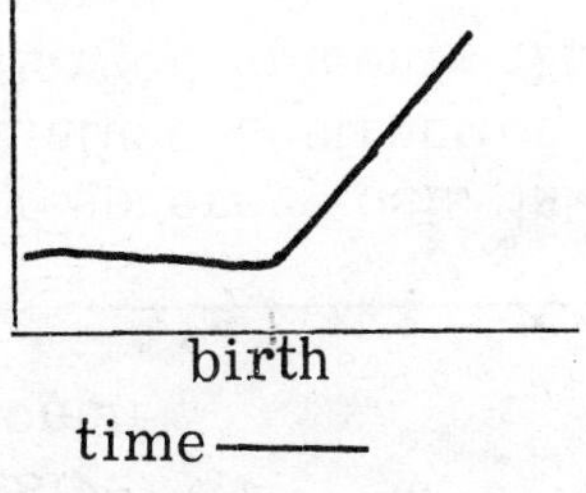

57. [✓] recessive
[✓] autosomal

---

58. Hereditary spherocytosis is a defect in red blood cells leading to their premature destruction by the spleen. This leads to anemia and an enlarged spleen. The most effective treatment is removal of the spleen.

A 17-year-old boy has anemia. His father and two of his father's three brothers have had splenectomies, but he does not know why.

Hereditary spherocytosis is:

____dominant	____autosomal
____recessive	____sex-linked

Is hereditary spherocytosis generally manifest congenitally?

____yes
____no

---

c. DIETARY RESTRICTION OF SUBSTANCES
- phenylalanine in phenylketonuria
- lactose in galactosemia
- purines in gout
- cholesterol in some lipid disorders

d. INCREASE EXCRETION OF SUBSTANCES
- cholesterol disorders (cholestyramine)
- gout (probenecid)
- hemochromatosis (bleed)
- Wilson's disease (chelating agent)

e. AVOID PRECIPITATING FACTORS
- glucose 6-phosphate dehydrogenase deficiency (drugs)
- hemophilia (trauma)
- diabetes (obesity)

3. F
T
Developmental abnormalities are structural and functional abnormalities which result from application of an injurious agent before birth.

---

4. The terms genetic and congenital have different but overlapping meanings.

Genetic means inherited due to the structure of DNA which is passed from generation to generation. Abnormal genes may or may not produce disease, and if disease is produced, it may or may not be detectable at birth.

Congenital means present at birth. In this text, we will use the word congenital only in reference to congenital disease, i.e., detectable abnormalities in structure and function present at birth.

Which is/are true?

____All genetic diseases are congenital diseases.

____Some genetic diseases are congenital diseases.

____All congenital diseases are genetic diseases.

____Some congenital diseases are genetic diseases.

---

62. B

---

63. At birth, the brains of babies with PKU are normal. Myelinization fails to continue normally, and the children become mentally retarded starting shortly after birth unless they are treated starting within weeks of birth. Treatment consists of a diet very low in phenylalanine.

INDICATE WHICH IS/ARE THE REASON(S) FOR BRAIN DAMAGE IN PKU:

a. High levels of phenylalanine (or one of its derivatives via the alternate pathways) cause improper myelinization.

b. The babies are less able to withstand the trauma of birth.

c. Due to lack of DOPA, the baby's brain cannot develop properly.

56. 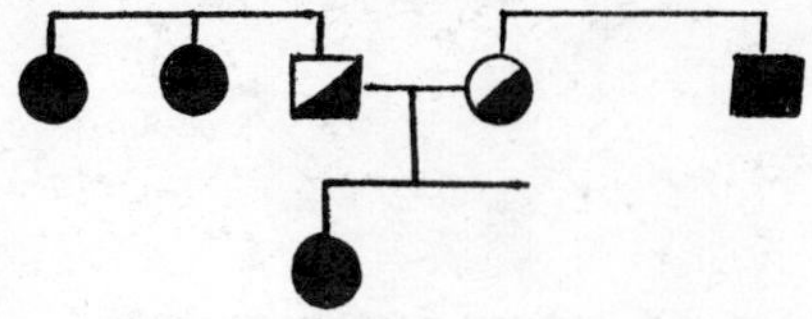

/✓/ recessive
1/4

---

57. If not recognized and treated, galactosemia causes a high rate of early deaths. A baby with galactosemia has a grandaunt and a cousin who died at a young age of a nutritional problem. No other information is available. This is a typical history for this disease.

Galactosemia is /_/ dominant or /_/ recessive

/_/ autosomal or /_/ sex-linked

---

g. DISEASES WHICH PRODUCE MINIMAL OR NO PROBLEMS
- most minor embryonic anomalies, e.g., double ureter, aberrant arteries, Meckel's diverticulum
- many genetic defects

pentosuria	Hageman factor deficiency
Gilbert's disease	beta-amino isobutyric aciduria
color-blindness	sickle cell trait
baldness	(and many others)

4. Classification by Method of Treatment

a. SURGICAL CORRECTION
- life-threatening embryonic anomalies
- socially unacceptable embryonic anomalies

b. SUPPLY MISSING PROTEIN OR METABOLITES

- diabetes mellitus	- cretinism
- agammaglobulinemia	- adrenogenital syndrome
- hemophilia	- Klinefelter's syndrome

4. ✓ Some genetic diseases are congenital diseases.
✓ Some congenital diseases are genetic diseases.

---

5. It may be difficult to decide whether a disease should be classified as a developmental abnormality.

If a disease is congenital, the injury must have occurred before birth, therefore, it is a developmental abnormality.

A disease which is not apparent for some time after birth may be a developmental abnormality if it was due to genetic or chromosome abnormalities or to intrauterine injury with delayed onset of manifestations.

MATCH THE FOLLOWING:

____ phocomelia (abnormal arm structure present at birth)	A. developmental abnormality
____ familial polyposis of the colon (genetically induced neoplastic lesions which cannot be detected until teen age)	B. insufficient information to classify
____ milk intolerance developing in two-month-old babies	

All ☐ congenital ☐ genetic diseases are classified in this text as developmental abnormalities.

---

63. a (Note: There is some question about this, but brain damage correlates better with blood levels of phenylalanine than anything else.)

---

64. The causative mechanism of PKU is ☐ intrauterine injury ☐ genetic ☐ chromosomal.

The manifestations of PKU are ☐ congenital ☐ noncongenital.

PKU manifestations appear as
☐ gross body deformities
☐ gross organ deformities
☐ diffuse or focal tissue changes
☐ physiologic or biochemical defects

55. 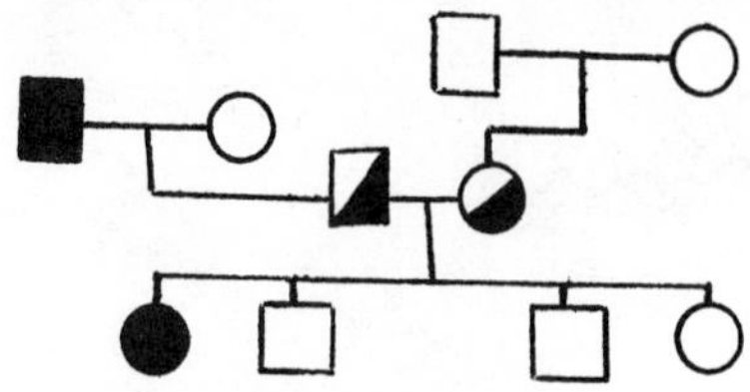

/✓/ recessive

---

56. Sickle cell disease is an hereditary disease of blacks. It is usually fatal by age 20.

A girl is found to have the disease. Two of her father's sisters and one of her mother's brothers died from the disease. FILL IN THE FAMILY TREE APPROPRIATELY:

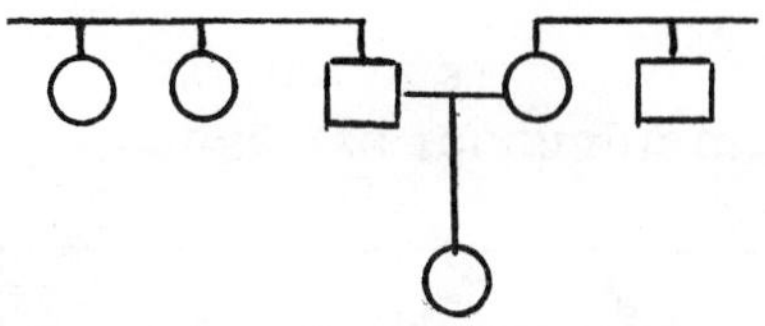

The inheritance pattern is /_/ dominant /_/ recessive.

It is possible to identify carriers of sickle cell genes by analysis of blood cells. Such people are said to have sickle cell trait (heterozygous carriers).
INDICATE THE CARRIERS IN THE DIAGRAM ABOVE BY BLACKENING HALF OF THE CIRCLE OR BOX.

The probability of the next child having the disease is ____________.

---

e. CAUSES OF PROBLEMS AT UNPREDICTABLE TIMES DEPENDING ON ENVIRONMENTAL FACTORS
   - hemophilia
   - glucose 6-phosphate dehydrogenase deficiency
   - trauma
   - drugs

f. CAUSES OF MILD TO MODERATE PROBLEMS WITH LATE ONSET
   - occasional embryonic anomalies, e.g., polycystic kidneys, mild congenital heart defect, absent kidney, Meckel's diverticulum which becomes inflammed
   - multifactorial genetic diseases
   - genetic diseases
     diabetes mellitus (most cases)
     gout

5. A
A
B
All [✓] congenital AND [✓] genetic diseases are classified in this text as developmental abnormalities.

---

6. A FAMILIAL disease is one in which two or more members of a family or extended family group are affected. Genes are only one of several mechanisms of transmitting disease among family members.

MATCH THE FOLLOWING:

____ a mother and son who both have tuberculosis

____ a father and son who both have hereditary spherocytosis

____ a maternal grandfather and grandson who are both color blind

A. genetic

B. familial

C. both genetic and familial

[ ] All [ ] some [ ] no familial diseases are classified as developmental abnormalities.

---

64. [✓] genetic
[✓] noncongenital
[✓] diffuse tissue changes (autopsy)
[✓] physiologic or biochemical (clinical)

---

65. Enzyme deficiencies can be manifest through many routes. Below is a diagram of some of these:

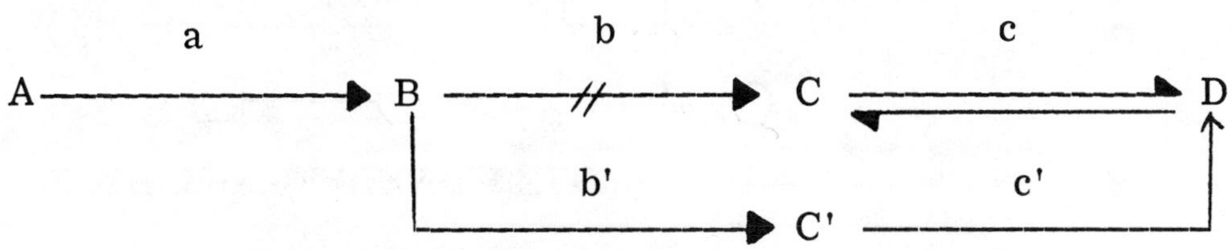

USE THE DIAGRAM TO MATCH THE FOLLOWING:

____ the alternate pathway b', c' can be used

____ substance B is not excretable; pathway b' does not exist

____ B is excretable by the kidney; pathway b' does not exist

A. storage of A or B may cause disease

B. lack of C or D may cause disease; A and B cause no trouble

C. there may be no observable abnormalities

54. 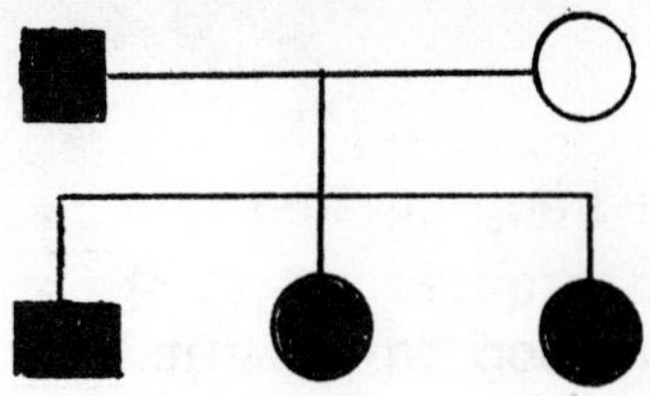

[✓] dominant

55. The grandfather (father's father) and first-born daughter both have a disease which is hereditary.

FINISH THE DIAGRAM BELOW:

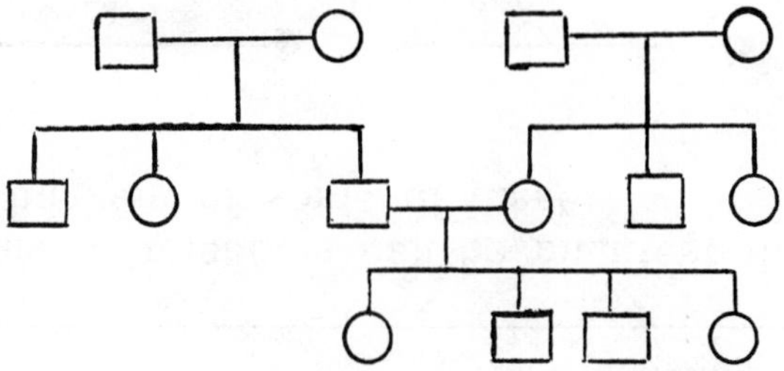

This is a [ ] dominant [ ] recessive trait.

INDICATE THE TWO PEOPLE WHO MUST BE HETEROZYGOUS FOR THE TRAIT (CARRIERS).

- genetic diseases
  - phenylketonuria
  - galactosemia
  - lipid storage diseases
  - glycogen storage diseases
  - juvenile diabetes mellitus
  - sickle cell anemia
  - agammaglobulinemia
  - cystic fibrosis
  - some forms of muscular dystrophy
  - osteogenesis imperfecta
  - osteopetrosis
  - congenital erythropoietic porphyria
  - thalassemia major
  - Fanconi syndrome
  - retinoblastoma
  - tuberous sclerosis

d. CAUSES OF SEVERE PROBLEMS STARTING AT PUBERTY TO EARLY ADULTHOOD

- Klinefelter's and Turner's syndromes
- genetic diseases
  - juvenile diabetes mellitus
  - Wilson's disease
  - Friedreich's ataxia
  - familial polyposis of colon

6. B
C
C
/✓/ Some familial diseases are classified as developmental abnormalities.

---

7. WHICH IS/ARE TRUE?

____All genetic (hereditary) diseases are familial.

____All familial diseases are hereditary.

---

65. C
A
B

---

66. A substance which accumulates due to a metabolic abnormality may be stored at its site of production or transported to other sites, such as reticuloendothelial cells (RES) for storage or the kidney for excretion.

MATCH THE FOLLOWING:

conditions	locus of storage
____substance unable to diffuse into blood	A. RES cells (macrophages)
____substance diffuses into blood; kidneys cannot excrete it	B. tissue in which substance is produced
____kidneys excrete substance	C. substance not stored

53. ✓ genetic

---

54.  = male 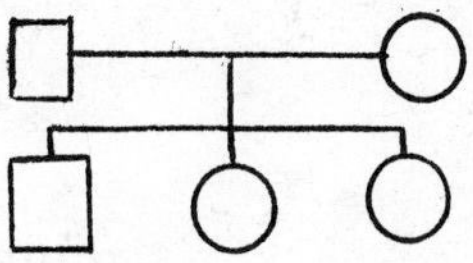 = marriage

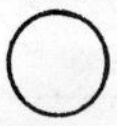 = female = children from the marriage in order of birth (left to right)

 = male with disease

 = female with disease

Assuming that the father and all of the children have the disease, FILL IN THE FAMILY TREE:

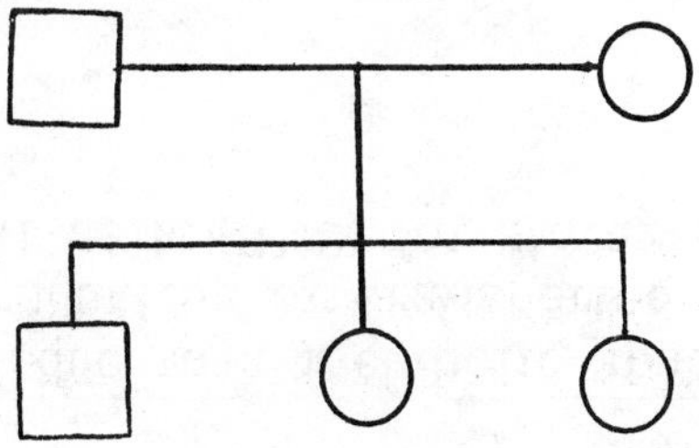

The disease is ▱ dominant ▱ recessive.

- fetal diseases of moderate severity, such as syphilis and erythroblastosis; severe congenital infections, such as cytomegalic inclusion disease; metabolic cretinism
- rarely, a genetic disease, e.g., hemophilia with bleeding following circumcision, some forms achrondroplasia, cystic fibrosis with meconium ileus (bowel obstruction due to thick, tenacious intestinal content), adrenogenital syndrome

c. CAUSES OF SEVERE PROBLEMS IN INFANCY AND CHILDHOOD
- Down's syndrome (social problems due to mental deficiency)
- embryonic anomalies with developed manifestations--e.g., congenital heart defects, meningomyelocele, hydrocephalus, anomalies which may partially block passageways leading to increased susceptibility to infection
- fetal diseases with late sequelae, e.g., mental retardation from brain damage in erythroblastosis, syphilis, toxoplasmosis

7. ✓ All genetic (hereditary) diseases are familial (at least potentially).

---

8. The first 8 weeks after fertilization, when most of the organs are being formed, is called the embryonic period. The next 32 weeks, during which growth is the primary activity, is called the fetal period.

INDICATE "T" TRUE OR "F" FALSE:

____The organism is called an embryo during the first 8 weeks.

____The organism is called a fetus during the rest of the prenatal (before birth) period.

____Most cell differentiation occurs during the fetal period.

____Cell growth occurs throughout both periods.

---

66. B
A
C

---

67. There are many enzymes involved in the metabolism of glucose. Deficiencies of various ones cause different storage patterns.

Glucose 6-phosphatase is present in liver and kidney and takes part in the following reaction:

glycogen → → glucose 6-phosphate —(glucose 6-phosphatase)→ glucose

Glucose 6-phosphate cannot diffuse across cell membranes. If glucose 6-phosphatase is deficient, where would you expect to find excess glycogen?

a. in the urine
b. in RES cells
c. in liver and kidney parenchymal cells

52. F
T
F
T
F

D. Genetic Abnormalities (29 frames)

When you complete this section, you will be able to select correct responses relating to the:

1. genetic abnormalities: pathogenesis, common features, classification, and examples.

53. Analysis of a family tree is often (but not always) helpful in determining whether a disease is genetic and, if so, its mode of inheritance. Although chromosome abnormalities involve heritable material, they usually occur accidentally during gametogenesis and produce sterile offspring.

Which of the following are likely to involve members in several generations of a family?

____embryonic and fetal abnormalities

____genetic abnormalities

____chromosome abnormalities

---

j. DISORDERS OF TRANSPORT

vitamin D-resistant rickets	renal tubular acidosis
renal glycosuria	Hartnup disease
cystinuria	cystic fibrosis (?)

3. Classification of Developmental Abnormalities by Severity

a. CAUSES ABORTION OR STILLBIRTH
- most autosomal chromosome abnormalities
- severe embryonic anomalies
- fetal diseases when severe, such as syphilis and erythroblastosis

b. CAUSES SEVERE PROBLEMS IN NEONATAL PERIOD
- some autosomal chromosome abnormalities
- occasional severe embryonic anomalies that survive to birth, e.g., anencephaly
- embryonic anomalies which affect organs which become functional at birth, e.g., tracheo-esophageal fistula, diaphragmatic hernia (bowel in chest cavity interferes with respiration), atresia of the intestine, imperforate anus, severe congenital heart defects, some cases of hydrocephalus

8. T
T
F
T

---

9. Cell growth = an increase in size or number of a given population of cells.

Cell differentiation = a seldom reversible change in the physical-chemical make-up of a cell or population of cells.

Involution = a decrease in the number of cells in a given (specialized) population.

MATCH THE EXAMPLES AND TERMS:

____the formation of the spinal column from the notochord	A. cell growth
____regression of the mesonephros	B. cell differentiation
____increasing length of the arm bud	C. involution

---

67. c. in liver and kidney parenchymal cells

---

68. Lysosomal maltase is present throughout the body but especially in muscles. It takes part in the following reaction:

$$\text{Glycogen} \xrightarrow{\text{lysosomal maltase}} \quad \longrightarrow \text{glucose}$$

If lysosomal maltase is absent, in which tissue would there be glycogen deposits? ____________________

51. ✓ chemical (altered blood sugar due to maternal diabetes)

✓ intrauterine injury (genetic effects of diabetes are always non-congenital)

✓ congenital

✓ gross body deformity
✓ gross organ deformity
✓ diffuse or focal tissue reactions (the organomegaly is due to diffuse enlargement of tissue rather than deformity)
✓ physiologic or biochemical defects (increased insulin)

---

52. INDICATE "T" TRUE OR "F" FALSE:

	frame reference
____ The susceptibility of tissues to injury remains constant throughout embryonic and fetal periods.	(34,37)
____ Injury during the embryonic period is likely to produce multiple gross malformations.	(37)
____ Injury during the fetal period is likely to produce multiple gross malformations.	(37)
____ The time of injury during the embryonic period is more important in determining the type of injury than the particular agent involved.	(38-40)
____ A wide variety of agents, such as the spirochetes of syphilis, mechanical trauma, and malnutrition, are likely to produce similar types of lesions when exposure occurs during the fetal period.	(43,46)

---

f. METALS
- Wilson's disease
- hemochromatosis

g. HEME AND PORPHYRINS
- congenital erythropoietic prophyria
- hepatic porphyria
- Gilbert's disease
- Dubin-Johnson syndrome

h. CONNECTIVE TISSUE, MUSCLE, AND BONE DISORDERS
- periodic paralysis
- muscular dystrophies
- Hurler's syndrome
- inherited type of amyloidosis
- hypophosphotasia
- osteogenesis imperfecta

i. BLOOD ELEMENT DISORDERS
- hereditary spherocytosis
- glucose 6-phosphate dehydrogenase deficiency
- hemophilia
- hemoglobinopathies
- agammaglobulinemia

9. B
C
A

---

10. MATCH THE FOLLOWING:

____obliteration of the posterior cardinal veins	A. cell growth
____the production of specialized axons by nerve cells	B. cell differentiation
____the increasing bulk of the tissue forming the myocardium	C. involution

---

68. muscles

---

69. Gangliosides are important structural lipids in neural tissue. A variety of enzyme defects block normal turnover of gangliosides. There are a few rare diseases associated with gangliosides.

MATCH DEFECT AND SYNDROME:

____accumulation of gangliosides incapable of crossing cell membranes	A. Tay-Sachs disease--storage in neurons
____accumulation of gangliosides capable of crossing cell membranes	B. Hurler's disease--neuro-lipids accumulate in RES cells

50. ✓ The fetus suffers greater injury from infection.

---

51. Children born of diabetic mothers often (1) are heavier than normal (more than 4 kg), (2) suffer from transient hypoglycemia after birth, and (3) have enlarged (hyperplastic) islets of Langerhans and generalized organomegaly. It is theorized these changes are caused by poor maternal blood sugar regulation, with the infant responding to the high blood sugar by producing insulin. The perinatal fatality rate is higher in these children.

CLASSIFY THE DEVELOPMENTAL ABNORMALITIES SEEN AT BIRTH IN CHILDREN OF DIABETIC MOTHERS:

cause	mechanism	onset	structural and functional abnormalities
___physical	___genetic	___congenital	___gross body deformity
___chemical	___chromosomal	___noncongenital	___gross organ deformity
___biological	___intrauterine		___diffuse or focal tissue reaction
___unknown	___injury		___physiologic or biochemical defects

---

b. AMINO ACID DISORDERS
- phenylketonuria
- familial goiter
- tyrosinosis
- alkaptonuria
- albinism
- maple syrup urine disease
- homocystinuria

c. LIPID DISORDERS
- familial hyperlipoproteinemias
- Tangier disease
- a-beta-lipoproteinemia
- Tay-Sachs disease
- metachromatic leukodystrophy
- Gaucher's disease
- Niemann-Pick disease
- Fabry's syndrome

d. STEROIDS
- adrenal-genital syndrome

e. PURINES AND PYRIMIDINES
- gout
- xanthinuria
- orotic aciduria

10. C
B
A

---

11. Induction is the transmission of a message by some chemical or physical means from one group of cells to another. This may cause involution, cell growth, or cell differentiation. In actual practice, the presence of induction is inferred when one of these responses occurs.

INDICATE IN WHICH EXAMPLES INDUCTION HAS OCCURRED:

____Notochord contact with the dorsal ectoderm causes formation of the neural tube.

____The mesonephros involutes.

____The leg bud grows.

---

69. A
B

---

70. A patient with cystic fibrosis has symptoms of malabsorption, with fatty stools caused by pancreatic insufficiency and frequent episodes of pneumonia due to bronchiolar obstruction. At this point, can you tell if this is a genetic disease traceable to a single protein abnormality?

____yes ____no

49. B
A
B
A

---

50. Cytomegalic inclusion disease is caused by a virus. It is usually asymptomatic in the adult, but in the fetus infected in utero, it causes widespread damage, including renal, hepatic, and neurologic injuries.

INDICATE WHICH OF THE FOLLOWING GENERALIZATIONS MADE EARLIER ARE ILLUSTRATED BY CYTOMEGALIC INCLUSION DISEASE:

____The fetus is more susceptible to poison than adults.

____The fetus is more susceptible to malnutrition than adults.

____The fetus suffers greater injury from infection than adults.

____The fetus suffers greater injury from radiation than adults.

A family practitioner caring for 1,000 people is likely to:
- have 2 patients with gout under his care.
- have 0 or several patients with spherocytosis under his care. (Although an average of 1/5 of physicians would have a patient with spherocytosis, these would not be evenly distributed.)
- have little chance of having a hemophiliac under his care (less than 1 in 50 physicians) but is likely to be seeing some patients with rare genetic diseases.
- be caring for 1 patient with Down's syndrome and have a 50% chance of caring for a patient with Klinefelter's syndrome.

2. Classification of Genetic Disease by Type of Substance Involved

a. CARBOHYDRATE DISORDERS

diabetes mellitus
pentosuria
fructosuria
glycogen storage diseases
oxalosis

11. ✓ Notochord contact with the dorsal ectoderm causes formation of the neural tube.

✓ The mesonephros involutes.

✓ The leg bud grows longer.

---

12. MATCH THE FOLLOWING:

Definition	Word
____present at birth	A. cell differentiation
____the structural or functional modification of a cell or group of cells	B. induction
____the transmission of a message from one group of cells to another	C. genetic
____inherited according to Mendelian laws	D. congenital
____the organism during the first 8 weeks after fertilization	E. embryo

---

70. Your answer is correct since it is your opinion. We would not have suspected that cystic fibrosis was a genetic disease without further information.

---

71. The pancreatic insufficiency and bronchiolar obstruction are due to an abnormal accumulation of mucoprotein which makes the secretions extremely tenacious and results in blocked secretory pathways.

Cystic fibrosis occurs in children and is usually fatal after a number of years, due to malnutrition or repeated pneumonia. It appears sporadically in families and is relatively common. It is likely to affect 1/4 of the children of an involved family.

Now, does cystic fibrosis sound like a genetic disease? ____yes ____no

If so, what is the inheritance pattern? ____________________

48. B
A
D
C

---

49. Three examples of diverse types of fetal injury will be presented.

In milder forms of erythroblastosis fetalis, maternal antibodies cross the placenta most extensively during the perinatal period, resulting in hemolysis and rising bilirubin levels. The unconjugated bilirubin is fat-soluble and crosses the immature blood-brain barrier to cause brain damage.

In more severe forms, maternal antibodies cross the placental barrier in the latter half of pregnancy, with resulting hemolysis, anemia, heart failure, and massive edema (hydrops).

MATCH THE FOLLOWING:

____fetal disease	A. milder forms of erythroblastosis fetalis
____disease at or just after birth	
____stillbirth likely	B. severe forms of erythroblastosis fetalis
____permanent brain damage may occur in first days after birth	

---

c. CHROMOSOMAL

- first trimester spontaneous abortions frequently have chromosome defects --not usually diagnosed
- Down's syndrome - 1:1,000 births
- Klinefelter's syndrome - 1:1,000 males

d. FROM ANOTHER VIEWPOINT

A family practitioner caring for 1,000 people is likely to:
- see several severe congenital embryonic anomalies each year and many minor anomalies.
- be very concerned with prevention of fetal diseases such as syphilis, erythroblastosis, and nutritional problems.
- have 20 diabetics within his population, 10 of whom have not been diagnosed.
- be concerned about many individuals who have a strong family history of heart disease, stroke, and cancer.

12. D
A
B
C
E

---

13. INDICATE "T" TRUE OR "F" FALSE:

	frame reference
____All developmental abnormalities are genetic.	(4)
____All developmental abnormalities are congenital.	(2, 3, 4, 5)
____All congenital abnormalities are familial.	(6)
____All familial diseases are developmental abnormalities.	(6, 7)
____All lesions produced by injury to the embryo are developmental abnormalities.	(1)
____All lesions produced by injury to the fetus are developmental abnormalities.	(1)
____All lesions produced by injury at birth are developmental abnormalities.	(1)

---

71. _✓_yes
autosomal recessive

---

72. The last series of frames have illustrated several mechanisms by which genetic diseases cause injury.

MATCH THE CONDITIONS WITH THE MECHANISMS:

____In phenylketonuria, an enzyme defect results in high blood levels of phenylalanine.
____In Tay-Sachs disease, an enzyme defect results in accumulation of ganglioside in neurons.
____In achondroplastic dwarfs, epiphyseal cartilage is abnormal.
____In cystic fibrosis, thick mucus accumulates in pancreatic ducts and bronchi, leading to pancreatic fibrosis and pneumonia.

A. enzyme defect; substrate does not leave the cell
B. enzyme defect; substrate enters blood
C. structural protein defect; gross body deformity results
D. defect unknown; accumulated material produces atrophy and secondary infection

47. A
B
B
A

---

48. The fetus also differs in many ways from the adult.

MATCH THE DIFFERENCES OF THE FETUS FROM THE ADULT WITH THE REASON FOR THESE DIFFERENCES:

Difference	Reason
____more susceptible to poisons	A. high rate of growth
____more susceptible to malnutrition	B. liver unable to conjugate and excrete many substances
____greater injury from radiation	C. retarded inflammatory reaction and undeveloped immunologic mechanisms
____greater injury from infection	D. large amounts of active, susceptible DNA

---

1. Frequency of Developmental Abnormalities

a. EMBRYONIC AND FETAL

- significant embryogenic anomalies (produce functional defects or social handicaps) - 4% of people
- insignificant embryonic anomalies - 15% of people
- fetal diseases - uncommon except for erythroblastosis

b. GENETIC

- multifactorial genetic diseases are very common--heart disease, strokes, cancer, hypertension, etc.
- diabetes mellitus (recessive, single-gene ?) - affects 2% of population
- relatively common single-gene diseases --few examples, e.g., gout - affects 0.2% of population
- uncommon single-gene disease--several examples, e.g., hereditary spherocytosis - affects 0.02% of population
- rare single-gene defects--many examples, e.g., hemophilia - affects 0.002% of population

13. F T
F T
F F
F

B. Classification of Developmental Abnormalities (14 frames)

When you complete this section, you will be able to select correct responses relating to the:

1. Classification of developmental abnormalities by
   a. cause: physical, chemical, biological or unknown.
   b. pathogenic mechanism: intrauterine injury, genetic, or chromosomal.
   c. onset of manifestations: congenital or noncongenital
   d. general type of structural and functional abnormalities: gross body deformities, gross organ deformities, diffuse or focal tissue reactions, or physiologic and/or biochemical defects only.

GO ON TO THE NEXT PAGE.

---

72. B
A
C
D

---

73. The most frequent genetic diseases are multifactorial, and it is difficult to establish clear lines of inheritance as shown in family trees.

The second largest group are disorders with incomplete penetrance and variable expressivity, such as diabetes mellitus. These also frequently fail to show typical family trees.

A large number of diseases are inherited in classic Mendelian patterns. They are rare as individual diseases.

MATCH THE FOLLOWING:

____ ____	multifactorial genetic	A. relatively common
____ ____	genetic disease with incomplete expressivity	B. relatively rare
____ ____	completely expressed genetic diseases with known structural or enzymatic protein defects	C. classic pedigrees D. vague and atypical pedigrees

46. A
B
A
B

---

47. MATCH THE FOLLOWING:

____large numbers of abnormalities with cause rarely evident

____few abnormalities with cause frequently apparent

____highly specific lesions often directly traceable to an injurious agent

____multiple gross anomalies with no directly observable cause

A. characteristic of embryonic injury

B. characteristic of fetal injury

---

106. family tree
karyotype (in selected cases)
time of onset of disease
exposure to drugs or disease during gestation
nature and distribution of lesions

F. Additional Data (0 frames)

PREAMBLE: There is no way you can learn all the features of all developmental abnormalities. Don't sweat it. Learn and remember what you can as you encounter these diseases. Since there are so many developmental abnormalities and most are rare, you will be encountering new ones for the rest of your life. You should be able to put them into general categories, and you should be able to look up more information about them.

GLANCE THROUGH THE FOLLOWING OUTLINES AND CONSIDER THE SPECTRUM OF DEVELOPMENTAL ABNORMALITIES. NO RESPONSES WILL BE REQUIRED.

GO ON TO NEXT PAGE

14. Developmental abnormalities can be classified in four ways:

1) cause of the abnormality: biological, chemical, physical, and (most frequently) unknown

2) pathogenic mechanism: intrauterine injury, genetic, and chromosomal. These can usually be identified and allow meaningful interpretation of the disease.

3) time of onset of manifestations: congenital or noncongenital

4) type of structural and functional abnormalities

Which classification system do you think is <u>most</u> useful?

____1) ____2) ____3) ____4)

Why?

---

73. A D
A D
B C

---

74. RANK THE FOLLOWING FROM MOST COMMON (1) TO LEAST COMMON (3):

____completely expressed genetic diseases

____incompletely expressed genetic diseases

____multifactorial genetic diseases

45. B
A
A
B

---

46. Embryonic abnormalities are often called congenital anomalies because of the anomalous (or abnormal) organogenesis, producing body or organ deformities which are always present and often evident at birth. There is usually not a trace of the reaction produced by the original injury.

Fetal diseases usually are classifiable by tissue reactions (e.g., syphilis is inflammatory, erythroblastosis is immunologically mediated necrosis of red cells, diabetes in the mother induces hyperplasia of islets of Langerhans in the fetus due to high glucose levels).

MATCH THE FOLLOWING:

____ knowledge of organogenesis helpful in predicting types of lesions
____ knowledge of pathogenesis of injury produced by various agents helpful in predicting types of lesions
____ mainly malformations due to unknown agents
____ variety of tissue reactions due to known agents

A. embryonic abnormalities
B. fetal abnormalities

---

105. B
C
A,B,C
A
A,B,C

---

106. LIST THE TYPES OF INFORMATION THAT ARE PARTICULARLY IMPORTANT IN CLASSIFYING DEVELOPMENTAL ABNORMALITIES:

____

____

____

____

____

14. We believe that classification of developmental abnormalities by pathogenic mechanism is most useful. Most causes of abnormal development are unknown; the time of onset is of interest, but by itself is of little value; and many developmental abnormalities produce similar structural and functional defects.

---

15. Physical, chemical, and biological agents cause abnormal development. In most cases of abnormal development, however, the disease cannot be classified by causative agents.

MATCH THE EXAMPLES AND CATEGORIES:

____deafness due to irradiation during gestation

____deafness due to Toxoplasma gondii infection in utero

____phocomelia (abnormally short limbs) due to maternal ingestion of thalidomide

____dextrocardia (transposition of the heart and associated structures)

A. physical
B. chemical
C. biological
D. unknown

---

74. 3
2
1

---

75. Of the classically inherited single gene defects, most of the diseases are autosomal recessive. Autosomal dominant disorders are the next most frequent in number of disorders. There are relative few sex-linked disorders, especially dominant ones.

LIST THE FOUR TYPES OF CLASSICALLY INHERITED DISORDERS IN ORDER OF GREATEST TO LEAST NUMBER OF KNOWN TYPES:

____

____

____

____

44. b. When a physician finds one anomaly in a newborn, he should be very thorough in looking for other anomalies.

---

45. At the end of the embryonic period, most of the cell differentiation has occurred, but the embryo is only 3 centimeters long, compared to 50 centimeters at birth. The weight during the same period goes from less than 10 grams to about 3,500 grams. During the fetal period, tissue migration takes place (mostly through differential growth rates).

MATCH THE FOLLOWING:

____growth

____differentiation

____organogenesis

____tissue migration

A. predominantly embryonic

B. predominantly fetal

---

104. F
T
T
F
F
F
T

---

105. If presented with a patient suspected of having a disease that might be classified as a developmental abnormality, you should now be able to classify the disease and, we hope, know how to find more detailed information about the specific disease.

Certain types of information are particularly useful in classifying developmental abnormalities. SEE IF YOU CAN MATCH THE TYPES OF INFORMATION WITH THE TYPE(S) OF ABNORMALITIES TO WHICH THEY ARE PERTINENT:

____family tree
____karyotype
____time of onset of disease
____exposure to drugs or disease during gestation
____nature and distribution of the lesions

A. embryonic and fetal abnormalities
B. genetic abnormalities
C. chromosome abnormalities

15. A
C
B
D

---

16. Abnormal development can occur as a result of genetic change, chromosome abnormality, or intrauterine injury.

Chromosomal changes are distinct from genetic change in that they usually are not hereditary and they involve massive numbers of genes. Intrauterine injury is the production of physical defects due to injury occurring during the embryonic or fetal periods.

Each of these types of injuries is caused by the application of an injurious agent at a specific time.

MATCH THE FOLLOWING:

Time	Type of Injury
____previous generations	A. intrauterine
____gametogenesis	B. chromosome abnormality
____intrauterine development	C. genetic change

---

75. autosomal recessive
autosomal dominant
sex-linked recessive
sex-linked dominant

---

76. Diabetes mellitus is the most common inherited disease which may be due to a single gene change. It is estimated that 10% of people will develop the disease if they live long enough. Two percent of the population have the disease at one point in time -- half are known cases and the other half can be picked up by population screening. Expressivity varies from severe juvenile to milder adult forms to no expression (normal phenotype). If one identical twin has diabetes, the other twin has a 50% chance of having the disease.

Diabetes mellitus
is ☐ common ☐ uncommon
has ☐ complete penetrance ☐ incomplete penetrance
has ☐ uniform expressivity ☐ variable expressivity
will ☐ skip generations ☐ not skip generations

43. B
A
C
D

---

44. Intrauterine changes are seldom single. Since the injurious agent is usually acting on the entire embryo or fetus, there are often multiple abnormalities.

INDICATE WHICH IS/ARE TRUE?

a. Single anomalies rule out the possibility of an intrauterine mechanism.

b. When a physican finds one anomaly in a newborn, he should be very thorough in looking for other anomalies.

103.

	Genetic diseases	Chromosome abnormalities	Embryonic and fetal abnormalities
gross body deformities	(X) few	X	X
gross organ deformities	(X) few	X	X
tissue reactions	X		(X) fetal types
physiologic or biochemical defects only	XXXX		

---

104. INDICATE "T" TRUE OR "F" FALSE:

	frame reference
____Chromosome abnormalities are usually familial.	(87)
____Chromosome abnormalities can be detected morphologically.	(84)
____Most chromosome abnormalities produce such gross defects that they are not compatible with fetal life.	(90)
____Autosomal dominant disorders are more numerous than autosomal recessive disorders.	(75)
____Sex-linked dominant disorders are more numerous than sex-linked recessive disorders.	(75)
____Incomplete or variable expressivity is unusual.	(73)
____Environmental factors play an important role in the expressivity of genetic diseases in general.	(77,78)

16. C
B
A

---

17. MATCH THE FOLLOWING:

Type of injury	Time	Characteristics
___ ___ genetic change	A. gametogenesis	1. hereditary
___ ___ chromosome abnormality	B. intrauterine development	2. not hereditary; massive numbers of genes involved
___ ___ intrauterine injury	C. previous generations	3. non-hereditary somatic defects

---

76. /✓/ common
/✓/ incomplete penetrance (does not always affect both identical twins)
/✓/ variable expressivity (mild to severe forms)
/✓/ will skip generations (because recessive)

---

77. There are a few diseases which appear to be controlled by several to many individual genes and to be affected by the environment. These multifactorial diseases are by far the most common genetic diseases.

MATCH THE FOLLOWING:

____ show Mendelian inheritance
____ show vague familial grouping
____ individual examples of these seen frequently by physicians
____ individual examples of these seen only uncommonly by physicians (except for diabetes)

A. single-factor genetic diseases

B. multifactorial genetic diseases

42. all of them

---

43. In contrast to embryonic injuries, the causes of fetal injuries are more often evident, the lesions are more specifically related to the cause, and the number of diseases are few.

MATCH THE FOLLOWING:

____Spirochetes of syphilis cross the placenta only in the second half of pregnancy and cause a characteristic chronic inflammation in many organs.

____Maternal iodine deficiency produces hypothyroidism (cretinism) in the fetus.

____Maternal antibodies cross the placenta and produce hemolysis (erythroblastosis fetalis).

____A child is born with heart deformities.

A. metabolic injury

B. infectious disease

C. allergic (hypersensitivity) reaction

D. defective embryogenesis--no cause evident

102.

	congenital	non-congenital
embryonic and fetal abnormalities	X	
autosomal chromosome diseases	X	
sex chromosome diseases		X
most genetic diseases		X
some genetic diseases	X	

---

103. The three mechanisms produce manifestations on different morphologic-functional levels.

MARK "X" TO INDICATE WHICH MAJOR FEATURES ARE ASSOCIATED WITH EACH MECHANISM:

	Genetic diseases	Chromosome abnormalities	Embryonic and fetal abnormalities
gross body deformities			
gross organ deformities			
tissue reactions			
physiologic or biochemical defects only			

17. C 1
A 2
B 3

---

18. NAME THE TYPE OF INJURY PRODUCED DURING EACH TIME PERIOD:

Time of Application of Injurious Agent

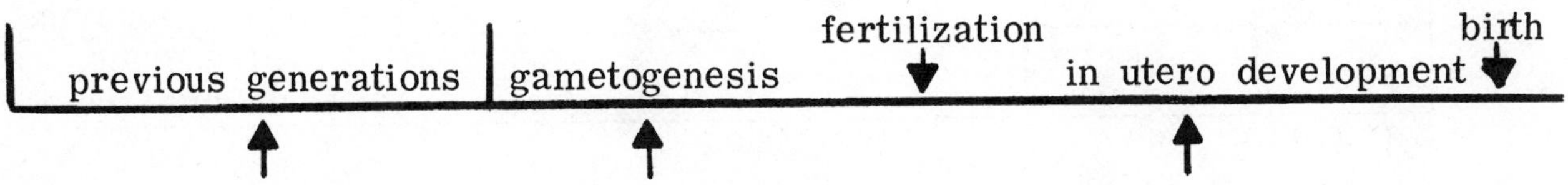

type of injury ______________ ________________ __________________

---

77. A
B
B
A

---

78. Coronary heart disease is the most common multifactorial disease. It seems to be influenced (as they all do) by both genetic and environmental factors.

MATCH THE FOLLOWING:

____smoking

____family history

____dietary habits (amount of cholesterol intake)

____obesity

A. genetic factors

B. environmental factors

Would you expect to be able to show a clear line of inheritance for this disease? ____yes ____no

41. A
B
A
B

---

42. Although many factors have been suspected to cause embryonic injury, there are very few cases in which the cause is known. Which of the following are reasonable explanations for this fact?

a. There are a great number of possible causes to be considered.

b. Identical malformations may arise from diverse causes.

c. Diverse malformations may arise from the same cause.

d. The cause may be clinically inconspicuous, e.g., mild rubella infection.

e. The time of injury is remote (7-8 months) from the time of discovery of the malformation.

---

101. F diabetes mellitus - genetic, noncongenital
B Down's syndrome - chromosomal, congenital
A imperforate anus - embryonic, congenital
F phenylketonuria - genetic, noncongenital
A one aplastic kidney - embryonic, congenital

---

102. INDICATE (IN GENERAL) WHEN LESIONS DUE TO THE VARIOUS MECHANISMS ARE MANIFESTED:

	congenital	non-congenital
embryonic and fetal abnormalities		
autosomal chromosome diseases		
sex chromosome diseases		
most genetic diseases		
some genetic diseases		

18. genetic chromosomal intrauterine

---

19. Each of these types of injury can be caused by physical, chemical, and biological agents. However, since the specific causes are usually not evident, it is easier to classify developmental abnormalities by the time of injury.

MATCH THE FOLLOWING:

____a developmental abnormality that has occurred in some members of a family for many generations	A. known physical, chemical, or biological agent
____increases in congenital heart disease are noted consistently to follow epidemics of rubella virus infections	B. specific causative agent unknown
____an abnormality involving large numbers of traits with predictable frequency in a population	

---

78. B
A (or B if diet is influenced by family)
B
B (or possibly A in some instances)
✓ no

---

79. In the disease sickle cell anemia, there is a defect in the structural protein of hemoglobin. The abnormality could be detected at birth by biochemical analysis of the hemoglobin protein or by noting the tendency of the cells to become "sickle shape" in vitro under low oxygen tension. The manifestations usually first appear in early childhood, when under stress associated with low oxygen tension, the cells begin to sickle, with plugging of the microcirculation (so-called sickle cell crisis). The parents both carry the sickle cell trait but do not develop sickle cell crises.

CLASSIFY SICKLE CELL ANEMIA:

inheritance pattern	type of defect	detectability of biochemical defect	onset of clinical manifestations
__autosomal recessive	__structural protein defect	__congenital	__congenital
__autosomal dominant	__enzymatic protein deficiency	__noncongenital	__noncongenital
__sex-linked recessive			
__sex-linked dominant			

40. ✓ Rubella is frequently unrecognized in adults.
✓ Congenital heart disease may be caused by other agents.

---

41. Thalidomide was used in Europe as a tranquilizer for several years. Many mothers who took this agent during a very specific time of pregnancy delivered children with hands attached to the shoulder by a single small bone (phocomelia) or with legs of similar structure.

COMPARE THALIDOMIDE AND RUBELLA AS INJURIOUS AGENTS:

____acts only at a specific time in embryogenesis

____may act at various times in embryogenesis

____produces injury only to a specific tissue

____may produce variable defects

A. thalidomide

B. rubella

---

100. B
A
B
C

---

101. We have now discussed the three basic mechanisms of abnormal development. We have also seen that the manifestations may be congenital, or non-congenital. Certain generalizations can be made relating these.

CHOOSE THE CORRECT LETTER:

____diabetes mellitus
____Down's syndrome
____imperforate anus
____phenylketonuria
____one aplastic kidney

	ONSET	
MECHANISM	congenital	non-congenital
embryonic and fetal injury	A	D
chromosomal	B	E
genetic	C	F

19. B
A
B

---

20. It is hard to pin down specific causative agents for genetic change and chromosome abnormalities. Obviously, controlled experiments are difficult. Evidence, however, points toward irradiation and a few toxic chemicals as occasional causes.

WHICH IS/ARE TRUE?

a. Irradiation is apparently capable of causing some developmental abnormalities.

b. There are probably numerous causes of all three types of injury which we do not know about yet.

---

79. ✓ autosomal recessive ✓ structural protein defect ✓ congenital ✓ noncongenital

---

80. CLASSIFY PHENYLKETONURIA:

cause	mechanism	onset	structural and functional abnormalities
___physical	___genetic	___congenital	___gross body deformity
___chemical	___chromosomal	___noncongenital	___gross organ deformity
___biological	___intrauterine injury		___diffuse or focal tissue reaction
___unknown			___physiologic or biochemical defects

39. ✓ The virus invades and kills susceptible cells. Rapid growth and differentiation make these cells susceptible during the indicated times.

---

40. Statistically there is a sharp rise in congenital heart disease after rubella epidemics. However, during these epidemics many mothers of infants with congenital heart defects have no history of rubella infection in early pregnancy. Furthermore, babies are born with congenital heart disease in years when rubella is not prevalent.

INDICATE WHICH STATEMENTS MIGHT HELP EXPLAIN THESE DATA:

____Rubella is frequently unrecognized in adults.

____Rubella is the only cause of congenital heart disease.

____Congenital heart disease may be caused by other agents.

---

99. F
T
T
T
F
T

---

100. At this point a few generalizations regarding family counseling should be made. You should now have the information needed to do this. MATCH THE FOLLOWING:

____A family has a child with a chromosome abnormality.

____One parent of a family has an autosomal dominant disease.

____An intrauterine injury has occurred to a child.

____A child is found to be homozygous for an autosomal recessive disease which neither parent manifests.

A. The chances are 1:2 that a child will have the disease.

B. The chances are no greater or only slightly greater than normal that the next child will have the disease.

C. The chances are 1:4 that the next child will have the disease.

20. Both a and b are true.

---

21. Developmental abnormalities may be classified on the basis of when the manifestation appears, as follows:

A congenital abnormality is a disease present and detectable at birth by morphologic, biochemical, or physiologic means.

A noncongenital abnormality is a disease which is neither present nor could it have been found at birth.

CLASSIFY THE FOLLOWING EXAMPLES:

____imperforate anus discovered on examination at birth	A. congenital (overt)
____horseshoe kidney present at birth but not discovered until autopsy	B. congenital (hidden)
____diabetes mellitus--an inherited disease which cannot be diagnosed at birth	C. noncongenital

---

80. ✓ unknown ✓ genetic ✓ noncongenital ✓ diffuse or focal tissue reactions (autopsy)
✓ physiologic or biochemical defect only (clinical)

---

81. INDICATE "T" TRUE OR "F" FALSE:

	frame reference
____Environment has relatively little influence on the occurrence of genetic disease.	(77,78)
____The more common genetic diseases can be traced to single abnormalities of genes.	(73)
____Dominant disorders are more numerous than recessive disorders.	(75)
____Manifestations of enzyme defects may result from decreased amount of product, storage of substrate at the site of production, or storage of substrate in other tissues.	(59,65, 66)
____All genetic diseases are rare.	(73,76)
____Incomplete or variable expressivity is unusual.	(73)

38. B
C
A

---

39. Rubella virus infection and maternal ingestion of thalidomide (a tranquilizer) are two well-established causes of embryonic injury.

We will first consider rubella. The injury varies with the time of the infection. Heart and eye defects are caused by infection early in the embryonic period and hearing defects are caused by later infection.

INDICATE WHICH OF THE FOLLOWING EXPLAINS WHY RUBELLA AFFECTS THESE ORGANS:

____The virus has a special selectivity for these cells only.

____The virus invades and kills susceptible cells. Rapid growth and differentiation make these cells susceptible during the indicated times.

---

98. Down's syndrome
[✓] yes
[✓] autosomes

---

99. INDICATE "T" TRUE OR "F" FALSE:

	frame reference
____Chromosome abnormalities are familial.	(87)
____Chromosome abnormalities are characterized by gross abnormalities in body structure.	(82, 89 90, 91)
____Chromosome abnormalities are characterized by abnormal karyotypes.	(84)
____Down's syndrome is usually evident at birth.	(89, 98)
____Klinefelter's syndrome is usually evident at birth.	(88, 92)
____Most chromosome abnormalities produce such gross defects that they are not compatible with fetal life.	(90)

21. A
B
C

---

22. Embryonic and fetal abnormalities must be congenital, because they are due to somatic injury during gestation.

Genetic alterations may be
1) nondisease, i.e., they may be present without producing any injury or even without being detected.
2) the cause of noncongenital developmental abnormalities if the disease produced is not detectable until some time after birth.
3) the cause of congenital disease if the disease is detected or potentially detectable at birth.

MATCH THE APPROPRIATE LETTER:

____always present at birth (may be hidden)
____sometimes present at birth
____sometimes produces noncongenital disease

A. intrauterine disease
B. genetic disease

---

81. F
F
F
T
F
F

E. Chromosome Abnormalities (25 frames)

When you complete this section, you will be able to select correct responses relating to the:

1. chromosome abnormalities: pathogenesis, classification, and features of common examples.

82. Chromosome abnormalities differ from genetic changes in that far greater numbers of genes are involved. The results are less predictable, and there is usually a far wider range of abnormalities in an individual due to the large number of genes involved.

INIDICATE WHETHER EACH DESCRIPTION IS CHARACTERISTIC OF GENETIC CHANGE (G) OR CHROMOSOME ABNORMALITY (C):

____many unrelated manifestations
____all manifestations traceable to a single defect
____show a Mendelian pattern of inheritance
____appear with a random distribution in the population
____abnormal chromosome squash

37. A (B)
B
C
A
B (A)
C

---

38. MATCH THE FOLLOWING:

____production of monsters	A. injury occurs during late embryogenesis
____major organ malformations	B. injury occurs during formation of germ layers
____minor anomalies	C. injury occurs in the middle of embryogenesis

---

97. Klinefelter's syndrome
✓ yes (due to two X chromosomes)

---

98. A newborn baby has the following abnormalities:

an abnormal face, with an epicanthal fold of skin obscuring the medial angle of each eye

abundant nuchal skin

a horizontal palmar crease

The diagnosis is ________________.

Is mental retardation likely? ☐ yes ☐ no

Karyotyping will reveal abnormal ☐ autosomes ☐ sex chromosomes.

22. A
B
B

---

23. Chromosomal changes are potentially detectable at birth by karyotyping. Autosomal changes produce gross structural abnormalities evident at birth; sex chromosome changes produce abnormalities related to sexual development at puberty.

MATCH THE FOLLOWING:

____ intrauterine disease evident at birth

____ intrauterine disease which is not evident at birth but produces complications as the individual grows up

____ gross deformities caused by abnormal autosomes

____ abnormal number of sex chromosomes

____ metabolic defects due to abnormal genes which are not biochemically detectable or manifest at birth

A. congenital (overt)

B. congenital (hidden)

C. noncongenital

---

82. C many unrelated manifestations
G all manifestations traceable to a single defect
G show a Mendelian pattern of inheritance
C appear with a random distribution
C abnormal chromosome squash

---

83. A fairly sharp distinction can be drawn between autosome and sex chromosome abnormalities. The sex chromosomes, as would be expected, are intimately involved in the control of both primary and secondary sex characteristics and frequently seem not to affect other functions. The autosome abnormalities seem to be more critical to life; most of them cause spontaneous abortion.

CHOOSE THE BEST ANSWER:

____ Most types are fatal.
____ Several types are compatible with life.
____ Many of the defects appear at puberty.
____ Most of the defects are present at birth.

A. autosome abnormalities
B. sex chromosome abnormalities

36. 2
5
6-10
2-10

---

37. Injuries occurring early in the embryonic period are likely to produce grotesque anomalies and abortion, but a few monsters survive to birth.

Gross organ malformations presumably are due to injuries occurring somewhat later in the embryonic period, and many do not produce difficulty until birth.

Lesser organ abnormalities and minor anomalies may be due to injury late in the embryonic period, and many do not produce serious illness.

MATCH THE FOLLOWING:

____anencephaly (aplasia of the brain and cranium)	A. monsters
____esophageal atresia (blind-ended esophagus)	B. major organ malformation
____Meckel's diverticulum of the ileum	C. minor anomalies
____often abort spontaneously	
____cause serious problems in neonatal period	
____often discovered incidentally	

---

96. trisomy 13
✓ no
very small

---

97. A male patient has the following:

small testes
gynecomastia
sterility
little facial hair

Which of the four chromosome syndromes we have considered do you think he has? ____________________

Buccal smear (cells scraped from the buccal mucosa) reveals cells with a Barr body. Is this consistent with the diagnosis you made?

____yes ____no

23. A
B
A
B
C

---

24. Developmental abnormalities can also be roughly classified by the type of structural and functional change present. This is useful because some correlation can be made between the types of changes and pathogenic mechanisms.

Gross body deformities are obvious structural defects evident on physical examination.

Gross organ deformities are obvious structural defects which would be evident on gross examination of the organ.

Diffuse or focal tissue reactions are the wide variety of degenerative or inflammatory lesions that are best characterized by histologic examination.

Physiologic or biochemical defects are used here to refer to abnormalities detectable only by physiologic or biochemical tests.

MATCH THE EXAMPLES AND CATEGORIES:

____cystine in the urine
____polycystic kidney
____phocomelia (short limbs)
____liver with large number of foamy macrophages in Gaucher's disease

A. gross body deformities
B. gross organ deformities
C. diffuse or focal tissue reactions
D. physiologic and/or biochemical defects only

---

83. A
B
B
A

---

84. Genes are not visible and must be detected by inference. Chromosomes can be visualized and analyzed if a cell in metaphase is squashed, stained, and photographed, and the photographed chromosomes are cut out and arranged into groups. The process is called karyotyping and the product is a karyotype. The usual technique involves culture of bone marrow cells or leukocytes. The cells are stimulated to divide and then stopped in metaphase by the drug colchicine.

MATCH THE FOLLOWING:

____basic defect present but cannot be directly visualized by karyotyping
____basic defect present and can be visualized by karyotyping
____basic cause acted during gestation and may not cause further damage
____diagnosis may involve cell culture and cytologic examinations

A. embryonic and fetal abnormalities
B. genetic abnormalities
C. chromosome abnormalities

35. Week 5 ✓ 6 ✓ 7 ✓ 8 ✓ 9 ✓ 10 ✓

---

36. Fertilization occurs about ____ weeks after the mother's last menstrual period.

The germ layers form primarily during the ____ week after the mother's last menstrual period.

Organogenesis and cell differentiation take place primarily during weeks _____-_____ after the mother's last menstrual period.

The embryonic period lasts from week ____ to ____ after the mother's last menstrual period.

---

95. B A
A C
C C
B A, B
C

---

96. A mother has a baby with small eyes, a hare lip, and six fingers on each hand. Which chromosome syndrome is most likely?

____

Are the chances greater than normal that her next child will have a similar set of abnormalities? _____yes _____no

What are the chances that this child will reach adulthood?

24. D
B
A
C

---

25. INDICATE THE TYPE OF EXAMINATION APPROPRIATE FOR DETECTION OF EACH OF THE FOLLOWING:

gross body deformity ______________________

gross organ deformity ______________________

diffuse or focal tissue reactions ______________________

physiologic or biochemical defects only ______________________

---

84. B
C
A
C

---

85. The number of sex chromosomes can often be determined by the simple technique of looking at cell nuclei for a clump of chromatin attached to the nuclear membrane. Such chromatin clumps correlate with the presence of two X chromosomes and are called Barr bodies. Smeared squamous cells from the mouth are usually used -- hence the name "buccal smear." No Barr bodies are seen with one X chromosome, and two Barr bodies are present with three X chromosomes.

MATCH THE FOLLOWING:

____may be detected by buccal smear
____may be detected by karyotyping
____usually incompatible with life or associated with gross defects at birth
____often compatible with life, with most striking changes noted at puberty

A. abnormal number of autosomes
B. abnormal number of sex chromosomes

34. ☑ embryonic

---

35. In clinical practice and hereafter in this text, times are given relative to the mother's last menstrual period rather than to fertilization. This adds about two weeks, i.e., the embryonic period ends about 10 weeks after the last menstrual period. The germ layers form during the fifth week after the mother's last menstrual period. After the germ layers are formed, organogenesis and cell differentiation take place. This happens primarily during the sixth through tenth weeks. Most injuries to the developing organism occur during the periods of formation of germ layers and organogenesis.

CHECK THE TIMES RELATIVE TO THE MOTHER'S LAST MENSTRUAL PERIOD WHEN THE EMBRYO IS HIGHLY SENSITIVE TO INJURIOUS AGENTS:

Week 1___ 2___ 3___ 4___ 5___ 6___ 7___ 8___ 9___ 10___ 11___ 12___

---

94. ✓ short stature
✓ failure of secondary sex characteristics to develop at puberty
✓ lack of menstruation
(There is no Barr body, because only one X chromosome is present.)

---

95. MATCH THE FOLLOWING:

____ "male"
____ "female"
____ either male or female
____ 44 autosomes, XXY
____ Trisomy 21
____ 44 autosomes, XO
____ mental retardation
____ usually observed at birth
____ frequently not discovered until puberty

A. Turner's Syndrome

B. Klinefelter's Syndrome

C. Down's Syndrome

25. gross body deformity: physical examination
gross organ deformity: gross organ examination
diffuse or focal tissue reactions: histologic examination
physiologic or biochemical defects only: physiologic or biochemical tests

---

26. From the following description CLASSIFY TAY-SACHS DISEASE:

Tay-Sachs disease occurs primarily in Jews from Northeastern Europe. The children are normal at birth. They develop progressive blindness, paralysis, and mental retardation, and die in a few years. Histologically, neurons have swollen, foamy cytoplasm due to accumulation of gangliosides.

cause	mechanism	onset	structural and functional abnormalities
____physical	____genetic	____congenital	____gross body deformity
____chemical	____chromosomal	____noncongenital	____gross organ deformity
____biological	____intrauterine injury		____diffuse or focal tissue reactions
____unknown			____physiologic or biochemical defects without other changes

---

85. B
A, B
A
B

---

86. Buccal smears are useful for detection of some:

____intrauterine injuries
____genetic disorders
____autosomal chromosome disorders
____sex chromosome disorders

Karyotyping is useful for detection of:

____intrauterine injuries
____genetic disorders
____autosomal chromosome disorders
____sex chromosome disorders

33.

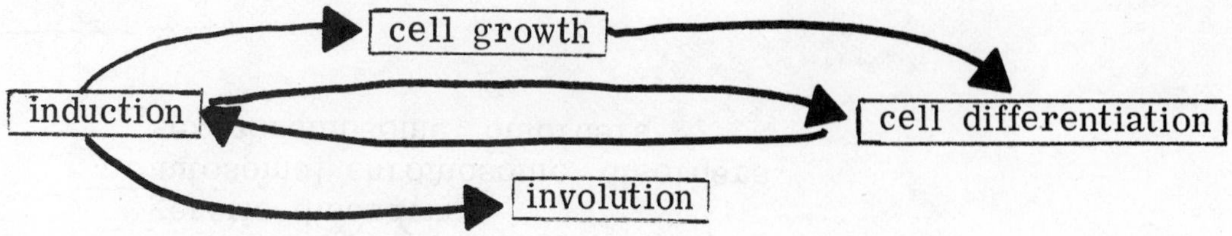

A
B
A

---

34. The prenatal organism is most sensitive to injury during germ layer formation, organogenesis, and cell differentiation.

This is the ☐ embryonic ☐ fetal stage.

---

93. b. patient complains of sterility
d. patient notes breast enlargement

---

94. "Females" with Turner's syndrome have fibrotic, poorly developed ovaries which never do produce much hormone. They have moderately abnormal bodies (smaller than siblings and a webbed appearance to the neck), but the majority of the manifestations appear at puberty, the time at which they are usually diagnosed.

INDICATE WHICH OF THE FOLLOWING WOULD BE USEFUL IN DIAGNOSING TURNER'S SYNDROME:

____short stature
____failure of secondary sex characteristics to develop at puberty
____lack of menstruation
____buccal smear in a female with one Barr body present

26. ✓ unknown ✓ genetic ✓ noncongenital ✓ diffuse or focal tissue reactions

---

27. INDICATE "T" TRUE OR "F" FALSE:

		frame reference
____	Most developmental abnormalities can be attributed to specific physical, chemical, and biological agents.	(14,15)
____	Developmental abnormalities are classified as genetic, chromosomal, or intrauterine injuries.	(14, 16-18)
____	Many developmental abnormalities are not apparent at birth.	(21,23)
____	A genetic disease which becomes manifest during adulthood is classified as a congenital abnormality.	(21,23)
____	Developmental abnormalities include a wide spectrum of structural and functional abnormalities.	(24)

---

86. Buccal smears are useful for detection of some sex chromosome disorders. Karyotyping is useful for detecting autosomal chromosome disorders and sex chromosome disorders.

---

87. Chromosomal changes in reproductive cells are assumed to occur by accident, since specific causes have not been established. Chromosomal changes also occur in somatic cells, including many neoplastic cells, but these changes do not lead to developmental abnormalities.
Chromosomal developmental abnormalities are not familial because the individuals with the abnormalities are not capable of reproduction.

Interruption of reproductive capabilities is likely to be advisable for parents of children with ☐ embryonic and fetal abnormalities ☐ genetic abnormalities ☐ chromosome abnormalities.

Interruption of reproductive capabilities is likely to be advisable for patients with ☐ embryonic and fetal abnormalities ☐ genetic abnormalities ☐ chromosome abnormalities.

32. b) Embryogenesis is a long sequence which is liable to modification throughout.

---

33. FILL IN THE EMPTY BOXES:

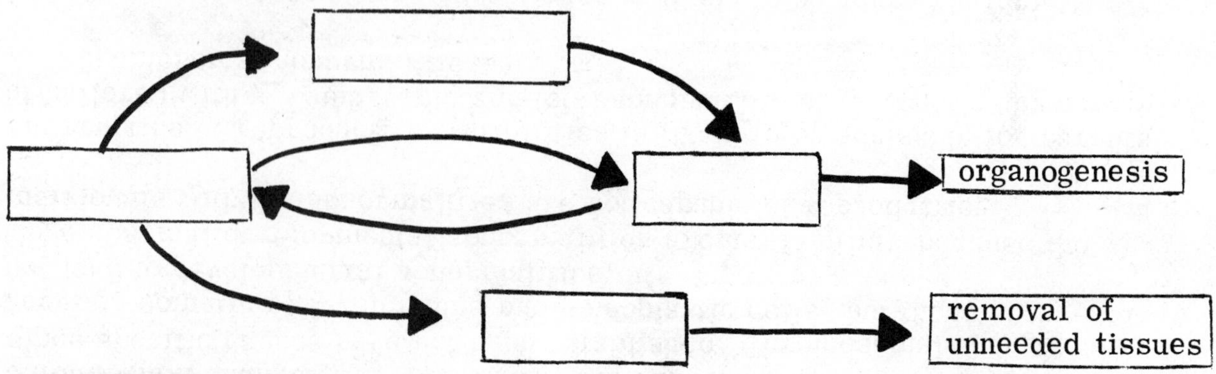

MATCH THE FOLLOWING:

____ microcephaly
____ double aortic arch
____ phocomelia (seal-like appendages)

A. defect of organogenesis
B. defect of involution

---

92. ✓ atrophic testes
✓ decreased facial hair
✓ presence of gynecomastia
c. puberty

---

93. Frequently these abnormalities go unnoticed, and the condition is discovered in adulthood.

Which findings may alert the physician to Klinefelter's syndrome?

a. abnormal buccal smear
b. patient complains of sterility
c. patient complains of frequent illness
d. patient notes breast enlargement

27. F
T
T
F
T

C. <u>Embryonic and Fetal Abnormalities</u> (25 frames)

When you complete this section, you will be able to select correct responses relating to the:

1. embryonic and fetal abnormalities: pathogenesis, common features, causes and examples

28. The organism's reaction is quite different during the embryonic period and the fetal period; thus each will be considered separately.

Embryogenesis is the growth in complexity from the newly fertilized egg to the differentiated fetus. This takes place during the first 8 weeks of life. This is a dynamic period, with several processes continuously interacting, as diagrammed below:

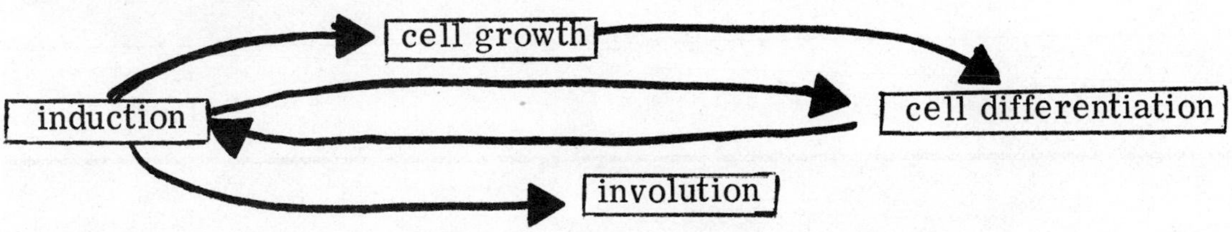

INDICATE THE PROCESSES THAT MAY RESULT FROM INDUCTION:
____cell growth ____cell differentiation ____involution

---

87. [✓] genetic abnormalities
[✓] genetic abnormalities

---

88. In chromosomal developmental abnormalities, the abnormal chromosomes occur by accident during gametogenesis and thus are transmitted to all or most of the cells of the involved individual. In the case of sex chromosome abnormalities, the manifestations may be delayed until the time of development of secondary sex characteristics, but a buccal smear done at any time would reveal the abnormality.

Autosomal chromosomal developmental abnormalities are:
____congenital, overt
____congenital, hidden
____non-congenital

Sex chromosome developmental abnormalities are:
____congenital, overt
____congenital, hidden
____non-congenital

31. cell differentiation, induction, cell differentiation

---

32. Do you think embryogenesis is a) "the straightforward unfolding of genetically predetermined patterns" or b) a long sequence which is liable to modification throughout?

a) ____

b) ____

---

91. Both are true.

---

92. Since Klinefelter's "males" have decreased levels of male hormones and relatively more female hormones, which of the following would you expect to see?

____normal testes
____atrophic testes

____increased facial hair
____decreased facial hair

____presence of gynecomastia (enlarged breasts)
____absence of gynecomastia

When do most of these manifestations become evident?

a. birth
b. shortly after birth
c. puberty
d. adulthood

28. ✓ cell growth ✓ cell differentiation ✓ involution

---

29. After differentiation has occurred, the cells often act to modify the nature of an adjacent group of cells. This is ____________________.

---

88. ✓ congenital, overt
✓ congenital, hidden

---

89. Down's syndrome (trisomy 21, or mongolism) is the most common autosomal chromosomal abnormality in live-born children. The following characteristics are common:

1. Abnormalities of the body: a fold of skin covering the medial corner of the eyes, a single palmar crease, severe mental retardation (IQ = 25-50).
2. There is seldom any family history of Down's syndrome.
3. It is seen more frequently with older mothers, women whose ova have been in the vulnerable meiotic prophase for many years.

Which of the following generalizations can be made:

____ There are many unrelated manifestations.
____ The disease is congenital.
____ The syndrome shows a Mendelian pattern of occurrence.
____ The injury probably occurs during gamatogenesis in the mother.

30. cell growth, cell differentiation, or involution

---

31. When the optic vessicle comes into contact with the surface epithelium, it induces the formation of an embryonic lens. After the lens differentiates, it induces the surface epithelium covering it to differentiate into cornea. This is an example of induction causing ________ ________, which causes further ________________, which causes further ____ ____________.

---

90. ✓ Few babies are born with chromosome abnormalities because most of these cause spontaneous abortion.

✓ Gross morphologic abnormalities are characteristic of trisomy 13.

---

91. Turner's and Klinefelter's syndromes are the two most common sex chromosome abnormalities.

A Turner's "female" (44 autosomes, one X chromosome) has poorly developed secondary sex characteristics associated with fibrotic ovaries.

A Klinefelter's "male" (44 autosomes, two X chromosomes, one Y chromosome) has poorly developed male secondary sex characteristics associated with small, non-functional testes.

WHICH IS/ARE TRUE?

____ The "female" with Turner's syndrome will have decreased levels of female sex hormones.

____ The "male" with Klinefelter's syndrome will have decreased levels of male sex hormones.

29. induction

---

30. Induction is the transmission of a message from one group of cells to another, which may cause _________ ______________, _________ ______________, or ______________.

TURN TEXT 180° AND CONTINUE.

---

89. ✓ There are many unrelated manifestations.
✓ The disease is congenital.
✓ The injury probably occurs during gamatogenesis in the mother.

---

90. Most autosomal alterations are fatal. This is evidenced by the large number of spontaneously aborted embryos with chromosome abnormalities and by the relatively few chromosome syndromes which have been described. As we have seen, trisomy 21 (Down's syndrome) is not fatal. Trisomy 13 is intermediate, being compatible with live birth but not with even moderate life span. A typical trisomy 13 baby might have microphthalmia (small eye), cleft palate, or polydactyly.

WHICH IS/ARE TRUE ?

____ Few babies are born with chromosome abnormalities because most of these cause spontaneous abortion.
____ Trisomy 13 is one of the autosomal abnormalities compatible with long life.
____ Gross morphologic abnormalities are characteristic of trisomy 13.

TURN TEXT 180° AND CONTINUE.

Unit 11. Hemodynamic Disorders: Mechanisms of Vascular Obstruction

Unit 11. HEMODYNAMIC DISORDERS: MECHANISMS OF VASCULAR OBSTRUCTION

OBJECTIVES

When you complete this unit, you will be able to select correct responses relating to the:

	starting page	frame numbers
A. Introduction	11.3	1-11

1. classification of hemodynamic disorders and subclassification of vascular obstruction.

B. Intrinsic Arterial Disease	11.25	12-67

1. definitions of arteriosclerosis, vasculitis, lymphangitis, and thrombophlebitis.
2. distinctions among atherosclerosis, arteriolosclerosis, and Mönckeberg's medial calcification in terms of
   - type and size of vessel involved
   - predisposing conditions
   - morphologic changes in vessels
   - results or complications of lesions
3. relationship of atherosclerosis to age, sex, and dietary habits.

C. Thrombosis	11.54	68-124

1. definitions of red thrombus, white thrombus, mural thrombus, septic thrombus, and postmortem clot.
2. causative role of changes in blood vessel walls, blood composition, and blood flow in thrombus formation.
3. steps in formation, propagation, organization, and recanalization of a thrombus.
4. mechanism and consequences of dissolution, retraction, and embolization of thrombi.

D. Embolization	11.71	125-180

1. distinctions among arterial embolism, venous embolism, and paradoxical embolism in terms of
   - common sources of emboli
   - path of transfer
   - common sites of enlodgement
2. definitions and common causes of Thrombotic emboli, fat emboli, air emboli, septic emboli, foreign-body emboli, bone marrow emboli, and amniotic fluid emboli.

PRETEST

UNIT 11. HEMODYNAMIC DISORDERS: MECHANISMS OF VASCULAR OBSTRUCTION

SELECT THE SINGLE BEST RESPONSE:

1. Subcategories of atherosclerosis INCLUDE
   (A) arteriosclerosis
   (B) arteriolosclerosis
   (C) both
   (D) neither

2. Arteriolosclerosis is characterized by involvement of vessels in the
   (A) heart
   (B) lung
   (C) kidney
   (D) brain

3. Atherosclerosis is more severe in
   (A) alcoholics vs. nonalcoholics
   (B) people with high dietary cholesterol vs. people with high serum cholesterol
   (C) hypertensives vs. nonhypertensives
   (D) Japanese vs. Americans

4. The tail of a venous thrombus is characterized by
   (A) "currant jelly" appearance
   (B) uniform red color
   (C) attachment to vessel wall
   (D) lines of Zahn
   (E) rubbery consistency

5. All of the following conditions involve thrombocytosis EXCEPT
   (A) atherosclerosis
   (B) postoperative state
   (C) following childbirth
   (D) polycythemia vera

6. Of the following, the most common source of arterial emboli is
   (A) pulmonary vein
   (B) pulmonary artery
   (C) left atrium
   (D) common carotid artery

7. Pulmonary emboli have all the following characteristics EXCEPT
   (A) commonly arise in leg veins
   (B) pass through the right heart before reaching the lung
   (C) consistently cause infarction in the lung
   (D) are usually thrombotic emboli

8. Air embolism
   (A) has its most serious effects in the left atrium
   (B) is often the result of surgical operations
   (C) occurs in divers while descending to the ocean floor
   (D) is lethal when more than 5 cc. of air enters the bloodstream

GO ON TO NEXT PAGE AND BEGIN THE UNIT.

A. Introduction (11 frames)

When you complete this section, you will be able to select correct responses relating to the:

1. classification of hemodynamic disorders and subclassification of vascular obstruction

1. The disorders to be dealt with in this unit are all disorders of the circulation of the blood. By combining the Greek words hemo- (blood) and dynamis (movement), these disorders may be called ______________ disorders.

1. hemodynamic

---

2. The disorders of circulation of the blood fall into three groups:

   vascular obstruction
   bleeding
   deranged blood flow

When blood flow in any part of the vascular system is hindered or blocked, we call this ______________ ________________.

When blood escapes from the vascular system, we have ______________.

When the blood is not adequately circulated to the entire body, we have ________________ blood ____________.

These disorders are all _________________ disorders.

---

91. fibrin
thrombin

---

92. As fibrin and platelets are added to the growing thrombus, leukocytes and erythrocytes in varying numbers are trapped.

INDICATE THE FOLLOWING ITEMS WHICH ARE IMPORTANT ELEMENTS OF A FRESH THROMBUS:

____platelets	____albumin
____globulins	____leukocytes
____erythrocytes	____mast cells
____fibrin	____endothelial cells

TURN TEXT 180^{0} AND CONTINUE.

2. vascular obstruction
bleeding
deranged (blood) flow
hemodynamic

---

3. MATCH THE FOLLOWING:

____Blood escapes from a vessel.

____A vessel is blocked.

____Blood circulation is inadequate.

A. vascular obstruction

B. bleeding

C. deranged blood flow

---

92. ✓ platelets
✓ erythrocytes
✓ fibrin
✓ leukocytes

---

93. Several changes in the blood itself can contribute to thrombus formation. SUPPLY THE MISSING INFORMATION:

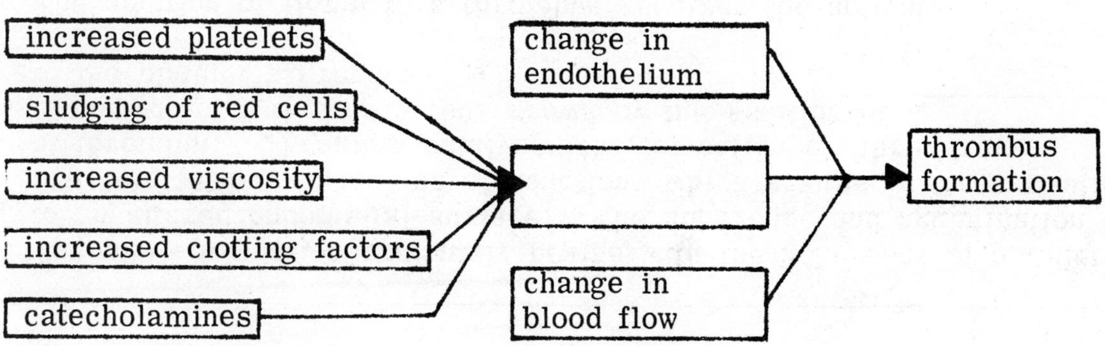

90. 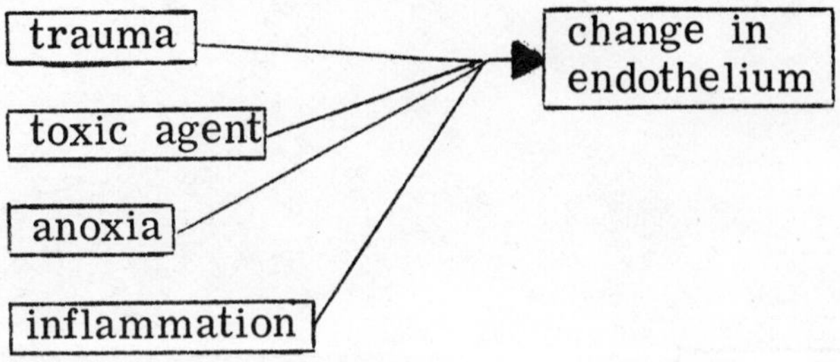

---

91. Thrombus formation ordinarily begins with the adherence of platelets to an altered endothelial surface. The adherence and agglutination of platelets initiates a series of reactions which results in the activation of thrombin. Thrombin catalyzes the formation of fibrin from fibrinogen. A thrombus thus grows by the addition of ______________ to the platelet aggregate.

The addition of fibrin to a thrombus requires the activation of ____________________ as an intermediate.

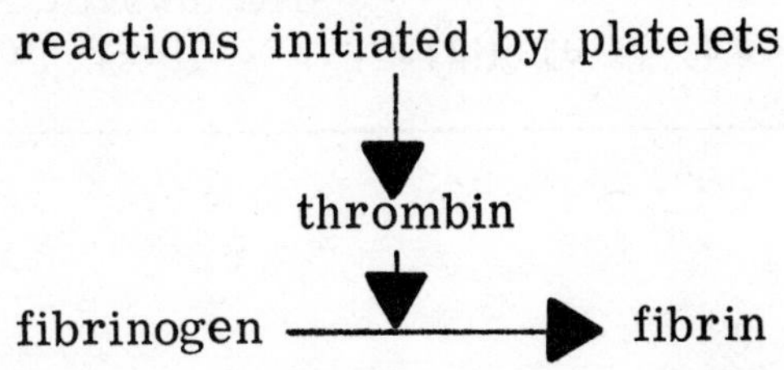

---

180. F
T
F
F
T

THIS IS THE END OF UNIT 11. TAKE THE POSTTEST ON PAGE xxxiv.

3. B
A
C

---

4. MATCH THE FOLLOWING (more than one letter may apply):

____a small artery ruptures into surrounding tissue	
____a failing heart is unable to pump enough blood	A. vascular obstruction
____a clot blocks a coronary artery	B. bleeding
____a blow ruptures numerous capillaries, resulting in a "bruise"	C. deranged blood flow
____loss of blood results in inadequate circulation	
____the thickened wall of a vessel narrows the lumen	

---

93. change in blood composition

---

94. We have seen the importance of platelets in thrombus formation. Certain clinical conditions which are associated with thrombosis involve an increase in the number of platelets (thrombocytes) present in the blood (thrombocytosis) and an increase in the adhesiveness of these platelets.

MATCH THE FOLLOWING:

____fewer platelets	A. increased chances of thrombosis
____more adhesive platelets	
____more platelets (thrombocytosis)	B. decreased chance of thrombosis

89. trauma
toxic
anoxic injury
inflammation

---

90. SUPPLY THE MISSING CAUSES OF ENDOTHELIAL DAMAGE:

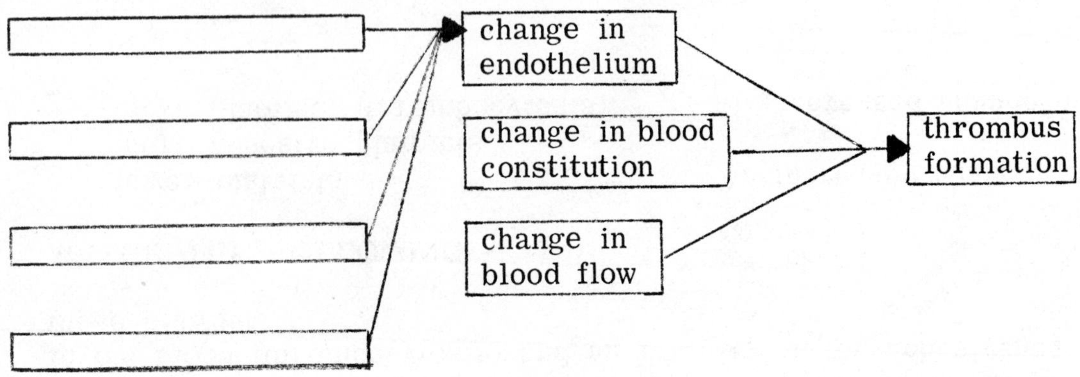

---

179. F
F
T
F
F

---

180. INDICATE "T" TRUE OR "F" FALSE:

	frame reference
____Fat embolism commonly occludes large pulmonary arteries.	(145)
____The most serious effects of fat embolism are in the brain.	(149)
____Fat embolism is always the result of trauma.	(151)
____Ten ml. of air injected into an arm vein is likely to be fatal.	(159)
____Childbirth involves a danger of pulmonary embolism.	(170)

4. B
C
A
B
B, C
A

---

5. Hemodynamic disorders may be local or systemic. Vascular obstruction and bleeding generally affect only limited parts of the body, and thus are ▱ local ▱ systemic disorders. Deranged blood flow generally affects the entire body and thus is a ▱ local ▱ systemic disorder.

---

94. B
A
A

---

95. Platelets may double or triple in number and increase in adhesiveness several days after major surgery and after childbirth. This period is associated with ▱ increased ▱ decreased risk of thrombosis.

88. C
D
A
B

---

89. Damage to the endothelium by a physical blow is an example of ______________.

A chemical compound which damages the endothelium is a/an ____________ agent.

When the endothelium is damaged by inadequate oxygenation, this is called ______________.

The body's own response to infection or irritation (which can damage the endothelium) is ______________.

---

178. T
F
F
T
F

---

179. INDICATE "T" TRUE OR "F" FALSE:

	frame reference
____A septic embolus is composed of tumor cells.	(127)
____Thrombotic emboli are formed free in a moving bloodstream.	(134, 135)
____Venous embolism and pulmonary embolism are virtually coextensive.	(134, 135)
____Venous emboli from the upper extremities are common.	(139)
____Fat embolism involves fat cells in the bloodstream.	(144, 153)

5. [✓] local
[✓] systemic

---

6. CLASSIFY THE FOLLOWING:

____bleeding

____vascular obstruction

____deranged blood flow

A. local disorder

B. systemic disorder

---

95. [✓] increased

---

96. In conditions in which red cells agglutinate into clumps--called sludging -- thrombosis is known to be more likely. It has been suggested that sludging of red cells in the vasa vasorum may cause anoxic damage to the endothelium, thus preparing the way for platelet adherence.

MATCH THE FOLLOWING:

____sludging increases likelihood of thrombosis

____adherence to endothelium initiates thrombosis

____increased following major surgery

A. platelets

B. red cells

87. 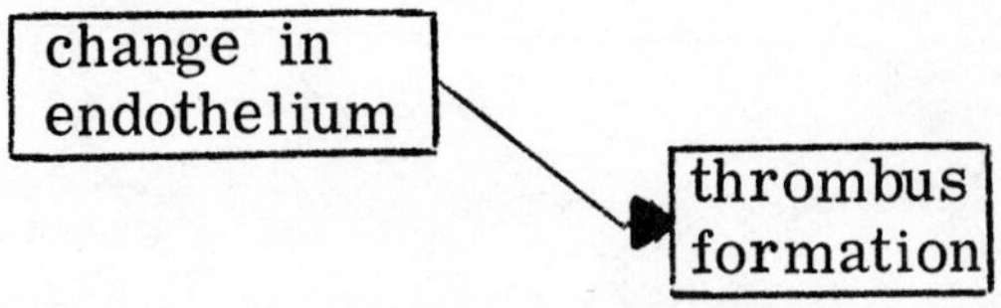

---

88. MATCH THE CAUSES OF ENDOTHELIAL DAMAGE ON THE RIGHT WITH THE DESCRIPTIONS OR EXAMPLES ON THE LEFT:

____inadequate blood supply	A. trauma
____tissue response to infection or injury	B. toxic agent
____damage by a blow	C. anoxia
____drug given intravenously	D. inflammation

---

177. B
A, B, C
A
B

---

178. INDICATE "T" TRUE OR "F" FALSE:

	frame reference
____Emboli more commonly arise in the venous than the arterial circulation.	(134, 139)
____Fat embolism is the most common type.	(134, 144)
____Venous emboli generally lodge in systemic veins.	(136)
____An arterial embolus may originate in a pulmonary vein.	(129)
____Paradoxical emboli must be minute in size.	(130)

6. A
A
B

---

7. There are three important mechanisms of vascular obstruction.

Intrinsic arterial diseases are deteriorations of the arterial wall.

Thrombosis is the process of blood clotting within a blood vessel, thus blocking the lumen.

Embolism occurs if a thrombus breaks free, or any other object enters the circulation, and blocks a vessel at some point distal to its origin.

MATCH THE FOLLOWING (more than one letter may apply):

____process in the vessel wall
____process in the vessel lumen
____may involve blood elements
____involves a stationary intravascular mass
____involves a detached intravascular object

A. intrinsic arterial disease

B. thrombosis

C. embolism

---

96. B
A
A

---

97. In polycythemia vera, there is an increased number of all types of blood cells, increased viscosity, and an increased likelihood of thrombosis. Increased viscosity of the blood ☐ increases ☐ decreases the likelihood of clotting.

MATCH THE FOLLOWING (more than one letter may apply):

____polycythemia vera

____following childbirth

____thrombosis more likely

____arteriosclerosis

A. red cells increased

B. platelets increased

C. both increased

D. neither increased

86. A
B
A

87. Thrombus formation due to endothelial changes can be initiated by trauma, toxic agents, anoxia, or vascular inflammation.

SUPPLY THE MISSING INFORMATION:

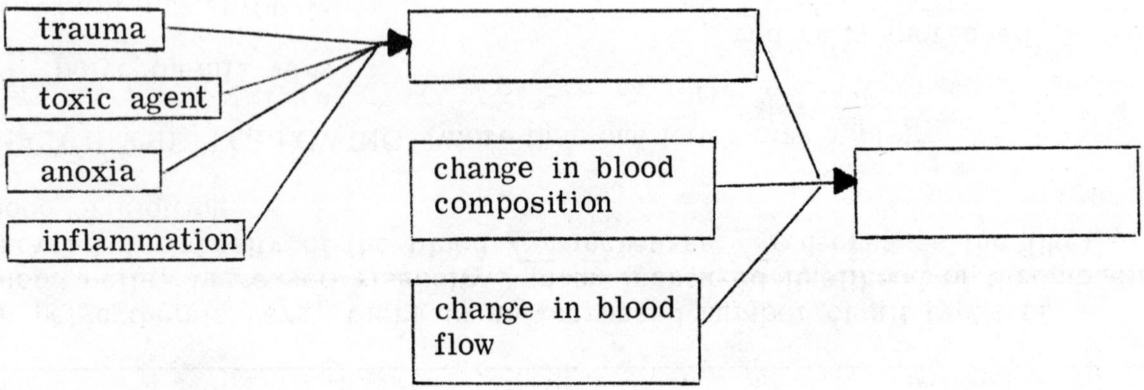

176. B
A
C
C
A
B

177. The effects of these emboli will depend on the size and type of material involved and the location of impaction.

MATCH THE EFFECTS ON THE LEFT WITH THE TYPE OF EMBOLI ON THE RIGHT:

____septicemia	A. tissue fragments
____pulmonary embolism	B. organisms
____metastatic cancer	C. foreign body
____widespread parasitic infestation	

7. A
   B,C
   B,C
   B
   C

---

8. FILL IN THE MISSING RESULT:

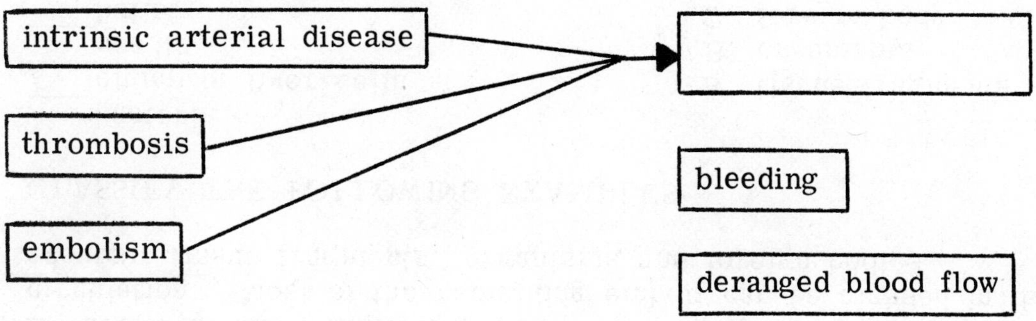

---

97. [✓] increases
    C
    B
    C
    D

---

98. In certain disease states, there is an increase in some of the humoral clotting factors. An increase of these clotting factors increases the speed of formation of fibrin, thus contributing to thrombus formation.

    Increased humoral _______________ factors contribute to the formation of _______________ from fibrinogen.

85.

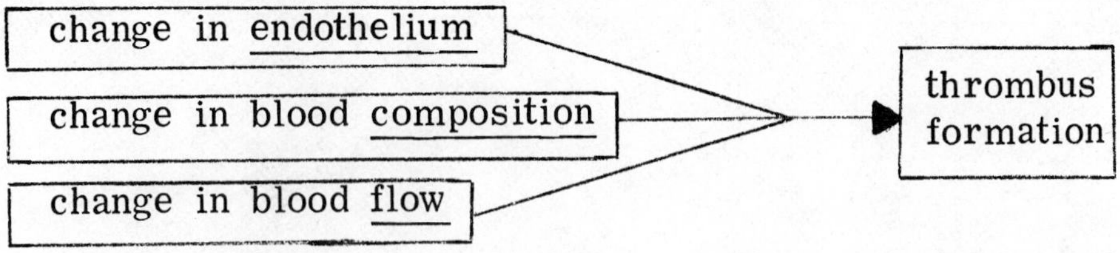

---

86. The normal endothelium presents a smooth surface to the blood flowing in the lumen. When the integrity of this endothelial surface is compromised, clotting can be initiated by the adherence of platelets to the damaged endothelium.

MATCH THE FOLLOWING:

____platelets do not adhere

____clotting may occur

____smooth surface

A. normal endothelium

B. damaged endothelium

---

175. ✓ kidney ✓ intestine
✓ spleen ✓ legs

---

176. A variety of other materials may occasionally embolize in the circulation. Most of the remaining emboli can be classed in three groups: tissue fragments, organisms, and foreign bodies.

CLASSIFY THE FOLLOWING EXAMPLES:

____bacteria
____clump of liver cells
____needle
____bullet
____tumor cells
____parasites

A. tissue fragments
B. organisms
C. foreign body

8. vascular obstruction

---

9. FILL IN THE MISSING MECHANISMS:

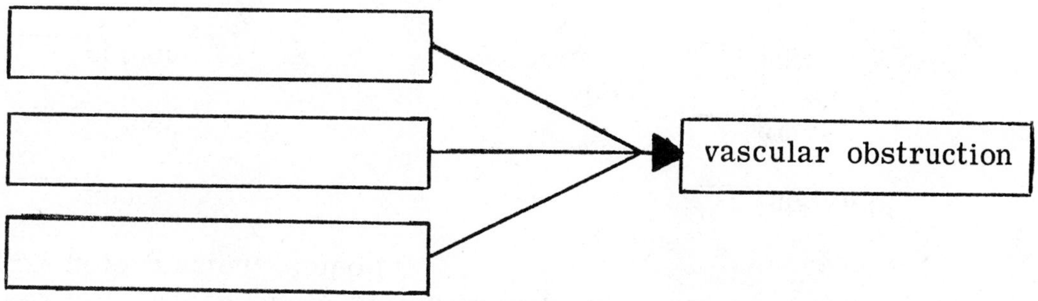

---

98. clotting (or coagulation)
fibrin

---

99. Disseminated intravascular clotting is a clinical syndrome in which widespread coagulation of the blood occurs because of an imbalance of procoagulation and anticoagulation factors. The release of clotting factors from damaged tissue or red cells can play an important part in this syndrome.

MATCH THE FOLLOWING CAUSES OF DISSEMINATED INTRAVASCULAR CLOTTING WITH THE MECHANISM INVOLVED:

____intravascular hemolysis
____snakebite (proteolytic enzymes)
____antigen-antibody complexes lodge in endothelium
____tissue thromboplastin released in crush injury

A. release of coagulation factors from damaged cells
B. endothelial damage

84. formation of a thrombus

85. SUPPLY THE MISSING INFORMATION:

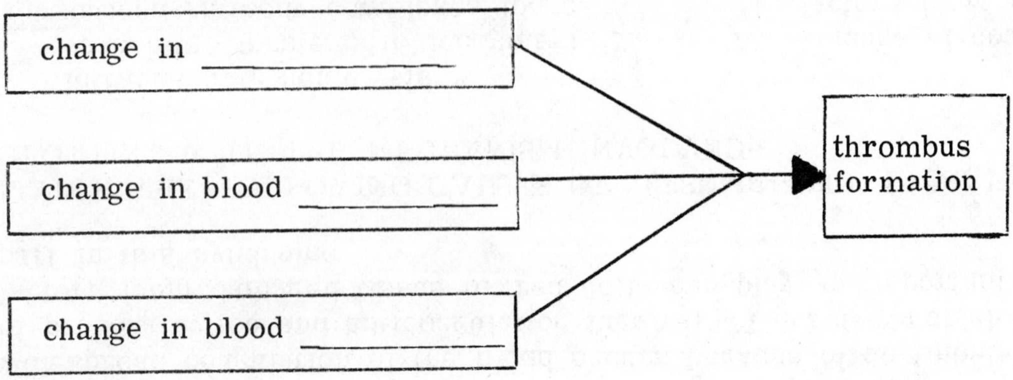

174. ✓ cholesterol crystals
✓ calcified material

175. Atheromatous emboli originate most commonly where atherosclerotic plaques are most common, the aorta and especially the abdominal aorta. Which of the following organs would be likely to be affected by atheromatous emboli?

____ lungs
____ kidney
____ spleen
____ intestine
____ arms
____ legs

9. 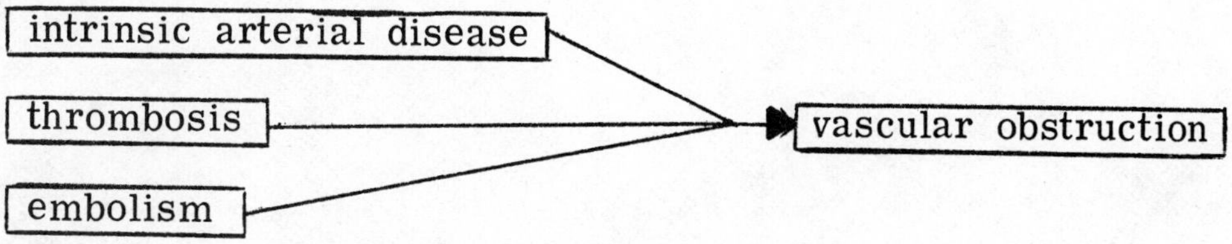

---

10. MATCH THE FOLLOWING:

____Blood coagulates in the femoral vein, obstructing it.	A. intrinsic arterial disease
____Fibrous tissue proliferates in the intima of an artery.	B. thrombosis
____Air enters a torn jugular vein and obstructs pulmonary capillaries.	C. embolism
____A fatty deposit thickens the intima of a coronary artery.	
____Fat droplets from the marrow of a broken bone are carried in the bloodstream to the renal glomeruli, where they lodge.	

---

99. A
B
B
A

---

100. When catecholamines are secreted in larger amounts or are infused, the blood coagulates more readily. It is believed that catecholamines (epinephrine, norepinephrine) stimulate the release of ADP (adenosine diphosphate) from platelets and cause platelet aggregation.

MATCH THE FOLLOWING:

____decreased secretion of epinephrine	A. blood coagulates more readily
____increased ADP released from platelets	B. blood coagulates less readily
____increased norepinephrine in blood	

83. A
C
B
C

84. These causative factors of thrombosis may be diagrammed thus:

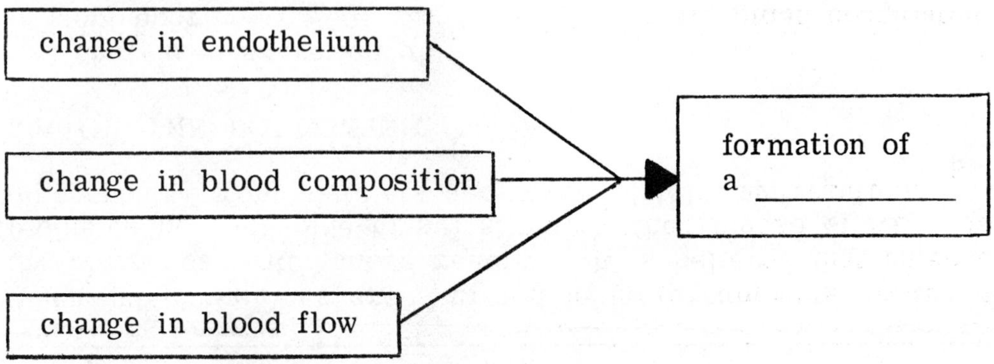

173. [✓] only small fragments are likely to enter the venous circulation, and will not damage the lung seriously.

174. Atheromatous embolism occurs when the contents of an atherosclerotic plaque are released into the bloodstream when a plaque is disrupted. Atheromatous emboli could be expected to contain:

____cholesterol crystals

____muscle fragments

____calcified material

10. B
A
C
A
C

---

11. INDICATE "T" TRUE OR "F" FALSE:

		frame reference
____	Hemodynamic disorders are classified into thrombosis, bleeding, and heart failure.	(2)
____	Bleeding is a category of deranged blood flow.	(2)
____	Vascular obstruction involves one basic mechanism.	(7)
____	Deranged blood flow is a systemic disorder.	(5)
____	Intrinsic arterial disease originates within the lumen of an artery.	(7)
____	Embolism and thrombosis usually produce local rather than systemic effects.	(5,7)

---

100. B
A
A

---

101. MATCH THE FOLLOWING CAUSES OF THROMBUS FORMATION WITH THEIR MECHANISM:

____increased platelets

____sludging of red cells

____trauma

____increased clotting factors

____inflammation

____anoxia

____increased catecholamines

A. changes in endothelium

B. changes in blood constituents

82. D
C
A
B

---

83. Three types of factors contribute to the formation of thrombi. They are damage to the vessel wall, changes in blood constituents, and changes in the rate of blood flow.

MATCH THE TYPE OF FACTOR ON THE RIGHT WITH THE EXAMPLES ON THE LEFT:

____ ulcerated endothelium	A. vessel wall
____ blood stasis	B. blood constituents
____ increased platelets	C. rate of flow
____ slowed bloodstream	

---

172. ☑ pulmonary

---

173. Bone marrow embolism is usually an incidental finding, rather than a source of serious consequences. This is probably because (CHOOSE ONE)

☐ marrow fragments would disperse readily in the circulation.

☐ only small fragments are likely to enter the venous circulation, and they will not damage the lung seriously.

11. F
F
F
T
F
T

B. <u>Intrinsic Arterial Disease</u> (56 frames)

When you complete this section, you will be able to select correct responses to the:

1. definitions of arteriosclerosis, vasculitis, lymphangitis and thrombophlebitis.
2. distinctions among atherosclerosis, arteriolosclerosis, and Mönckeberg's medial calcification in terms of
   - type and size of vessel involved
   - predisposing conditions
   - morphologic changes in vessels
   - results or complications of lesions
3. relationship of atherosclerosis to age, sex, and dietary habits

12. The arterial system is subject to a variety of disease processes. A number of these tend to cause obstruction of blood flow because they involve hardening and especially thickening of the arterial wall. The thickened wall narrows the lumen.

MATCH THE FOLLOWING:

____ narrowing of the lumen	A. hardening
____ reduction of flexibility	B. thickening

---

101. B
B
A
B
A
A
B

---

102. Two basic types of change in blood flow contribute to thrombosis. FILL IN THE EMPTY BOX:

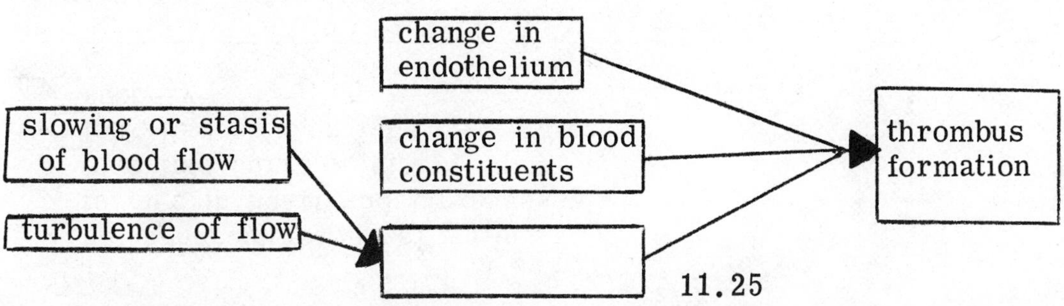

81. ✓ not adherent to vessel walls
✓ formed in heart and large vessels
✓ look like currant jelly
✓ look like chicken fat
✓ rubbery

---

82. MATCH THE FOLLOWING:

____ formed after death	A. mixed thrombus
____ white in color	B. red thrombus
____ lines of Zahn	C. platelet thrombus
____ erythrocytes trapped in clot	D. postmortem clot

---

171. amniotic fluid
☑ during

---

172. Bone marrow embolism may occur in the venous circulation after the fracture of bones containing red marrow. The mechanism is much like that of fat embolism, with which it is sometimes associated.

Bone marrow fragments will be found in the ☐ systemic ☐ pulmonary arteries.

12. B
A

---

13. The name for this group of diseases comes from the Greek roots for "artery" (arterio-) and "hardening" (sclerosis). Hardening of the arteries is thus called ____________________.

---

102. change in blood flow

---

103. The two types of changes in blood flow have to do with changes in the rate and the dynamics of flow. FILL IN THE EMPTY BOXES:

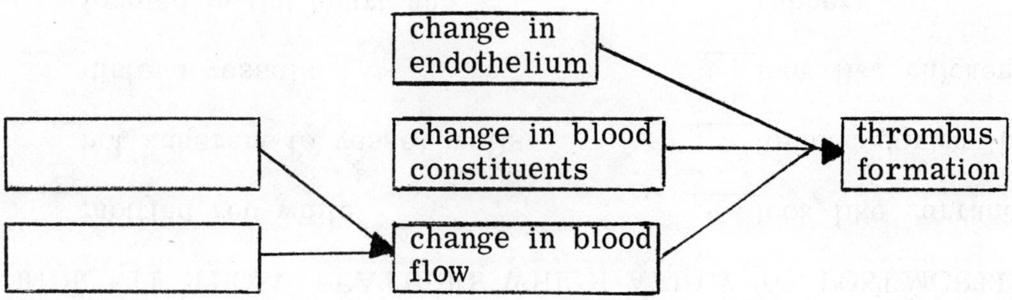

80. A
B
A, B

---

81. Postmortem clots, unlike thrombi, are not adherent to vessel walls. Thrombi also tend to distend the vessel, while postmortem clots do not.

INDICATE THOSE FEATURES WHICH APPLY TO POSTMORTEM CLOTS:

____mottled red-white	____look like currant jelly
____not adherent to vessel walls	____formed during life
____distend vessels	____look like chicken fat
____formed in the heart and large vessels	____rubbery

---

170. pulmonary

---

171. A possible complication of childbirth is embolism of ______________ fluid. Considering the mechanism involved, it seems most likely that such embolism would occur ☐ before ☐ during ☐ after labor.

13. arteriosclerosis

---

14. Arteriosclerosis includes:
    1. atherosclerosis
    2. arteriolosclerosis (or arteriolar sclerosis)
    3. Mönckeberg's medial calcification

Arteriosclerosis is a generic term for a number of diseases, all of which involve ______________ and ______________ of the arterial wall.

Arteriosclerosis is ☐ one ☐ several disease(s).

---

103. 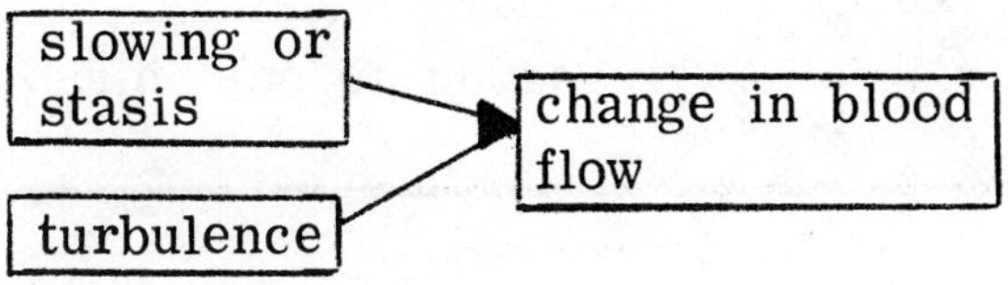

---

104. Serious slowing or stasis of flow in a vessel may result in the depletion of nutrients and oxygen, and cause endothelial changes thus making platelet adherence possible.

In which of the following situations is this mechanism likely?

____ downstream from an occlusive venous thrombus
____ mild aortic stenosis
____ incompetent valves permit pooling in the legs

79. A
B
A, B

---

80. Postmortem clots may be a homogeneous dark red and rubbery--a "currant jelly" clot--or may be a clear yellowish color where the red cells have settled out before coagulation--a "chicken fat" clot. Both types often occur together.

____blood coagulates after death with red cells included

____plasma coagulates after red cells have settled out

____type of postmortem clot

A. "currant jelly" clot

B. "chicken fat" clot

---

169. brain (and/or heart)

---

170. Amniotic fluid embolism is a relatively uncommon complication of childbirth, which can cause sudden death. Amniotic fluid components are forced into the maternal circulation by uterine contractions. Because the material enters the systemic veins, their effects will be produced primarily in the ____________________ arteries.

14. hardening (and) thickening

[✓] several

---

15. Arteriosclerosis leads to obstruction of the lumen of arteries because the walls of the artery are

[ ] hardened
[ ] thickened

---

104. ✓ downstream from an occlusive venous thrombus
✓ incompetent valves permit pooling in the legs

---

105. Disease conditions in which circulation is decreased to the entire body can promote thrombus formation.

INDICATE THOSE CONDITIONS IN WHICH THE CHANGE IN BLOOD FLOW PROMOTING THROMBUS FORMATION IS SYSTEMIC RATHER THAN LOCAL OR REGIONAL:

____ portal hypertension
____ inadequate total blood volume
____ heart failure
____ immobilization of a leg by a cast
____ thrombosis of the inferior mesenteric artery

78. Zahn

---

79. During postmortem examinations, the pathologist must distinguish between thrombi formed during life and blood clots that have developed after death. Post mortem clotting occurs in the heart and major vessels a few hours after death.

MATCH THE FOLLOWING:

____formed during life	A. thrombus
____formed after death	
____found at autopsy	B. postmortem clot

---

168. ☑ throughout the body

---

169. In decompression sickness, as in arterial air embolism, the fatal cases are generally due to the obstruction of vessels in the ______________________.

15. [✓] thickened

---

16. The most important of the degenerative arterial diseases is atherosclerosis. This term means literally "fatty-hardening." The root athero- therefore means ________________.

INDICATE THE GENERAL NAME AND FIRST SUBCATEGORY OF HARDENING AND THICKENING OF ARTERIES:

____

1. ________________________

---

105. ✓ inadequate total blood volume
✓ heart failure

---

106. Normally, the cells of the blood are separated from the endothelium by a thin plasma layer. Turbulent flow allows formed elements of the blood to come in contact with the vessel wall. This makes adherence of the platelets possible, leading to thrombus formation.

In which of the following places could turbulent flow contribute to thrombus formation?

____ descending aorta (normal)

____ fibrillating atrium

____ in an aortic aneurysm

77. C
A
B

---

78. The variegated appearance of a mixed thrombus is due to the lines of ________________.

---

167. [✓] slowly
[✓] less

---

168. The effects of decompression are due to the gas bubbles formed in the vessels and in tissues, especially adipose tissue, in which nitrogen is quite soluble.

The gas bubbles formed during decompression occur [ ] locally [ ] throughout the body.

16. fatty (or "fat")
arteriosclerosis
1. atherosclerosis

---

17. Atherosclerosis involves the accumulation of deposits of lipids in the intima of large arteries.

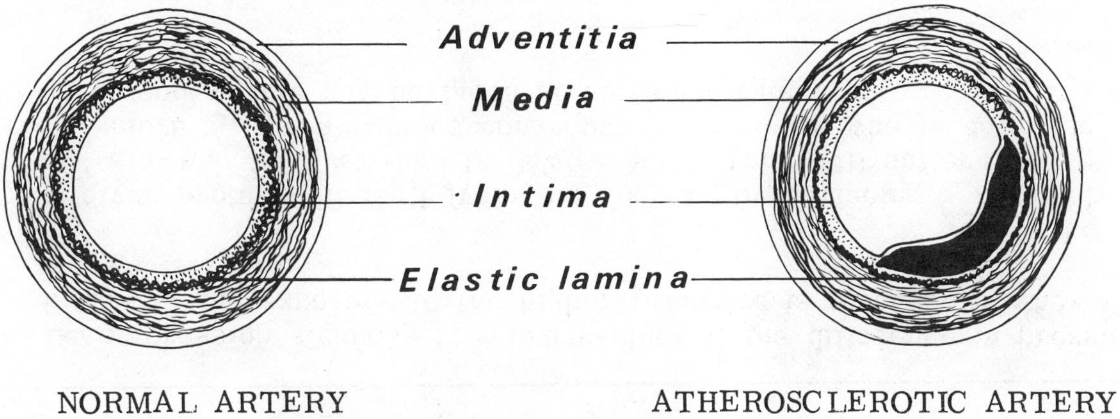

In the diseased artery, the wall is ☐ thickened ☐ thinned and the lumen is ☐ dilated ☐ narrowed .

The significant lesion is in the ____________________.

---

106. __✓__ fibrillating atrium
__✓__ in an aortic aneurysm

---

107. Venous blood travels more slowly than arterial blood. Veins also contain more valves and more branchings, which contribute to turbulence. The fact that thrombosis is much more common in veins than in arteries is probably due to

____ the relatively slower blood flow

____ more turbulent flow

76. B
A
D
C
E

---

77. More common than red or white thrombus are mixed thrombi. A mixed thrombus has a distinctive appearance because of strands of grayish-white fibrin and platelets alternating with masses of agglutinated red cells and leukocytes. These alternating red and white strands are referred to as lines of Zahn.

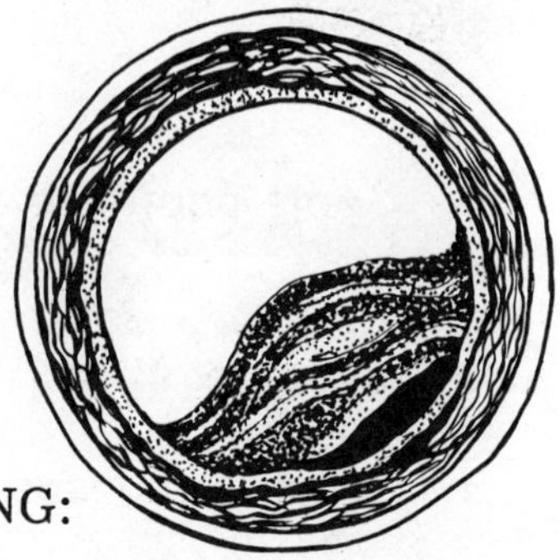

Mixed thrombus with lines of Zahn

MATCH THE FOLLOWING:

____lines of Zahn	A. white thrombus
____composed of platelets	B. red thrombus
____uniform color from red cells	C. mixed thrombus

---

166. A
B
B

---

167. Decompression sickness is more serious if the difference in pressure is great, the exposure to the higher pressure is extended, or the pressure change is rapid.

A diver protects himself from the "bends" by surfacing ☐ rapidly ☐ slowly. A diver who is down a short time will suffer ☐ more ☐ less serious consequences than one who is down for an extended time and surfaces at the same rate.

17. [✓] thickened
[✓] narrowed
intima

---

18. LABEL THIS DIAGRAM:

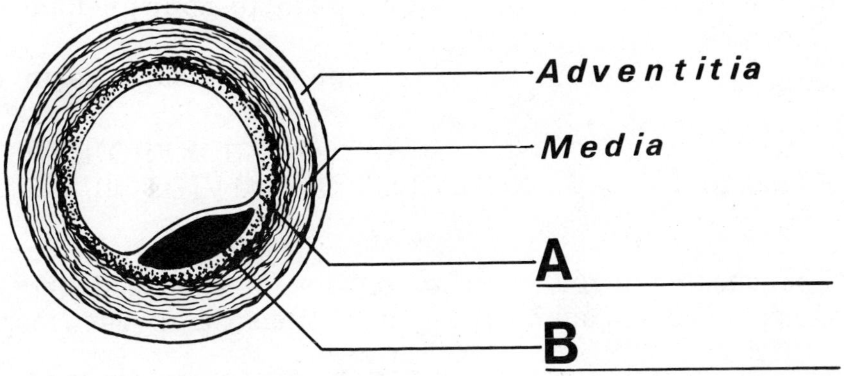

---

107. ✓ the relatively slower blood flow
✓ more turbulent flow

---

108. INDICATE "T" TRUE OR "F" FALSE:

____ Platelets are added to a thrombus only after a fibrin base has been laid down.
____ Prothrombin and thrombin have antagonistic actions on blood clotting.
____ Prolonged stasis in the bloodstream is very likely to result in thrombosis.
____ Very few agents are capable of damaging vascular endothelium.
____ Arterial thrombi are more common than venous thrombi.

75. B
A
A
B

---

76. MATCH THE FOLLOWING:

____blood flow completely obstructed

____thrombus composed mostly of platelets

____thrombus that contains many trapped red and white cells

____blood flow not completely obstructed

____plaque on lining of heart

A. white thrombus
B. occlusive thrombus
C. non-occlusive thrombus
D. red thrombus
E. mural thrombus

---

165. B
A

---

166. The decrease in pressure causing decompression sickness may be from high pressure to normal or from normal pressure to low pressure.

MATCH THE FOLLOWING SITUATIONS WITH THE TYPE OF PRESSURE CHANGE INVOLVED:

____a diver surfaces rapidly

____a high-altitude aircraft cabin develops a leak

____a spacecraft is pierced by a meteorite

A. high pressure lowered to normal

B. normal pressure lowered to subatmospheric

18. 1. intima
    2. lipid deposit

---

19. As the aorta and the common iliac arteries are the most commonly involved arteries in atherosclerosis, you would guess that the vessels involved are generally ☐ small ☐ large arteries.

---

108. F
F
T
F
F

---

109. The fate of a thrombus: After a thrombus is formed a variety of things may happen to it. FILL IN THE EMPTY BOX:

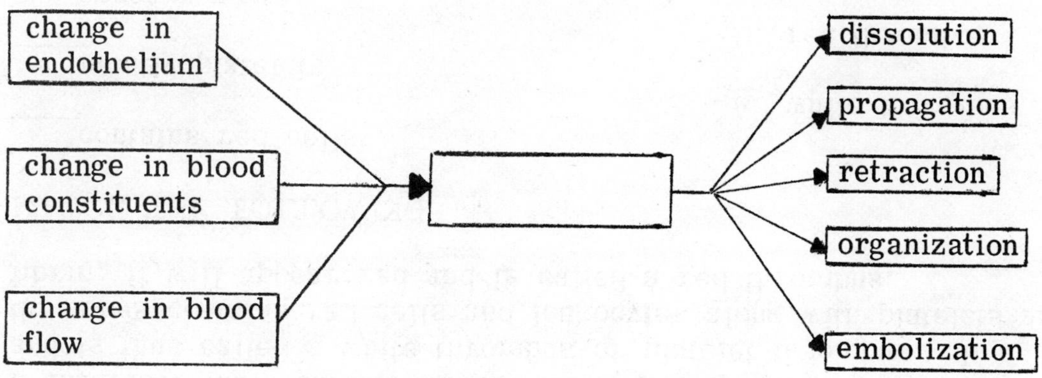

74. vegetation
A
B

---

75. A thrombus that consists almost entirely of platelets appears white and is thus called a white thrombus, or platelet thrombus. If a thrombus contains red cells and leukocytes along with platelets and fibrin, it will appear red and is called a red thrombus.

MATCH THE FOLLOWING:

____contains red cells

____mostly platelets

____appears white

____appears red

A. white thrombus

B. red thrombus

---

164. ✓ coronary artery ✓ cerebral artery

---

165. Another type of gas embolism occurs when dissolved gas in the blood and tissue comes out of solution because the ambient pressure is rapidly lowered. The effects of this are called decompression sickness.

MATCH THE FOLLOWING:

____exogenous source of gas emboli

____endogenous source of gas emboli

A. decompression sickness

B. air embolism

19. [✓] large

---

20. Atherosclerosis is a disease of elastic and large muscular arteries. It predominantly involves arteries in the systemic circuit including the aorta and its major branches to visceral organs, to the head, and to the lower extremities.

Which of the following arteries would you expect to be commonly involved in atherosclerosis, based on the above principle?

____common iliac arteries
____renal arterioles
____common carotid arteries
____coronary arteries
____splenic artery
____pulmonary arteries
____vena cavae

---

109. [thrombus formation]

---

110. Dissolution of a small thrombus may occur before organization can take place. This occurs by the activity of fibrinolysin (plasmin), a plasma-proteolytic enzyme activated by a factor in tissue extracts. Fibrinolysin attacks particularly the fibrin in a thrombus.

CHECK THOSE QUALITIES OR ACTIVITIES ASSOCIATED WITH FIBRINOLYSIN:

____breaks down fibrin
____inactivates thrombin
____proteolytic enzyme
____may dissolve a thrombus
____activates the healing process in a thrombus

73. mural

---

74. A thrombus is "septic" if it contains pathogenic microorganisms. Rheumatic damage to heart valves is often followed by bacterial endocarditis with septic mural thrombi. A thrombus without organisms present is "bland."

A septic mural thrombus on a heart valve is an example of ________________.

MATCH THE FOLLOWING:

____thrombus on a heart valve, containing colonies of Staphylococcus aureus

____thrombus over the site of a myocardial infarct, containing no microorganisms

A. septic mural thrombus
B. bland mural thrombus

---

163. [✓] above

---

164. Arterial air embolism may be fatal with smaller amounts of air than is the case in venous air embolism. This occurs by the occlusion of arteries in vital organs.

CHOOSE THE MOST LIKELY LOCATIONS OF FATAL AIR EMBOLISM:

____bronchial artery ____cerebral artery

____coronary artery ____lingual artery

____portal vein

20. ✓ common iliac arteries
✓ common carotid arteries
✓ coronary arteries
✓ splenic artery

The pulmonary arteries are not usually involved, probably because of the lower pressure in the pulmonary circulation.

---

21. Early atherosclerotic lipid deposits are predominantly intracellular. The lipid-containing cells are called foam cells (because of the lipid-filled vacuoles) or lipophages (literally "fat-eaters"). These cells have many characteristics of smooth muscle cells, and are thus also called myointimal cells.

CHECK THOSE CHARACTERISTICS OR NAMES WHICH APPLY TO THE FAT-FILLED CELLS OF ATHEROSCLEROSIS:

____ foamy appearance
____ lipophages
____ endothelial cells
____ smooth muscle characteristics
____ appear like fibroblasts
____ myointimal cells

---

110. ✓ breaks down fibrin
✓ proteolytic enzyme
✓ may dissolve a thrombus

---

111. The enzyme primarily involved in the dissolution of a thrombus is ____________________.

72. mural
✓ aorta
✓ left ventricle

---

73. Irregular thrombi can form on heart valves. These are called vegetations. Vegetations, because attached to the walls of a vessel, are a type of ________________ thrombus.

---

162. ☑ pulmonary
paradoxical

---

163. If air does reach the systemic circulation, because of its relative density it will tend to rise into the main branches of the aortic arch. Thus, arterial air embolism is most likely to affect areas of the body ☐ below ☐ above the level of the heart.

21. ✓ foamy appearance ✓ smooth muscle characteristics
✓ lipophages ✓ myointimal cells

---

22. Early, reversible intracellular lipid deposits--called intimal streaking--commonly occur even in early childhood but do not always develop into more complex fibrotic plaques. Fibrotic plaques rarely occur before the third decade.

MATCH THE FOLLOWING:

____intimal streaking

____fibrotic plaques

____affects all ages

____affects only mature persons

____intact lipophages predominate

A. early lesion

B. complicated lesion

---

111. fibrinolysin (or plasmin)

---

112. Propagation, the formation of an extended thrombus, occurs when the initial thrombus creates conditions favorable for the development of further thrombus. Which of the following conditions would contribute to propagation of a thrombus?

____blood flow is slowed or stopped downstream from a venous thrombus

____an occlusive venous thrombus releases thrombin

____plasmin is activated in large amounts

____a metabolic disorder has seriously decreased the fibrinogen content of the blood

71. ✓ composed of blood elements
✓ adheres to the wall of a vessel or the heart

---

72. Plaque-like thrombi are commonly found in the chambers of the heart, especially the left side, and in large systemic arteries. These are called ________________ thrombi.

Which of the following are likely locations for such thrombi?

____aorta

____pulmonary vein

____left ventricle

____pulmonary artery

---

161. ☑ paradoxical

---

162. Air in a systemic artery may originate as air entering a ☐ systemic ☐ pulmonary vein or as air passing through some arteriovenous communication from the pulmonary artery. The latter is a case of ________________ embolism.

22. A
B
A
B
A

---

23. Large superficial aggregations of lipophages gradually interfere with the nourishment of underlying tissue. Lipophages deep in the mass break down, releasing their contents extracellularly. Degradation of these lipoproteins results in the formation of some cholesterol crystals.

MATCH THE EFFECTS ON THE RIGHT WITH THE CAUSES ON THE LEFT:

____degradation of lipoproteins	A. extracellular fat deposits
____breakdown of lipophages	B. cholesterol crystals

---

112. ✓ blood flow is slowed or stopped downstream from a venous thrombus
✓ an occlusive venous thrombus releases thrombin

---

113. A thrombus will not propagate unless there is relative stasis of blood flow or turbulence. The tail of a propagating thrombus develops in the direction of the heart (in arteries or veins) and may attain several centimeters in length. The tail, unlike the initial thrombus, is a homogeneous dark red and is not ordinarily attached to the vessel wall.

MATCH THE FOLLOWING:

____lines of Zahn	A. initial thrombus
____attached to wall	B. tail of thrombus
____homogeneous red in color	
____grows toward heart	
____mixed thrombus	
____not likely to develop without stasis	

70. [✓] occlusive

---

71. A thrombus which adheres as a sort of plaque to the wall of the heart or a blood vessel is called a mural thrombus. A mural thrombus is often non-occlusive but may grow into an occlusive thrombus.

Which of the following qualities apply to all mural thrombi?

____composed of blood elements

____occludes blood flow

____adheres to the wall of a vessel or the heart

---

160. [✓] small
pulmonary

---

161. Some air may pass through the pulmonary circulation and enter systemic arteries. This becomes a case of [ ] arterial [ ] paradoxical embolism.

23. B
    A

---

24. The accumulation of lipids also interferes with the normal smoothness of the endothelium, thus allowing the adherence of platelets and fibrin. When these accumulations of platelets and fibrin are organized, a fibrotic cap is gradually formed over the intimal deposit.

LABEL THESE DIAGRAMS 1, 2, & 3 IN THE ORDER OF THEIR DEVELOPMENT:

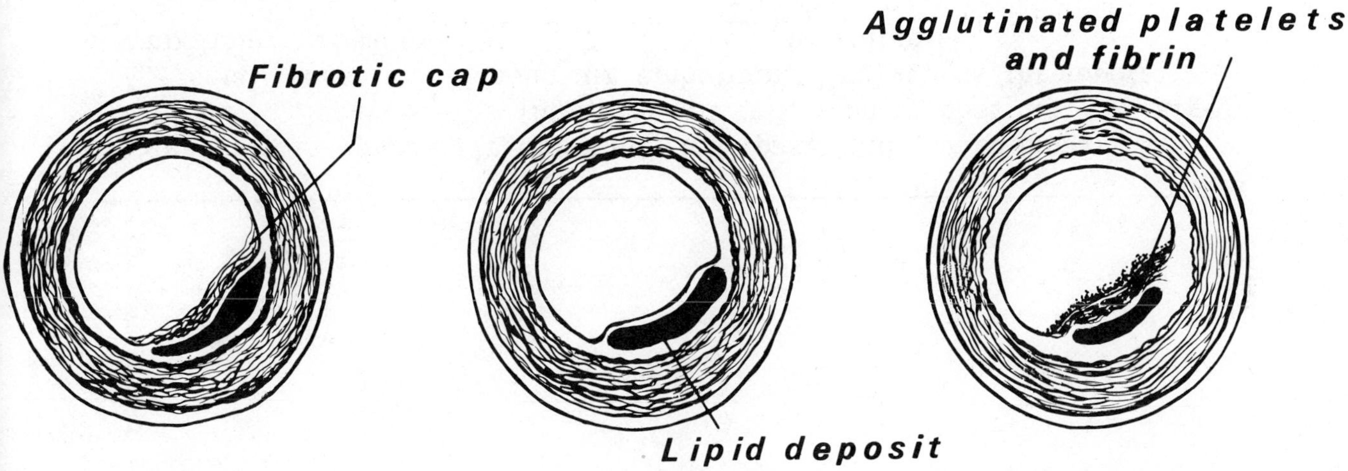

_____ _____ _____

---

113. A
     A
     B
     B
     A
     B

---

114. Retraction of a thrombus involves the shrinking of the thrombus to as little as one-half its original volume. Platelets are primarily responsible for retraction (by means of a contractile protein, thrombosthenin). Retraction is more pronounced in a thrombus composed primarily of platelets. Retraction may reopen a channel closed by an occlusive thrombus. Thrombin which is released during retraction may, however, promote propagation of the thrombus if it is not dispersed rapidly enough.

INDICATE THOSE RESULTS WHICH MAY BE ASSOCIATED WITH RETRACTION OF A THROMBUS:

____reopening of a channel
____disappearance of the thrombus
____propagation of the thrombus
____shrinking of platelets in the thrombus

69. ✓ formed from elements of the blood
✓ formed during life
✓ solid mass

---

70. Thrombi are classified as occlusive or non-occlusive, depending on whether or not blood flow in the affected vessel is completely obstructed.

A thrombus which fills the lumen of a vessel is a(n) ▱ occlusive ▱ non-occlusive thrombus.

---

159. B
A
B
A
A
B

---

160. Some air in venous air embolism will pass into the pulmonary arteries. Because it is fluid, the air will tend to obstruct ▱ large ▱ small vessels. Venous air embolism, like venous thrombotic embolism, produces ____________________ embolism.

24. __3__ __1__ __2__

---

25. ORDER THESE STEPS IN THE FORMATION OF A FIBROTIC PLAQUE (1, 2, 3, 4, 5):

____alteration of the anticoagulant properties of endothelium

____breakdown of lipophages and release of their contents

____adherence of platelets and fibrin

____formation of intracellular lipid deposit

____organization of platelet fibrin deposit

---

114. _✓_ reopening of a channel
_✓_ propagation of the thrombus
_✓_ shrinking of platelets in the thrombus

---

115. The factors in a thrombus which are primarily responsible for retraction of the thrombus are the ________________.

Retraction may ☐ obstruct ☐ open a vascular channel.

68. ✓ a lump of platelets and fibrin block a coronary artery
✓ a large red mass develops on the endocardium at the site of an infarct

---

69. INDICATE THE CHARACTERISTICS WHICH APPLY TO THROMBI:

____forms in tissue spaces

____formed from elements of the blood

____formed during life

____formed in veins only

____solid mass

---

158. [✓] different from

---

159. The lethal dose in venous air embolism has been considered to be about 100 to 150 ml. This varies according to the rate of entry, the general condition of the person, and the position of the person.

DECIDE WHICH OF THE FOLLOWING CONDITIONS WOULD REQUIRE MORE OR LESS THAN AVERAGE AMOUNTS OF AIR TO BE LETHAL:

____upright position
____prone position
____weakened patient
____healthy patient
____slow entry of air
____rapid entry of air

A. more air required

B. less air required

25. 3
2
4
1
5

---

26. A fibrotic plaque is not usually a clinical problem, but a variety of complications may ensue which may have clinical significance. Some of these are:

calcification of the plaque
hemorrhage into the plaque
thrombosis over an ulcerated plaque
atrophy of the subjacent muscle layer
disruption of the plaque

A complicated plaque is ☐ less ☐ more clinically significant than a simple fibrotic plaque.

MATCH EACH COMPLICATION ON THE RIGHT WITH ITS CAUSE ON THE LEFT:

____ coagulation of blood over altered endothelium
____ rupture of vasa at periphery of plaque
____ reduced circulation to subjacent media
____ deposit of minerals in the fibrotic cap
____ entrance of moving blood from the lumen into a break in the plaque

A. calcification
B. hemorrhage into plaque
C. thrombosis
D. atrophy of muscle layer
E. disruption of plaque

---

115. platelets
☑ open

---

116. All or part of a thrombus may break away and be carried to another part of the circulatory system. This process is called embolization. Embolization is likely where a thrombus is not firmly attached to the vessel wall or where some process within the thrombus is tending to break it up.

Which of the following situations are likely to result in embolization?

____ the tail of a propagating venous thrombus
____ a mural thrombus overlying an atherosclerotic area of the aorta
____ a septic vegetation on the aortic valve
____ an occlusive thrombus in a coronary artery

67. T
F
F
F
F

C. Thrombosis (57 frames)

When you complete this section, you will be able to select correct responses relating to the:

1. definitions of red thrombus, white thrombus, mural thrombus, septic thrombus, and postmortem clot
2. causative role of changes in blood vessel walls, blood composition, and blood flow in thrombus formation
3. steps in formation, propagation, organization, and recanalization of a thrombus
4. mechanism and consequences of dissolution, retraction, and embolization of thrombi

68. A thrombus is a solid or semisolid mass formed in a vessel during life from the constituents of circulating blood. The process of thrombus formation is called thrombosis.

INDICATE THE DESCRIPTIONS BELOW WHICH ARE EXAMPLES OF THROMBI:

____drawn blood coagulates in a test tube
____blood clots where it has flowed from an open wound
____a lump of platelets and fibrin block a coronary artery
____a large red mass develops on the endocardium at the site of an infarct
____blood coagulates in the heart several hours after death

---

157. V V
A A
V V, A
A V

---

158. When air enters a systemic vein (venous air embolism) in sufficient amounts, death may ensue. Death occurs because of a froth trap established in the outflow tract of the right ventricle, making the pumping action of the heart ineffective by the froth's compressibility. This situation occurs more readily if the patient is in an upright position and if air enters quickly. The mechanism of death in venous air embolism is ☐ the same as ☐ different from the mechanism in venous thrombotic embolism.

26. ☑ more
C
B
D
A
E or B

---

27. MATCH EACH COMPLICATION ON THE RIGHT WITH ITS EFFECT OR MANIFESTATION ON THE LEFT:

____ expansion of the plaque with blood
____ distention of the weakened vessel wall (aneurysm)
____ release of plaque contents into the lumen
____ plaque becomes brittle, inelastic
____ occlusion of the lumen

A. calcification
B. hemorrhage into the plaque
C. thrombosis
D. atrophy of muscle layer
E. disruption of the plaque

---

116. ✓ the tail of a propagating venous thrombus (not firmly attached)
✓ a mural thrombus overlying an atherosclerotic area of the aorta (rapidly moving bloodstream may disrupt it)
✓ a septic vegetation on the aortic valve (bacterial action breaks it up)

---

117. When a thrombus is disrupted and part of it moves freely in the circulation, we have ____________________.

This process ☐ will ☐ will not ordinarily have serious consequences.

66. F
T
T
F
F

---

67. INDICATE "T" TRUE OR "F" FALSE:

	frame reference
____Mönckeberg's sclerosis and medial calcification are names for the same process.	(54)
____Medial calcification affects all ages.	(57)
____Monckeberg's sclerosis is a serious obstructive disorder.	(58)
____Vasculitis means inflammation of a vein.	(59, 60)
____Vasculitis is the most common obstructive vascular disease.	(62)

---

156. A
B
A
B

---

157. Air embolism is a possible consequence of certain medical and surgical procedures. Those procedures involving the lung or left heart would lead to arterial air embolism; most others, to venous air embolism.

CLASSIFY THE FOLLOWING PROCEDURES AS POSSIBLY LEADING TO (A) ARTERIAL OR (V) VENOUS AIR EMBOLISM:

____neck operations	____cesarean section
____pulmonary resection	____induction of pneumothorax
____intravenous therapy	____cardiac operations
____lung aspiration	____brain operations

27. B
D
E
A
C (and sometimes B and E)

---

28. MATCH THE FOLLOWING:

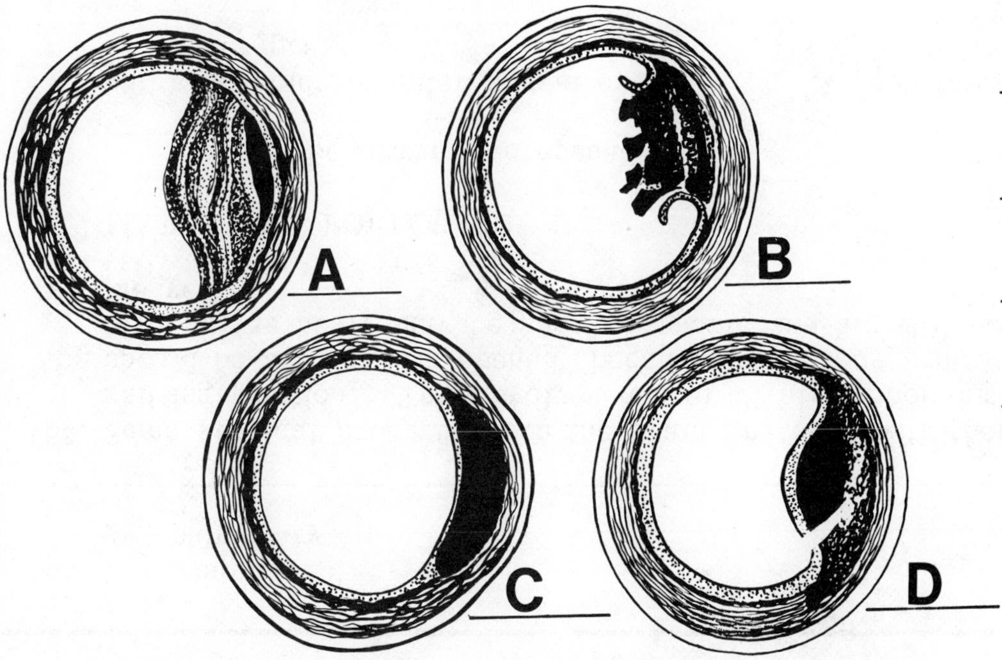

____hemorrhage into the plaque

____thrombosis over the plaque

____atrophy of the subjacent muscle

____disruption of the plaque

---

117. embolization
[✓] will

---

118. When a thrombus remains intact, the elements which make it up soon undergo certain changes. The cellular elements break down and the thrombus becomes decolorized and homogeneous (hyalinized). Softening may occur in the center of a large thrombus due to the release of proteolytic enzymes from leukocytes.

INDICATE THOSE CHANGES WHICH CAN OCCUR IN A THROMBUS:

____hyalinization

____decolorization

____softening

____inflammation

____edema

65. T
F
F
T
F

---

66. INDICATE "T" TRUE OR "F" FALSE:

	frame reference
____Arteriolosclerosis affects arteries of all sizes.	(44)
____Intimal hyaline deposition is a normal concomitant of aging.	(47)
____Hypertension has different effects in renal arterioles and in small arteries proximal to these arterioles.	(50)
____Arteriolosclerosis does not ordinarily affect blood flow in the vessels involved.	(49)
____Visceral arteries are usually those first affected by Monckeberg's sclerosis.	(54)

---

155. ☑ systemic
☑ pulmonary

---

156. Some surgical procedures on the brain are done with the patient in a sitting position. This involves danger of air embolism if a vein should be accidentally opened, because the venous pressure above the level of the heart may be subatmospheric and air will be drawn into the vein.

MATCH THE FOLLOWING:

____air may be drawn into opened vein

____air would not enter a vein except under pressure

____above level of the heart

____below the level of the heart

A. subatmospheric venous pressure

B. supra-atmospheric venous pressure

28. D
A
C
B

---

29. Of these complications, any which increase the size of the plaque or associated mass or which release foreign matter into the bloodstream can result in obstruction of blood flow.

Which of these is/are most likely to result in obstruction?

____calcification

____hemorrhage into the plaque

____thrombosis over the plaque

____atrophy of the subjacent muscle

____disruption of the plaque

---

118. ✓ hyalinization
✓ decolorization
✓ softening

---

119. A large thrombus that does not undergo dissolution or embolization will ordinarily undergo healing. The process of healing is a process of organization. Endothelial cells from the periphery of the thrombus spread over the exposed surface of the thrombus and invade the thrombus forming new capillaries and endothelium-lined spaces. Fibroblasts also invade the thrombus, forming fibrous tissue.

MATCH THE FOLLOWING:

____cover the exposed surface of a thrombus

____form new capillaries

____form fibrous tissue

A. endothelial cells

B. fibroblasts

64. F
T
F
F
T
F

---

65. INDICATE "T" TRUE OR "F" FALSE:

	frame reference
____ Lipophages in atheromatous plaques resemble smooth muscle cells.	(21)
____ Intracellular fat deposits are often irreversible.	(30)
____ Calcification is a property of early atherosclerotic plaques.	(26)
____ An atherosclerotic plaque may initiate a thrombus.	(26)
____ Serum cholesterol varies directly with cholesterol intake.	(34)

---

154. ✓ reduce local tissue pressure

---

155. Air embolism occurs if air is forced or drawn into the circulatory system. Unless injected under pressure, air is most likely to enter a vein where subatmospheric pressure can occur. As in thrombotic embolism, air embolism is classified as venous or arterial.

Venous air embolism involves air entering a ☐ systemic ☐ pulmonary vein.

Arterial air embolism involves air entering a ☐ systemic ☐ pulmonary vein.

29. ✓ hemorrhage into the plaque
✓ thrombosis over the plaque
✓ disruption of the plaque

---

30. It is not yet clear to what extent atherosclerotic plaques are reversible. With favorable conditions, some intracellular and extracellular lipid may disappear from a plaque at any stage. Some parts of a plaque will not regress, however. Among these are: crystalline cholesterol, elastin-bound lipid, and the fibrotic or calcified cap. Which of the following are potentially reversible in an atherosclerotic plaque?

____cholesterol crystals

____extracellular lipoprotein

____fibrotic cap

____intracellular lipoprotein

---

119. A
A
B

---

120. The cells primarily involved in the organization of a thrombus are ____________________ cells and ____________________.

63. ✓ thrombosis
✓ intimal proliferation
[✓] rare

---

64. INDICATE "T" TRUE OR "F" FALSE:

	frame reference
____Arteriosclerosis and atherosclerosis are synonymous.	(16)
____Thickening of the arterial wall tends to produce obstruction.	(12)
____Hardening of the arteries is a distinct disease process.	(13)
____Atherosclerosis begins as fat deposits in the medial layer of an artery.	(17)
____Intimal streaking with fat deposits is not a clinically serious problem.	(22)
____Orientals have an unusually high incidence of atherosclerosis.	(37)

---

153. A
A
B

---

154. Given the three necessary factors for fat embolism, which of the following is the most plausible way to decrease the likelihood of fat embolism?

____immobilize any freed fat
____repair disrupted veins
____reduce local tissue pressure

30. _✓_ extracellular lipoprotein
_✓_ intracellular lipoprotein

---

31. At which of these stages of development of an atherosclerotic deposit is it probably still possible for the lesion to disappear completely, assuming adequate changes in plasma lipids?

____ intimal streaking

____ considerable extracellular lipoprotein

____ extracellular cholesterol crystals

____ fibrotic cap

____ ulcerated fibrotic cap

____ calcified plaque

---

120. endothelial
fibroblasts

---

121. During organization, the thrombus gradually becomes a mass of vascularized connective tissue. The vascular spaces formed by the endothelium may extend and coalesce, reestablishing blood circulation through the originally occlusive thrombus. This process is called recanalization.

MATCH THE FOLLOWING:

____ formation of fibrous tissue in a thrombus
____ formation of vascular channels in a thrombus
____ replacement of the thrombotic elements with scar tissue

A. organization

B. recanalization

62. [✓] can

[✓] is not

---

63. INDICATE THOSE RESULTS OF VASCULAR INFLAMMATION WHICH CAN RESULT IN OBSTRUCTION OF BLOOD FLOW:

____thrombosis
____dilation
____intimal proliferation
____medial necrosis

Primary vasculitis is a [ ] common [ ] rare cause of vascular obstruction.

---

152. _✓_ tibia _✓_ femur

---

153. Fat embolism, according to the most likely theory, involves these three factors:

release of fluid fat from ruptured cells
disrupted and open veins
increased local tissue pressure, forcing the fat into the venous system

MATCH EACH OF THESE FACTORS WITH ITS CAUSE:

____release of fat from ruptured cells	A. trauma itself
____disrupted veins	B. edema or hemorrhage
____increased tissue pressure	

31. ✓ intimal streaking
✓ considerable extracellular lipoprotein

---

32. The incidence of atherosclerosis is related to factors of age, sex, diet, and possibly hereditary factors. In general, atherosclerosis becomes more serious with age.

Which of the following is most likely to have serious atherosclerosis?

____30-year-old man with average diet

____50-year-old man with average diet

---

121. A
B
A

---

122. INDICATE "T" TRUE OR "F" FALSE:

	frame reference
____A thrombus may form either in a blood vessel or in tissue spaces.	(68)
____The most common form of thrombus is a mixed thrombus.	(77)
____A postmortem clot is indistinguishable from a red thrombus.	(81)
____A vegetation on a heart valve is a form of mural thrombus.	(73)
____Mural thrombi are almost always occlusive.	(71)
____Leukocytes give the white color to white thrombi.	(75)

61. A
C
B

---

62. Primary vasculitis is rare, but serious complications may ensue when it occurs. An inflamed vessel may undergo medial necrosis, thrombosis, local dilation or rupture, and scarring with endarterial proliferation. Of these results, thrombosis and endarterial proliferation (proliferation of the intima) can obstruct blood flow.

Vasculitis ☐ can ☐ cannot be an obstructive vascular disorder. Because vasculitis does not generally cause hardening of the arteries, it ☐ is ☐ is not considered a subclass of arteriosclerosis.

---

151. N T
T T
N N
N T

---

152. The most common and important cause of fat embolism is disruption of fatty marrow because of the fracture of long bones. Bones which are likely to involve fat embolism when fractured include:

____clavicle	____femur
____tibia	____skull
____rib	____mandible

32. ✓ a 50-year-old man with average diet

---

33. At least premenopausally, women have less atherosclerosis than men of the same age. Which of these is most likely to have severe atherosclerosis?

____40-year-old man

____40-year-old woman

____30-year-old woman

---

122. F
T
F
T
F
F

---

123. INDICATE "T" TRUE OR "F" FALSE:

	frame reference
____An occlusive thrombus always remains occlusive.	(109)
____A thrombus invariably remains where it was formed.	(116)
____Fibroblasts and mast cells are the primary cells involved in the organization of a thrombus.	(119)
____Thrombin promotes the retraction of a thrombus.	(91)
____Propagation of a thrombus occurs readily in a rapidly flowing bloodstream.	(112)
____The tail of a propagating venous thrombus often becomes an embolus.	(116)

60. arteritis
phlebitis
aortitis
lymphangitis

---

61. Vasculitis can result from a variety of intravascular and perivascular infections, immunologic reactions, and irritants.

MATCH THE FOLLOWING CAUSES OF VASCULITIS:

____septicemia (blood-borne infection)	A. infection
____ulceration into gastroduodenal artery by acid (peptic ulcer)	B. immunologic reactions
____antibody complexes lodge in vascular basement membrane	C. irritants

---

150. [✓] is not

---

151. The causes of fat embolism include a variety of traumatic and non-traumatic lesions.

DESIGNATE THE FOLLOWING CAUSES OF FAT EMBOLISM AS "T" TRAUMATIC OR "N" NON-TRAUMATIC:

____fatty liver	____fracture of bones
____laceration of adipose tissue	____contusion of adipose tissue
____inflammation of marrow	____decompression sickness
____diabetes mellitus	____childbirth

33. ✓ 40-year-old man

---

34. High serum cholesterol levels seem to correlate with increased atherosclerosis, but dietary cholesterol does not correlate well with serum cholesterol levels.

Which of the following criteria has the most prognostic value in dealing with atherosclerosis?

____high cholesterol intake

____high serum cholesterol

---

123. F
F
F
F
F
T

---

124. INDICATE "T" TRUE OR "F" FALSE:

	frame reference
____Retraction of a thrombus may reopen a vascular channel.	(114)
____Significant retraction is more likely in a mixed thrombus than in a red thrombus.	(114)
____Endothelialization of the surface of a thrombus helps prevent propagation.	(119)
____Embolization of a thrombus remains just as likely after organization has begun.	(116,119)

59. vasculitis

60. Similarly, inflammation of arteries is called ____________.

Inflammation of veins (the Greek root phleb-) is called ____________.

Inflammation of the aorta is called ____________.

Inflammation of lymph vessels (the Latin root lymph- and the Greek root angi-) is called ____________.

149. ☑ the serious consequences of occlusion of even small vessels

150. In the kidney, fat embolism may be marked, especially in the glomerular capillaries, but parenchymal changes are not obvious and kidney failure does not result.

Fat embolism in the kidney ☐ is ☐ is not ordinarily a clinical problem.

34. ✓ high serum cholesterol

---

35. Dietary saturated fats (rather than cholesterol) appear to increase serum cholesterol, whereas a significant proportion of polyunsaturated fats in the diet appears to lower serum cholesterol.

MATCH THE FOLLOWING:

____increased serum cholesterol	A. polyunsaturated fats in diet
____decreased serum cholesterol	B. saturated fats in diet

---

124. T
T
T
F

D. Embolization (56 frames)

When you complete this section, you will be able to select correct responses relating to the:

1. distinctions among arterial embolism, venous embolism, and paradoxical embolism in terms of
   - common sources of emboli
   - path of transfer
   - common sites of enlodgement
2. definitions and common causes of thrombotic emboli, fat emboli, air emboli, septic emboli, foreign-body emboli, bone marrow emboli, and amniotic fluid emboli

125. The third important mechanism of vascular obstruction is embolism. Embolism is a partial or complete obstruction of any part of the vascular system by any mass carried there in the circulation. The transported material is called an embolus.

MATCH THE FOLLOWING:

____an obstructive process involving a detached mass in the circulatory system	A. embolus
____a free mass in the vascular system	B. embolism

58. [✓] hardening
[✓] does not
Mönckeberg's medial calcification

---

59. In addition to the arteriosclerotic diseases, arteries and other vessels are subject to various inflammatory lesions. Vascular inflammation (from the Latin root vascul-, meaning vascular, and the Latin root itis, meaning inflammation) is known as ____________________.

---

148. [✓] fat arrives here first and in greatest quantity
[✓] numerous small vessels may be occluded

---

149. The other organ which may be seriously affected by fat embolism is the brain.

The serious effects in the brain are due to:

[ ] the arrival of fat in large quantities
[ ] the serious consequences of occlusion of even small vessels
[ ] the occlusion of large vessels

35. B
A

---

36. Which of the following diets is MOST likely to contribute to atherosclerosis?

____vegetarian diet (low content of saturated fats)

____average American diet

____diet with average total fat, but higher proportion of polyunsaturated fats

____diet with a high percentage of caloric intake as ethanol

---

125. B
A

---

126. Emboli may be solid, liquid, or gaseous.

MATCH THE FOLLOWING:

____air

____tumor cells

____detached thrombus

____fat globules

A. solid embolus
B. liquid embolus
C. gaseous embolus

57. ✓ 60-year-old man

---

58. Medial calcification results primarily in ☐ thickening ☐ hardening of the arterial wall and thus ☐ does ☐ does not readily result in vascular obstruction.

The calcification involved in atherosclerotic plaques and in Mönckeberg's sclerosis can be seen on radiographic films. If a film shows continuous radiopaque bands in the legs, the disease is ______________________.

---

147. ☑ paradoxical

---

148. Because of the small size of the vessels involved, fat embolism does not have serious effects on most organs. The lungs are one of the two exceptions.

The lungs may be seriously affected because:

☐ large arteries are occluded
☐ fat arrives here first and in greatest quantity
☐ numerous small vessels may be occluded

36. __✓__ average American diet

---

37. The incidence of atherosclerosis in Japan is about one-tenth that among whites, blacks, and naturalized Japanese Americans. This is probably due to:

____ a greater proportion of females in the population

____ diet lower in fats

____ racially determined genetic factors

____ climatic conditions

---

126. C
A
A
B

---

127. Emboli also may be bland or septic, depending on whether they contain pathogenic organisms.

MATCH THE FOLLOWING:

____ embolus from mural thrombus in bacterial endocarditis

____ embolus from mural thrombus in myocardial infarct

A. bland embolus
B. septic embolus

56. Mönckeberg's
B
A
C

---

57. The frequency of medial calcification is directly related to age. In which of the following persons is medial sclerosis most likely?

____50-year-old man

____40-year-old man

____60-year-old man

---

146. ☑ pulmonary
☑ venous

---

147. Because of the fluidity of fat droplets, some may readily pass through small pulmonary arteriovenous shunts or the pulmonary capillaries themselves and enter the systemic circulation. We then have ☐ venous ☐ arterial ☐ paradoxical embolism.

37. _✓_diet lower in fats

---

38. Diabetes mellitus raises serum cholesterol levels. Therefore, we would expect diabetics to have a(n) ☐ decreased ☐ increased chance of developing atherosclerosis.

---

127. B
A

---

128. Part of a thrombus over an atherosclerotic plaque dislodges and is impacted in a renal artery. This embolus is:

____solid

____liquid

____gaseous

____septic

____bland

55. medial
☑ muscular
A
B
C
A
C
A

---

56. Medial calcification is also called ____________________'s sclerosis.

MATCH THE FOLLOWING:

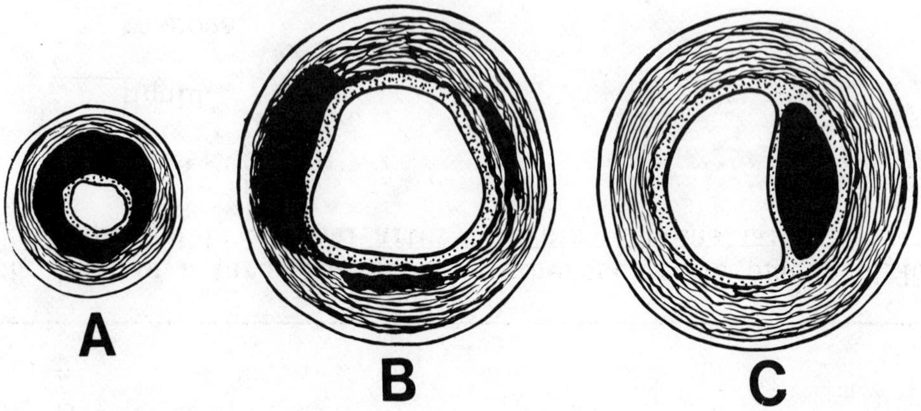

___medial calcification

___arteriolosclerosis

___atherosclerosis

---

145. ✓ capillaries
✓ arterioles

---

146. Fat would usually enter the circulation via systemic veins. Thus, the most common location of obstructive embolism would be the ☐ systemic ☐ pulmonary arterioles and capillaries.

Fat embolism usually is manifest as ☐ venous ☐ arterial embolism.

38. /✓/ increased

---

39. Systemic hypertension is associated with an increased incidence of atherosclerotic disease. The added stress on the vessel walls apparently contributes to the development of atherosclerotic plaques. Which of the following is most likely to develop atherosclerosis?

____50-year-old "normal" male

____50-year-old hypertensive male

____50-year-old hypertensive female

---

128. _✓_ solid
_✓_ bland

---

129. Emboli are also classified according to their point of origin. Emboli which arise between the systemic capillary bed and the pulmonary bed are called venous emboli. Emboli which arise between the pulmonary capillary bed and the systemic capillary bed are called arterial emboli.

CLASSIFY THE FOLLOWING SOURCES OF EMBOLI AS (A) ARTERIAL OR (V) VENOUS:

____right atrium	____pulmonary vein
____aorta	____right ventricle
____femoral vein	____left atrium

54. ✓ radial arteries
✓ temporal arteries
✓ tibial arteries

arteriosclerosis
1. atherosclerosis
2. arteriolosclerosis
3. Mönckeberg's medial calcification

---

55. Mönckeberg's sclerosis involves calcification of the ________________ layer of ☐ muscular ☐ elastic arteries of the head, neck, and extremities.

MATCH THE ARTERIES WITH THE DISEASES MOST LIKELY TO AFFECT THEM:

____aorta
____renal arterioles
____brachial artery
____renal artery
____tibial arteries
____coronary arteries

A. atherosclerosis
B. arteriolosclerosis
C. Mönckeberg's medial calcification

---

144. ☑ liquid

---

145. Because the embolic fat is fluid, the occluded vessels are very small.

Which of the following would you expect to be subject to occlusion by fat embolism?

____capillaries
____arterioles
____small arteries
____main branch arteries
____aorta

39. _✓_ 50-year-old hypertensive male

---

40. Clinical evidence suggests that hereditary factors play an important role in the development of atherosclerosis. Which of the following is/are indicative of increased chances of atherosclerotic disease?

____ family history of coronary artery disease
____ family history of stroke
____ family history of diabetes

---

129. V A
A V
V A

---

130. An embolus that arises in the venous circulation but enters the arterial side, or vice versa, is called a paradoxical embolus. Paradoxical embolism requires an arteriovenous communication or an embolus small or flexible enough to pass through pulmonary capillaries. Which of the following conditions could account for paradoxical embolism?

____ atrial septal defect
____ patent ductus arteriosus
____ pulmonary arteriovenous shunt
____ ventricular septal defect
____ patent foramen ovale
____ systemic arteriovenous fistula

53. A
B
A

---

54. The third form of hardening of the arteries involves the muscular arteries of the head, neck, and extremities. It is called Mönckeberg's sclerosis. Medial calcification is likely to affect which of the following arteries?

____radial arteries

____temporal arteries

____pulmonary arteries

____tibial arteries

____mesenteric arteries

INDICATE THE GENERIC TERM AND SUBCATEGORIES OF HARDENING AND THICKENING OF ARTERIES: ________________

1. ________________
2. ________________
3. ________________

---

143. ☑ does

---

144. Next to thrombotic embolism, fat embolism is the most common. This involves fluid fat (not cells) entering into the bloodstream and occluding small vessels.

Fat embolism is a form of ☐ solid ☐ liquid ☐ gas embolism.

40. ✓ family history of coronary artery disease
✓ family history of stroke
✓ family history of diabetes

---

41. CHECK WHICH ARE INDICATIVE OF GREATER DANGER OF ATHEROSCLEROSIS:

____ female
____ diabetic
____ low-fat diet
____ over 40
____ family history of heart disease
____ alcoholic
____ hypertensive
____ temperate climate
____ low serum cholesterol

---

130. ✓ atrial septal defect
✓ patent ductus arteriosus
✓ pulmonary arteriovenous shunt
✓ ventricular septal defect
✓ patent foramen ovale
✓ systemic arteriovenous fistula

---

131. MATCH THE FOLLOWING:

____ embolus arising in a systemic vein and lodging in a systemic artery
____ embolus arising in a systemic vein and lodging in a pulmonary artery
____ embolus arising in a systemic artery and lodging in a systemic artery
____ embolus arising in the left atrium and lodging in a systemic artery

A. arterial embolus
B. venous embolus
C. paradoxical embolus

52. B
B
A

---

53. MATCH THE ETIOLOGIC AGENTS OF ARTERIOLOSCLEROSIS ON THE RIGHT WITH THE APPROPRIATE LOCATIONS ON THE LEFT:

____renal arterioles A. hypertension

____visceral arterioles B. aging

____intrarenal arteries

---

142. ✓ renal lobar artery
✓ intracerebral artery
✓ posterior tibial artery

---

143. The effects of arterial embolism depend on the organ, size of artery, and type of circulation involved.

The location of an embolus ☐ does ☐ does not influence the seriousness of its effects.

41. ✓ diabetic
✓ over 40
✓ family history of heart disease
✓ hypertensive

---

42. INDICATE "T" TRUE OR "F" FALSE:

____ Diabetics have more atherosclerosis than non-diabetics.

____ Polyunsaturated fats in the diet raise serum cholesterol.

____ Atherosclerosis is not influenced by heredity.

____ Serum cholesterol levels have prognostic value in dealing with atherosclerosis.

---

131. C
B
A
A

---

132. An embolus will lodge at the point in its movement where the vessel diameter becomes as small as the embolus. This occurs almost exclusively in arteries.

A venous embolus will lodge in a ☐ systemic ☐ pulmonary artery.

An arterial embolus will lodge in a ☐ systemic ☐ pulmonary artery.

51. [✓] intrarenal arteries
[✓] hypertension

---

52. MATCH THE PROCESSES INVOLVED IN ARTERIOLOSCLEROSIS ON THE RIGHT WITH THE APPROPRIATE LOCATIONS ON THE LEFT:

____renal arterioles

____splenic arterioles

____intrarenal arteries

A. medial hypertrophy, intimal proliferation
B. hyaline degeneration

---

141. ✓ mural thrombus in the left ventricle
✓ vegetations on the aortic valve
✓ mural thrombus on a plaque in the aorta
✓ thrombus in the left atrium

---

142. Arterial emboli most frequently occlude arteries in the spleen, kidneys, brain, and lower extremities, though other organs may be involved.

CHECK THOSE ARTERIES WHICH ARE AMONG THE MORE COMMON SITES OF ARTERIAL EMBOLISM:

____renal lobar artery
____radial artery
____intracerebral artery
____posterior tibial artery
____coronary artery
____hepatic artery

42. T
F
F
T

---

43. A second type of hardening of the arteries, or ____________________, is called arteriolosclerosis or arteriolar sclerosis. The name suggests that this disease does not affect all arteries, but primarily ____________________.

---

132. [✓] pulmonary
[✓] systemic

---

133. Emboli arising in the splanchnic veins will be carried to the liver. Thus an embolus which arises in the splenic vein or the superior mesenteric vein will lodge in
____ a systemic artery
____ a pulmonary artery
____ either
____ neither

50. A. media (hypertrophic)
    B. (internal) elastic lamina (hyperplastic)
    C. endothelium (hyperplastic)

---

51. Hyperplasia of the elastic lamina and endothelium in hypertension may give the arteries an "onionskin" appearance in cross-section with concentric full-circumference involvement.

This "onionskin" appearance occurs in ☐ precapillary arterioles
☐ intrarenal arteries

It is associated with ☐ aging
☐ hypertension

---

140. ✓ femoral vein ✓ cavernous sinus
✓ right atrium ✓ popliteal vein

---

141. Arterial thrombotic emboli usually arise in the left heart or the aorta and lodge in systemic arteries more distal in the circulation. Which of the following are likely sources of arterial emboli?

____ mural thrombus in the left ventricle
____ vegetations on the aortic valve
____ atherosclerotic plaque in the pulmonary vein
____ mural thrombus on a plaque in the aorta
____ thrombus in the left atrium
____ thrombus in the right atrium

43. arteriosclerosis
arterioles

---

44. Arteriolosclerosis primarily affects small visceral arteries. Thus, you would expect to find it in the

____spleen	____pancreas
____legs	____arms
____kidney	____adrenals

---

133. ✓ neither. It will lodge in the portal vein, the one important exception to arteries as the usual point of impaction of emboli.

---

134. Emboli are also classified according to the type of material composing the embolus. Approximately 95% of all emboli originate as detached parts of thrombi. Thrombotic emboli are ☐ less ☐ more common than other types of emboli.

49. B A
The most characteristic lesion of hypertension is arteriolosclerosis of the kidney.

---

50. In addition to the intimal hyaline deposits in renal arterioles, hypertension produces several effects in the intrarenal arteries proximal to the arterioles. LABEL THE DIAGRAM:

hypertrophy of the muscular media
hyperplasia of the elastic lamina
hyperplasia of the endothelial lining

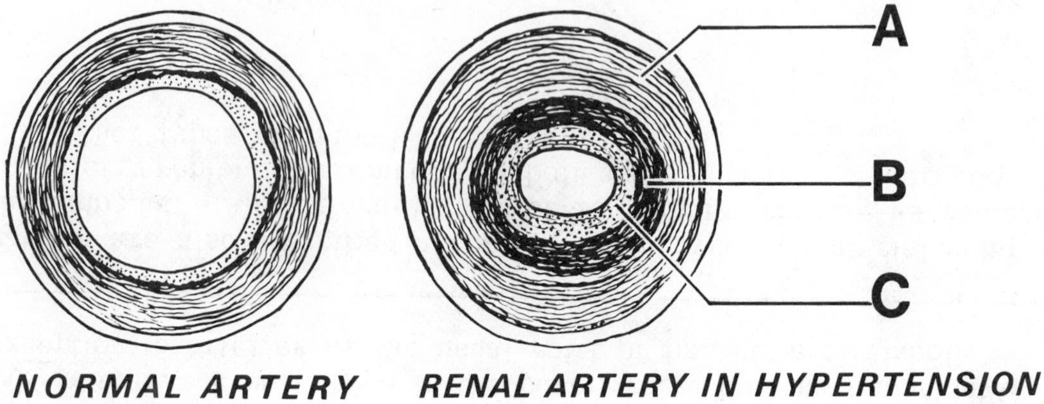

---

139. 3
2
1
[✓] most
[✓] is not

---

140. Following the leg veins in frequency as sources of venous emboli are the pelvic veins, the right atrium, right ventricle, and the cavernous sinus. Emboli from the upper extremities rarely occur naturally but are sometimes associated with the use of intravenous catheters.

INDICATE THE COMMON SOURCES OF VENOUS EMBOLI:

____femoral vein	____basilic vein
____right atrium	____cavernous sinus
____portal vein	____popliteal vein
____inferior vena cava	____renal vein

44. ✓ spleen
✓ kidney
✓ pancreas
✓ adrenals

---

45. Arteriolosclerosis generally involves focal hyaline deposits beneath the intimal layer. Under certain circumstances, however, it involves endothelial proliferation or intimal musculoelastic proliferation. This information leads you to suspect that arteriolosclerosis is

____ a single clearly defined disease process

____ at least two processes which affect the arterial intima

---

134. [✓] more

---

135. An embolus composed of agglutinated platelets, fibrin, and blood cells is a ____________ embolus. Such an embolus is all or part of a detached ____________.

48. B arteriosclerosis
A 1. atherosclerosis
B 2. arteriolosclerosis
B
B

---

49. Hypertension may contribute to arteriolosclerosis in other organs, but its most serious effect is on the kidney, where hyaline deposits may thicken the intima, replace the media, and interfere with blood flow.

MATCH THE FOLLOWING:

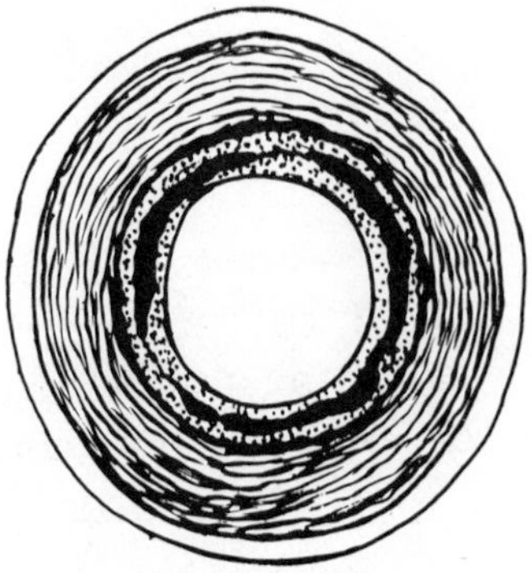
____

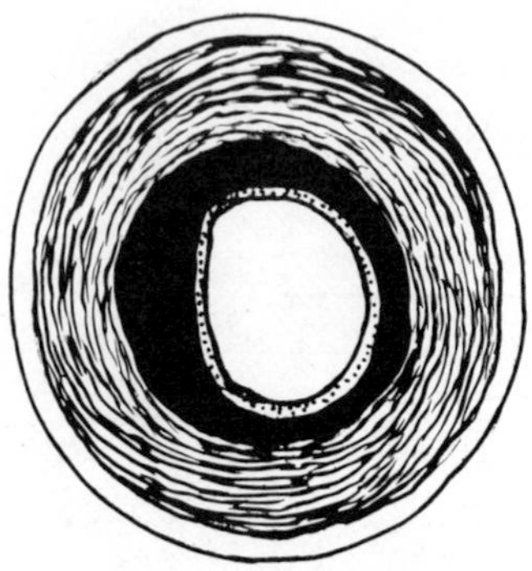
____

A. renal arteriolosclerosis related to hypertension

B. visceral arteriolosclerosis related to aging

The most characteristic lesion of hypertension is arteri_ _ _sclerosis of the ____________.

---

138. B
A
C
[✓] do not

---

139. Approximately 95% of all thrombotic venous emboli arise from thrombi in the veins of the legs. Pulmonary embolism is often the first manifestation of venous thrombosis.

ORDER THE FOLLOWING EVENTS (1, 2, 3):

____pulmonary embolism
____venous embolism
____venous thrombosis

Leg veins are the [ ] most [ ] least common source of venous emboli.

Thrombosis in leg veins often [ ] is [ ] is not symptomatic.

45. _✓_ at least two processes which affect the arterial intima

---

46. At least two etiologic factors of arteriolosclerosis are known: aging and systemic hypertension.

Which person is most likely to have arteriolosclerosis?

____60-year-old normotensive man

____60-year-old hypertensive man

____30-year-old normotensive man

---

135. thrombotic
thrombus

---

136. Thrombotic venous emboli lodge in the pulmonary artery or its branches. This results in pulmonary embolism. Obstruction of pulmonary circulation is <u>the</u> significant complication of ▱ venous ▱ arterial embolism.

47. C B A

---

48. Intimal hyaline deposits associated with aging alone are common in the spleen, pancreas, adrenals, and uterus, but are generally insignificant in the kidneys. Prolonged hypertension, however, uniformly produces serious hyaline arteriolosclerosis in the kidneys almost exclusively.

MATCH THE FOLLOWING ORGANS WITH ARTERIOLOSCLEROSIS TO THE ETIOLOGIC AGENT ASSOCIATED WITH IT:

____spleen
____kidney   A. prolonged hypertension
____uterus
____pancreas   B. aging
____adrenals

INDICATE THE GENERIC NAME AND FIRST TWO SUBCATEGORIES OF HARDENING AND THICKENING OF ARTERIES:

____

1. ________________
2. ________________
3. ________________

---

137. ✓ right heart failure
✓ sudden death
✓ decreased systemic circulation

---

138. Moderate-size pulmonary emboli may or may not result in infarction and hemorrhage. They may be silent or produce transient symptoms. Emboli in small branches of the pulmonary artery are commonly found incidentally at autopsy.

MATCH THE EVENT ON THE LEFT WITH THE POSSIBLE OUTCOME ON THE RIGHT:

____main pulmonary artery occluded by embolus

____large branch of pulmonary artery occluded by embolus

____small branch of pulmonary artery occluded by embolus

A. infarction or transient symptoms
B. death
C. no clinical consequences

Pulmonary emboli usually ☐ do ☐ do not produce pulmonary infarcts.

46. ____60-year-old hypertensive man

---

47. Thickening of the intima with connective tissue is a normal concomitant of aging. Included in the thickened intima may be focal hyaline deposits derived from mural fibrin deposits or filtered accumulations of plasma proteins.

MATCH THESE DIAGRAMS WITH THE LABELS:

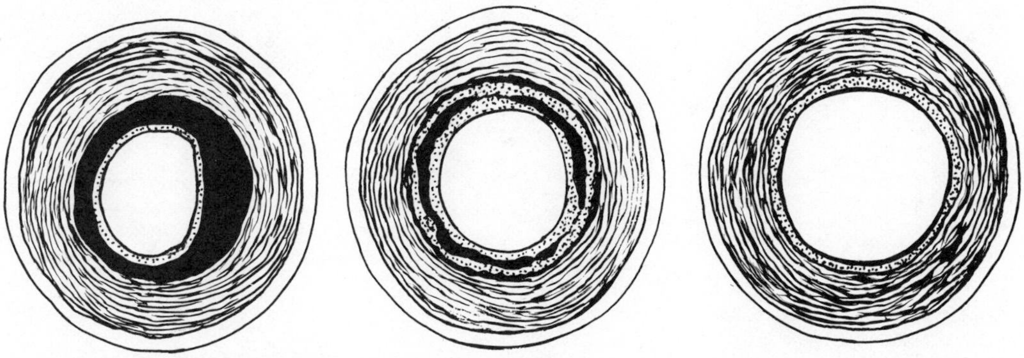

________ ________ ________

A. arteriole of a young person
B. normal arteriole of an older person
C. arteriole of older person with arteriolosclerosis

TURN TEXT 180° AND CONTINUE.

---

136. [√] venous

---

137. Massive pulmonary embolism, blocking a large part of the pulmonary circulation, may result in sudden or delayed death, probably from right heart failure and/or decreased systemic circulation.

CHECK THOSE ITEMS WHICH ARE POSSIBLE RESULTS OF MASSIVE PULMONARY EMBOLISM:

____no clinical manifestations
____right heart failure
____sudden death
____systemic hypertension
____decreased systemic circulation

TURN TEXT 180° AND CONTINUE.

Unit 12. Hemodynamic Disorders: Effects of Vascular Obstruction

Unit 12. HEMODYNAMIC DISORDERS: EFFECTS OF VASCULAR OBSTRUCTION

OBJECTIVES

When you complete this unit, you will be able to select correct responses relating to the:

	starting page	frame numbers
A. Ischemia	12.3	1-25

1. definition of hypoxia and ischemia.
2. factors which contribute to the seriousness of ischemic damage.
3. effects of partial ischemia.

B. Infarction	12.42	26-56

1. definition of infarct and infarction.
2. differences between arterial and venous infarcts and among pale infarcts, red infarcts, and gangrene in terms of:
   - causative mechanisms
   - common locations
   - morphologic appearance
   - manifestations and outcome
3. manifestations of vascular occlusion, infarcts, and vasculitis.

C. Natural History of Infarcts	12.31	57-84

1. natural history of infarcts of the heart, brain, kidney, spleen, intestine, and lung in terms of:
   - frequency
   - manifestations
   - morphology
   - mechanisms
   - complications and outcome

PRETEST

UNIT 12. HEMODYNAMIC DISORDERS: EFFECTS OF VASCULAR OBSTRUCTION

SELECT THE SINGLE BEST RESPONSE

1. Which of the following generally causes hypoxia BUT NOT ischemia?
   (A) anemia
   (B) embolism
   (C) thrombosis
   (D) atherosclerosis
   (E) external pressure occluding an artery

2. Ischemic damage is most likely with
   (A) gradual occlusion of a functional end artery
   (B) occlusion of a leg vein
   (C) moderate atherosclerosis of a coronary artery
   (D) sudden occlusion of an anastomotic artery
   (E) sudden occlusion of a functional end artery

3. The term <u>infarct</u> is best used to indicate a type of
   (A) degeneration
   (B) heart attack
   (C) lesion
   (D) process

4. Hemorrhagic infarcts are associated with
   (A) venous occlusions
   (B) organs with extensive collateral circulation
   (C) both
   (D) neither

5. All of the following may result from venous occlusion EXCEPT
   (A) wet gangrene
   (B) ischemic necrosis
   (C) anemia infarct
   (D) breakdown of hemoglobin to hemosiderin
   (E) coagulation necrosis

6. Vasculitis is characterized by
   (A) redness, heat, swelling, and pain
   (B) cyanosis, edema, and loss of sensation
   (C) pallor, coldness, and absent pulsations
   (D) dull aches and pressure tenderness

7. The natural history of cerebral infarcts is characterized by
   (A) healing by resolution and regeneration
   (B) widely varying clinical manifestations
   (C) unresolved coagulation necrosis
   (D) hemorrhage due to venous occlusion
   (E) sudden death in most instances

8. An infarct of which organ is most likely to be fatal if untreated?
   (A) bowel
   (B) heart
   (C) brain
   (D) lung
   (E) kidney

GO ON TO NEXT PAGE AND BEGIN THE UNIT.

A. Ischemia (25 frames)

When you complete this section, you will be able to select correct responses relating to the:

1. definitions of hypoxia and ischemia.
2. factors which contribute to the seriousness of ischemic damage.
3. effects of partial ischemia.

1. The obstruction of a blood vessel may decrease or stop the flow of blood to the tissues supplied by that vessel. These tissues are thus deprived of their full needs in terms of: (INDICATE THE APPROPRIATE TERMS)

____nutrients

____waste removal

____oxygen

Of these, the most immediately crucial is ________________.

1. ✓ nutrients
✓ waste removal
✓ oxygen
Of these, the most immediately crucial is oxygen.

---

2. Local or regional hypoxia due to decreased blood flow is called ischemia. Ischemia involves inadequate oxygenation of tissues (hypoxia). The inadequate oxygenation resulting from ischemia may be partial (hypoxia) or complete (anoxia).

MATCH THE FOLLOWING DEFINITIONS:

____inadequate blood flow	A. hypoxia
____inadequate oxygen supply	B. ischemia
____no oxygen supply	C. anoxia

---

43. ____ these areas are constantly exposed to bacteria

---

44. An infarct with proliferating putrefactive bacteria is called ________________.

TURN TEXT 180° AND CONTINUE.

2. B
A
C

---

3. Ischemia is not the only cause of hypoxia. For example, in anemia, the blood is deficient in red cells and may be unable to carry enough oxygen. Thus there may be ☐ ischemia ☐ hypoxia without ☐ ischemia ☐ hypoxia.

---

44. gangrene

---

45. When putrefactive bacteria proliferate in a pale infarct, as in an extremity infarcted by arterial occlusion, the result is dry gangrene. In dry gangrene of an extremity, the extremity mummifies, turns black, and eventually will slough. Most often, the toes, the foot, and the lower leg are involved by dry gangrene.

A patient presents with an edematous, cyanotic, painless foot. Is this a case of dry gangrene?

42. B
B
B

---

43. Exposure of an infarct to invasion by putrefactive bacteria may lead to gangrene. Gangrene is the invasion and proliferation of anaerobic putrefactive bacteria in dead tissue. Gangrene commonly occurs in infarcted extremities and infarcted bowel.

Gangrene occurs in extremities and in bowel infarcts because:

____these areas are supplied by functional end arteries

____the reticuloendothelial system is not well developed

____these areas are constantly exposed to bacteria

---

84. T
T
F
T
T

THIS IS THE END OF UNIT 12. TAKE THE POSTTEST ON PAGE xxxvi.

3. /✓/ hypoxia
/✓/ ischemia

---

4. Inadequate local perfusion of blood is called _____ __________.

Inadequate oxygenation of tissue, whether generalized, regional, or local, is called ________________, or ____________________.

Anemia can be a cause of /_/ ischemia /_/ hypoxia but is not a direct cause of /_/ ischemia /_/ hypoxia.

---

45. No. The symptoms are pathognomonic for venous occlusion. If it becomes gangrenous, it would be wet gangrene rather than dry gangrene.

---

46. Signs and symptoms are useful for indicating the probable site of an infarct, but often are not specific for infarcts vs. some other disease process.

Various enzymes are released into the general circulation by dying cells. Serum enzyme determinations may be useful in determining the likelihood of necrosis vs. some other process, and the types of enzymes released may suggest the type of tissue involved.

MATCH THE FOLLOWING:

____most useful to indicate whether there is necrotic tissue in the body

____useful to indicate the location of the problem

A. signs and symptoms

B. serum enzyme tests

41. A
C
B

---

42. The development of a hemorrhagic infarct is similar except for the color caused by red cells and their decomposition products. A red infarct will vary from red to black as it develops, because of the hemoglobin breakdown products present.

MATCH THE FOLLOWING:

____extensive pigment present	A. pale infarct
____can turn black	B. red infarct
____extravasated red cells	

---

83. T
T
F
T
T

---

84. INDICATE "T" TRUE OR "F" FALSE:

	frame reference
____Splenic infarcts easily go undiagnosed.	(70)
____A dense, wedge-shaped scar in the kidney would suggest an old infarct.	(68,71)
____Bowel infarction is usually not serious because of the functional reserve of the bowel.	(72)
____The fibrinolytic mechanism helps protect the lung from infarction.	(77)
____The symptoms and signs of pulmonary embolism may be very non-specific.	(80)

4. ischemia
hypoxia or anoxia
☑ hypoxia but not ☑ ischemia

---

5. The most common cause of ischemia is vascular obstruction due to intrinsic disease, such as atherosclerosis, thrombosis, or embolism. Other important but less common causes of ischemia include local vasospasm, external pressure on a vessel, and selective shunting of blood away from the vascular supply of a vessel. The ischemic effects of these mechanisms are similar to the effects of intrinsic vascular obstruction.

CLASSIFY THE EXAMPLES:

____ High doses of ergot alkaloids used for migraine headaches may produce necrosis of fingers and toes due to vascular contraction.

____ Chronic blood loss reduces the red blood cell count to one-half normal.

____ With acute blood loss, blood flow to the renal arteries is reduced more than to other visceral vessels.

____ Severe atherosclerosis of the iliac arteries reduces blood flow to the lower extremities.

____ Tissue necrosis follows the prolonged application of a tight tourniquet to the thigh.

A. intrinsic vascular obstruction

B. vasospasm

C. external pressure

D. selective shunting

E. hypoxia without ischemia

---

46. B
A, B (sometimes)

---

47. Serum glutamic oxaloacetic transaminase (SGOT), glutamic pyruvic transaminase (SGPT), lactic dehydrogenase (LDH), and creatine phosphokinase (CPK) are the most useful enzymes as an adjunct in the diagnosis of infarcts. These enzymes are released from necrotic cells and appear in the serum. Serum levels of these enzymes may be elevated for several hours to several days following development of an infarct. Not all serum enzyme changes are related to necrosis.

Which is/are true?

a. Elevated serum enzymes are diagnostic of an infarct.

b. Elevated serum enzymes are helpful in substantiating the presence of an infarct.

c. Serum alkaline phosphatase is usually elevated in infarcts.

40. ✓ necrosis without immediate loss of architecture
✓ homogeneity of cell contents

---

41. Within a week, granulation tissue will begin to form at the periphery of an infarct. Within weeks to several months, the entire infarct will have been replaced by dense scar tissue, unless the infarct is very large.

MATCH THE FOLLOWING:

____ no evident granulation tissue	A. first few days after infarction
____ dense scar tissue	B. first week through second month
____ granulation tissue forming	C. after three months

---

82. ✓ myocardial infarction
✓ pulmonary embolism

---

83. INDICATE "T" TRUE OR "F" FALSE:

	frame reference
____ Myocardial infarcts are pale and undergo coagulation necrosis.	(58)
____ An arrhythmia is a dangerous complication of a myocardial infarct.	(61)
____ Cardiac tamponade is an example of an arrhythmia.	(63)
____ Cerebral tissue undergoes liquefaction necrosis.	(66)
____ The manifestations of cerebral infarction are widely variable.	(67)

5. B
E
D
A
C

---

6. Raynaud's disease is an example of a syndrome involving ischemia resulting from vasospasm. Exposure to cold initiates a vasospastic response in the fingers, which results in ischemia, with blanching and numbness. It occurs predominantly in young women.

Which of the following may be associated with Raynaud's disease?

____ischemia

____hypoxia

____vascular obstruction

____vasospasm

The changes in Raynaud's disease are caused by /_7 a functional change /_7 organic disease within vessels.

---

47. b. elevated serum enzymes are helpful in substantiating the presence of an infarct

---

48. Edema with cyanosis is considered pathognomonic for venous occlusion. Pain and some loss of sensation and function are common also.

Which of the following sets of signs and symptoms would be adequate to diagnose venous occlusion?

____pain and loss of sensation in a hand

____cyanosis, edema, and loss of sensation in a leg

____edema and pain in a foot

39. ✓ is a tissue response to necrosis
✓ occurs around an infarct
✓ involves vascular congestion

---

40. Microscopically, an infarct in most tissues is seen to undergo coagulative necrosis. Tissue architecture remains recognizable, but the cells take on a homogeneous, eosinophilic appearance. Nuclei shrink and eventually decolorize.

Which of the following are characteristics of most infarcts?

____necrosis without immediate loss of architecture

____basophilic change

____homogeneity of cell contents

____retention of evident nuclei

---

81. B
A

---

82. If a hospitalized patient suddenly develops symptoms of chest pain and breathing distress and dies within a few minutes, the clinician is not likely to be certain of the cause of death, since the picture would easily fit both pulmonary embolism and myocardial infarction.

If the patient was ill with other pulmonary or cardiac problems, this differential diagnosis may be even more involved.

Sudden death with thoracic symptoms will suggest to the clinician (uncomplicated):

____myocardial infarction

____cerebrovascular accident

____pulmonary embolism

6. _✓_ ischemia
_✓_ hypoxia
_✓_ vasospasm
[✓] functional change

---

7. Vascular obstruction can have more or less serious effects, depending on the extent and degree of ischemia, rate of development, and the sensitivity of the cells involved. Which of the following factors would help determine the extent and degree of ischemia?

____degree of occlusion of a vessel

____size of the vessel involved

____rapidity of occlusion

____amount of collateral circulation

---

48. _✓_ cyanosis, edema, and loss of sensation in a leg

---

49. It is estimated that less than ten percent of venous thromboses result in edema, cyanosis, and stagnant anoxia, and that only a few of these will progress to infarction and gangrene.

PLACE THE FOLLOWING IN THE ORDER OF THEIR FREQUENCY OF OCCURRENCE (1, 2, 3):

____gangrene due to venous occlusion

____venous thrombosis

____edema and cyanosis

38. /✓/ hemorrhagic

---

39. After 12 to 24 hours, a pale infarct is surrounded by a red, congested area, with an inflammatory cell response beginning in the surrounding tissue.

Inflammation:

____is a tissue response to necrosis

____occurs around an infarct

____is the first visible change in an infarct

____involves vascular congestion

---

80. A
A
B

---

81. An important sign used to distinguish pulmonary embolism from some other circulatory disturbances is jugular venous pressure. In pulmonary embolism, pulmonary blood flow is impeded, and pressure backs up through the right heart to the systemic circulation. One of the most easily observed results is increased pressure in the neck veins, often with noticeable distention and pulsation. This sign is non-specific, however, since it can also be present in right heart failure of other cause. It is most useful for distinguishing pulmonary embolism from hypovolemic shock, which has some similar manifestations.

MATCH THE FOLLOWING:

____increased jugular venous pressure	A. hypovolemic shock
____low jugular venous pressure	B. pulmonary embolism

7. ✓ degree of occlusion of a vessel
✓ size of the vessel involved
✓ rapidity of occlusion
✓ amount of collateral circulation

---

8. The size of the obstructed artery determines the extent of the resulting ischemia.

MATCH THE FOLLOWING:

____ extensive ischemia	A. small artery obstructed
____ small area of ischemia	B. large artery obstructed
____ complete organ ischemia	

---

49. 3
1
2

---

50. With acute arterial occlusion, there is usually sudden severe pain, probably associated with vascular spasm following the obstructive process. In slowly developing arterial occlusion, there is often no pain.

MATCH THE FOLLOWING:

____ sudden arterial occlusion	A. little pain
____ gradual arterial occlusion	B. severe pain

37. B
A
B

---

38. Infarct literally means "stuffed with blood." The term must have been associated originally with /_/ pale /_/ hemorrhagic infarcts.

---

79. A, B
A, B
B

---

80. Pulmonary embolism is often not recognized clinically because the signs and symptoms are variable and non-specific. The "usual" symptoms of serious pulmonary embolism are sudden respiratory distress, with hyperventilation, dyspnea, tachycardia, and a subjective feeling of breathlessness and anxiety. If infarction is involved there may be hemoptysis (coughing up blood). A small infarct, on the other hand, may produce no distinct manifestations.

MATCH THE FOLLOWING:

____may cause dyspnea	A. massive pulmonary embolism
____may cause sudden death	B. minor pulmonary embolism
____may be overlooked	

8. B
A
B

---

9. An incompletely occluded vessel will not cause complete ischemia.

Which of the following obstructive processes is generally completely occlusive and thus would be expected to cause complete ischemia by itself?

____arterial embolism

____mural thrombosis

____atherosclerosis

---

50. B
A

---

51. In an extremity, arterial occlusion is generally associated with coldness, pallor, loss of pulsations, and loss of sensation. Pain may or may not be present.

Which of the following sets of signs and symptoms would indicate arterial occlusion?

____pain, heat, swelling, redness

____swelling, tenderness, cyanosis, diminished pulsations

____pallor, coldness, absent pulsations, pain

36. pale
artery

---

37. An infarct which remains filled with considerable extravasated blood is called a red, or hemorrhagic, infarct. Hemorrhagic infarcts are the rule in venous obstruction; they also may occur in arterial obstruction where there is collateral blood supply or a dual blood supply.

MATCH THE FOLLOWING:

____filled with extravasated blood	A. pale infarct
____contains little blood	B. red infarct
____caused by venous obstruction	

---

78. B
A
A

---

79. Massive pulmonary embolism will produce pulmonary hypertension and may result in death because of right heart failure or because of decreased systemic circulation. If the patient survives and repeated emboli are organized in the pulmonary arteries, the work load of the right ventricle may be greatly increased, with resulting hypertrophy.

MATCH THE FOLLOWING:

____increased work load on the right ventricle	A. acute pulmonary embolism
____pulmonary hypertension	B. residual healed embolic obstructions
____hypertrophy of the right ventricle	

9. ✓ arterial embolism

---

10. On the other hand, an occluded vessel need not cause ischemia if there is adequate collateral circulation to the area.

Which of the following conditions could involve occlusion without ischemia to the area supplied?

____area supplied only by the occluded artery

____highly anastomotic blood supply

____dual blood supply to the area

---

51. ✓ pallor, coldness, absent pulsations, pain

---

52. MATCH THE FOLLOWING SIGNS AND SYMPTOMS WITH THE CONDITIONS WITH WHICH THEY ARE ASSOCIATED:

____pallor

____cyanosis

____edema

____absent pulsations

____pain

A. arterial occlusion

B. venous occlusion

35. ✓ arterial occlusion
✓ blanching of the infarcted tissue

---

36. An infarct that becomes lighter than the surrounding tissue is called a ____________ infarct. Such an infarct is generally caused by the occlusion of a(n) ____________.

---

77. ✓ emboli are stopped by the lungs
✓ the lungs help prevent embolic damage to other tissues

---

78. It has been estimated that in a normally healthy person, fifty percent or more of the pulmonary circulation would have to be blocked before pulmonary embolism would very likely be fatal. Circulation in the remaining system can double without pulmonary arterial pressure increasing significantly or edema being produced.

MATCH THE FOLLOWING:

____ may be fatal in a healthy patient

____ mild to serious effects

____ no significant pulmonary hypertension

A. less than 50% of pulmonary circulation obstructed

B. more than 50% of pulmonary circulation obstructed

10. __✓__ highly anastomotic blood supply
__✓__ dual blood supply to the area

---

11. An end artery is one which is the sole supply to its area of distribution. Occlusion of an end artery will result in /_/ partial /_/ complete ischemia to its area of distribution. Occlusion of an end artery is likely to be /_/ insignificant /_/ damaging.

---

52. A
B
B
A
A, B (variable)

---

53. The manifestation of inflammatory processes in arteries and veins is a dull ache associated with tenderness upon pressure.

Which of the following sets of symptoms is suggestive of a vasculitis?

____stabbing pain through the left side into the left arm, with weakness and faintness

____dull, deep pain in the extremities on movement and corresponding to pulsations

____local swelling in the left forearm with pain on pressure

34. B
B
A

---

35. When an infarct is caused by occlusion of an end artery, venous blood is carried away from the area, leaving the infarct lighter in color than the surrounding viable tissue. Such an infarct is called a pale infarct. An infarct which occurs as the result of venous occlusion or an arterial occlusion where collateral circulation continues to bring blood to the area will not be pale.

A pale infarct involves:

____arterial occlusion

____extravasated blood in the infarct

____a dual blood supply

____blanching of the infarcted tissue

---

76. [√] red

---

77. A thrombotic embolus in a pulmonary artery rapidly activates the fibrinolytic mechanism, which dissolves thrombotic masses by breaking down the fibrin in them. In one study, ninety percent of pulmonary emboli disappeared within the first four hours. Lung tissue is not so sensitive that infarction is likely with less than four hours of ischemia.

The lung has been called a filter for the circulating system. This statement implies that:

____emboli pass readily through the pulmonary circulation

____emboli are stopped by the lungs

____the lungs help prevent embolic damage to other tissues

11. /✓/ complete
/✓/ damaging

---

12. Some important end arteries supply the kidney, spleen, retina, and basal ganglia in the brain.

Which of the following disorders could result from end artery obstruction, based on the examples above?

____neurologic disorders

____shortness of breath

____blindness

____hepatic insufficiency

---

53. ✓ dull, deep pain in the extremities on movement and corresponding to pulsations

---

54. MATCH THE FOLLOWING SETS OF SYMPTOMS AND SIGNS WITH THE PROBABLE DIAGNOSES:

____sudden severe pain, with loss of pulsations in a foot	A. arterial occlusion
____dull pain and tenderness in the arms and legs	B. venous occlusion
____swollen, cyanotic foot	C. vasculitis

33. B
A, B
B

---

34. The first changes to appear in an infarct are functional. Grossly visible morphologic changes may take as long as 24 hours to appear in some tissues. The first gross changes will be blanching in the infarcted area and congestion in the viable tissue bordering the infarct.

MATCH THE FOLLOWING:

____ grossly visible changes	A. earliest change
____ congested border	B. later change
____ functional changes	

---

75. ✓ It is more common than lung infarction.
✓ It is the result of venous embolism.
✓ Pulmonary emboli are often quickly dissolved.

---

76. Because the lung has a dual blood supply, if infarction occurs, the result is likely to be a ☐ pale ☐ red infarct.

12. ✓ neurologic disorders
✓ blindness

---

13. A functional end artery is one which is not the sole supplier of an area, but collateral circulation is inadequate to prevent ischemia if it is occluded suddenly. Also, occlusion of small arteries and arterioles is less likely to cause ischemia.
INDICATE THE CHARACTERISTICS WHICH APPLY TO FUNCTIONAL END ARTERIES:

____ sole supply to an area

____ some collateral circulation present

____ ischemia results if occluded suddenly

____ rich anastomotic blood supply

____ occlusion of arterioles does not produce ischemia

---

54. A
C
B

---

55. INDICATE "T" TRUE OR "F" FALSE:

	frame reference
____ An infarct is the result of ischemia.	(26)
____ Most infarcts result from arterial occlusion.	(28)
____ An infarct usually initiates an inflammatory response.	(39)
____ Most infarcted tissues undergo coagulative necrosis.	(40)
____ The extremities are one of the common sites for gangrene.	(43)

32. __✓__ abundant blood in the area but not flowing.

---

33. MATCH THE FOLLOWING:

____ stagnant anoxia	A. arterial occlusion
____ ischemia	B. venous occlusion
____ rarely leads to infarct	

---

74. __✓__ gangrene within 48 hours
__✓__ severe abdominal discomfort
__✓__ death within days if surgery is not done

---

75. While pulmonary embolism is quite common, infarction of the lung is much less common. There are two reasons for this. Most important is that the lung has a dual blood supply. Second is that the fibrinolytic mechanism is especially active in the pulmonary arteries. Where embolism is not serious enough for death to occur in a short time, a thrombotic embolus is likely to be dissolved before infarction can occur.

Which of the following are true of pulmonary embolism?

____ It is more common than lung infarction.

____ It is the result of venous embolism.

____ It generally results in death or serious disability.

____ Pulmonary emboli are often quickly dissolved.

13. ✓ some collateral circulation present
✓ ischemia results if occluded suddenly
✓ occlusion of arterioles does not produce ischemia

---

14. Functional end arteries supply the myocardium, bowel, parts of the brain, and the extremities.

Based on these examples, which of the following disorders could result from the obstruction of functional end arteries?

____renal insufficiency

____neurologic disorders

____myocardial infarct

____liver infarct

____ischemia of calf muscles

---

55. T
T
T
T
T

---

56. INDICATE "T" TRUE OR "F" FALSE:

	frame reference
____Infarction may result from arterial or venous obstruction.	(28)
____Edema commonly occurs with arterial occlusion.	(48)
____Pain is more likely in acute ischemia than chronic ischemia.	(50)
____Atherosclerosis alone is a common cause of sudden arterial occlusion.	(30)
____Vasculitis involves a dull pain or tenderness over the affected vessels.	(53)

31. [✓] rarely

---

32. Where venous obstruction leads to infarction, the mechanism of infarction is stagnant anoxia. The ischemia of venous infarcts is associated with:

____high oxygen content

____very little blood in the area involved

____abundant blood in the area but not flowing

---

73. A
B
A
A, B

---

74. Bowel infarcts are hemorrhagic even when they result from arterial occlusion, because of the anastomotic blood supply. The infarcted section of bowel first becomes red and then develops to some shade of green or black as the extravasated and stagnant blood breaks down. The infarct softens under bacterial action and will rupture unless removed surgically.

Given a patient with infarction of a segment of small bowel, which of these conditions would you expect?

____death within 2 hours

____gangrene within 48 hours

____severe abdominal discomfort

____death within days if surgery is not done

____uneventful recovery with medication only

14. ✓ neurologic disorders
✓ myocardial infarct
✓ ischemia of calf muscles

---

15. The degree of ischemia produced by vascular occlusion is also influenced by the rapidity with which the occlusion occurs. A slowly occlusive disorder may allow time for the collateral circulation to hypertrophy and take over supplying blood to the area. This process might take, at the least, several weeks.

The collateral circulation is most likely to have a chance to develop in ☐ thrombosis ☐ embolism ☐ atherosclerosis.

This process is most likely to be important if the artery involved is a(n) ☐ end artery ☐ functional end artery ☐ highly anastomotic artery.

---

56. T
F
T
F
T

C. Natural History of Infarcts (28 frames)

When you complete this section, you will be able to select correct responses relating to the:

1. natural history of infarcts of the heart, brain, kidney, spleen, intestine, and lung in terms of:
   - frequency
   - manifestations
   - morphology
   - mechanisms
   - complications and outcome

57. Myocardial infarction is a common cause of death in the U.S. The most common mechanism of infarction is arterial obstruction, usually by atherosclerosis with or without thrombosis.
Partial obstruction, usually resulting from atherosclerosis, causes ischemia and can cause infarction if there is an episodic decrease in general blood flow or an increased need of oxygen by the myocardium.

MATCH THE FOLLOWING MECHANISMS OF MYOCARDIAL INFARCTION WITH THEIR CAUSES:

____ arterial occlusion	A. atherosclerosis with increased activity (stress)
____ partial occlusion with decreased blood flow	B. atherosclerosis with thrombosis
____ partial occlusion with increased need for oxygen	C. atherosclerosis with decreased blood pressure

30. A
B
B
A

---

31. Venous obstruction must be extensive to result in infarction, as anastomotic vessels would usually carry away venous blood around an occlusion.

Venous thrombosis ☐ usually ☐ rarely results in infarction.

---

72. A, B, C
C
A
A

---

73. Bowel infarction may be the result of venous or arterial occlusion. Venous occlusion most commonly results from entrapment of bowel and its mesentery in a hernia sac or by a fibrous adhesion resulting from a previous abdominal operation. Arterial occlusion is most commonly due to atherosclerosis or embolism in the superior mesenteric artery.

MATCH THE FOLLOWING:

____ hernial strangulation	A. venous occlusion
____ thrombi dislodged from a mural thrombus in the heart	B. arterial occlusion
____ results in stagnant anoxia	
____ may cause bowel infarction	

15. [✓] atherosclerosis
[✓] functional end artery

---

16. In general, the venous system is more highly anastomotic than the arterial system. Occlusive venous thrombosis tends to be

[ ] more serious

[ ] less serious

than occlusive arterial thrombosis.

---

57. B
C
A

---

58. A myocardial infarct is generally a pale infarct of irregular shape. It may involve all or only part of the thickness of the wall. The shape and thickness of the infarct are variable because the muscle layers of the ventricles are supplied by separate branches of the coronary arteries. The areas of the myocardium most often infarcted are the wall of the left ventricle and parts of the interventricular septum.

INDICATE THOSE CHARACTERISTICS WHICH APPLY TO MYOCARDIAL INFARCTS:

____regular circular shape

____hemorrhagic

____pale

____involve right ventricle most commonly

____irregular shape

____variable thickness

29. ✓ the alternate supply will prevent ischemia in the tissues

---

30. Sudden arterial occlusion is usually due to embolism or thrombosis. Thrombosis is often associated with atherosclerotic plaques. Slow arterial occlusion is usually due to one of the arteriosclerotic processes.

MATCH THE FOLLOWING (more than one letter may apply):

____atherosclerosis without thrombosis

____thrombosis

____embolism

____arteriolosclerosis

A. slow arterial occlusion

B. rapid arterial occlusion

---

71. A, B
A, B
B, C
A, B, C

---

72. Bowel infarction is a surgical emergency and will invariably result in death if the lesion is not resected. Infarcted bowel is constantly exposed to bacteria in the intestine, leading to gangrene. Gangrenous bowel will eventually rupture, causing peritonitis and death.

MATCH THE FOLLOWING (more than one letter may apply):

____commonly fatal

____neurologic symptoms

____gangrene

____requires surgery

A. bowel infarction

B. myocardial infarction

C. cerebral infarction

16. [✓] less serious

---

17. The degree of ischemic damage also depends on the sensitivity of various cells to ischemia. In general, metabolically active cells, which require more nutrients and oxygen and produce metabolic wastes more rapidly, are more sensitive to ischemic damage.

MATCH THE FOLLOWING:

____metabolically active cell	A. not easily damaged by ischemia
____metabolically inactive cell	B. easily damaged by ischemia

---

58. _✓_ pale
_✓_ irregular shape
_✓_ variable thickness

---

59. Myocardial infarcts are often asymptomatic and diagnosed by functional changes or at autopsy by the presence of old scars. Pain is the most important clinical manifestation. When severe chest pain is associated with radiation to the left arm, it is highly suggestive of myocardial infarct. Other, less distinct pain patterns may be caused by myocardial ischemia or other diseases in other organs.

MATCH THE FOLLOWING:

____severe "heartburn" with some fatigue and weakness	A. symptoms probably due to myocardial infarction
____stabbing pain in the left chest and arm	B. symptoms possibly due to myocardial infarct
____nerve conduction defects demonstrated by electrocardiogram	C. functional evidence of myocardial injury

28. ____ prolonged hypoxia
_✓_ degenerative changes proceeding to cell death

---

29. Arterial obstruction in tissues with a dual blood supply only rarely leads to infarction. This is because

____ tissues with dual supply are probably not sensitive to ischemia

____ the alternate supply will prevent ischemia in the tissues

____ dual blood supply is the definition of an end artery, which is especially vulnerable

---

70. A
A
B
B

---

71. Renal and splenic infarcts undergo coagulation necrosis and heal by shrinkage and replacement with dense scar tissue.

MATCH THE FOLLOWING (more than one letter may apply):

____ undergoes coagulation necrosis	A. renal or splenic infarct
____ heals with dense fibrous tissue	B. myocardial infarct
____ generally a serious incident	C. cerebral infarct
____ may be unrecognized clinically	

17. B
A

---

18. Heart muscle, neurons, and kidney tubule epithelial cells are highly active metabolically. They are therefore /_/ sensitive /_/ insensitive to ischemic damage.

---

59. B
A
C

---

60. Changes in the electrical activity of the heart, associated with myocardial ischemia and infarction often are observable in the electrocardiogram (ECG). The location and size of an infarct can often be estimated. The ECG often is helpful in distinguishing an infarct from ischemia or coronary insufficiency. If you suspect a myocardial infarct in a patient, what would you recommend in order to make a diagnosis?

____aspirin

____bed rest

____electrocardiogram

____oxygen

____serum enzyme tests

27. necrotic
    B
    A

---

28. An infarct may be the result of arterial or venous occlusion, or, in some cases, of no occlusive process at all. Extended severe, local hypoxia is the only prerequisite. Most infarcts, however, are the result of ischemia caused by arterial occlusion.

INDICATE THE NECESSARY CONDITIONS FOR INFARCTION:

____thrombosis

____prolonged hypoxia

____venous occlusion

____degenerative changes proceeding to cell death

____atherosclerosis

---

69. ✓ looking for a possible extrarenal cause

---

70. Splenic infarcts may present with pain in the upper left quadrant. Splenic infarcts generally heal by replacement with fibrous tissue. Serious complications are unlikely, since the spleen is not essential to life.

MATCH THE FOLLOWING:

____myocardial infarct

____cerebral infarct

____kidney infarct

____splenic infarct

A. common cause of death

B. not directly life-threatening

18. [✓] sensitive

---

19. Gradual, partial ischemia produces degenerative changes and atrophy in the tissues supplied.

Indicate the factors involved in partial ischemia:

____hypoxia

____atrophy

____degenerative changes

____no residual circulation

____inadequate circulation

---

60. _✓_ electrocardiogram
_✓_ serum enzyme tests

---

61. Less than one-fifth of patients with myocardial infarcts die of that particular episode. The mortality rate is considerably higher, however, if cardiac arrhythmias (indicative of conduction disturbances) are present.

Which of these patients with a myocardial infarct is MOST LIKELY to die of this episode?

____symptoms were minor, infarct discovered by ECG

____moderate pain but evidence of atrioventricular conduction interference

____disabling pain, evidence of moderate-size anteroseptal infarct, but no arrhythmia

26. B
A

---

27. The process by which an infarct develops is infarction. An infarct is a localized area of ______________ tissue.

MATCH THE FOLLOWING:

____a lesion	A. infarction
____a process	B. infarct

---

68. A, B, C
A, B
C
A, B

---

69. The symptoms of renal infarct are generally mild and non-specific. Some pain and hematuria may occur. No serious complications are likely, because of the large functional reserve of the kidneys. If an embolic cause is suspected, it is more important to find and deal with this.

A suspected renal infarct should be dealt with by:

____removing the affected organ

____treating with dialysis

____looking for a possible extrarenal cause

____doing nothing

19. _✓_ hypoxia
_✓_ atrophy
_✓_ degenerative changes
_✓_ inadequate circulation

---

20. Chronic, incomplete ischemia in an extremity due to partial narrowing of the lumen of major arteries may cause atrophy of skeletal muscle, with weakness and pain on exertion (ischemic pain).

A patient complains of recurrent weakness and pain in his legs when he walks more than a block. Could this be a case of chronic ischemia?

Atrophy is often the result of ☐ partial ☐ complete ischemia due to ☐ atherosclerosis ☐ an embolus in ☐ an artery ☐ a vein.

---

61. _✓_ moderate pain but evidence of atrioventricular conduction interference

---

62. If the heart is able to carry out its function adequately following an infarct, recovery is likely. Cardiac function is compromised if the conduction system is involved or if so much of the myocardium is infarcted that adequate pumping is impossible. In the first case, serious arrhythmias result. In the second, myocardial insufficiency may lead to heart failure and shock. In either case, the prognosis is serious.

MATCH THE FOLLOWING:

____ arrhythmias

____ myocardial insufficiency

A. conduction system involved in the infarct
B. massive infarction of heart muscle
C. serious prognosis

25. T
F
T
T
T

B. Infarction (31 frames)

When you complete this section, you will be able to select correct responses relating to the:

1. definitions of infarct and infarction
2. differences between arterial and venous infarcts and among pale infarcts, red infarcts and gangrene in terms of:
   - causative mechanisms
   - common locations
   - morphologic appearance
   - manifestations and outcome
3. manifestations of vascular occlusion, infarcts, and vasculitis

26. Sudden, complete ischemia, when maintained long enough, will result in necrosis of the area involved. The necrotic area is called an infarct.

MATCH THE FOLLOWING:

____area of tissue necrosis	A. ischemia
____inadequate blood supply to tissue	B. infarct

---

67. A, B
A, B
A
B
A

---

68. Infarcts in the kidney and spleen are relatively common and rarely serious. Most often they are the result of embolism, usually derived from cardiac mural thrombi. Renal and splenic infarcts are classic pale infarcts, triangular in shape, with the narrow end pointing to the obstructed artery and the wide edge near the capsule.

MATCH THE FOLLOWING (more than one letter may apply):

____pale	A. splenic infarct
____triangular in shape	B. renal infarct
____may be immediately fatal	C. myocardial infarct
____often caused by embolus	

20. yes
[✓] partial [✓] atherosclerosis [✓] artery

---

21. In parenchymatous organs, gradual ischemia results in the loss of parenchymal cells and their replacement by fibrous or adipose tissue while stromal cells are spared.

Parenchymal cells disappear because:

____they do not receive enough oxygen

____they are more sensitive than the stromal cells

____they are destroyed by fibroblasts

____they are more active metabolically than stromal cells

---

62. A,C
B,C

---

63. As the infarcted tissue softens and is broken down by inflammatory cells, a myocardial infarct may rupture (usually about 7 to 10 days after infarction), filling the pericardium with blood. This may result in external pressure on the heart, thus preventing filling of the heart (cardiac tamponade). Rupture is an uncommon cause of death in myocardial infarction.

MATCH THE FOLLOWING:

____blood in the pericardial sac	A. hemopericardium
____fluid pressure around the heart which prevents filling	B. cardiac tamponade

24. F
F
T
T
F

---

25. INDICATE "T" TRUE OR "F" FALSE:

	frame reference
____Collateral circulation can be very important, even in functional end arteries.	(13)
____If vascular occlusion occurs rapidly, it causes less damage, in general, than if it occurs slowly.	(13)
____Very active cells are more sensitive to ischemia than inactive ones.	(17)
____In some tissues, ischemia results in selective degeneration of cells.	(19)
____Ischemic pain may result from accumulated metabolites.	(22)

---

66. A
A
B

---

67. Like myocardial infarcts, brain infarcts may be asymptomatic, may present highly suggestive findings, or may present with suggestive but non-specific findings. Asymptomatic brain infarcts are common at autopsy in old people and are normally associated with severe atherosclerosis of the cerebrovascular system.

Unlike myocardial infarcts, cerebral infarcts are usually not painful but rather are manifest by neurologic deficits. One of the most characteristic modes of presentation is hemiplegia (paralysis of one side of the body). Also, sudden death is uncommon. Death may occur within a few days if the infarct is massive or involves the respiratory center, but more often patients survive with their functional deficit (some improvement occurs as degenerating cells recover).

MATCH THE FOLLOWING:

____often occurs without patient's being aware of it
____symptoms may be highly suggestive or quite non-specific
____death may occur suddenly (before patient can be brought to the hospital)
____usually manifest by functional deficit
____usually manifest by pain

A. myocardial infarction

B. cerebral infarction

21. ✓ they do not receive enough oxygen
✓ they are more sensitive than the stromal cells
✓ they are more active metabolically than stromal cells

---

22. Ischemia can cause severe pain in the area. The pain is probably a result of irritation of nerve endings in the oxygen-starved area by accumulated acidic metabolites, notably lactic acid. Reflex vascular spasm has also been suggested as the cause of some ischemic pain.

Which of the following are possible causes of ischemic pain?

____accumulated lactic acid

____vasodilation

____vascular spasm

---

63. A
B

---

64. Within approximately three months, the infarcted myocardium will have been completely replaced by dense scar tissue.

Which of these properties will an infarct have after three months?

____contractility

____hypercellularity

____denseness

____fibrous quality

23. ✓ increased demand on the myocardium
✓ decreased perfusion of the myocardium

---

24. INDICATE "T" TRUE OR "F" FALSE:

	frame reference
____ Ischemia and anoxia are interchangeable terms.	(2)
____ Ischemia is always the result of luminal obstruction of blood vessels.	(5)
____ Atherosclerosis without thrombosis rarely causes complete obstruction.	(9)
____ Collateral circulation acts as insurance against ischemia.	(10)
____ No important organs are supplied by end arteries.	(11,12)

---

65. A, B
A, B
A, B
A, B
A, B

---

66. Infarcted brain tissue is softened and removed by phagocytic cells, leaving a fluid-filled cavity lined by glial cells. Brain tissue does not regenerate functional neurons.

MATCH THE FOLLOWING:

____ undergoes liquefaction — A. cerebral infarction

____ cavity remains — B. myocardial infarction

____ replaced by fibrous connective tissue

22. _✓_ accumulated lactic acid
_✓_ vascular spasm

---

23. Angina pectoris is an example of ischemic pain. It occurs as brief episodes of substernal pain upon inadequate perfusion of the myocardium, usually during stress. Angina would be increased by:

____increased coronary perfusion

____increased demand on the myocardium

____increased relaxation

____decreased perfusion of the myocardium

TURN TEXT 180° AND CONTINUE.

---

64. _✓_ denseness
_✓_ fibrous quality

---

65. Cerebral infarction is a common cause of death or severe disability. Brain cells are very sensitive to anoxia, and some parts of the brain are supplied by end arteries or functional end arteries. Thrombosis associated with atherosclerosis is the most common mechanism of cerebral infarction. Embolism, hemorrhage, and other disease processes can also result in brain infarction.

MATCH THE FOLLOWING:

____important cause of death — A. cerebral infarction

____often involves occlusion of functional end arteries — B. myocardial infarction

____serious disability may result

____organ very sensitive to ischemia

____maybe caused by atherosclerosis

TURN TEXT 180° AND CONTINUE.

Unit 13. Hemodynamic Disorders: Bleeding Disorders

Unit 13. HEMODYNAMIC DISORDERS: BLEEDING DISORDERS

OBJECTIVES

When you complete this unit, you will be able to select correct responses relating to the:

		starting page	frame numbers
A.	Types of Hemorrhage	13.3	1-15

1. definitions of hemorrhage, hematoma, petechia, ecchymosis, purpura
2. symptoms, signs, and laboratory abnormalities in both acute and chronic hemorrhage

B.	Causes of Hemorrhage	13.33	16-58

1. comparison of the following mechanisms of hemorrhage:

   local vessel wall lesions
   clotting (coagulation) disorders
   abnormalities of platelets
   generalized vascular defects

   in terms of:

   type of hemorrhage produced
   common sites of bleeding
   causes

C.	Outcome of Hemorrhage	13.36	59-74

1. steps in the normal hemostatic mechanisms and their roles in the control of bleeding
2. outcome of hemorrhage into tissues and body spaces

PRETEST

UNIT 13. HEMODYNAMIC DISORDERS: BLEEDING DISORDERS

SELECT THE SINGLE BEST RESPONSE:

1. Which of the following statements relating to the classification of hemorrhage is true?
   (A) Purpura is a specific type of hemorrhage.
   (B) Petechiae are larger than ecchymoses.
   (C) Hematomas are likely to result from capillary rupture.
   (D) Purpura may involve petechiae and ecchymoses.

2. Common manifestations of chronic hemorrhage include
   (A) shock
   (B) anemia
   (C) both
   (D) neither

3. Local lesions of vessels likely to be associated with chronic hemorrhage include
   (A) aneurysms
   (B) lacerations
   (C) fractures
   (D) ulcerated neoplasms

4. Hemorrhagic diathesis is by definition
   (A) a local disorder
   (B) bleeding by diapedesis
   (C) predisposing to hemorrhage
   (D) always manifest
   (E) a coagulation factor deficiency

5. A patient presents with a bleeding tendency with normal prothrombin and partial thromboplastin times, increased bleeding time, and a positive tourniquet test. The difficulty most likely involves
   (A) vitamin K deficiency
   (B) liver disease
   (C) thrombocytopenia
   (D) hypofibrinogenemia
   (E) decreased fibrinolysin

6. A patient is found to have a deficiency of prothrombin and several associated clotting factors. Likely causes of this disorder include
   (A) extensive chronic liver damage
   (B) vitamin K deficiency
   (C) both
   (D) neither

7. In the process of thrombosis, which of the following events occurs third?
   (A) platelet agglutination
   (B) plasmin activation
   (C) fibrin formation
   (D) vascular contraction

8. Red blood cells which have hemorrhaged into tissue spaces will
   (A) be mostly reabsorbed into capillaries in the area by diapedesis
   (B) undergo caseous necrosis
   (C) break down and be engulfed by macrophages
   (D) remain intact for several weeks
   (E) be engulfed by polys

GO ON TO NEXT PAGE AND BEING THE UNIT

A. Types of Hemorrhage (15 frames)

When you complete this section, you will be able to select correct responses relating to the:

1. definitions of hemorrhage, hematoma, petechia, ecchymosis, purpura

2. symptoms, signs, and laboratory abnormalities in both acute and chronic hemorrhage

1. The second major class of hemodynamic disorders has to do with blood escaping from the cardiovascular system. This type of disorder is called a _______________ disorder.

74. F
T
T
T
F
T

THIS IS THE END OF UNIT 13. TAKE THE POSTTEST ON PAGE xxxviii.

1. bleeding (hemorrhagic)

---

2. The technical term for bleeding is hemorrhage. Hemorrhage may occur in two ways: by rupture of a vessel of any size or by passage of erythrocytes through apparently unruptured vessel walls. The latter is called hemorrhage by diapedesis (literally, "putting a foot through").

   MATCH THE FOLLOWING:

   ____vessel wall is disrupted — A. rupture

   ____erythrocytes pass through intact vessel wall — B. diapedesis

37. A, B
A, B
A, B
B
A

---

38. There are other rare hemophilia-like diseases caused by genetic deficiencies of other coagulation factors. In general, all of these diseases involve persistent bleeding with minor trauma and a prolonged coagulation time. Inheritance of these is generally autosomal recessive.

MATCH THE FOLLOWING:

____autosomal recessive inheritance	A. classic hemophilia
____sex-linked recessive inheritance	B. hemophilia B
____persistent bleeding from trauma	C. hemophilia-like diseases
____plasma coagulation factor deficiency	

TURN TEXT 180° AND CONTINUE.

---

73. B
A

---

74. INDICATE "T" TRUE OR "F" FALSE:

	frame reference
____All hemorrhages, regardless of size, require medical attention.	(67)
____Hemothorax can cause respiratory problems.	(68,70)
____Hemorrhage into the trachea can cause respiratory problems.	(71)
____Cerebral hemorrhage is a serious threat to life.	(69)
____Several pigments, including melanin, are residues of hemorrhage.	(73)
____Fibrosis is a possible result of hematoma formation.	(72)

2. A
   B

---

3. The technical term for bleeding is ______________.

---

38. C
    A, B
    A, B, C
    A, B, C

---

39. Hypoprothrombinemia is almost always due to an acquired deficiency of prothrombin and related factors (V, VII, IX, X). The common manifestation is slow, oozing hemorrhage associated with trauma and involving failure of fibrin formation. Ecchymoses of the skin and bleeding from the mucous membranes in various parts of the body may occur in severe cases.

    MATCH THE FOLLOWING:

    ____massive hemorrhage — A. hypoprothrombinemia

    ____slow, oozing hemorrhage — B. hemophilia

    ____hereditary disease

    ____usually acquired

36. ✓ intractable hemorrhage on slight trauma
✓ prolonged coagulation time
✓ hemarthrosis

---

37. Hemophilia B, a very rare disease, is caused by a deficiency of factor IX (Christmas factor). Its manifestations are similar to those of classic hemophilia. Like classic hemophilia, it is inherited as a sex-linked recessive.

MATCH THE FOLLOWING (more than one letter may apply):

____sex-linked recessive inheritance	A. Hemophilia A
____involves prolonged coagulation time	B. Hemophilia B
____afflicts males primarily	
____deficiency of factor IX	
____deficiency of antihemophilic factor	

---

72. B
A
B

---

73. The debris from breakdown of extravasated red blood cells will eventually be phagocytized by reticuloendothelial cells; the pigments derived from bilirubin (hemosiderin and hematoidin) may stain the tissue for some time, as in a "black eye."

MATCH THE FOLLOWING:

____residues indicating old sites of hemorrhage	A. reticuloendothelial cells
____phagocytize the debris of extravasated blood cells after hemorrhage	B. hemosiderin and hematoidin

3. hemorrhage

---

4. Hemorrhage can be classified as capillary, venous, arterial, or cardiac, depending on its origin.

MATCH THE FOLLOWING:

EXAMPLES	ORIGIN OF HEMORRHAGE
____pulsatile spurting of blood	A. capillary
____tiny hemorrhages in any tissue	B. venous
____pericardium fills with blood	C. arterial
____rapid, non-pulsatile bleeding	D. cardiac
____oozing of blood from a gash	

---

39. B
A
B
A

---

40. Congenital hypoprothrombinemia is extremely rare. The acquired form can result from several conditions. As the prothrombin complex of factors is produced in the liver, liver disease may result in hypoprothrombinemia. Another cause is deficiency of vitamin K, which is essential to the synthesis of prothrombin and factors VII, IX, and X. A third cause is overdosage of anticoagulants (vitamin K antagonists).

MATCH THE FOLLOWING:

____vitamin K deficiency	A. congenital hypoprothrombinemia
____liver disease	B. acquired hypoprothrombinemia
____autosomal recessive inheritance	
____uncontrolled anticoagulant therapy	

35. ✓ deficiency of fibrinogen
✓ deficiency of coagulation factor VIII
✓ deficiency of prothrombin

---

36. Classic hemophilia (hemophilia A) is an uncommon hereditary deficiency of factor VIII (antihemophilic factor) which results in a defect in the formation of plasma thromboplastin. This defect is inherited as a sex-linked recessive. Manifestations include persistent hemorrhage with slight trauma and bleeding into joints, subcutaneous tissue, muscles, and the genitourinary tract. Usual laboratory findings include prolonged coagulation time and normal bleeding time. Bleeding time is a measure of capillary bleeding. In hemophilia, capillary bleeding is adequately controlled because platelet and vasoconstrictive mechanisms are intact.

INDICATE THOSE CONDITIONS ASSOCIATED WITH CLASSIC HEMOPHILIA:

____sex-linked dominant inheritance
____intractable hemorrhage on slight trauma
____deficiency of Stuart factor
____prolonged coagulation time
____hemarthrosis
____occurs equally in males and females

---

71. A
B
A, B
A

---

72. Small amounts of extravasated blood may be absorbed without causing any tissue changes. Larger masses of blood may be partially replaced by fibrous tissue. A capsule may even be formed around a large hematoma.

MATCH THE FOLLOWING:

____may become encapsulated — A. small hematoma

____may be absorbed without residual damage — B. large hematoma

____may be replaced by fibrous tissue

4. C (or D)
A
D
B
A (B,C)

---

5. Bleeding may be spontaneous or traumatic, depending on whether or not obvious trauma caused the bleeding.

MATCH THE FOLLOWING:

____ a bruise develops after a blow to the eye.	A. spontaneous bleeding
____ bleeding from the nose upon bending over	B. traumatic bleeding
____ Mr. Z suffers a ruptured spleen in a cycle accident	

---

40. B
B
A
B

---

41. Vitamin K is a fat-soluble vitamin ingested in the diet and also synthesized by intestinal bacteria. Deficiency may result from inadequate intake, inadequate intestinal biosynthesis, or inadequate absorption because of lipid digestion defects.

Which of the following conditions could result in hypoprothrombinemia because of vitamin K deficiency?

____ bile duct obstruction

____ inadequate diet

____ pancreatic disease, with deficient lipase production

____ bowel sterilization by antibiotics

34. A, B
A
A

---

35. Specific humoral factors are involved in a sequence of reactions leading to the formation of fibrin. Deficiencies or complete absence of these may result in a hemorrhagic diathesis.

Which of the following would be examples of this type of disorder?

____deficiency of fibrinogen

____deficiency of platelets

____deficiency of coagulation factor VIII

____excess of thrombin

____deficiency of prothrombin

---

70. B
A
B
A
A

---

71. Blood in the trachea or bronchi can cause death by asphyxiation due to mechanical blockage and/or bronchospasm.

MATCH THE FOLLOWING:

____hemothorax

____may cause asphyxiation

____respiratory difficulty

____atelectasis

A. blood in the pleural cavity

B. bleeding into the trachea or bronchi

5. B
   A
   B

---

6. Hemorrhage is classified as internal or external, depending on whether or not the blood is visible outside the body.

MATCH THE FOLLOWING (more than one letter may apply):

___bleeding from a cut on the hand	A. external hemorrhage
___bleeding from a ruptured mesenteric artery	B. internal hemorrhage
___bleeding into the lung, some of which leaves the body by coughing	
___bleeding into the thigh muscles	

---

41. _✓_ bile duct obstruction
    _✓_ inadequate diet
    _✓_ pancreatic disease, with deficient lipase production
    _✓_ bowel sterilization by antibiotics

---

42. Liver disease may result in a deficiency of the prothrombin complex (the vitamin K-related factors) but may also result in deficiencies in factor V and fibrinogen.

MATCH THE FOLLOWING:

___deficiency of prothrombin	A. liver disease
___deficiency of prothrombin-related factors	B. vitamin K deficiency
___deficiency of fibrinogen	
___deficiency of factor V	

33. ✓ platelet count
✓ platelet function tests

---

34. Very rarely, an excess of platelets (thrombocythemia) may be associated with a hemorrhagic diathesis, though it is more commonly associated with a thrombotic tendency. It is believed that the high concentration of platelets inhibits the production of plasma thromboplastin and thus prevents thrombin formation (or blood coagulation).

MATCH THE FOLLOWING:

____associated with hemorrhagic diathesis — A. thrombocythemia

____thrombotic tendency — B. thrombocytopenia

____inhibits production of thromboplastin

---

69. B
A

---

70. Blood in the pleural spaces will decrease the effective volume of the lung, collapsing part of the lung (atelectasis) and decreasing total ventilation.

MATCH THE FOLLOWING:

____blood in the pericardial sac — A. hemothorax

____blood in the pleural cavity — B. hemopericardium

____decreases pumping ability of the heart

____decreases ventilation

____may cause atelectasis

6. A
   B
   A, B
   B

---

7. Hemorrhages may be of varying size. Tiny hemorrhagic spots, generally from disruption of capillaries, are called petechiae. Larger blotchy areas of extravasated blood are called ecchymoses and usually result from leakage from small veins or large numbers of capillaries.

   MATCH THE FOLLOWING:

   ____blotchy hemorrhage — A. petechia

   ____tiny hemorrhagic spot — B. ecchymosis

   ____capillary hemorrhage

---

42. A, B
    A, B
    A
    A

---

43. The final important clotting factor which may lead to hemorrhagic disorders if deficient is fibrinogen. The deficiency of fibrinogen may be partial (hypofibrinogenemia) or complete (afibrinogenemia). It also may be congenital or acquired. Clotting time will be prolonged, although bleeding time may be normal.

    MATCH THE FOLLOWING (more than one letter may apply):

    ____complete lack of fibrinogen — A. hypofibrinogenemia

    ____leads to hemorrhagic problem — B. afibrinogenemia

    ____reduced amount of fibrinogen

    ____delayed clotting time

32. B
B
A

---

33. Thrombocytopathic purpura has clinical features similar to those of the thrombocytopenic purpuras. How, then, would you distinguish these diseases?

____bleeding time

____tourniquet test

____platelet count

____platelet function tests

---

68. D
C
A
B

---

69. In cerebral hemorrhage, considerable pressure may be built up because of the inability of the skull to expand.

MATCH THE FOLLOWING:

____tissues do not expand to relieve pressure

____tissues expand to relieve pressure

A. hemorrhage into soft tissues

B. hemorrhage within the skull

7. B
A
A (B)

---

8. A hematoma is a local mass of blood, usually clotted, that forms a tumor-like mass in a tissue. It is more likely than the other types to be a result of arterial rupture.

MATCH THE FOLLOWING:

____clotted blood forms a mass in the gluteus medius muscle	A. hematoma
____numerous capillary hemorrhages into the dermis	B. petechiae
____the skin appears blotchy from areas of extravasated blood	C. ecchymosis

---

43. B
A, B
A
A, B

---

44. The congenital form of fibrinogen deficiency is very rare, and its cause is unknown. The acquired form has a variety of causes, which fall into three groups: those involving faulty synthesis, those involving defibrination by disseminated intravascular coagulation, and those involving pathological fibrinolytic activity.

MATCH THE FOLLOWING (more than one letter may apply):

____fibrinogen used up in pathologic coagulation	A. faulty synthesis
____fibrinogen destroyed before it can be used	B. defibrination
____not enough fibrinogen produced	C. fibrinolysis
____acquired fibrinogen deficiency	

31. A, B, C
C
B
A

---

32. If platelets are normal in number but deficient in morphology or function, the result may be the same as in thrombocytopenia. Platelet abnormality, as distinguished from inadequate numbers of platelets, is known as thrombocytopathy or thrombasthenia.

MATCH THE FOLLOWING:

____functionally abnormal platelets	A. thrombocytopenia
____thrombasthenia	B. thrombocytopathy
____inadequate numbers of platelets	

---

67. A
B
A

---

68. Massive local hemorrhage may produce mechanical effects that interfere with normal function. This is the case in bleeding into subdural spaces, the pleural cavity, the pericardium, the trachea or bronchi, and joint spaces.

MATCH THE FOLLOWING:

____may compress the brain	A. hemothorax
____may reduce joint movement	B. hemopericardium
____may compress lung	C. hemarthrosis
____may cause cardiac tamponade	D. subdural hematoma

8. A
B
C

---

9. The term <u>purpura</u> refers to a number of conditions involving spontaneous hemorrhages of widely varying size and type.

MATCH THE FOLLOWING:

____massive blood clot in tissue spaces	A. purpura
____tiny hemorrhages	B. hematoma
____condition with varying hemorrhagic manifestations	C. petechiae

---

44. B
C
A
A, B, C

---

45. Faulty synthesis of fibrinogen is due to disease of the liver, where fibrinogen is formed.

INDICATE THOSE CONDITIONS WHICH MAY BE THE RESULT OF LIVER DISEASE:

____thrombocytopenia

____deficiency of prothrombin

____deficiency of prothrombin-related factors

____hypofibrinogenemia

30. A, B
A, B
A
A, B

---

31. The third type of thrombocytopenic purpura, thrombotic thrombocytopenic purpura, results when platelets are used up in thrombotic activity. This is a rare disease of unknown cause. It is characterized by purpura, hemolytic anemia, and neurologic manifestations of small-vessel thrombi in the brain.

MATCH THE FOLLOWING (more than one letter may apply):

____manifested by superficial hemorrhage	A. thrombotic thrombocytopenic purpura
____faulty production of platelets	B. thrombocytopenic purpura immunologic
____antibodies against platelets	C. secondary thrombocytopenic purpura
____platelets consumed by thrombotic activity	

---

66. F
T
T
F
F
T

---

67. Small, local hemorrhages are usually insignificant; however, if they involve a vital structure, such as the optic nerve or the brainstem, serious consequences may develop.

MATCH THE FOLLOWING:

____ecchymosis involving the eyelids ("black eye")	A. insignificant medically
____hemorrhage into the medulla oblongata	B. possible serious consequences
____bleeding from abrasions	

9. B
C
A

---

10. Hemorrhage may be acute or chronic. Acute hemorrhage involves the loss of relatively large amounts of blood from the cardiovascular system in a short time. Chronic hemorrhage involves continued loss of blood from the cardiovascular system over a long time.

MATCH THE FOLLOWING:

____loss of large amounts of blood

____continuing loss of blood

____occurs in a short time

A. acute hemorrhage

B. chronic hemorrhage

---

45. ✓ deficiency of prothrombin
✓ deficiency of prothrombin related factors
✓ hypofibrinogenemia

---

46. Hypofibrinogenemia as a result of defibrination occurs whenever there is diffuse intravascular clotting to use up the fibrinogen. Diffuse intravascular clotting can occur whenever tissue coagulation factors enter the bloodstream or when there is extensive endothelial damage or hemolysis.

Which of the following conditions may result in defibrination?

____severe septicemia producing extensive capillary injury

____proteolytic enzymes from snake venon causing red blood cell destruction

____incompatible transfusion with lysis of red blood cells

____amniotic fluid, which is rich in tissue thromboplastic, accidentally crosses the placenta and enters the maternal circulation at the time of childbirth

29. A
B
B
A

---

30. The laboratory abnormalities in thrombocytopenic purpura immunologic and secondary thrombocytopenic purpura are similar in the most commonly used tests. Coagulation time (a test of fibrin formation) is normal, bleeding time (a test of platelet activity) is prolonged, and platelet count is low. The tourniquet test of capillary fragility is often positive. Differential diagnosis is made on the basis of other manifestations in secondary thrombocytopenia.

MATCH THE FOLLOWING (more than one letter may apply):

____low platelet count	A. secondary thrombocytopenic purpura
____positive tourniquet test	B. thrombocytopenic purpura immunologic
____additional manifestations unrelated to platelets	
____prolonged bleeding time	

---

65. D
A
B
C

---

66. INDICATE "T" TRUE OR "F" FALSE:

	frame reference
____Local reactions to stop bleeding are extravascular in orgin.	(59)
____Platelet adherence results in the formation of a plug to close the source of bleeding.	(60,62)
____Coagulation disorders do not produce capillary hemorrhages.	(60)
____The hemostatic mechanism is synonymous with the clotting (coagulation) mechanism.	(59,60)
____Serotonin promotes the agglutination of platelets.	(63)
____Fibrinolysin is important in restoring vascular continuity after control of bleeding.	(65)

10. A, B
B
A

---

11. Massive acute hemorrhage may cause circulatory collapse and death from hypoxia to vital parts of the body. The resulting anoxia may also initiate the mechanisms of secondary hypovolemic shock, which may or may not be fatal, depending on the amount of blood loss and the rapidity and adequacy of treatment.

The immediate effects of massive acute hemorrhage primarily relate to which of the following?

____amount of fluid in the vascular system

____relative proportion of fluid and cells in the blood

____decreased oxygen supply to tissues

____clotting of blood in the vascular system (thrombosis)

---

46. all of them

---

47. The clinical picture in the defibrination syndrome (diffuse intravascular coagulation; consumption coagulopathy) includes a bleeding tendency and organ damage due to the disseminated coagulation. Brain and kidney are especially likely to be damaged. The laboratory will find delayed clotting time.

MATCH THE FOLLOWING:

____diffuse coagulation

____organ damage by tiny thrombi

____liver disease

____delayed clotting time

A. faulty fibrin synthesis

B. defibrination syndrome

28. ✓ anti-cancer drugs which kill labile cells
✓ lymphocytic leukemia
✓ massive whole-body irradiation

---

29. Platelet deficiency is sometimes the result of an immunologic mechanism involving the production of antibodies against platelets. This is now called thrombocytopenic purpura immunologic, although the old term, idiopathic thrombocytopenic purpura, is still used at times.

MATCH THE FOLLOWING:

____idiopathic thrombocytopenic purpura	A. thrombocytopenic purpura immunologic
____chemical poisoning	B. secondary thrombocytopenia
____lymphoma	
____anti-platelet antibodies	

---

64. C
A
B

---

65. A final part of the hemostatic mechanism is the role of fibrinolysin (plasmin) in dissolving the clot after it has done its job. Fibrinolysin is activated from profibrinolysin in the plasma by the presence of fibrin. Fibrinolysis may be important for reopening vascular channels which were not totally disrupted by trauma but were closed off by the hemostatic reaction.

MATCH THE FOLLOWING:

____"cleanup" after hemostatic mechanisms	A. vessel contraction
____vessel response to disruption	B. platelet adherence and agglutination
____formation of hemostatic plug	C. fibrin formation
____reinforcement and enlargement of the hemostatic plug	D. fibrinolysis

11. ✓ amount of fluid in the vascular system
✓ decreased oxygen supply to tissues

---

12. The decreased blood pressure that results from the loss of large amounts of blood will initiate a complex set of compensatory reactions which work together to increase blood pressure and blood volume. Three processes are involved: vasoconstriction, decreased renal filtration, and mobilization of fluid from the tissues into the vascular system.

MATCH THE FOLLOWING:

MECHANISMS	EFFECTS
____ vasoconstriction	A. increases blood pressure
____ decreased renal filtration	B. increases blood volume
____ mobilizing fluid into the vascular system	

---

47. B
B
A
A, B

---

48. A third cause of fibrinogen deficiency is pathologic fibrinolytic activity. Fibrinolytic activity occurs when a plasma enzyme, plasmin (fibrinolysin), is activated from its inactive form, plasminogen (profibrinolysin), by an activator present in tissue extracts (cyto-fibrinolysokinase). Plasmin lyses fibrin and also digests fibrinogen.

MATCH THE FOLLOWING:

____ lyses fibrin	A. plasmin
____ same as fibrinolysin	B. plasminogen
____ an inactive plasma enzyme	
____ digests fibrinogen	

27. A
B
A
A
B

---

28. Defective formation of platelets by bone marrow is called secondary thrombocytopenia. This can occur whenever there is extensive loss of productive marrow, either by replacement by non-productive tissue as in leukemias and lymphomas, or by damage to the marrow by drugs and chemicals, whole-body irradiation, or chronic infection.

Which of the following conditions could result in secondary thrombocytopenia?

____amputation of both legs
____anti-cancer drugs which kill labile cells
____lymphocytic leukemia
____massive whole-body irradiation

---

63. B
A
A, B

---

64. The third phase of hemostasis involves the formation of fibrin.

The initial hemostatic plug of platelets is reinforced and augmented by the formation of fibrin. This is initiated by substances released from platelets or present in the damaged tissues at the site of hemorrhage.

MATCH THE FOLLOWING:

____decreased diameter of bleeding vessel	A. platelets adhere and agglutinate
____formation of a hemostatic plug	B. fibrin formation
____blood clot added to the hemostatic plug	C. vessel contraction

12. A
B
B

---

13. The primary consideration in chronic blood loss is the depletion of iron stores, leading to an iron-deficiency anemia, and consequent systemic hypoxia when severe.

MATCH THE FOLLOWING:

____circulatory collapse	A. acute blood loss
____shock	B. chronic blood loss
____iron-deficiency anemia	

---

48. A
A
B
A

---

49. Increased plasmin activity occurs in many of the same situations as does defibrination, notably as a complication of pregnancy or of pulmonary surgery.

Pulmonary tissue, placental tissue, and amniotic fluid have a high level of fibrinolytic activity.

Which of the following facts would you expect to follow from the previous observation?

____90% of pulmonary emboli dissolve within four hours.

____Purpuric manifestations sometimes follow after pulmonary surgery.

____Amniotic fluid embolism results in fibrinolytic activity as well as defibrination.

26. B
    A
    C

---

27. The thrombocytopenic purpuras are of three basic types. Platelets may be deficient in number if not produced in adequate numbers, if destroyed by an immunologic mechanism, or if consumed in large numbers by thrombotic activity.

MATCH THE FOLLOWING:

____widespread thrombotic activity

____major surgery

____massive bone marrow destruction

____anti-platelet antibodies

____childbirth

A. thrombocytopenia

B. thrombocytosis

---

62. B
    A
    B

---

63. Another role of platelets is the release of serotonin, a vasoconstrictor which contributes to continued vascular contraction.

MATCH THE FOLLOWING:

____agglutination of platelets

____mediated by serotonin

____platelets play an important role

A. vasoconstriction

B. hemostatic plug

13. A
A
B

---

14. INDICATE "T" TRUE OR "F" FALSE:

	frame reference
____Petechiae are the result of bleeding from capillaries.	(7)
____Hematoma means bleeding into a joint capsule.	(8)
____Spontaneous hemorrhage is often the result of trauma.	(5)
____The manifestations of purpura are midway in size between petechiae and ecchymoses.	(9)
____Hemorrhage by diapedesis is a disorder of the feet.	(2)

---

49. all of them

---

50. The third type of condition associated with a hemorrhagic diathesis involves generalized vascular defects without striking derangement in blood coagulation mechanisms. These are to be distinguished from the more localized vascular defects observed in trauma and vascular diseases.

MATCH THE FOLLOWING:

____traumatic injury

____atherosclerosclerotic plaque

____capillary damage associated with septicemia

____diffuse capillary weakness due to vitamin C deficiency

A. localized vascular defect

B. generalized vascular defect

25. diathesis
platelets
clotting (or coagulation)
vessels

---

26. Several types of platelet disorders can cause a hemorrhagic diathesis. Because platelets are essential to the maintenance of capillary integrity, a deficiency of platelets (thrombocytopenia) will result in an increased likelihood of capillary hemorrhages.

MATCH THE FOLLOWING:

____pechechia

____capillary integrity maintained

____hematoma

A. normal platelet count

B. thrombocytopenia

C. large artery cut

---

61. vascular contraction
platelets
fibrin
(or equivalent)

---

62. The first phase of hemostasis is vascular smooth muscle contraction. The second phase involves the adherence of platelets to the damaged edges of the vessel. These platelets promote agglutination of more platelets (by releasing ADP) until a hemostatic plug has been formed.

MATCH THE FOLLOWING:

____formation of a hemostatic plug

____counteracts hemorrhage by decreasing diameter of the vessel

____part of the hemostatic mechanism mediated by ADP

A. vessel contraction

B. platelet adherence and agglutination

14. T
F
F
F
F

---

15. INDICATE "T" TRUE OR "F" FALSE:

	frame reference
____Internal hemorrhage could easily go undiscovered.	(5, 6, 13)
____Hematoma is a kind of cancer.	(8)
____Chronic hemorrhage is an immediate threat to life.	(13)
____The body has numerous ways of compensating for loss of blood.	(12)
____Acute hemorrhage may result in shock.	(11)

---

50. A
A
B
B

---

51. One of the generalized vascular defects is an autosomal dominant hereditary disease: hereditary hemorrhagic telangiectasia (Rendu-Osler-Weber disease). Multiple dilated venules and capillaries (telangiectases) are present in the skin and mucous membrane. The telangiectases often do not appear until the third decade of life or later. Epistaxis (nose-bleed) is the most common type of bleeding, followed by gastrointestinal hemorrhage and hemorrhage from other mucous membranes.

MATCH THE FOLLOWING:

____autosomal dominant inheritance	A. hereditary hemorrhagic telangiectasia
____sex-linked recessive inheritance	
____coagulation defect	B. hemophilia
____vascular defect	
____involves a hemorrhagic diathesis	

24. A
B
A (B)

---

25. A hemorrhagic tendency is called a hemorrhagic ______________.
Such a tendency is produced by disorders of ______________,
disorders of humoral ______________ factors, and disorders of
blood ______________.

---

60. A
B
A
B

---

61. LIST THREE FACTORS INVOLVED IN THE HEMOSTATIC MECHANISM:

____

____

____

15. T
F
F
T
T

B. Causes of Hemorrhage (43 frames)

When you complete this section, you will be able to select correct responses relating to the:

1. comparison of the following mechanisms of hemorrhage:
   local vessel wall lesions
   clotting (coagulation) disorders
   abnormalities of platelets
   generalized vascular defects

   in terms of:
   type of hemorrhage produced
   common sites of bleeding
   causes

16. Local vascular damage is a common cause of hemorrhage. On the other hand, bleeding may sometimes be due to systemic disorders involving either elements within the blood or the vascular system itself.

MATCH THE FOLLOWING:

____weakened vessel walls throughout the body	A. local lesion
____unbalanced blood clotting mechanism	B. systemic disorder
____torn vessel	

---

51. A
B
B
A
A, B

---

52. Vitamin C (ascorbic acid) is required for capillary wall integrity. A deficiency of this vitamin (scurvy) results in increased capillary fragility and bleeding manifestations.

MATCH THE FOLLOWING:

____hereditary disease	A. scurvy
____involves capillary fragility	
____nutritional deficiency	B. hereditary hemorrhagic telangiectasia
____bleeding manifestations	

23. A
B
✓ cancer of the colon
✓ cancer of the bronchus

---

24. The systemic disorders which are associated with hemorrhage are platelet abnormalities, abnormalities of the humoral coagulation factors, and disorders of the blood vessels. These produce a generalized hemorrhagic tendency, called a hemorrhagic diathesis (di-ath' e-sis).

MATCH THE FOLLOWING:

____ a generalized disorder which increases the likelihood of bleeding	A. hemorrhagic diathesis
____ the escape of blood from the vascular system at one or more locations	B. hemorrhage associated with systemic disorder
____ caused by decreased platelets, coagulation abnormalities, and generalized disorders of blood vessels	

---

59. A
B
B

---

60. Vascular contraction and platelet agglutination are sufficient to control bleeding from small vessels. Fibrin formation, the end product of the coagulation mechanism, is necessary for the body to control bleeding from large vessels.

MATCH THE FOLLOWING:

____ bleeding may occur from small vessels	A. platelet deficiency
____ bleeding will not occur from small vessels	B. coagulation defect
____ likely to produce petechiae	
____ likely to produce hematomas	

16. B
B
A

---

17. Local vascular damage may be the result of physical trauma or may occur spontaneously as a result of various disease processes.

CLASSIFY THE FOLLOWING CAUSES OF HEMORRHAGE AS RELATING TO "T" TRAUMA OR "D" DISEASE:

____stab wound	____aneurysm
____lacerations	____fracture
____arteriosclerosis	____abrasions
____contusions	

---

52. B
A, B
A
A, B

---

53. Anaphylactoid purpura (Schönlein-Henoch purpura) is an allergic disorder which involves a purpura secondary to alterations of the small blood vessels. This purpura is distinguished from other allergic purpuras by the presence of gastrointestinal symptoms, joint symptoms, and renal involvement.

MATCH THE FOLLOWING:

____Schönlein-Henoch purpura	A. vitamin C deficiency
____scurvy	B. anaphylactoid purpura
____immunologic reaction	

22. B
A
A, B

---

23. Hemorrhage may also result from the erosion of blood vessels by ulcers or neoplasms. Neoplasms on surfaces of body passageways are most likely to cause serious blood loss, because there is no tissue pressure to control the bleeding.

MATCH THE FOLLOWING:

____occur on surface of body passageways by definition — A. ulcers
____occur in many locations but are particularly likely to bleed when on surface of body passageway — B. neoplasms

Which of the following neoplasms are likely to cause anemia because of hemorrhage?

____cancer of the colon
____cancer of the thyroid
____cancer of the bronchus
____cancer of bone

---

58. T
T
F
F
T
T

C. Outcome of Hemorrhage (16 frames)

When you complete this section, you will be able to select correct responses relating to the:

1. steps in the normal hemostatic mechanisms and their roles in the control of bleeding
2. outcome of hemorrhage into tissues and body spaces

59. Three factors are involved in the control of bleeding from injured blood vessels: Smooth muscle contraction results in narrowing and retraction of the injured vessel; platelets accumulate at the site of injury to the vessel; and fibrin is formed when needed.

MATCH THE FOLLOWING:

____smooth muscle contraction in vessels
____platelets
____fibrin

A. narrow(s) lumen of vessel
B. plug(s) lumen of vessel

17. T stab wound
T lacerations
D arteriosclerosis
T contusions

D(T) aneurysm
T fracture
T abrasions

---

18. Physical trauma can result in discontinuity of vessels and extravasation of blood. The seriousness of the resulting hemorrhage depends on the size and type of vessel involved and the rapidity with which intrinsic hemostatic mechanisms (or external intervention, in the case of large vessels) bring the bleeding to a stop.

Which of the following are characteristics usually associated with traumatic hemorrhage?

___ Hemorrhage follows immediately upon the trauma.

___ Seriousness varies greatly.

___ The result is chronic hemorrhage.

___ Natural hemostatic mechanisms are activated to control the bleeding.

---

53. B
A
B

---

54. The sensitizing agent in Schönlein-Henoch purpura can be a variety of things but is commonly bacteria (especially streptococci) or certain foods. The body's pathologic immunologic response to these agents damages the small blood vessels.

MATCH THE FOLLOWING:

___ involves a continuing hemorrhagic diathesis due to structural defect

___ can be initiated by bacterial infection

___ can be caused by dietary deficiency

___ inherited disorder

A. anaphylactoid purpura

B. hereditary hemorrhagic telangiectasia

C. scurvy

21. A, B
A
B

---

22. Seven to ten days following myocardial infarction, the necrotic wall of the heart may rupture and cause massive hemorrhage into the pericardium. This distention of the pericardium with blood is called hemopericardium. The resulting external pressure on the heart, preventing normal pumping action, is cardiac tamponade. Cardiac tamponade is almost always fatal.

MATCH THE FOLLOWING:

____external pressure interferes with the heart's action	A. hemopericardium
____blood in the pericardial sack	B. cardiac tamponade
____could be caused by a stab wound	

---

57. F
T
T
F
T

---

58. INDICATE "T" TRUE OR "F" FALSE:

	frame reference
____Vitamin K is essential for elaboration of certain clotting factors.	(40)
____Hypofibrinogenemia results in prolonged clotting time.	(43)
____Defibrination is the result of liver disease.	(46)
____Fibrinolysis and defibrination are two words for the same thing.	(46, 48)
____Plasmin is responsible for dissolution of fibrin and fibrinogen.	(48)
____Lack of vitamin C can lead to bleeding disorders.	(52)

18. ✓ Hemorrhage follows immediately.
✓ Seriousness varies greatly.
✓ Natural hemostatic mechanisms are activated.

---

19. The walls of atherosclerotic vessels are generally brittle and therefore more subject to rupture by ordinary body movements, changes in blood pressure, or trauma to the weakened vessel.

MATCH THE FOLLOWING:

____may be due to trauma	A. traumatic bleeding
____may seem spontaneous	B. hemorrhage from vascular lesions due to disease
____likely to be external	

---

54. B
A
C
B

---

55. Finally, generalized vascular damage may lead to purpura when there is a direct toxic effect on the endothelium from anoxia, chemicals, or septicemia.

MATCH THE FOLLOWING:

____anoxia	A. toxic purpura
____septicemia	B. anaphylactoid purpura
____may involve bacteria	

20. ✓ often associated with cerebral hemorrhage
✓ generally involve the circle of Willis

---

21. Aneurysms of the thoracic and abdominal aorta are the second most common type of aneurysm. These may develop from syphilitic mesaortitis, atherosclerosis, or intimal defects. At least three-fourths of people with aortic aneurysms die from rupture and hemorrhage within 5 years of diagnosis.

MATCH THE FOLLOWING:

____a common cause of death by hemorrhage

____leads to subarachnoid hemorrhage

____may follow atherosclerotic lesions

A. berry aneurysm

B. aortic aneurysm

---

56. F
T
F
T
F
F

---

57. INDICATE "T" TRUE OR "F" FALSE:

	frame reference
____Secondary thrombocytopenia is a deficiency of secondary thrombocytes.	(28)
____Thrombotic thrombocytopenic purpura involves excessive coagulation and hemorrhage.	(31)
____Classic hemophilia occurs more often in males than females.	(36)
____All the defects in coagulation factors are sex-linked.	(38)
____Liver disease can cause coagulation defects.	(40, 42)

19. A, B
B
A

---

20. Aneurysms are a common cause of hemorrhage. Berry aneurysms of the cerebral arteries (especially the anterior half of the circle of Willis at the base of the brain) are the most common type of aneurysm. Rupture of these aneurysms is the most common cause of subarachnoid hemorrhage and is frequently fatal.

INDICATE THOSE QUALITIES ASSOCIATED WITH BLEEDING FROM BERRY ANEURYSMS:

____usually innocuous

____often associated with cerebral hemorrhage

____generally involve the circle of Willis

TURN TEXT 180° AND CONTINUE.

---

55. A
A
A, B

---

56. INDICATE "T" TRUE OR "F" FALSE:

	frame reference
____Physical trauma results in a systemic hemorrhagic diathesis.	(17, 18, 24)
____External intervention may be required to stop bleeding from a large artery.	(18)
____The most common aneurysms are aortic aneurysms.	(20)
____Aortic aneurysms are generally fatal if untreated.	(21)
____Cardiac tamponade is a kind of arrhythmia.	(22)
____A hemorrhagic diathesis is a kind of surgical procedure.	(24)

TURN TEXT 180° AND CONTINUE.

Unit 14. Hemodynamic Disorders: Derangements of Blood Flow

Unit 14. HEMODYNAMIC DISORDERS: DERANGEMENTS OF BLOOD FLOW

OBJECTIVES

When you complete this unit, you will be able to select correct responses relating to the:

	starting page	frame numbers
A. Shock	14.3	1-44

1. distinctions between hypotension and shock
2. distinctions among the following types of shock in terms of definition, mechanisms, and common causes:
   - cardiogenic shock
   - hypovolemic shock
   - normovolemic shock
   - hemorrhagic shock
   - neurogenic shock
   - anaphylactic shock
   - septic shock
   - irreversible shock
3. structural and functional effects of shock and their mechanisms

	starting page	frame numbers
B. Heart Failure	14.16	45-74

1. distinction between acute and chronic and between left-sided and right-sided heart failure in terms of structural and functional changes

	starting page	frame numbers
C. Edema	14.52	75-97

1. mechanisms of edema formation in lymphatic obstruction, venous obstruction or stasis, vascular injury, and altered osmotic pressure

PRETEST

UNIT 14. HEMODYNAMIC DISORDERS: DERANGEMENTS OF BLOOD FLOW

SELECT THE SINGLE BEST RESPONSE:

1. NECESSARY conditions for the existence of shock include
   (A) hypovolemia
   (B) loss of tone in peripheral vasculature
   (C) inadequate perfusion of tissues
   (D) myocardial depression
   (E) bleeding

2. Pooling or sequestration of blood in the vascular system is characteristic of which type(s) of shock?
   (A) neurogenic
   (B) anaphylactic
   (C) both
   (D) neither

3. Which type of shock is almost always reversible?
   (A) septic
   (B) hypovolemic
   (C) neurogenic
   (D) anaphylactic

4. Features of profound shock include
   (A) massive edema
   (B) slow pulse rate
   (C) slow, deep respirations
   (D) urinary urgency
   (E) acidosis

5. A feature of acute left-sided heart failure is
   (A) centrilobular necrosis of the liver
   (B) hemosiderin-laden alveolar macrophages
   (C) pitting, dependent edema
   (D) alveolar transudation
   (E) left ventricle hypertrophy

6. Lesions descriptive of left-sided heart failure include
   (A) centrilobular congestion of the liver
   (B) hemosiderin-laden macrophages in pulmonary alveoli
   (C) both
   (D) neither

7. Which of the following pairs of mechanisms of edema both usually produce transudates rather than exudates?
   (A) increased capillary permeability and lymphatic obstruction
   (B) salt and water overload and hypoproteinemia
   (C) inflammation and heart failure
   (D) lymphatic obstruction and increased venous pressure
   (E) increased venous pressure and increased capillary permeability

8. The nephrotic syndrome results in
   (A) lymphedema
   (B) inflammatory edema
   (C) edema due to altered plasma osmotic pressure
   (D) edema due to increased capillary hydrostatic pressure

GO ON TO NEXT PAGE AND BEGIN THE UNIT

A. <u>Shock</u> (44 frames)

When you complete this section, you will be able to select correct responses relating to the:

1. distinctions between hypotension and shock
2. distinctions among the following types of shock in terms of definition, mechanisms, and common causes:
   - cardiogenic shock
   - hypovolemic shock
   - normovolemic shock
   - hemorrhagic shock
   - neurogenic shock
   - anaphylactic shock
   - septic shock
   - irreversible shock
3. structural and functional effects of shock and their mechanisms

1. Under some circumstances, arterial blood pressure may drop below the normal range. This is called hypotension, and may be due to a decrease in blood volume, a decrease in peripheral resistance, or a decrease in work done by the heart. Hypotension may or may not involve inadequate perfusion and tissue damage. Which of the following situations may directly produce hypotension?

____massive hemorrhage
____extensive atherosclerosis
____peripheral vasodilation
____myocardial damage
____hyperemia

1. ✓ massive hemorrhage
✓ peripheral vasodilation
✓ myocardial damage

---

2. A patient sometimes has blackouts upon standing from a sitting position He is told that his compensatory reflexes are not responding efficiently. The blackouts are from ☐ hypoxia, ☐ congestion, ☐ infarction of the brain, and are caused by ☐ hypertension ☐ hypotension ☐ acrophobia.

---

49. B
A
C

---

50. If these compensatory mechanisms fail to maintain adequate cardiac output, a state of cardiac decompensation exists. Clinical heart failure is present only when decompensation exists.

MATCH THE FOLLOWING:

____compensatory mechanisms fail to maintain adequate cardiac output

____compensatory mechanisms succeed in maintaining adequate cardiac output

A. cardiac compensation

B. cardiac decompensation

TURN TEXT 180° AND CONTINUE.

---

97. T
T
T
T
T
T

THIS IS THE END OF UNIT 14. TAKE THE POSTTEST ON PAGE xl.

2. [√] hypoxia
[√] hypotension

---

3. Hypotension can produce inadequate perfusion of tissues, especially the brain. Syncope (fainting) is a salutary response in many instances, since adequate perfusion may be restored when the brain is on the same level as the heart rather than above it.

MATCH THE FOLLOWING:

____may result from hypotension

____may lead to syncope

____may result from syncope

A. inadequate perfusion of brain

B. adequate perfusion of brain

---

50. B
A

---

51. The term acute heart failure is used to express several degrees of acuteness of onset or severity of heart failure.

MATCH THE FOLLOWING EXAMPLES OF ACUTE HEART FAILURE WITH THEIR NAMES:

____sudden permanent cessation of heart-beat due to cardiac conduction defect

____acute myocardial injury, resulting in inability to maintain normal blood pressure

____an episode of stress or injury to the heart produces increased pulmonary pressure, resulting in transudation of fluid into pulmonary alveoli with acute respiratory distress

A. cardiogenic shock

B. cardiac death

C. acute pulmonary edema

48. Heart failure is the inability of the heart to maintain normal circulation to meet the body's needs (or equivalent).
Shock is a condition of acutely reduced blood flow and inadequate perfusion of tissues (or equivalent).

---

49. The body will attempt to compensate for the inadequate cardiac output. The most important adjustments are increased heart rate, cardiac dilatation, and cardiac hypertrophy. When these adjustments maintain adequate output, a state of compensation is achieved.

MATCH THE FOLLOWING COMPENSATORY MECHANISMS WITH THEIR EFFECTS:

____increased stroke volume	A. increased heart rate
____increased stroke rate	B. cardiac dilatation
____increased force of contraction	C. cardiac hypertrophy

---

96. F
T
T
F
F
F

---

97. INDICATE "T" TRUE OR "F" FALSE:

	frame reference
____Inflammatory edema is a result of increased capillary permeability.	(86, 88)
____Liver disease may cause altered plasma osmotic pressure.	(84)
____The nephrotic syndrome causes edema primarily because of loss of protein.	(85)
____Increased capillary permeability involves the movement of excess protein into the tissues.	(86)
____Elephantiasis is a manifestation of obstruction of lymphatics.	(91)
____Aldosterone promotes the active reabsorption of sodium.	(94)

3. A
A
B

---

4. Hypotension may lead to shock, a condition in which there is an acute reduction of blood flow and an inadequate perfusion of the tissues. Shock involves hypotension, but the reverse is not necessarily true.

MATCH THE FOLLOWING (use only one response for each item):

____reduced arterial blood pressure	A. hypotension
____acutely reduced blood flow and inadequate tissue perfusion with anoxia	B. shock
____a physical finding	
____a disease condition	

---

51. B
A
C

---

52. Chronic heart failure is gradual in onset, is of milder degree than acute heart failure, often fluctuates in severity, and is always characterized by elevated venous pressure.

MATCH THE FOLLOWING:

____a very unstable condition which must lead to improvement or death	A. acute heart failure
____may be stabilized with suboptimal perfusion	B. chronic heart failure
____severe pulmonary edema	
____pulmonary congestion with variable edema	
____gradual onset	
____rapid onset	

47. A
B
B
B
A

---

48. Heart failure is ______________________________

____.

Shock is ______________________________________

____.

---

95. all of them

---

96. INDICATE "T" TRUE OR "F" FALSE:

	frame reference
____Edema involves an increased volume of intracellular fluid.	(75)
____Capillary endothelium is freely permeable to electrolytes.	(77)
____Albumin is important in maintaining fluid homeostasis.	(83)
____Normal lymph contains no proteins.	(79)
____Decreased capillary pressure will result in edema.	(81)
____Cardiac failure lowers the plasma osmotic pressure.	(81)

4. A
B
A
B

---

5. A systemic circulatory derangement in which there is an acutely reduced perfusion of tissues with consequent anoxia is ______________. Low arterial blood pressure with or without adequate tissue perfusion is called ________________.

---

52. A
B
A
B
B
A

---

53. The manifestations of congestive heart failure vary depending on the severity of passive venous congestion in the pulmonary and systemic veins. Left-sided heart failure is heart failure with manifestations associated with passive congestion of the pulmonary veins. Right-sided heart failure is heart failure with manifestations associated with passive congestion of the systemic veins.

INDICATE THE LESIONS THAT MIGHT BE DUE TO (L) LEFT-SIDED HEART FAILURE AND TO (R) RIGHT-SIDED HEART FAILURE:

____distention of jugular veins
____pulmonary edema
____centrilobular congestion of the liver
____edema of the ankles

46. B
A
B
A

---

47. The term congestive heart failure derives from the fact that the characteristic elevation of blood pressure results in venous congestion in various parts of the body. The term heart failure is often used to refer particularly to congestive heart failure.

MATCH THE FOLLOWING:

____acute reduction in blood flow and inadequate perfusion of tissues	A. shock
____inability to maintain normal circulatory dynamics and to meet demands of the body	B. heart failure
____often subacute or chronic	
____passive congestion of veins	
____severely defective tissue perfusion	

---

94. A
A
B

---

95. Sodium and water retention occurs in a variety of clinical conditions, including congestive heart failure, hepatic cirrhosis and the nephrotic syndrome. It is likely that this mechanism is a secondary cause of edema in these conditions, since each involves other mechanisms which may result in edema.

In cardiac failure, for example, which of the following mechanisms of edema may be involved?

____increased capillary hydrostatic pressure due to increased venous pressure
____increased capillary permeability due to anoxic damage
____decreased glomerular filtration because of decreased renal blood flow
____increased aldosterone secretion because of decreased renal blood flow

5. shock
hypotension

---

6. STATE IN YOUR OWN WORDS THE DIFFERENCES BETWEEN HYPOTENSION AND SHOCK.

____

____

____

____

____

____

---

53. R
L
R
R

---

54. Heart failure with manifestations associated with tissues supplied by systemic veins is called ________ -sided heart failure.

Heart failure with manifestations associated with tissues supplied by pulmonary veins is called ________ -sided heart failure.

45. B
A

---

46. Most forms of heart failure are "stabilized," with circulation maintained at a suboptimal level with altered circulatory dynamics and inability to respond to all of the needs of the body. The principal equilibrating force is a rise in venous pressure. Venous pressure rises to the level that will increase cardiac filling and effective contraction to the point where cardiac output maintains circulation.

MATCH THE FOLLOWING:

____characterized by hypotension	A. heart failure in general
____characterized by increased venous pressure	B. cardiogenic shock
____immediately life-threatening	
____may reach a state of equilibrium with suboptimal circulation	

---

93. R
E
E
R
E

---

94. Aldosterone is a hormone secreted by the adrenal cortex under the influence of angiotensin. Aldosterone acts on the kidney tubule, causing it to reabsorb sodium (and water) and secrete potassium. Aldosterone is present in increased amounts in cases of congestive heart failure, hepatic cirrhosis, and the nephrotic syndrome, though it is not known exactly why this is so. Aldosterone seems to be a mechanism involved in edema formation in heart, kidney, and liver diseases. Other mechanisms which may be involved in the retention of sodium and water are a decreased glomerular filtration rate and increased secretion of antidiuretic hormone.

MATCH THE FOLLOWING:

____aldosterone	A. fluid actively reabsorbed by tubules
____antidiuretic hormone	B. filtration decreased, resulting in less fluid loss
____lowered glomerular fluid flow	

6. Hypotension is a physical finding--a decreased blood pressure.
In addition to decreased blood pressure, shock is characterized by decreased blood flow and inadequate perfusion of tissues, with tissue anoxia (or equivalent).

---

7. The mechanisms of shock are basically the same as the mechanisms of hypotension and can be diagrammed as follows:

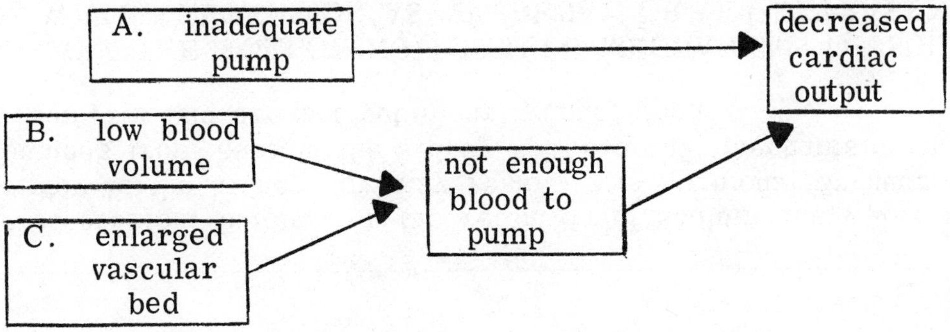

CLASSIFY THE MECHANISMS (A, B, OR C) OF THESE CLASSIC CAUSES OF SHOCK:

____severe fright, with pooling of blood in splanchnic bed

____severe blood loss following injury

____an extensive myocardial infarction

---

54. right
left

---

55. Either the right heart or the left heart may fail. In either case, the dominant clinical manifestations of heart failure are associated with the effects of elevated venous pressure.

MATCH THE FOLLOWING:

____elevated pulmonary venous pressure	A. right-heart failure
____elevated systemic venous pressure	B. left-heart failure

44. T
T
T
F
F
T

B. Heart Failure (30 frames)

When you complete this section, you will be able to select correct responses relating to the:

1. distinction between acute and chronic and between left-sided and right-sided heart failure in terms of structural and functional changes

45. The heart may function inadequately without producing the profound immediately life-threatening failure of function exemplified by cardiogenic shock. In the broad sense, heart failure is the inability of the heart to maintain the normal circulatory dynamics and to meet the demands of the body.

MATCH THE FOLLOWING:

____pumping failure manifest by falling blood pressure	A. heart failure in general
____inadequate pumping of variable severity	B. cardiogenic shock

---

92. A
B

---

93. The mechanism involved in the retention of sodium and water may be intrinsic to the kidney or may result from hormonal or neural influences from outside the kidney. The actual mechanisms involved are complex and are not yet clearly understood.

CLASSIFY THE FOLLOWING POSSIBLE MECHANISMS OF SODIUM AND WATER RETENTION AS "R" RENAL OR "E" EXTRARENAL IN ORIGIN:

____decreased glomerular filtration rate
____decreased inactivation of aldosterone by the liver
____increased secretion of antidiuretic hormone
____enhanced tubular reabsorption of sodium
____hypersecretion of aldosterone

7. C
B
A

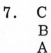

8. FILL IN THE BOXES WITH THE THREE BASIC MECHANISMS LEADING TO SHOCK:

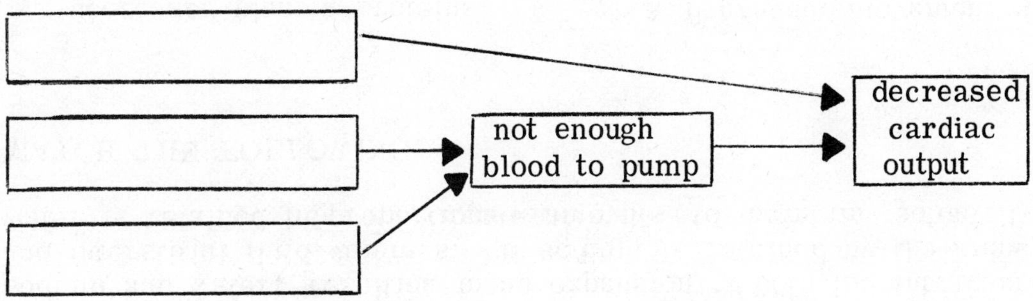

---

55. B
A

---

56. When the left heart is failing, pulmonary venous pressure is elevated. The manifestations of this condition are associated with the passive congestion and edema of the lungs. In severe cases of left-sided heart failure, pulmonary arterial pressure may also be elevated and right-sided heart failure may follow.

MATCH THE FOLLOWING:

____ may be secondary to the failure of the other side of the heart	A. right-sided heart failure
____ results in elevation of pulmonary venous pressure	B. left-sided heart failure
____ manifested by difficulty breathing (dyspnea) and liquid-air bubbles (rales) heard in the lung bases	

43. T
F
F
T
T
T

---

44. INDICATE "T" TRUE OR "F" FALSE:

	frame reference
____Tissue anoxia may accentuate the basic circulatory disorders in shock.	(24)
____Peripheral vasoconstriction and increased heart rate are compensatory changes in shock.	(26)
____Angiotensin and catecholamines are vasoconstrictive agents.	(28, 29)
____Irreversible shock is fatal about three-fourths of the time.	(33)
____Shock often results in a metabolic alkalosis.	(39)
____The kidney is the most commonly damaged organ in shock.	(41)

---

91. B
B
A

---

92. A final important cause of edema is the progressive retention of sodium and water, resulting in an expansion of both the intravascular and interstitial fluid volumes. If sodium is retained by the kidney, water is retained in proportionate amounts to maintain isotonicity.

MATCH THE FOLLOWING:

____decreased plasma proteins	A. decreased movement of water out of extracellular fluid
____increased renal retention of sodium and water	B. increased movement of water into extracellular fluid

8. inadequate pump

low blood volume

enlarged vascular bed

---

9. FILL IN THE BOXES:

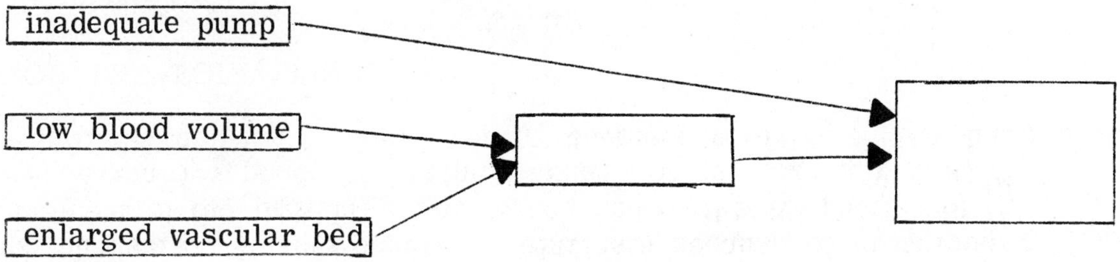

---

56. A
B
B

---

57. The physiology of congestive heart failure is actually more complex than simple passive congestion. There is usually some degree of inadequate perfusion of tissue, which adds to the injury in areas of severe congestion, and secondary changes with salt and water retention add to the volume overload.

This unit will not deal extensively with these complex physiologic changes but rather will emphasize the lesions and major functional changes associated with passive congestion.

The effects of heart failure ☐ are ☐ are not simply due to passive congestion.

The morphologic lesions of heart failure ☐ can ☐ cannot be associated with congestion of the pulmonary and systemic veins.

42. B is in shock.

---

43. INDICATE "T" TRUE OR "F" FALSE :

	frame reference
____Shock generally involves hypotension.	(4)
____Hypotension is a pathognomonic sign of shock.	(4)
____Neurogenic shock is a result of damage to the myocardium.	(14)
____Cardiogenic shock may be a form of normovolemic shock.	(12)
____Blood volume may decrease because of dehydration.	(18)
____Compensatory changes in shock may result in a return to normal circulation.	(33)

---

90. B
A
A, B
A, B

---

91. Lymphedema may result from the excision of regional lymph nodes, as is done in a radical mastectomy, or from tumor infiltration into lymph channels. It also occurs in filariasis because of inflammatory involvement of the inguinal lymph nodes and of the lymphatics of the lower extremities produced by the filarial worms. In filariasis, the legs and scrotum can become greatly distended with lymph (elephantiasis).

MATCH THE FOLLOWING:

____filariasis

____tumor invasion

____radical mastectomy

A. excision of lymph nodes

B. obstruction of lymphatic channels

9. | not enough blood to pump | | decreased cardiac output |

---

10. MATCH THE FOLLOWING:

Causes of Shock	Mechanisms of Shock
____extensive blood loss due to hemorrhage	A. inadequate pump
____acute failure in myocardial contraction	B. low blood volume
____pooling of blood in peripheral vessels	C. enlarged vascular bed
____serious dehydration from diarrhea	

---

57. [✓] are not
[✓] can

---

58. Acute left-heart failure may present with dyspnea (difficulty breathing) or orthopnea (difficulty breathing in a reclining position) and rales (sounds heard in the chest due to air-liquid mixing in alveoli).

MATCH THE MANIFESTATIONS OF ACUTE LEFT-HEART FAILURE WITH THEIR CAUSES:

____dyspnea	A. increased pulmonary venous pressure with edema formation
____orthopnea	
____shock	B. decreased systemic circulation
____lung rales	

41. A
B

---

42. The patient in shock generally presents with these manifestations: weakness, pallor, cold moist skin, shallow respiration, rapid weak pulse, hypotension, and oliguria. Advanced shock may involve apathy, stupor, and coma, and may result in death.

Which of the following patients is/are in shock?

A is flushed, feverish, and incoherent, and has a rapid pulse, labored breathing, and general malaise.

B is pale and cold-skinned, and has a rapid weak pulse, shallow respiration, and general weakness.

C has a rapid pulse, weakness, and shooting pains from the sternum into the left arm.

---

89. A
B
A, B
A, B
A, B

---

90. A fourth cause of edema is obstruction of lymphatic channels. When this normal channel for the removal of interstitial fluid and proteins is obstructed or otherwise inadequate, the fluid collects in the tissues. This condition is called lymphedema and is a basically localized condition. The edema fluid in lymphedema is high in protein.

MATCH THE FOLLOWING:

____results from increased capillary permeability	A. lymphedema
____results from lymphatic obstruction	B. inflammatory edema
____a local form of edema	
____high protein content in edema fluid	

10. B
A
C
B

---

11. LIST THREE MECHANISMS OF SHOCK:

____

____

____

---

58. A
A
B
A

---

59. The morphologic changes of left-heart failure are in the lungs and pleural spaces. Passive congestion is the dilation of veins and capillaries due to the increased venous pressure. Edema involves the transudation of fluid into the alveolar spaces of the lungs, also because of the increased pressure. Pleural effusion (also called hydrothorax) involves the transudation of fluid into the pleural spaces because of increased venous pressure in capillaries of the pleura. "Heart-failure cells," which may be present after a period of chronic heart failure, are macrophages filled with hemosiderin from broken-down extravasated red cells.

MATCH THE FOLLOWING WITH MOST DIRECT CAUSE:

____ pulmonary congestion	A. increased venous pressure
____ pulmonary edema	B. transudation of fluid
____ pleural effusion	C. extravasation of blood with phagocytosis
____ "heart-failure cells"	

40. A
A
B
B

---

41. The kidney is especially likely to be damaged in shock. Reduced perfusion, along with the resulting tubular degeneration, results in renal insufficiency with oliguria (decreased urine output) or anuria (no urine output) and retention of nitrogenous wastes.

MATCH THE FOLLOWING:

Effects	Causes
____tubular degeneration	A. hypoxia
____elevated blood urea nitrogen	B. reduced urine formation

---

88. C
A, B
A, B

---

89. Edema associated with inflammation is usually localized to the area of inflammation. More generalized release of histamine due to allergic mechanisms or sometimes to neurogenic stimuli may produce edema in multiple sites, such as skin, intestine, and respiratory tract. The latter type of edema is called angioneurotic edema, and the wheals on the skin are called urticaria or hives.

MATCH THE FOLLOWING:

____local edema at site of injury	A. inflammatory edema
____may involve skin, intestine, and respiratory tract	B. angioneurotic edema
____may be caused by histamine release	
____involves increased capillary permeability	
____exudate rather than transudate	

11. inadequate pump
low blood volume
enlarged vascular bed

---

12. Cardiogenic shock is shock due to inadequate pumping action by the heart itself.

Hypovolemic shock is shock due to low blood volume.

Normovolemic shock is shock associated with normal blood volume. The term is usually used to describe shock due to an enlarged vascular bed, but it also may include cardiogenic shock.

MATCH THE FOLLOWING (more than one letter may apply):

Cause of Shock	Type of Shock
____severe toxic myocarditis	A. cardiogenic shock
____prolonged exposure to hot sunlight, with voluminous sweating	B. hypovolemic shock
____massive bleeding from duodenal ulcer	C. normovolemic shock
____severe emotional situation	

---

59. A
B
B
C

---

60. Right-sided heart failure is usually the result of left-sided heart failure, but it may occur alone. Right-sided heart failure raises systemic venous pressure, resulting in venous congestion and edema in various parts of the system. Subcutaneous edema (especially in the lower extremities), hydrothorax (secondary to congestion of the parietal pleura), generalized venous congestion, and cyanosis are among the manifestations of right-sided heart failure.

MATCH THE FOLLOWING:

____involves lung parenchyma	A. right-sided heart failure
____primarily involves organs other than lung	B. left-sided heart failure
____may produce pleural effusion (hydrothorax)	
____commonly leads to the other of the two	

39. B
A
B

---

40. The morphologic changes in shock are also the result of decreased oxygen availability. Degeneration and necrosis occur especially in parenchymatous organs. Congestion, edema, and petechial hemorrhages sometimes occur in various places because of damaged capillaries.

CLASSIFY THE FOLLOWING EFFECTS OF SHOCK:

Effects	Causes
____centrilobular necrosis of the liver	A. inadequate oxygenation tissues
____tubular necrosis of the kidney	
____pulmonary congestion and edema	B. capillary damage
____petechiae on the serosa of body cavities	

---

87. A, B
C
C
A, B

---

88. Local edema is a component of the inflammatory response. Capillary and venule permeability is increased by chemical mediators, histamine, and the plasma kinins. Inflammatory edema results from infections, burns, allergic reactions, irritation, and mechanical injury.

MATCH THE FOLLOWING (more than one letter may apply):

____passes into tissue spaces in edema	A. histamine
____increases capillary permeability	B. plasma kinins
____released or activated by tissue damage	C. albumin

12. A,C
B
B
C

---

13. Cardiogenic shock is ________________________________.

Hypovolemic shock is ________________________________.

Normovolemic shock is ________________________________.

Hypovolemic and normovolemic shock ☐ are ☐ are not mutually exclusive situations.

Normovolemic and cardiogenic shock ☐ are ☐ are not mutually exclusive situations.

---

60. B
A
A, B
B

---

61. The effects of right-heart failure are due to elevated venous pressure in the systemic veins and occur throughout the body (excluding the lungs, unless the left heart is also involved). Generalized effects of this increased pressure include venous congestion, edema, and cyanosis. Venous congestion causes cyanosis, a blue-to-purple appearance of the skin due to deoxygenated blood in superficial vessels. It also causes distinct changes in parenchymatous organs such as the liver and spleen. Edema may be generalized but is most noticeable in subcutaneous tissues, especially in dependent parts of the body. Pitting edema refers to the observation that pressure on edematous tissues produces an indentation which does not disappear immediately.

MATCH THE FOLLOWING:

____cyanosis	A. right-heart failure
____venous congestion	
____edema	B. left-heart failure
____pitting edema	

38. A
B
A

---

39. The metabolic disturbances of shock are the effects on cellular activity of a decreased availability of oxygen. One important effect is a shift from aerobic to anaerobic metabolism, with a resultant increase in acidic products (lactate, pyruvate) and a systemic metabolic acidosis.

MATCH THE FOLLOWING:

____anaerobic metabolism
____aerobic metabolism
____acidic products

A. normal oxygen availability
B. inadequate oxygen availability

---

86. A
A (B)
A
B

---

87. Edema due to increased capillary permeability is most often due to local inflammation, but may be systemic due to generalized capillary damage. The edema fluid in these conditions is high in proteins (an exudate).

MATCH THE FOLLOWING (more than one letter may apply):

____usually systemic or regional
____usually localized
____edema fluid with high protein content
____edema fluid with low protein content

A. increased capillary hydrostatic pressure
B. decreased plasma osmotic pressure
C. vascular injury

13. Cardiogenic shock is shock due to inadequate pumping action of the heart itself.
Hypovolemic shock is shock due to low blood volume. (or equivalent)
Normovolemic shock is shock associated with normal blood volume.
[✓] are
[✓] are not

---

14. Hemorrhagic shock is a subtype of hypovolemic shock in which the low blood volume is due to bleeding.

Neurogenic shock is a subtype of non-cardiogenic normovolemic shock due to functional changes in the nervous mediation of the peripheral vascular bed. By common parlance, "functional" in this context means not associated with structural change.

MATCH THE FOLLOWING:

____ due to a structural lesion
____ not due to a structural lesion
____ associated with extensive myocardial infarction
____ low blood volume
____ enlarged vascular bed

A. hemorrhagic shock
B. neurogenic shock
C. both A and B
D. neither A nor B

---

61. A
A, B
A, B
A

---

62. Venous congestion due to right-heart failure has distinctive morphologic effects on the liver. In the liver, congestion is most prominent in the centrilobular areas (around the central veins). When chronic, the centrilobular congestion is often so severe and so distinctly demonstrated that a neophyte may mistakenly call it hemorrhage. In severe prolonged heart failure, centrilobular degeneration and atrophy due to necrosis often accompany this congestion. The changes are called chronic passive congestion of the liver. The speckled appearance resembles a nutmeg, hence the name "nutmeg" liver.

MATCH THE FOLLOWING:

____ small yellow liver, with necrosis rimmed by fatty metamorphosis at center of each lobule
____ slightly enlarged red liver, with blood-filled vessels and sinusoids but no necrosis or distinct demarcation
____ slightly enlarged liver, with small dark red areas intertwined with light areas, and packed red cells centrilobularly, with degeneration and hemosiderin pigment
____ an irregular area of blood dissecting through the liver associated with trauma

A. acute passive congestion of liver
B. chronic passive congestion of liver
C. hemorrhage in liver
D. carbon tetrachloride poisoning

37. A
B

---

38. Numerous other, more complex explanations have been offered for the progression of shock to irreversibility. In general, anoxia is the causative factor and some effect on the microvasculature is the important precipitating factor in the progression of shock.

MATCH THE FOLLOWING:

____anoxic damage to microvasculature A. reduces venous return primarily

____depression of the myocardium B. reduces cardiac output primarily

____depression of the vasomotor center

---

85. 4
5
1
2
3

---

86. A third cause of edema is increased capillary permeability. Agents which damage capillary endothelium will allow proteins to pass into the interstitial fluid. This decreases plasma osmotic pressure, increases tissue osmotic pressure, and prevents the return of fluid to the vascular system. If lymphatic channels are unable to carry off the excess fluid, edema results.

MATCH THE FOLLOWING:

____endothelial damage A. inflammation

____increased lymph volume B. hypoproteinuria

____protein leak into tissue at site of edema formation

____protein does not leak into tissue at site of edema formation

14. A
B
D
A
B

---

15. Neurogenic shock is also called primary shock, because it is not secondary to (or due to) any structural change. However, neurogenic or primary shock may be associated with injuries. For example, a person injured in a car accident may go into shock due to "fright."

MATCH THE FOLLOWING:

____ initial reaction to severe injury which usually improves rapidly	A. neurogenic shock
____ more delayed reaction to injury which may lead to death if untreated	B. hemorrhagic shock
____ primary functional disorder	

---

62. D
A
B
C

---

63. The congestive effects of right-heart failure may be exacerbated by salt and water retention mediated through the kidney. At least two mechanisms are involved. Decreased renal blood flow decreases the glomerular filtration rate. Decreased renal flow also activates the renin-angiotensin-aldosterone system, which results (through the effects of aldosterone on renal tubules) in increased retention of sodium and water.

Congestive heart failure is associated with

☐ increased ☐ decreased fluid reaching renal tubules

☐ increased ☐ decreased sodium excretion

☐ increased ☐ decreased glomerular filtration rate

☐ increased ☐ decreased aldosterone secretion

36. A (B)
B

---

37. Some investigators consider cerebral ischemia an important factor in irreversible shock. Cerebral ischemia would involve the vasomotor center, which, if depressed, would cause dilatation of the peripheral circulation and accentuation of the inadequate venous return and cardiac output. Again, a vicious cycle is obvious.

MATCH THE FOLLOWING:

____reduces circulation primarily by reducing venous return	A. depression of vasomotor center
____reduces circulation primarily by reducing cardiac output	B. depression of myocardium

---

84. osmotic
[✓] decreased
[✓] into the tissues
[✓] generalized
[✓] transudate

---

85. The nephrotic syndrome is a clinical state characterized by proteinuria, hypoproteinemia, and edema. It involves increased glomerular capillary permeability. Protein which passes into the glomerular filtrate is not reabsorbed by the tubules and is lost in the urine.

ORDER (1, 2, 3, 4, 5) THE FOLLOWING EVENTS IN THE NEPHROTIC SYNDROME:

____decreased plasma osmotic pressure

____edema

____increased glomerular capillary permeability

____proteinuria

____hypoproteinemia

15. A
B
A

---

16. Primary (neurogenic) shock may occur following trauma or may result from pain of various sorts, or from strong emotional responses. It is generally transient and not a serious threat to health or life.

Primary shock involves a ______________ stimulus resulting in the ______________ of splanchnic vessels and a(n) ______________ in venous return to the heart.

---

63. [✓] decreased fluid reaching renal tubules
[✓] decreased sodium excretion
[✓] decreased glomerular filtration rate
[✓] increased aldosterone secretion

---

64. When both sides of the heart are failing, the salient clinical features usually are associated with right-sided failure. These are pitting edema of the lower extremities, passive congestion and enlargement of the liver and spleen, and, in severe cases, generalized cyanosis.

INDICATE THE TYPE OF HEART FAILURE PRIMARILY RESPONSIBLE FOR EACH OF THE FOLLOWING:

____dyspnea, orthopnea

____ankle edema, enlarged liver and spleen

____cyanosis

____hydrothorax

A. left-sided heart failure

B. right-sided heart failure

C. either right- or left-sided heart failure

35. B
A

---

36. Another mechanism which may be involved in irreversible shock is depression of the myocardium because of the decreased perfusion and resulting myocardial ischemia. The effect is to reduce further blood pressure and flow to the body. The vicious cycle involved is obvious.

MATCH THE FOLLOWING:

____causes reduced cardiac output	A. depression of the myocardium
____causes reduced effective blood volume	B. anoxic damage to capillaries

---

83. B
A
A

---

84. Serious liver dysfunction can decrease the production of albumin, resulting in hypoproteinemia. If this is serious enough, edema will result. The edema fluid in hypoproteinemia is low in proteins, unlike some other types of edema.

Hypoproteinemia results in edema because the plasma ________ pressure is ☐ increased ☐ decreased, resulting in a net movement of fluid ☐ into the tissues ☐ into the plasma. The edema in this case would be ☐ local ☐ generalized. The edema fluid is a ☐ transudate ☐ exudate.

16. Primary shock involves a neurogenic stimulus resulting in the dilation (dilatation) of splanchnic vessels and a(n) decrease in venous return to the heart.

---

17. Secondary shock (or true shock) is a more serious disorder and often tends toward progressive circulatory failure, tissue damage, and death.

MATCH THE FOLLOWING:

____a transient disorder — A. primary shock

____a serious disorder — B. secondary shock

____progressive circulatory failure

____temporarily reduced perfusion

____may be fatal

---

64. A
B
B
C

---

65. Because the manifestations of heart failure are so closely tied up with venous congestion and its effects, the clinical syndrome is often referred to as ______________ heart failure.

34. A
B
B
A
A

---

35. Anoxic damage to capillaries and other small vessels may result in vasodilation and/or increased permeability. Either of these effects will reduce the effective circulating blood volume and accentuate the conditions which precipitated shock in the first place.

MATCH THE FOLLOWING:

____decreases actual blood volume	A. vasodilation
____decreases venous return because of peripheral pooling	B. increased permeability

---

82. A
B
A
[✓] transudate

---

83. Edema may result from a decrease in plasma osmotic pressure. The important osmotically active elements in the plasma are proteins, especially albumin. With inadequate albumin present, the osmotic pressure of the plasma will not draw enough fluid back into the capillaries. The net fluid loss to the interstitium leads to edema. Decreased plasma proteins may result from inadequate synthesis by the liver or from loss of proteins through the kidney, intestine, or skin.

MATCH THE FOLLOWING:

____glomerulonephritis	A. inadequate production of plasma proteins
____hepatic cirrhosis	B. loss of proteins through the kidney
____malnutrition	

17. A
B
B
A
B

---

18. When shock results from a decrease in actual blood volume, this may have several causes: loss of whole blood from the site of a wound or operation; loss of plasma from a burn site; loss of fluid by vomiting, diarrhea, or sweating; or escape of fluid into the interstitial compartment due to widespread increase in vascular permeability.

Which of the following are examples of decrease in actual blood volume which may result in shock?

____ massive embolism
____ massive bleeding from a duodenal ulcer
____ cholera, with massive diarrhea and vomiting
____ intravascular infection
____ prolonged exposure to hot sun, with voluminous sweating

---

65. congestive

---

66. The causation of heart failure may be outlined as follows:

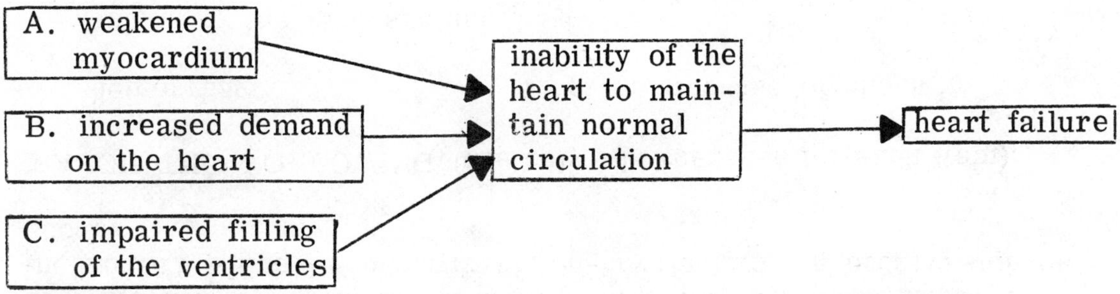

CLASSIFY THE FOLLOWING CAUSES OF HEART FAILURE (A, B, or C FROM ABOVE):

____ cardiac tamponade
____ systemic hypertension
____ myocardial infarct
____ myocarditis
____ pulmonary embolism

33. B
A
A
B

---

34. The pathologic circulatory changes in shock are maintained and augmented by the anoxia they produce. Anoxic damage to tissues is the factor which must explain the progress of shock to irreversibility, but the exact mechanism is unknown. The most likely possibilities are anoxic damage to the microcirculatory system, the myocardium, and the vasomotor center. These are the factors which introduce a vicious cycle into the progression of shock.

MATCH THE FOLLOWING (use only one response for each item):

____hemorrhage	A. original cause of shock
____anoxia of the myocardium	
____anoxia of capillaries	B. possible cause of irreversibility in shock
____septicemia	
____myocardial infarction	

---

81. B
A
A
C

---

82. Increased capillary blood pressure--and the resulting edema--may be localized or generalized, depending on the cause.

CLASSIFY THE FOLLOWING TYPES OF EDEMA:

____venous thrombosis	A. localized edema
____right-heart failure	B. generalized edema
____postural edema	

The edema fluid due to increased capillary hydrostatic pressure is a ▱ transudate ▱ exudate.

18. ✓ massive bleeding from a duodenal ulcer
✓ cholera, with massive diarrhea and vomiting
✓ prolonged exposure to hot sun, with voluminous sweating

---

19. Cardiogenic shock may be due to
1) filling defects, as in cardiac tamponade, where external pressure prevents the proper filling of the atria.
2) emptying defects, as in myocardial insufficiency due to massive infarction, or diffuse myocarditis.
3) acute mechanical obstructions, such as an embolus occluding the right ventricle, which prevent both filling and emptying.

CLASSIFY THE FOLLOWING EXAMPLES OF CAUSES OF CARDIOGENIC SHOCK:

____ myocardial infarction

____ massive venous embolism or air embolism

____ cardiac tamponade

A. filling defect

B. emptying defect

---

66. C A
B B and/or C
A

---

67. INDICATE THE TYPES OF CAUSES OF HEART FAILURE:

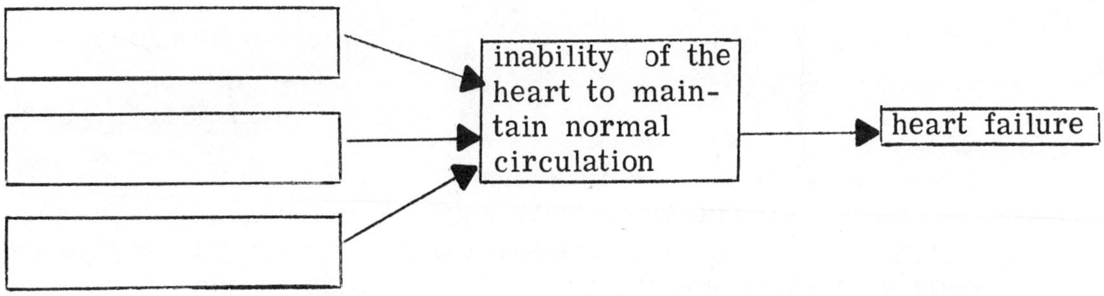

32. A
A, B
B

---

33. In some patients, if the original cause of shock has been controlled, the compensatory mechanisms may reestablish adequate circulation and the patient recovers. This is reversible shock. In other cases, the circulation degenerates to the point where no kind of treatment will restore adequate circulation, and the patient deteriorates and dies. This is irreversible shock.

MATCH THE FOLLOWING:

____compensation fails	A. reversible shock
____compensation succeeds	B. irreversible shock
____may result in recovery	
____follows a fatal course	

---

80. ✓ increased capillary hydrostatic pressure
✓ increased capillary permeability

---

81. Capillary hydrostatic pressure higher than normal overpowers the osmotic attraction of fluid back into the capillaries. Edema results. The most common cause of increased capillary hydrostatic pressure is elevated venous pressure. Elevated venous pressure can result from venous obstruction, cardiac failure, or gravitational effects related to posture. The edema fluid due to increased capillary pressure is low in proteins (a transudate).

CLASSIFY THE FOLLOWING CAUSES OF INCREASED CAPILLARY PRESSURE:

____inadequate cardiac output after myocardial infarction	A. venous obstruction
____thrombosis of the femoral vein	B. heart failure
____pressure of a pregnant uterus on the inferior vena cava	C. gravitational effect
____ankle edema because of incompetent valves in leg veins associated with varicose veins	

19. B
A, B
A

---

20. An example of secondary non-cardiogenic normovolemic shock that deserves special mention is anaphylactic shock.

Anaphylactic shock is an allergic reaction in which massive releases of histamine or histamine-like substances produce shock due to vasodilation and pooling of blood in the vascular system.

MATCH THE FOLLOWING (more than one letter may apply):

____normovolemic	A. anaphylactic shock
____primary shock	B. neurogenic shock
____treatment primarily directed toward vasoconstriction	C. cardiogenic shock
____treatment should be directed toward hemostasis	D. hemorrhagic shock
____treatment should be directed toward improved cardiac contraction	

67.

weakened myocardium

increased demand

impaired filling of the ventricles

---

68. Heart muscle which is weakened beyond the level of its functional reserve results in inadequate pumping, especially under stress conditions. One or both sides of the heart may be weakened, depending on the nature of the process involved.

MATCH THE FOLLOWING:

CAUSE	MECHANISM
____myocarditis	A. heart failure brought on by weakened myocardium
____prolonged systemic hypertension	B. heart failure brought on by increased demands on the heart
____myocardial infarct	
____too much fluid transfused into the vascular system	

31. A
A
A, B

---

32. MATCH THE FOLLOWING:

____secretion of catecholamines

____renin-angiotensin-aldosterone system

____secretion of antidiuretic hormone

A. mechanism tending to increase blood pressure

B. mechanism tending to increase blood volume

---

79. B
A

---

80. Net movement of fluid between the plasma and the interstitial fluid will result from changes in any of the factors involved in homeostasis. Important among these are: an increase in capillary hydrostatic pressure, a decrease in plasma osmotic pressure, an increase in capillary permeability, and obstruction of lymphatic channels. A fifth cause of edema is the retention of sodium and water, expanding both the interstitial and intravascular fluid volumes.

Which of the following will cause edema?

____increased capillary hydrostatic pressure

____increased plasma osmotic pressure

____increased capillary permeability

20. A,B,C
B
A,B
D
C

---

21. Anaphylactic shock may be triggered by a variety of agents to which a patient has been previously sensitized, such as drugs (most commonly penicillin), bee stings, inhalants and certain foods. It may be lethal. Adrenalin (epinephrine), a powerful vasoconstrictor, is useful in treatment and should be readily available to susceptible persons.

MATCH THE FOLLOWING (more than one letter may apply):

____primary shock
____secondary shock
____usually innocuous
____may be life-threatening
____normovolemic
____hypovolemic

A. anaphylactic shock
B. neurogenic shock
C. hemorrhagic shock

---

68. A
B
A
B

---

69. Mechanical overload of the heart by increased pumping demand on it may lead to heart failure. The overload may involve undue resistance to ejection, or conditions which demand increased cardiac output.

MATCH THE FOLLOWING CAUSES OF MYOCARDIAL OVERLOAD WITH THEIR MECHANISM:

____aortic stenosis (narrowing of aortic valve)
____massive pulmonary embolism
____systemic hypertension
____aortic insufficiency (failure of aortic valve to prevent reflux)
____arteriovenous fistula (shunting of blood from artery to vein)

A. resistance to ejection
B. demand for increased output

30. B
A
A

---

31. When there is hypovolemia, another set of mechanisms attempts to restore blood volume. These mechanisms include the increased secretion of aldosterone (stimulated by angiotensin) and antidiuretic hormone, both of which influence kidney tubules to retain fluid. Another mechanism, arteriolar vasoconstriction, lowers capillary pressure, resulting in fluid movement into the plasma throughout the body, AND decreases the glomerular filtration rate, thus conserving fluid volume.

MATCH THE FOLLOWING (more than one letter may apply):

____aldosterone	A. mechanism operative on the kidney to restore blood volume
____antidiuretic hormone	
____arteriolar vasoconstriction	B. mechanism operative outside the kidney

---

78. water
electrolytes
proteins
☑ higher
☑ lower

---

79. Not quite all of the fluid which leaves the capillaries is able to return to them. The lymphatic vessels allow the drainage of this fluid from the tissues, along with proteins that have entered the interstitial fluid, and return this fluid to the venous system. The net movement of fluid between plasma and interstitial fluid should be zero. If there is net movement of fluid from the plasma to the interstitial compartment, the result is edema.

MATCH THE FOLLOWING:

____positive net movement of fluid between plasma and interstitium	A. homeostasis
____no net movement of fluid between plasma and interstitium	B. edema formation

21. B
A,C
B
A,C
A,B
C

---

22. Septic shock is shock associated with bacteremia. The exact mechanisms of septic shock are poorly understood. Many instances of septic shock are attributed to bacterial endotoxin because shock is found more frequently with bacteremia due to gram-negative organisms which contain endotoxin in their cell walls and because intravenous injection of endotoxin will produce shock.

Septic shock is a form of :

____cardiogenic shock

____hypovolemic shock

____normovolemic shock

---

69. A
A
A
B
B

---

70. The conditions which increase the work load of the heart and thus lead to heart failure are often limited initially to either the pulmonary or systemic circulation, and thus the heart failure produced is primarily left- or right-sided.

MATCH THE FOLLOWING CAUSES OF HEART OVERLOAD WITH THE TYPE OF HEART FAILURE THEY WILL PRODUCE:

____congenitally narrowed aortic valve
____pulmonary embolism
____incompetent mitral valve (allows regurgitation)
____incompetent pulmonic valve
____systemic hypertension

A. left-heart failure

B. right-heart failure

29. ✓ increased arterial pressure
✓ increased functional blood volume
✓ decreased capillary pressure

---

30. The compensatory vasoconstriction affects primarily the skin and abdominal organs, thus in effect redistributing the blood flow to the heart and brain, which are more immediately vital for life.

MATCH THE FOLLOWING:

____ decreased perfusion of the brain	A. compensatory vasoconstriction in shock
____ increased perfusion of the brain	B. circulatory changes of shock
____ decreased perfusion of skin	

---

77. A
B

---

78. The capillary endothelium allows the free passage of ____________ and ______________ but not ____________.

Plasma at the arterial end of a capillary has a ☐ higher ☐ lower hydrostatic pressure and a ☐ higher ☐ lower concentration of osmotically active particles than plasma at the venous end of the capillary.

22. _✓_ normovolemic shock

23.

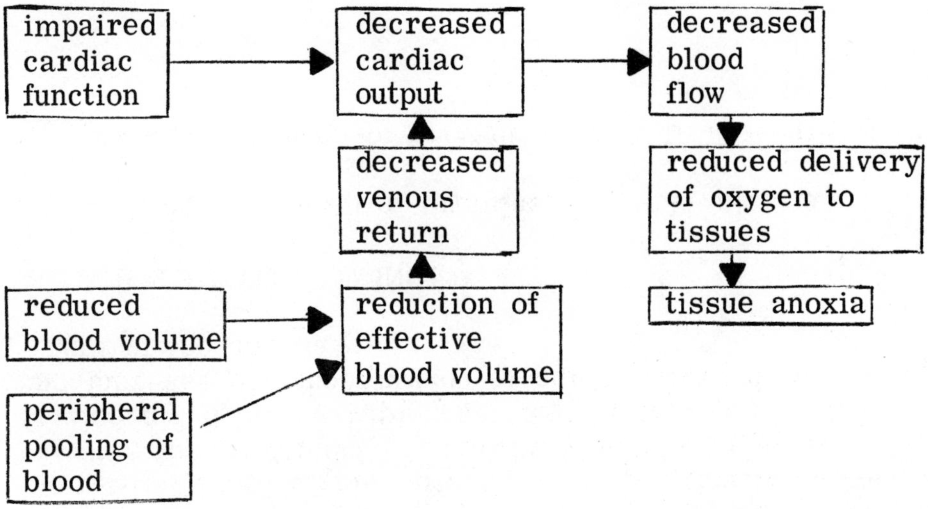

The "first" effect common to all cases of shock is decreased __________ ____________.

The "final" common effect in shock is ____________ ____________.

---

70. A
B
A
B
A

---

71. Cardiac failure due to impaired filling is generally the result of some external constriction.

MATCH THE FOLLOWING:

____pulmonary stenosis	A. impaired filling
____cardiac tamponade	B. increased load on the heart
____constrictive pericarditis	
____pulmonary fibrosis, with increased vascular resistance	

28. A
A, B

---

29. The hypoxic kidney also produces humoral factors which cause vasoconstriction. Among these are renin, which activates angiotensin in the plasma, and a vasomotor excitor material (VEM). Angiotensin causes arteriolar vasoconstriction, which decreases capillary pressure, leading to a shift of fluid into the vessels from the tissue compartment. This will aid in restoration of blood volume in hypovolemic shock.

Which of the following are effects of renal humoral factors produced in response to hypoxia?

____decreased arterial pressure
____increased arterial pressure
____increased functional blood volume
____decreased capillary pressure

---

76. A
B

---

77. Capillary endothelium allows free movement of water and electrolytes but normally allows the passage of very little protein. The concentration of proteins in the plasma is much higher than in the interstitial fluid. This difference in osmotically active molecules explains the movement of fluid back into the plasma. This movement is also aided by the rapid decrease of capillary hydrostatic pressure and increase of concentration of osmotically active particles along the length of the capillary.

MATCH THE FOLLOWING:

____high concentration of proteins A. plasma

____low concentration of proteins B. interstitial fluid

23. cardiac output
tissue anoxia

---

24. If tissue anoxia is allowed to continue, the circulation may deteriorate even further. The mechanisms of this further deterioration are complex and may involve:

1) anoxic damage to the vasculature, resulting in vasodilation and/or increased vascular permeability
2) ischemia of the heart muscle, further decreasing cardiac output
3) cerebral ischemia depressing the vasomotor center, resulting in vasodilation

Each of these changes introduces a vicious cycle aspect to the shock.

MATCH THE FOLLOWING ANOXIC CHANGES WITH THEIR MOST IMMEDIATE EFFECTS:

____ anoxia of the vasculature
____ ischemia of the heart muscle
____ cerebral ischemia

A. decreased cardiac output
B. reduction of effective blood volume

---

71. B
A
A
B

---

72. The causes of acute heart failure are processes which rapidly weaken the myocardium, put increased demand on it, or prevent ventricular filling. The causes of chronic heart failure are generally gradually developing processes which result in chronically inadequate cardiac action.

MATCH THE FOLLOWING CAUSES OF HEART FAILURE WITH THE TYPE OF FAILURE THEY ARE LIKELY TO PRODUCE:

____ myocardial infarct
____ aortic stenosis
____ systemic hypertension
____ cardiac tamponade (from a ruptured infarct)
____ massive pulmonary embolism

A. acute heart failure
B. chronic heart failure

27. B
A, B
A, B

---

28. In shock, neural influences increase heart rate and cause vasoconstriction. These effects are mediated by the carotid and aortic pressoreceptors and the cardiac and vasomotor centers of the brain. Catecholamine secretion by the adrenals is a second major mechanism leading to vasoconstriction.

MATCH THE FOLLOWING:

____increased heart rate	A. neural influence
____vasoconstriction	B. catecholamines

---

75. A
B
B
A

---

76. Tissue fluid is normally kept in a homeostatic condition by a set of complex factors. Fluid and electrolyte exchange occurs constantly between the plasma and interstitial fluid via the semipermeable capillary endothelium. Fluid moves out of the capillaries at their arterial end because of capillary hydrostatic pressure, and back into the capillaries at the venous end because of a net plasma osmotic pressure.

MATCH THE FOLLOWING:

____causes fluid movement out of the capillaries at their arterial end	A. capillary hydrostatic pressure
____causes fluid movement back into the capillaries at the venous end	B. plasma osmotic pressure

24. B
A
B

---

25. Introducing these cyclic aspects into our diagram, we have:

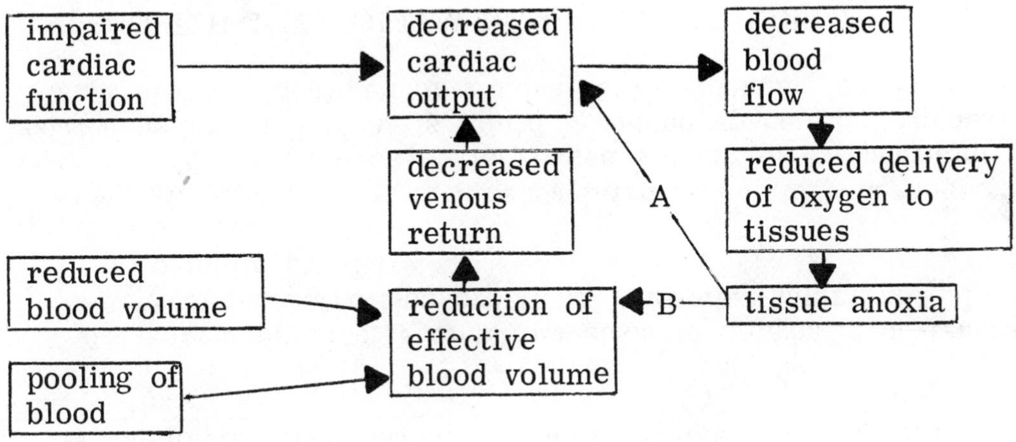

MATCH THE PROCESSES BELOW WITH THEIR PLACE (A, B) IN THE DIAGRAM:

____myocardial ischemia
____anoxia of the microvasculature
____ischemia of the vasomotor center

---

72. A
B
B
A
A

---

73. INDICATE "T" TRUE OR "F" FALSE:

	frame reference
____Congestive heart failure is generally more acutely serious than shock.	(45)
____Cardiac failure may cause shock.	(45, 51)
____Acute heart failure may be manifest by hypotension and/or elevated venous pressure.	(46, 51)
____In compensated heart failure, cardiac output is normal, but there may be increased heart rate, cardiac dilatation, or cardiac hypertrophy.	(49)
____The major lesions of chronic heart failure are associated with venous congestion.	(53)
____Pulmonary edema is a manifestation of right-sided heart failure.	(54)

26. B
A
A
B

---

27. From another point of view, the cause of the shock could be considered as a failure of the normal compensatory mechanism.

INDICATE THE COMPENSATORY MECHANISM(S) MOST LIKELY TO BE EVIDENT FOR THE FOLLOWING TYPES OF SHOCK:

____cardiogenic shock due to myocardial infarct with a conduction defect
____hemorrhagic shock due to a severed popliteal artery
____neurogenic shock during the recovery period

A. increased cardiac rate
B. vasoconstriction

---

74. F
F
F
T
F
T

C. Edema (23 frames)

When you complete this section, you will be able to select correct responses relating to the:

1. mechanisms of edema formation in lymphatic obstruction, venous obstruction or stasis, vascular injury, and altered osmotic pressure

75. Besides shock and heart failure, a third circulatory derangement is edema. Edema involves an increased volume of extracellular, extravascular fluid, that is, fluid in tissue spaces and serous cavities. Edema may be localized or generalized, depending on the cause.

CATEGORIZE THE FOLLOWING CAUSES OF EDEMA:

____inflammation of a hand
____right-sided heart failure
____electrolyte imbalance
____lymphatic obstruction

A. local edema
B. generalized edema

25. A
B
B

---

26. In response to hypotension and tissue hypoxia, the system attempts to compensate. Neural and humoral influences initiate acceleration of the heart rate and peripheral vasoconstriction in an attempt to return arterial pressure and circulation to normal.

MATCH THE FOLLOWING:

____increased heart rate

____decreased cardiac output

____peripheral pooling of blood

____peripheral vasoconstriction

A. circulatory changes leading to shock

B. compensatory changes to combat shock

TURN TEXT 180° AND CONTINUE.

---

73. F
T
T
T
T
F

---

74. INDICATE "T" TRUE OR "F" FALSE:

		frame reference
____	Left-sided heart failure is often secondary to right-sided heart failure.	(60)
____	The physiologic changes of heart failure can all be simply explained on the basis of venous congestion.	(57)
____	"Heart-failure cells" are characteristic of right-sided heart failure.	(59)
____	Chronic heart failure may produce centrilobular degeneration and necrosis in the liver.	(62)
____	Massive pulmonary embolism produces heart failure by weakening the myocardium.	(66)
____	Shunting of blood may produce heart failure by increasing demands on the heart.	(69)

TURN TEXT 180° AND CONTINUE.

Posttests for Units 1-14

Directions

Select the single best response. If you do not know the answer, make a guess.

Answers to all the posttests are found in the following section, beginning on page xliii.

POSTTESTS
UNIT 1: INTRODUCTION TO PATHOLOGY

1. Study of which of the following is more germane to Pathology than to other basic medical science disciplines?
   (A) effects of acid on digestion of meat
   (B) effects of acid on the staining reaction of parietal cells
   (C) effects of acid on esophageal mucosa
   (D) effects of pH on absorption from the intestine

2. Which indicates the correct use of the term etiology?
   (A) Pathology is concerned with the etiology of syphilis.
   (B) The etiology of syphilis is the spirochete *Treponema pallidum*.
   (C) both
   (D) neither

3. A lesion is defined as a
   (A) disease
   (B) structural abnormality
   (C) functional deficit
   (D) area of necrosis
   (E) localized defect

4. Cell death and cell degeneration are usually followed immediately by
   (A) inflammation
   (B) repair
   (C) atrophy
   (D) necrosis
   (E) hyperplasia

5. Which is classified as a disturbance of growth rather than as abnormal development?
   (A) atrophy
   (B) aplasia
   (C) both
   (D) neither

6. Which of the following is an example of growth disturbance and/or neoplasia?
   (A) changes in muscle after its blood supply is blocked
   (B) increase in thickness of epithelial layer of skin
   (C) congenital absence of one lung
   (D) response of tissue to a biological agent

7. Which of the following is an example of inflammation?
   (A) cellular and vascular response to an electrical burn
   (B) death of tissue surrounding a cut
   (C) enlargement of the left ventricle
   (D) obstruction of the pancreatic duct, causing a decrease in the number of acinar cells

8. A lesion characterized by decreased organ size due to decreased size of cells is classified as
   (A) a congenital defect
   (B) a growth disturbance
   (C) necrosis
   (D) inflammation

POSTTESTS

9. An infection is defined as
   (A) invasion of the body by microorganisms
   (B) invasion and multiplication of organisms in the body
   (C) the presence of organisms in the body
   (D) invasion of the body by organisms and reaction of the body to the organisms

10. Hyperplasia is an increase in tissue volume due to
    (A) increase in cell number
    (B) increase in cell size
    (C) both
    (D) neither

11. Which of the following is a sign?
    (A) a patient's report of pain in the abdomen
    (B) high blood glucose levels
    (C) a severe headache
    (D) a physician's observation of abdominal tenderness

12. Which of the following might be considered either a sign or a symptom, depending on context?
    (A) tenderness in the navel
    (B) leukocytes in the navel
    (C) pain in the navel
    (D) mass in the navel

13. The term pathogenesis refers to
    (A) the mechanism by which structural abnormalities cause functional abnormalities,
    (B) the means by which a disease produces manifestations
    (C) the mechanism by which injurious agents cause structural and functional abnormalities which in turn cause other abnormalities and manifestations
    (D) the mechanism by which a disease produces functional abnormalities and manifestations

14. A pathognomonic manifestation is one which
    (A) indicates a specific diagnosis
    (B) is present in only the most advanced diseases
    (C) is present in most diseases and aids in diagnosis
    (D) often indicates that a disease is in the resolution phase

15. Which of the following procedures is performed in a pathologist's laboratory?
    (A) blood glucose determination
    (B) culture of the blood
    (C) both
    (D) neither

16. Which of the following procedures is performed in a clinical pathology laboratory?
    (A) white blood cell count
    (B) examination of cells from the uterine cervix for cancer
    (C) both
    (D) neither

Answers to this posttest are found on page xliv.

POSTTESTS
UNIT 2: INFLAMMATION: THE VASCULAR AND CELLULAR RESPONSE TO INJURY

1. By definition the process of acute inflammation includes
   (A) vascular proliferation
   (B) fibroblastic reaction
   (C) both
   (D) neither

2. Chemical mediators of inflammation include
   (A) amines
   (B) polypeptides
   (C) both
   (D) neither

3. Which is capable of causing pain and is a long-acting mediator of the vascular response of inflammation?
   (A) histamine
   (B) negative chemotactic agent
   (C) positive chemotactic agent
   (D) bradykinin

4. Manifestations of inflammation resulting from increased vascular permeability include
   (A) heat and redness
   (B) pain and swelling
   (C) both
   (D) neither

5. Which of the cardinal signs of inflammation result(s) from increased blood volume?
   (A) redness
   (B) redness and heat
   (C) redness, heat, and swelling
   (D) redness, heat, swelling, and pain

6. All of the following are thought to be causes of pain in an inflamed area EXCEPT
   (A) pressure of the exudate
   (B) acidic breakdown products
   (C) histamine
   (D) bradykinin

7. An exudate is characterized by
   (A) low protein content
   (B) high red blood cell content
   (C) high specific gravity
   (D) brown color

8. Which of the following statements relating to the process of inflammation is true?
   (A) Capillary dilation and increased permeability are caused by different substances.
   (B) The release of chemical mediators of inflammation immediately follows injury.
   (C) Capillary dilation causes exudation.
   (D) Kinins are vasoactive amines.

9. Short-acting mediators of inflammation are
   (A) kinins
   (B) produced by polys
   (C) released by mast cells
   (D) activated from blood plasma

10. Which statement relating to vascular permeability is true?
   (A) The degree of capillary permeability varies with different inflammatory reactions.
   (B) Capillaries are permeable to plasma proteins under normal conditions.
   (C) Arterioles greatly increase in permeability during inflammation.
   (D) Transudates are more viscous than exudates.

11. If the following events were put in sequence as they occur in an inflammatory reaction, which would occur third?
   (A) migration of leukocytes
   (B) margination of leukocytes
   (C) tissue injury
   (D) increased blood volume, leading to heat and redness

12. Which is out of order in relation to movement of leukocytes in inflammation?
   (A) emigration ⟶ migration
   (B) accumulation ⟶ migration
   (C) margination ⟶ adhesion
   (D) adhesion ⟶ emigration

13. Which of the following statements concerning debris is FALSE?
   (A) It causes tissue damage.
   (B) It often remains in the tissue long after inflammation has ceased.
   (C) The removal of debris and fluid is called resolution.
   (D) It is dissolved by enzymes released from polys and can then be carried away by plasma fluid.

14. The cells which appear second in an acute inflammatory focus are
   (A) mononuclear phagocytes
   (B) lymphocytes
   (C) neutrophils
   (D) eosinophils

15. The site of digestion of damaged tissue or injurious agents is
   (A) intracellular
   (B) intercellular
   (C) both
   (D) neither

16. The function of polymorphonuclear leukocytes and mononuclear leukocytes in inflammation is
   (A) release of chemical mediators
   (B) digestion of injurious agents
   (C) both
   (D) neither

Answers to this posttest are found on page xliv.

POSTTESTS

UNIT 3: INFLAMMATORY CELLS: STRUCTURE AND FUNCTION

1. Aggregates of small, dark-staining (hematoxaphilic) cells with little cytoplasm in an inflammatory site are likely to be
   (A) polys
   (B) macrophages
   (C) eosinophils
   (D) lymphocytes

2. Aggregates of large, pale-staining cells in an inflammatory site are likely to be
   (A) polys
   (B) macrophages
   (C) eosinophils
   (D) lymphocytes

3. In routine microscopic sections of tissue stained with hematoxylin and eosin, the granules of basophils and mast cells are
   (A) red
   (B) blue
   (C) neutrophilic
   (D) not evident

4. Langhans' cells characteristically are
   (A) very large oval cells with central, segmented nuclei
   (B) formed in an inflammatory site containing debris too large to be phagocytized
   (C) large irregular cells with multiple peripherally arranged nuclei
   (D) large irregular cells with many centrally located nuclei

5. Which inflammatory cells have eccentric nuclei and abundant basophilic cytoplasm?
   (A) lymphocytes
   (B) plasma cells
   (C) both
   (D) neither

6. Large multinucleated cells with nuclei arranged in a horseshoe around central cytoplasm are called
   (A) Langhans' giant cells
   (B) foreign-body giant cells
   (C) both
   (D) neither

7. Cells in an H & E section with one- or two-lobed nuclei and prominent cytoplasmic granules are
   (A) neutrophils
   (B) eosinophils
   (C) basophils
   (D) giant cells

8. Basophils
   (A) are the primary source of histamine release in inflammation
   (B) contain histamine but do not play a major role in inflammation
   (C) appear only in the late stages of inflammation
   (D) are chemotropic in response to chemical agents such as turpentine

9. Neutrophils
   (A) reproduce rapidly in an inflammatory site
   (B) live for only a few days in the tissues
   (C) are the predominant cell type in prolonged inflammations
   (D) are continually synthesizing and releasing digestive enzymes in an inflammatory site

10. Which cells survive in an acid pH and phagocytose debris?
    (A) neutrophils
    (B) macrophages
    (C) both
    (D) neither

11. Lymphocytes
    (A) actively migrate from the blood to the tissues early in inflammation
    (B) actively proliferate in the acute stages of inflammation
    (C) appear late in inflammation
    (D) produce digestive enzymes which help remove debris

12. Plasma cells
    (A) appear in the blood during chronic infections
    (B) appear only in inflammations caused by bacteria
    (C) are transformed into lymphocytes
    (D) appear in the tissues late in an inflammatory reaction

13. During an inflammatory reaction, the pH of the area
    (A) steadily decreases
    (B) generally increases
    (C) always increases
    (D) may either increase, decrease, or remain about the same

14. The role of neutrophils and mononuclear phagocytes in inflammation can be characterized by all of the following EXCEPT
    (A) neutrophils arrive at the inflammatory site about 12 hours after injury
    (B) mononuclear phagocytes can function in acid media
    (C) dissolution of debris is an important function of polys
    (D) polys are important in destruction of microbial invaders

15. Opsonification refers to the
    (A) removal of extracellular debris by specific digestive enzymes
    (B) process by which antibodies make bacteria more susceptible to phagocytosis
    (C) enzymatic destruction of large particles of foreign material over a long period of time
    (D) destruction of the fibrin barrier formed around some bacterial infection sites

16. Agranulocytosis refers to a condition in which
    (A) all white blood cells are reduced in number
    (B) granulocytes are ineffective in phagocytizing invaders
    (C) neutrophils are greatly decreased in number
    (D) neutrophils do not form enzyme-containing granules

Answers to this posttest are found on page xliv.

POSTTESTS

UNIT 4: FACTORS WHICH MODIFY INFLAMMATION

1. Which of the following does not ordinarily affect the invasiveness of bacteria?
   (A) stimulation of fibrin formation in blood vessels and lymphatics
   (B) production of spreading factors
   (C) production of toxins
   (D) susceptibility to phagocytosis

2. Acute inflammations do NOT vary in the
   (A) duration of the reaction
   (B) order of events of the cellular response
   (C) composition of the exudate
   (D) degree of localization

3. Which of the following is FALSE?
   (A) Viruses are potent pyogenic agents.
   (B) Pathogenic bacteria which enter the blood often cause severe infections.
   (C) Some bacteria can be ingested by phagocytes but not digested.
   (D) The amount, duration of exposure, and pathogenicity of an agent modify the inflammatory response.

4. Which are normally pyogenic?
   (A) chemicals
   (B) viruses
   (C) both
   (D) neither

5. An agent which the body's defenses cannot overcome will always cause
   (A) serous exudation
   (B) fibrinous exudation
   (C) acute inflammation
   (D) chronic inflammation

6. Which characterizes the relationship of bacteria to the phagocytic process?
   (A) Once an organism has been ingested by a phagocyte, it is no longer capable of injuring the host.
   (B) Leukocytosis-promoting factor increases bacterial susceptibility to phagocytosis.
   (C) Not all organisms which are ingested by phagocytes are killed.
   (D) Opsonification protects bacteria from phagocytosis.

7. The term <u>pyogenic</u> refers to the ability of certain substances to cause
   (A) fever
   (B) increased poly production
   (C) both
   (D) neither

8. The formation of a thick fluid composed of large numbers of dead and living polys and partially liquified debris is likely to involve all of the following as pathogenic factors except
   (A) polys
   (B) viruses
   (C) enzymes
   (D) chemotactic agents

9. In the list below, select the pair of injurious agents which differ in pathogenicity.
   (A) ultraviolet light and x-rays
   (B) 10^2 staphylococci and 10^7 staphylococci
   (C) 1 hour of sunlight and 3 hours of sunlight
   (D) an iron at 200° and boiling water

10. Which of the following is true of pyogenic agents?
   (A) They produce widespread edema and mononuclear infiltrate.
   (B) They attract large numbers of polys.
   (C) They often cause multiple small hemorrhages.
   (D) They produce pyrogens.

11. Which is LEAST predictable in its influence on inflammation reactions?
   (A) physiologic condition of the host
   (B) location in the body
   (C) toxicity of agent
   (D) invasiveness of agent

12. The physiologic condition of an individual
   (A) is quantitatively related to nutritional status
   (B) affects the frequency and severity of inflammatory diseases
   (C) primarily affects the type of inflammatory disease that occurs
   (D) is too vague a concept to be important

13. The general physiologic condition of a host
   (A) does not generally influence the pattern of an inflammatory reaction very much
   (B) is determined by age, nutrition, and presence or absence of disease
   (C) is an important factor only in inflammations due to pyogenic agents
   (D) is important only when it influences the efficiency of the cellular defensive response

14. The outcome of an inflammatory response is influenced by the
   (A) vascularity of the tissue
   (B) presence of naturally occurring glycoprotein complexes
   (C) both
   (D) neither

15. An injurious agent would cause the most extensive damage in
   (A) muscle tissue
   (B) a joint space
   (C) dense connective tissue
   (D) loose connective tissue

16. An inflammation would probably spread most rapidly in
   (A) skeletal muscle
   (B) lung
   (C) spleen
   (D) kidney

Answers to this posttest are found on page xliv.

POSTTESTS

UNIT 5: CLASSIFICATION AND COMPLICATIONS OF INFLAMMATION

1. Which is/are generally associated with an inflammation becoming chronic ?
   (A) increasing prominence of the cardinal signs
   (B) fibroblastic proliferation
   (C) both
   (D) neither

2. Which are the characteristic cells of acute inflammation ?
   (A) lymphocytes and plasma cells
   (B) polys (neutrophils)
   (C) histiocytes
   (D) eosinophils

3. Acute inflammations are by definition always of
   (A) short duration
   (B) severe intensity
   (C) both
   (D) neither

4. Which are the characteristic cells of granulomatous inflammation ?
   (A) plump macrophages
   (B) lymphocytes and plasma cells
   (C) polys (neutrophils)
   (D) eosinophils

5. Epithelioid cells are
   (A) transformed epithelial cells
   (B) the primary cell of epithelial tumors
   (C) transformed macrophages
   (D) outer layer cells of an eosinophilic granuloma

6. Which is most characteristic of chronic inflammation of tuberculous type ?
   (A) collections of plasma cells and lymphocytes
   (B) collections of macrophages
   (C) proliferation of capillaries and fibroblasts
   (D) collections of eosinophils

7. Which of the following most closely resembles blood plasma ?
   (A) serous exudate
   (B) sanguinous exudate
   (C) fibrinous exudate
   (D) catarrhal exudate

8. Catarrhal exudates
   (A) occur only on mucous membranes
   (B) are usually followed by hemorrhagic exudation
   (C) usually contain large numbers of erythrocytes
   (D) contain large numbers of polys

POSTTESTS

9. Which type of exudate is associated with leakage of the smallest particles from vessels?
   (A) catarrhal
   (B) serous
   (C) fibrinous
   (D) purulent

10. An ulcer is a
   (A) ramifying defect containing dead tissue and leukocytes
   (B) diffuse mixture of dead mucosal cells, bacteria, and inflammatory exudate on a mucosal surface
   (C) spherical defect containing dead tissue and leukocytes
   (D) defect in an epithelial lined surface

11. A pseudomembranous inflammation is characterized by a
   (A) defect in an epithelial lined surface
   (B) diffuse mixture of dead mucosal cells, bacteria, and inflammatory exudate on a mucosal surface
   (C) spherical defect containing dead tissue and leukocytes
   (D) ramifying defect containing dead tissue and leukocytes

12. An abscess is a
   (A) defect in an epithelial lined surface
   (B) diffuse mixture of dead mucosal cells, bacteria, and inflammatory exudate on a mucosal surface
   (C) spherical defect containing dead tissue and leukocytes
   (D) ramifying defect containing dead tissue and leukocytes

13. Carbuncles
   (A) usually develop in internal organs
   (B) involve hemorrhagic exudation
   (C) have multiple points of discharge
   (D) generally develop into granulomatous inflammations

14. Cellulitis
   (A) often is a result of empyema
   (B) usually spreads via lymphatics
   (C) is a poorly limited, diffuse inflammation
   (D) generally develops in highly cellular organs

15. In which of the following areas could pseudomembranous inflammation take place?
   (A) pleural cavity
   (B) intestinal tract
   (C) skin
   (D) meninges

16. Which indicates inflammation?
   (A) typhlitis
   (B) synovioma
   (C) prostatism
   (D) carotenemia

Answers to this posttest are found on page xliv.

POSTTESTS
UNIT 6: SYSTEMIC MANIFESTATIONS OF INFLAMMATION

1. By definition, fever occurs when
   (A) body temperature rises due to stimuli reaching the thermoregulatory center
   (B) oral temperature exceeds 37.7^{o} C
   (C) body heat production exceeds heat loss
   (D) a patient notices symptoms associated with elevated temperature

2. Which is true?
   (A) Vasodilation is manifested by a drop in skin temperature.
   (B) Elevation of body temperature due to exercise is fever.
   (C) Vasoconstriction and shivering are primary mechanisms of increased heat loss.
   (D) Pyrexia is caused by a resetting of the body's thermostat at a higher level.

3. Which is true?
   (A) The thermoregulatory center increases or decreases body temperature in response to pyrogens.
   (B) The effect of pyrogens on the thermoregulatory center is similar to that of heat.
   (C) During the cold stage of fever, heat production is less than heat loss.
   (D) Deep thermal receptors in the hypothalamus are influenced by blood temperature.

4. Shivering is a mechanism to
   (A) increase heat production
   (B) decrease heat production
   (C) increase heat loss
   (D) decrease heat loss

5. Which cells are associated with pyrogen production?
   (A) lymphocytes
   (B) plasma cells
   (C) eosinophils
   (D) neutrophils

6. Copious sweating generally occurs in which stage(s) of fever?
   (A) cold stage
   (B) hot stage
   (C) defervescence
   (D) all stages

7. Which is a systemic manifestation of inflammation resulting from fever?
   (A) alkalosis
   (B) ketosis
   (C) high blood glucose
   (D) positive nitrogen balance

8. What is the significance of fever?
   (A) It is usually harmful.
   (B) It may be harmful or innocuous
   (C) It is always harmful.
   (D) It is an important part of the body's defense mechanism.

9. A white cell count of 25,000/cu. mm. is
   (A) within the normal range
   (B) pathognomonic for leukemia
   (C) leukocytosis
   (D) leukopenia

10. Leukocytosis is most commonly due to abnormality in the number of circulating
   (A) monocytes and granulocytes
   (B) neutrophils and lymphocytes
   (C) eosinophils
   (D) polys

11. Prolonged leukocytosis is associated with
   (A) necrosis of the bone marrow
   (B) inflammation of the bone marrow
   (C) release of immature cells from bone marrow
   (D) the release of leukocytosis-promoting factor

12. Leukopenia
   (A) is caused by leukopenia-promoting factor
   (B) is the direct result of hyperplasia of the bone marrow
   (C) occurs in overwhelming prolonged infections
   (D) occurs in most inflammations

13. Erythrocyte sedimentation rate is increased in association with
   (A) elevated plasma fibrinogen and gamma globulin levels
   (B) decreased plasma fibrinogen and gamma globulin levels
   (C) acute inflammation but not with chronic inflammation
   (D) chronic inflammation but not with acute inflammation

14. An elevated gamma globulin level
   (A) is often associated with chronic inflammation
   (B) is usually associated with lymphocytosis caused by bacterial infections
   (C) causes a decrease in erythrocyte sedimentation rate
   (D) is due to plasma cell hypertrophy

15. Elevated fibrinogen levels are
   (A) not related to erythrocyte sedimentation rate
   (B) associated with increased erythrocyte sedimentation rate
   (C) often used to diagnose internal inflammation
   (D) usually preceded by elevated gamma globulin levels

16. Lymphadenitis involves
   (A) hyperplasia of the reticular phagocytic cells
   (B) infiltration of the node by polys
   (C) both
   (D) neither

Answers to this posttest are found on page xlv.

POSTTESTS
UNIT 7: NECROSIS

1. Which indicate(s) irreversible cell damage?
   (A) pyknosis, karyolysis, karyorrhexis
   (B) permeability of the cell membrane to large molecules such as trypan blue
   (C) both
   (D) neither

2. Which of the following is/are used to distinguish irreversible from reversible cell damage?
   (A) nuclear changes
   (B) swelling or eosinophilia of cytoplasm
   (C) both
   (D) neither

3. A histologic examination of a section of tissue reveals swollen cells with cloudy cytoplasm, increased eosinophilia, and nuclei pushed to the periphery. These changes are most characteristic of
   (A) degeneration
   (B) autolysis
   (C) coagulation necrosis
   (D) liquefaction necrosis

4. Which is/are true?
   (A) Necrosis and cell death are interchangeable terms.
   (B) Somatic death is a form of necrosis.
   (C) both
   (D) neither

5. Which is LEAST helpful in distinguishing postmortem autolysis from necrosis?
   (A) polymorphonuclear leukocyte infiltrate
   (B) karyorrhexis, karyolysis, and pyknosis
   (C) a zone of congestion
   (D) a grossly wedge-shaped lesion

6. Microscopically, autolysis and degeneration are usually distinguished by changes in
   (A) cytoplasm
   (B) nuclei
   (C) both
   (D) neither

7. Choose the correct statement concerning a high-power view of the center of a renal infarct compared to a high-power view of a severely autolyzed kidney without necrosis.
   (A) The two views may look the same microscopically.
   (B) Cytoplasmic changes will be more striking in the autolyzed kidney without necrosis.
   (C) Nuclear changes will be more striking in the autolyzed kidney without necrosis.
   (D) The autolyzed kidney without necrosis will exhibit liquefaction.

8. Enzymes play an important role in causing cell death in which of the following situations?
   (A) myocardial infarct
   (B) brain infarct
   (C) caseous necrosis
   (D) gas gangrene
   (E) autolysis

9. X-rays cause necrosis by
   (A) producing DNA injury
   (B) precipitating cell proteins
   (C) both
   (D) neither

10. Ischemia to a solid organ may result in
   (A) degeneration only
   (B) degeneration and necrosis only
   (C) necrosis and autolysis only
   (D) degeneration, necrosis, and autolysis

11. A localized, slightly soft, and slightly yellow lesion in a solid organ has red margins, grossly. Microscopically, it exhibits autolysis in the center, and congestion and acute inflammation at the margins. Which type of necrosis is present?
   (A) coagulation
   (B) caseous
   (C) gangrenous
   (D) liquefaction

12. Which of the following fit(s) descriptions of liquefaction necrosis?
   (A) a fluctuant, subcutaneous mass that ruptures and exudes yellow, creamy material
   (B) a defect near the surface of the brain containing clear fluid
   (C) both
   (D) neither

13. Macrophages, epithelioid, and giant cells are associated with
   (A) liquefaction necrosis
   (B) coagulation necrosis
   (C) caseous necrosis
   (D) gangrenous necrosis

14. Which commonly cause liquefaction necrosis?
   (A) pyogenic bacteria
   (B) tubercle bacilli
   (C) both
   (D) neither

15. Enzymatic fat necrosis is most closely associated with
   (A) pancreatic necrosis
   (B) fatty metamorphosis of the liver
   (C) dystrophic calcification
   (D) amyloidosis

16. Which is associated with slow decomposition of tissue by saprophytic bacteria?
   (A) gas gangrene
   (B) wet gangrene
   (C) dry gangrene
   (D) fibrinoid necrosis

Answers to this posttest are found on page xlv.

POSTTESTS
UNIT 8: HEALING

1. Repair and physiologic replacement are by definition
   (A) basic pathologic processes
   (B) both involved in healing
   (C) both involved with cell proliferation
   (D) primarily connective tissue processes

2. Cells which are incapable of mitosis in postnatal life are called
   (A) labile
   (B) stable
   (C) both
   (D) neither

3. Which is the correct order from greatest to least regenerative capacity?
   (A) nerve, smooth muscle, cardiac muscle
   (B) smooth muscle, nerve, cardiac muscle
   (C) cardiac muscle, smooth muscle, nerve
   (D) cardiac muscle, nerve, smooth muscle

4. Which types of cells are classified as permanent cells?
   (A) glial cells
   (B) osteocytes
   (C) both
   (D) neither

5. In which of the following are both tissues composed of stable cells?
   (A) gland parenchyma and bone marrow
   (B) nerve tissue and myocardium
   (C) bone and adipose tissue
   (D) glial cells and surface epithelium

6. The formation of fibrous scar tissue occurs during the process of
   (A) disorderly regeneration
   (B) organization
   (C) both
   (D) neither

7. Anoxic damage to proximal kidney tubules due to shock heals by
   (A) resolution alone
   (B) orderly regeneration
   (C) disorderly regeneration
   (D) organization

8. Disorderly regeneration would be expected to occur in which of the following situations in the liver?
   (A) centrilobular necrosis
   (B) abscess
   (C) widespread multilobular damage
   (D) surgical removal of part of a lobe

9. Two weeks after an abdominal operation, histologically the scar would appear
   (A) acellular, avascular, disorderly fibrous
   (B) acellular, avascular, orderly fibrous
   (C) cellular, vascular, orderly fibrous
   (D) cellular, vascular, disorderly fibrous

10. Which of the following occurs with healing of a broken bone but is NOT typical of organization at other sites of injury?
   (A) formation of granulation tissue
   (B) fibroblastic infiltration
   (C) fibroblastic differentiation into osteoblasts
   (D) formation of a clot in the injured area

11. A four centimeter nodule found in the periphery of the lung consists of central amorphous eosinophilic material surrounded by a layer of dense, relatively acellular fibrous tissue containing a few lymphocytes. The age of this lesion is most likely
   (A) 1 day
   (B) 1 week
   (C) 1 month
   (D) 1 year

12. Approximately how long does it take after a myocardial infarct for the scar to reach full strength?
   (A) 1 week
   (B) 2 weeks
   (C) 1 month
   (D) several months

13. After treatment with a cancer chemotherapeutic agent, a patient's white blood count drops to 2,000 cells/mm^3. After discontinuing the agent, the bone marrow is likely to undergo
   (A) resolution only
   (B) orderly regeneration
   (C) disorderly regeneration
   (D) organization

14. Healing of a wound by first intention may involve all of the following EXCEPT
   (A) an inflammatory reaction
   (B) fibroblastic proliferation
   (C) epithelial proliferation
   (D) exposed granulation tissue

15. Which is most likely to produce significant delay in healing?
   (A) presence of necrotic tissue
   (B) moderate protein deficiency
   (C) diabetes mellitus
   (D) vitamin B_{12} deficiency

16. A biopsy of an operative incision which is healing poorly shows granuloma formation. What is the most likely cause?
   (A) staphylococcus infection
   (B) streptococcus infection
   (C) *Clostridium tetani* infection
   (D) suture reaction

Answers to this posttest are found on page xlv.

POSTTESTS
UNIT 9: DEGENERATION

1. Acute cell degeneration is characterized by dysfunction of the cell
   (A) cytoplasm
   (B) nucleus
   (C) both
   (D) neither

2. Which statement most correctly describes the relationship between degeneration and necrosis?
   (A) The mechanisms of chronic degeneration are generally similar to those of necrosis.
   (B) Agents which produce necrosis can also produce degeneration without necrosis.
   (C) All agents which produce degeneration can also produce necrosis.
   (D) Each type of degeneration is associated with a corresponding type of necrosis.

3. Which of the following is suggested when the morphologic features of chronic degeneration are associated with a fibrous reaction?
   (A) a specific lysosomal defect
   (B) a relative degree of anoxia
   (C) imperceptible necrosis
   (D) bacterial infection

4. Which of the following is an example of degeneration associated with lipid accumulation?
   (A) amyloidosis
   (B) mucoid accumulation
   (C) xanthoma
   (D) Mallory bodies

5. Which type of degeneration is characterized by extracellular lipid deposits?
   (A) fatty metamorphosis
   (B) adiposity
   (C) mineral oil granuloma
   (D) xanthoma

6. Which is true?
   (A) Insoluble lipids only accumulate extracellularly.
   (B) Glycogen appears as dense, fluffy masses in H & E sections.
   (C) Protein deposits tend to have specific appearances depending on the protein involved.
   (D) Extracellular accumulations of water are not usually called degenerations.

7. Which is/are characteristically deposited intracellularly?
   (A) amyloid
   (B) glycogen
   (C) both
   (D) neither

8. Which of the following characterizes the accumulation of cholesterol in tissue?
   (A) It is not present in routine tissue sections because it is water-soluble.
   (B) Its crystals are dissolved from routine tissue sections, leaving cleft-like spaces which are specific for cholesterol.
   (C) It is only deposited extracellularly.
   (D) Tissue deposits are almost always in the form of crystals.

POSTTESTS

9. Which occur(s) in the liver?
   (A) adiposity
   (B) fatty metamorphosis
   (C) both
   (D) neither

10. Which is associated with acute changes in solid organs such as kidney, liver, and heart?
   (A) adiposity
   (B) cloudy swelling
   (C) mucoid change
   (D) calcification

11. Which is/are usually reversible?
   (A) hydropic change
   (B) amyloid deposition
   (C) both
   (D) neither

12. Which is usually due to specific metabolic defects?
   (A) glycogen degeneration
   (B) mucoid degeneration
   (C) adiposity
   (D) fibrinoid degeneration

13. Dystrophic calcification is defined by
   (A) elevated serum calcium levels
   (B) occurrence at sites of injury
   (C) both
   (D) neither

14. Atherosclerosis is a complex degenerative process involving all of the following EXCEPT
   (A) intracellular cholesterol deposits
   (B) intracellular hyaline change
   (C) extracellular cholesterol deposits
   (D) extracellular hyaline change

15. Reduced protein synthesis is likely to produce
   (A) atherosclerosis
   (B) fatty metamorphosis
   (C) both
   (D) neither

16. Hyalin is a
   (A) specific protein which appears to be made of fine fibrils when examined by electron microscopy
   (B) lipoprotein residue from intracellular digestion
   (C) both
   (D) neither

Answers to this posttest are found on page xlv.

POSTTESTS
UNIT 10: DEVELOPMENTAL ABNORMALITIES: EMBRYONIC AND FETAL, GENETIC AND CHROMOSOMAL

1. Familial disorders are
   (A) the same as genetic disorders
   (B) usually congenital
   (C) commonly associated with chromosomal abnormalities
   (D) sometimes caused by infectious agents

2. The fetal period comprises the
   (A) period of organogenesis
   (B) last 3 months of pregnancy
   (C) both
   (D) neither

3. Involution is
   (A) the cause of aplasia and hypoplasia
   (B) due to a genetic abnormality
   (C) the most common cause of congenital abnormalities
   (D) controlled by the phenomenon of induction

4. Defects of organogenesis are characterized as
   (A) congenital
   (B) caused by injury due to physical agents during the fetal period
   (C) both
   (D) neither

5. Congenital heart disease and other gross organ defects are produced by injury during
   (A) gametogenesis
   (B) the fetal period
   (C) both
   (D) neither

6. Which types of abnormalities are usually familial?
   (A) chromosomal
   (B) embryonic
   (C) both
   (D) neither

7. Which may be detected on preparations of dividing cells (karyotyping)?
   (A) genetic disorders
   (B) embryonic injuries
   (C) both
   (D) neither

8. Which is a good example of a hidden congenital abnormality?
   (A) double ureter
   (B) omphalocele
   (C) diabetes mellitus
   (D) a female heterozygous for hemophilia

9. Abortion because of a possible embryonic defect might be considered if the mother had rubella
   (A) 2 weeks after the last menstrual period
   (B) 8 weeks after the last menstrual period
   (C) 16 weeks after the last menstrual period
   (D) 32 weeks after the last menstrual period

10. The cause can often be determined for lesions with onset during the
   (A) embryonic period
   (B) fetal period
   (C) both
   (D) neither

11. Injuries during the fetal period are most likely to interfere with which of the following?
   (A) involution
   (B) cell differentiation
   (C) cell growth
   (D) organogenesis

12. Which is an example of a genetic structural protein defect?
   (A) an achondroplastic dwarf
   (B) mental retardation in phenylketonuria
   (C) both
   (D) neither

13. Genetic diseases rarely are the cause of
   (A) storage diseases
   (B) metabolic deficiencies
   (C) tissue damage from toxic metabolites
   (D) gross organ deformities

14. Most genetic diseases have
   (A) typical pedigrees
   (B) normal karyotypes
   (C) both
   (D) neither

15. Of the following, which probably accounts for the greatest percentage of abortions?
   (A) genetic abnormalities
   (B) chromosomal abnormalities
   (C) embryonic injuries
   (D) fetal injuries

16. Sex chromosome disorders are usually associated with
   (A) sterility
   (B) changes which do not become evident until puberty
   (C) both
   (D) neither

Answers to this posttest are found on page xlv.

POSTTESTS

UNIT 11: HEMODYNAMIC DISORDERS: MECHANISMS OF VASCULAR OBSTRUCTION

1. Subcategories of atherosclerosis INCLUDE
   (A) arteriosclerosis
   (B) arteriolosclerosis
   (C) both
   (D) neither

2. The evolution of an atherosclerotic plaque is characterized by
   (A) initial intracellular deposition of lipid
   (B) initial involvement of intima and muscularis
   (C) initial involvement of arterioles
   (D) reversibility by ulceration of the fibrotic cap
   (E) irreversibility of all stages

3. Arteriolosclerosis is characterized by involvement of vessels in the
   (A) heart
   (B) lung
   (C) kidney
   (D) brain

4. The lesion most intimately associated with hypertension is
   (A) atherosclerosis
   (B) arteritis
   (C) phlebitis
   (D) medial calcification
   (E) arteriolosclerosis

5. Atherosclerosis is more severe in
   (A) alcoholics vs. nonalcoholics
   (B) people with high dietary cholesterol vs. people with high serum cholesterol
   (C) hypertensives vs. nonhypertensives
   (D) Japanese vs. Americans

6. Which is characterized by a slightly friable mass composed of irregular red and gray layers which distends a blood vessel?
   (A) tumor embolus
   (B) atherosclerosis
   (C) postmortem clot
   (D) thrombus

7. The tail of a venous thrombus is characterized by
   (A) "currant jelly" appearance
   (B) uniform red color
   (C) attachment to vessel wall
   (D) lines of Zahn
   (E) rubbery consistency

8. Which of the following changes in blood predisposes to thrombosis?
   (A) decreased fibrinogen
   (B) decreased thrombin
   (C) increased albumin
   (D) decreased platelets
   (E) increased catecholamines

9. All of the following conditions involve thrombocytosis EXCEPT
   (A) atherosclerosis
   (B) postoperative state
   (C) following childbirth
   (D) polycythemia vera

10. Of the following, an occlusive thrombus of the femoral vein is LEAST likely to undergo
   (A) embolization
   (B) propagation
   (C) hemorrhage
   (D) organization
   (E) recanalization

11. Of the following, the most common source of arterial emboli is
   (A) pulmonary vein
   (B) pulmonary artery
   (C) left atrium
   (D) common carotid artery

12. Which is a paradoxical embolus?
   (A) embolus arising in a systemic vein and lodging in a systemic artery
   (B) embolus arising in a systemic vein and lodging in a pulmonary artery
   (C) embolus arising in a systemic artery and lodging in a systemic artery
   (D) embolus arising in the left atrium and lodging in a systemic artery

13. Pulmonary emboli have all the following characteristics EXCEPT
   (A) commonly arise in leg veins
   (B) pass through the right heart before reaching the lung
   (C) consistently cause infarction in the lung
   (D) are usually thrombotic emboli

14. Which statement concerning the natural history of venous thrombi of the legs is true?
   (A) They usually produce prominent local signs and symptoms.
   (B) They are the most common source of pulmonary emboli.
   (C) They are most commonly caused by venous obstruction.
   (D) They are usually white thrombi.

15. Air embolism
   (A) has its most serious effects in the left atrium
   (B) is often the result of surgical operations
   (C) occurs in divers while descending to the ocean floor
   (D) is lethal when more than 5 cc. of air enters the bloodstream

16. Types of embolism most commonly due to fractures of bones include
   (A) fat embolism
   (B) bone marrow embolism
   (C) both
   (D) neither

Answers to this posttest are found on page xlvi.

UNIT 12: HEMODYNAMIC DISORDERS: EFFECTS OF VASCULAR OBSTRUCTION

1. Which of the following generally causes hypoxia BUT NOT ischemia?
   (A) anemia
   (B) embolism
   (C) thrombosis
   (D) atherosclerosis
   (E) external pressure occluding an artery

2. Occlusion of which of the following vessels is most likely to produce an infarct?
   (A) major branch of portal vein
   (B) pulmonary lobar artery
   (C) renal arcuate artery
   (D) arteriole in the myocardium
   (E) saphenous vein

3. Ischemic damage is most likely with
   (A) gradual occlusion of a functional end artery
   (B) occlusion of a leg vein
   (C) moderate atherosclerosis of a coronary artery
   (D) sudden occlusion of an anastomotic artery
   (E) sudden occlusion of a functional end artery

4. A patient presents with gradually progressive weakness of the legs and pain on mild exertion. His legs are slightly pale, and the skin is thin and shiny. He is probably suffering from
   (A) atherosclerosis
   (B) venous thrombosis
   (C) arterial emboli
   (D) left heart failure
   (E) gangrene

5. The term <u>infarct</u> is best used to indicate a type of
   (A) degeneration
   (B) heart attack
   (C) lesion
   (D) process

6. Which statement describing infarcts is FALSE?
   (A) A red infarct generally results from venous occlusion.
   (B) Dry gangrene occurs primarily in pale infarcts.
   (C) An intestinal infarct is hemorrhagic even if it results from arterial occlusion.
   (D) Dry gangrene often involves internal organs.
   (E) Pale infarcts result from artery occlusion.

7. Hemorrhagic infarcts are associated with
   (A) venous occlusions
   (B) organs with extensive collateral circulation
   (C) both
   (D) neither

8. Which of the following describes the appearance of the usual pale infarct?
   (A) Light microscopic changes are evident almost immediately.
   (B) A small infarct will be resolved by 3 to 8 days.
   (C) The infarcted area exhibits liquefaction necrosis.
   (D) An acute inflammatory response is evident within 24 hours.
   (E) Large amounts of hemosiderin are evident in the infarcted area.

9. All of the following may result from venous occlusion EXCEPT
   (A) wet gangrene
   (B) ischemic necrosis
   (C) anemia infarct
   (D) breakdown of hemoglobin to hemosiderin
   (E) coagulation necrosis

10. A venous infarct of the lower extremity is characterized by
   (A) loss of sensation, swelling, cyanosis
   (B) pain, pallor, and edema
   (C) pain, dryness, and cyanosis
   (D) pallor, dryness, and loss of sensation

11. Vasculitis is characterized by
   (A) redness, heat, swelling, and pain
   (B) cyanosis, edema, and loss of sensation
   (C) pallor, coldness, and absent pulsations
   (D) dull aches and pressure tenderness

12. Myocardial infarcts are often
   (A) asymptomatic
   (B) caused by emboli
   (C) caused by Mönckeberg's medial sclerosis
   (D) regenerated

13. The natural history of cerebral infarcts is characterized by
   (A) healing by resolution and regeneration
   (B) widely varying clinical manifestations
   (C) unresolved coagulation necrosis
   (D) hemorrhage due to venous occlusion
   (E) sudden death in most instances

14. Infarcts of which organ(s) are pale, triangular, and rarely serious in themselves?
   (A) kidney
   (B) spleen
   (C) both
   (D) neither

15. An infarct of which organ is most likely to be fatal if untreated?
   (A) bowel
   (B) heart
   (C) brain
   (D) lung
   (E) kidney

16. Red infarcts characteristically occur in
   (A) lung
   (B) intestine
   (C) both
   (D) neither

Answers to this posttest are found on page xlvi.

UNIT 13: HEMODYNAMIC DISORDERS: BLEEDING DISORDERS

1. Which of the following statements relating to the classification of hemorrhage is true?
   (A) Purpura is a specific type of hemorrhage.
   (B) Petechiae are larger than ecchymoses.
   (C) Hematomas are likely to result from capillary rupture.
   (D) Purpura may involve petechiae and ecchymoses.

2. Major changes associated with acute hemorrhage include generalized
   (A) vasodilation
   (B) thrombosis
   (C) both
   (D) neither

3. Common manifestations of chronic hemorrhage include
   (A) shock
   (B) anemia
   (C) both
   (D) neither

4. In a patient with a bleeding duodenal ulcer of 2 months' duration, you are most likely to find
   (A) hypovolemic shock
   (B) hypertension
   (C) anemia
   (D) fresh blood in the stool
   (E) generalized vasoconstriction

5. Local lesions of vessels likely to be associated with chronic hemorrhage include
   (A) aneurysms
   (B) lacerations
   (C) fractures
   (D) ulcerated neoplasms

6. Significant arterial aneurysms develop most frequently in the
   (A) aorta and pulmonary arteries
   (B) renal artery and cerebral arteries
   (C) pulmonary arteries and superior mesenteric artery
   (D) aorta and cerebral arteries
   (E) aorta and the left coronary artery

7. Hemorrhagic diathesis is by definition
   (A) a local disorder
   (B) bleeding by diapedesis
   (C) predisposing to hemorrhage
   (D) always manifest
   (E) a coagulation factor deficiency

8. Deficiency in platelets is most often manifest by
   (A) hematomas
   (B) petechiae
   (C) both
   (D) neither

9. A patient presents with a bleeding tendency with normal prothrombin and partial thromboplastin times, increased bleeding time, and a positive tourniquet test. The difficulty most likely involves
   (A) vitamin K deficiency
   (B) liver disease
   (C) thrombocytopenia
   (D) hypofibrinogenemia
   (E) decreased fibrinolysin

10. Deficiency of antihemophilic globulin is manifested by
   (A) bleeding into joints
   (B) petechial hemorrhage
   (C) both
   (D) neither

11. A patient is found to have a deficiency of prothrombin and several associated clotting factors. Likely causes of this disorder include
   (A) extensive chronic liver damage
   (B) vitamin K deficiency
   (C) both
   (D) neither

12. A patient with isolated hypofibrinogenemia will have
   (A) increased bleeding time
   (B) increased clotting time
   (C) increased prothrombin time
   (D) increased partial thromboplastin time
   (E) positive tourniquet test

13. In the process of thrombosis, which of the following events occurs third?
   (A) platelet agglutination
   (B) plasmin activation
   (C) fibrin formation
   (D) vascular contraction

14. Select the response below which best explains the function of blood platelets in regard to the vascular system.
   (A) They serve as the chief source of thromboplastin in the clotting process following hemorrhage.
   (B) By adhering to diseased areas of vessel walls, they protect the vessel from further injury.
   (C) They initiate control of hemorrhage by forming an adhesive mass which tends to quickly plug defects in vessel walls and promote clot formation.
   (D) Disintegrating platelets liberate thrombin to initiate the clotting process.

15. Red blood cells which have hemorrhaged into tissue spaces will
   (A) be mostly reabsorbed into capillaries in the area by diapedesis
   (B) undergo caseous necrosis
   (C) break down and be engulfed by macrophages
   (D) remain intact for several weeks
   (E) be engulfed by polys

16. A large hematoma in a skeletal muscle will
   (A) resolve completely within one week
   (B) serve as a substrate for bacterial growth in most cases
   (C) cause necrosis of surrounding tissue
   (D) necessitate surgical removal to prevent permanent disability
   (E) leave deposits of fibrous tissue and pigment for weeks

Answers to this posttest are found on page xlvi.

POSTTESTS
UNIT 14: HEMODYNAMIC DISORDERS: DERANGEMENTS OF BLOOD FLOW

1. NECESSARY conditions for the existence of shock include
   (A) hypovolemia
   (B) loss of tone in peripheral vasculature
   (C) inadequate perfusion of tissues
   (D) myocardial depression
   (E) bleeding

2. Neurogenic, septic and cardiogenic shock are all characterized by
   (A) equal prognoses if untreated
   (B) need for blood transfusion
   (C) peripheral vasodilation at onset
   (D) normal blood volume in early stages
   (E) progression to irreversible shock

3. Pooling or sequestration of blood in the vascular system is characteristic of which type(s) of shock?
   (A) neurogenic
   (B) anaphylactic
   (C) both
   (D) neither

4. Which type of shock is hypovolemic?
   (A) hemorrhagic
   (B) cardiogenic
   (C) both
   (D) neither

5. Which type of shock is almost always reversible?
   (A) septic
   (B) hypovolemic
   (C) hemorrhagic
   (D) neurogenic
   (E) anaphylactic

6. Following a severe episode of profound shock, which is most likely?
   (A) reduced urine output
   (B) gangrene of the leg
   (C) generalized edema
   (D) disseminated intravascular coagulation

7. Features of profound shock include
   (A) massive edema
   (B) slow pulse rate
   (C) slow deep respirations
   (D) urinary urgency
   (E) acidosis

8. Cardiac decompensation implies
   (A) a history of myocardial infarction
   (B) left-ventricle hypertrophy
   (C) inadequate cardiac output
   (D) systemic arterial hypertension

POSTTESTS

9. A feature of acute left-sided heart failure is
   (A) centrilobular necrosis of the liver
   (B) hemosiderin-laden alveolar macrophages
   (C) pitting dependent edema
   (D) alveolar transudation
   (E) left ventricle hypertrophy

10. Characteristic features of right-sided heart failure (as opposed to left-sided) INCLUDE
   (A) causes elevated pulmonary venous pressure
   (B) more common than left-sided failure
   (C) most commonly results from left-sided failure
   (D) usually associated with pulmonary atherosclerosis
   (E) more commonly acute than left-sided failure

11. Lesions descriptive of left-sided hart failure include
   (A) centrilobular congestion of the liver
   (B) hemosiderin-laden macrophages in pulmonary alveoli
   (C) both
   (D) neither

12. At autopsy a patient was found to have hemosiderin-laden alveolar macrophages, "nutmeg" liver, hydrothorax,and ankle edema. The patient had
   (A) left heart failure
   (B) right heart failure
   (C) both
   (D) neither

13. Which of the following pairs of mechanisms of edema both usually produce transudates rather than exudates?
   (A) increased capillary permeability and lymphatic obstruction
   (B) salt and water overload and hypoproteinemia
   (C) inflammation and heart failure
   (D) lymphatic obstruction and increased venous pressure
   (E) increased venous pressure and increased capillary permeability

14. Widespread edema (rather than localized edema) is likely in
   (A) lymphatic obstruction
   (B) capillary damage
   (C) inflammation
   (D) hypoalbuminemia

15. The nephrotic syndrome results in
   (A) lymphedema
   (B) inflammatory edema
   (C) edema due to altered plasma osmotic pressure
   (D) edema due to increased capillary hydrostatic pressure

16. Transudates commonly result from
   (A) increased hydrostatic pressure
   (B) altered osmotic pressure
   (C) both
   (D) neither

Answers to this posttest are found on page xlvi.

Answers to Posttests

Each test contains 16 items. A score of 13 or higher indicates mastery of the material in the unit.

Next to the answers to each question are the numbers of the frames in which the material is presented.

Answers to pretest items can also be found here if you remember that the pretest items are the same as the odd-numbered items in the posttest for the unit.

ANSWERS TO POSTTESTS

UNIT 1

	Best Response	Frame Reference
1.	C	4,7
2.	A	11
3.	B	21
4.	A	37,41
5.	A	44, 57
6.	B	44,48
7.	A	37
8.	B	44
9.	D	33
10.	A	48
11.	D	70
12.	D	70,72
13.	C	75,76
14.	A	79
15.	C	75,100
16.	A	98,100

UNIT 2

	Best Response	Frame Reference
1.	D	6,16
2.	C	18,23
3.	D	23,47
4.	B	29, 50
5.	B	27
6.	C	47
7.	C	32,35,38
8.	B	16,23,27
9.	C	19,20
10.	A	34,38,40
11.	B	61
12.	B	61
13.	B	75,76
14.	A	67
15.	C	80,83
16.	B	75,77,83

UNIT 3

	Best Response	Frame Reference
1.	D	13
2.	B	14,22
3.	D	4,20
4.	C	34,35
5.	B	18
6.	A	34,35
7.	B	6,7
8.	B	90
9.	B	49
10.	B	64,65
11.	C	80
12.	D	78
13.	A	64
14.	A	51,64, (Unit 2-58)
15.	B	88
16.	C	70

UNIT 4

	Best Response	Frame Reference
1.	C	21
2.	B	1,2
3.	A	16
4.	D	15,16
5.	D	2
6.	C	26
7.	D	12,13
8.	B	13-16
9.	A	6,8
10.	B	13-15
11.	A	37
12.	B	37,41
13.	B	37
14.	A	48
15.	B	49,50
16.	B	48,49

UNIT 5

	Best Response	Frame Reference
1.	B	29,33
2.	B	28
3.	A	7
4.	A	39
5.	C	39,42
6.	B	42
7.	C	59,63
8.	A	73
9.	B	59,63
10.	D	112
11.	B	76
12.	C	91
13.	C	104
14.	C	109
15.	B	76
16.	A	123

ANSWERS TO POSTTESTS (Continued)

	Best Response	Frame Reference	Best Response	Frame Reference
UNIT 6				
	1. A	2,5,6	9. C	69,70
	2. D	5,6,11	10. D	70,76
	3. D	24,27	11. C	77
	4. A	13,14	12. C	91
	5. D	36	13. A	109
	6. C	51,52	14. A	100
	7. B	55,57	15. B	109
	8. B	64	16. C	119,120
UNIT 7				
	1. C	10,12,13	9. A	62
	2. A	7,8	10. D	69,72
	3. A	7	11. A	69,74
	4. D	19,21,25	12. C	82
	5. B	26,29,31,35	13. C	86,87
	6. B	35,37	14. A	82
	7. A	35	15. A	97
	8. D	61	16. C	104
UNIT 8				
	1. C	20	9. D	77
	2. D	24	10. C	90,91,92
	3. B	36	11. D	77,78,102
	4. D	29	12. D	77,89
	5. C	29	13. B	47
	6. C	60,106	14. D	121,123,124
	7. B	48-53	15. A	125,128,130
	8. C	106-111	16. D	125,127
UNIT 9				
	1. A	2,3	9. B	81,82
	2. B	20,23	10. B	41,42
	3. C	14,15	11. A	8,35,119
	4. C	100	12. A	55
	5. C	98	13. B	141
	6. D	34	14. B	103,118
	7. B	52,113,116	15. B	90,75
	8. B	66,68,73	16. D	110
UNIT 10				
	1. D	6	9. B	35
	2. D	8	10. B	42,43
	3. D	9,11	11. C	45
	4. A	34-37, 46	12. A	59, 61,72
	5. D	37	13. D	72
	6. D	16,17	14. B	73,84
	7. D	84	15. B	90
	8. A	21,22,23	16. C	91,92,93

ANSWERS TO POSTTESTS (Continued)

Best Response	Frame Reference	Best Response	Frame Reference
UNIT 11			
1. D	14, 16, 43	9. A	95, 97
2. A	17, 21, 30	10. C	109
3. C	48	11. C	141
4. E	48	12. A	130
5. C	34, 37, 39	13. C	138, 139
6. D	77, 81	14. B	139
7. B	113	15. B	156-161
8. E	100	16. C	152-172
UNIT 12			
1. A	3	9. C	37, 42
2. C	8, 10, 12, 16	10. A	48
3. E	13, 14, 15	11. D	53
4. A	20	12. A	57, 59
5. C	27	13. B	65, 66, 67
6. D	32, 35, 45, 74	14. C	68
7. B	5	15. A	72
8. D	39, 40	16. C	74, 76
UNIT 13			
1. D	7, 8, 9	9. C	30
2. D	11, 12	10. A	36
3. B	13	11. C	40
4. C	13	12. B	43
5. D	5	13. C	62, 64, 65
6. D	20, 21	14. C	61, 63
7. C	24	15. C	72
8. B	26	16. E	71, 72
UNIT 14			
1. C	4	9. D	58, 59
2. D	12, 14, 22	10. C	56, 58, 60, 64
3. C	14, 20	11. B	59
4. A	7, 10, 12	12. C	59
5. D	16	13. B	81, 84, 86, 90
6. A	41	14. D	83, 84
7. E	39, 41, 42	15. C	83, 85
8. C	50	16. C	81, 83, 84

Appendix: Evaluation Data by Unit

Unit	Mean Scores, % Pretest/Posttest	% of students rating unit good or excellent	% of students who preferred program to other methods	average completion time, hours
1. INTRODUCTION TO PATHOLOGY	50/90	90	95	1.8
2. INFLAMMATION: THE VASCULAR AND CELLULAR RESPONSE TO INJURY	39/93	92	95	1.7
3. INFLAMMATORY CELLS: STRUCTURE AND FUNCTION	51/92	84	95	1.7
4. FACTORS WHICH MODIFY INFLAMMATION	50/90	81	97	1.2
5. CLASSIFICATION AND COMPLICATIONS OF INFLAMMATION	38/94	81	97	2.2
6. SYSTEMIC MANIFESTATIONS OF INFLAMMATION	53/95	88	97	1.8
7. NECROSIS*	31/85	67	80	2.8
8. HEALING	42/89	86	84	2.7
9. DEGENERATION*	45/88	55	80	3.2
10. DEVELOPMENTAL ABNORMALITIES: EMBRYONIC AND FETAL, GENETIC AND CHROMOSOMAL	34/85	86	89	2.7

* before revisions

Unit	Mean Scores, % Pretest/Posttest	% of students rating unit good or excellent	% of students who preferred program to other methods	average completion time, hours
11. HEMODYNAMIC DISORDERS: MECHANISMS OF VASCULAR OBSTRUCTION	35/89	87	85	3.0
12. HEMODYNAMIC DISORDERS: EFFECTS OF VASCULAR OBSTRUCTION	56/88	89	87	1.7
13. HEMODYNAMIC DISORDERS: BLEEDING DISORDERS	53/88	73	80	2.0
14. HEMODYNAMIC DISORDERS: DERANGEMENTS OF BLOOD FLOW	44/90	88	85	2.3

Index